LINDA ~~EASTWOOD~~

8.3rd .95

To Linda

Thank you for your support and commitment to our programmes.

The Pichn Canada Team

B[illegible]

A NEW KIND *of* RAY

A NEW KIND *of* RAY

The Radiological Sciences in Canada • Les Sciences Radiologiques au Canada

1895–1995

100 YEARS

EDITED BY

JOHN E ALDRICH AND BRIAN C LENTLE

UNIVERSITY OF BRITISH COLUMBIA

VANCOUVER, CANADA

Published in Vancouver, British Columbia, Canada for
The Canadian Association of Radiologists
Suite 510, 5101 rue Buchan
Montréal, Quebec, H4P 2R9
Canada

ISBN 0-9699557-0-7

Editors John E Aldrich and Brian C Lentle
Designer Ken Hughes
Illustrator Lorry Hughes
Typesetting Iris and Mervin Schindel
Printer Friesen Printers
Printing Consultants Impressions Marketing
Printed in Canada

Text typeset in Stone Serif and Stone Sans Serif

To our wives and children:

Sylvia, Graham, Jenny and Martin;

Jean, Susan and Stephen.

Preface

There is nothing which you know which is of no use.
— Robertson Davies

We have been collecting the material for this volume for nearly twenty years. The catalyst in bringing it into print was the centennial of Röntgen's discovery of x-rays. We have had no illusions about editing a best-selling volume, and it was only the generosity of a number of corporate and individual sponsors, listed separately, that finally allowed publication. Not least, the Council of the Canadian Association of Radiologists(CAR), in collectively stating the will not to let a once-in-a-hundred-years occasion pass unnoticed, was crucial in bringing this volume to fruition.

The book owes much to many people. Many of the contributors kept faith when publication was uncertain. Our wives, Sylvia and Jean, both worked with us and waited. Many individuals were helpful beyond simple courtesy. Mr Ken Hughes of the Emily Carr Institute of Art and Design was instrumental in bringing the project to completion and is responsible for the design of the book. Lorry Hughes created the illustrations that precede each part of the text. The advice and support of Dr C Stuart Houston was immensely valuable. We owe particular debts to Mr John Berthiaume and the Committee on Commercial Liaison of CAR, Mr Joe Sardi, Ms Suzanne Charette and her staff at the Canadian Association of Radiologists' head office, Mr Chris Eden of Eden Arts, Dr David Gray, Dr John Radomsky, Dr Jacques Sylvestre, Dr Stephanie Wilson, Dr Ian Sutherland, Dr Harald Stolberg, Dr Claude Nahmias, Dr Guy Duckett, Dr Gordon Potts, Mr Bill Forrest, Ms Diane Sauvé, Ms Phyllis Wasylyshyn, Ms Linda Harrison, Dr Stephane Carignan, Ms Susan (Lentle) Campbell and particularly Drs Ronald Burr and Wally Roy, both previous presidents of the Canadian Association of Radiologists. Ms Rita Hudec and Executive Director Dr Richard Lauzon, both of the Canadian Association of Medical Radiation Technologists, and Ms Marjorie Sorrell of the Ontario Association of Medical Radiation Technologists went out of their way to meet or correspond with us and be helpful. Help was also generously given by Ms Mo Gupta of the Vancouver Hospital, Ms Pat Smith of the Atomic Energy Control Board of Canada, Mr Alan Crawford of the Bank of Canada and Mr Drew Gillies of the National Film Board. Jean Lentle, Virginia Zepeda-Vidal and Diane Bozzer kindly did much of the word processing.

We owe the most to those who have made this volume possible—the contributors. Not all of them knew they were preparing text for this purpose. Some articles were written with great commitment for this particular volume; some are reprinted with permission from other publications. Others were written because of the foresight of earlier archivists sometimes twenty or thirty years ago or more. These pieces have been kept on file in the hope that such a publication as this might materialize. Wherever possible we have sought permission to publish from the authors, their family or executors. However, particular thanks are due to the late Dr EM Crawford, a former secretary of the Canadian Association of Radiologists, and Dr RG (Bob) Fraser, a former president, whose names figure prominently among those who have preserved the history of the association, and who have, therefore, made our lives so much easier.

Dr Jocelyne Lapointe, with customary graciousness, served to repair the deficiencies in our use of French. She has also translated text, worked tirelessly and given us invaluable information and advice, and we are indebted to her for her kind interest and her support. Mr David Zieroth and Mr Robert Adams of *A to Z Writing and Editing* have expertly done a final edit of the English text, and Dr Jocelyne Lapointe has completed a similar task *vis à vis* the French text. Ms Jane Rowlands of the Department of Biomedical Communications at the University of British Columbia provided the graphics, and the entire staff of Biomedical Communications at the Vancouver Hospital and Health Sciences Centre were of enormous help. It is trite but nevertheless true to say that to these people is owed much of whatever credit is due for this volume: its limitations are entirely our responsibility.

We are by nature collectors rather than academically trained historians and that has been our *modus operandi.* This is not a critical history but a celebration: a celebration of a collective undertaking by engineers, computer scientists, nurses, physicians, physicists, radiopharmacists, secretaries, technologists and others, on behalf of all of our patients. It is a celebration of the past but also of the future, the future of specialties which change more quickly than most and which are already responding to the need to redefine the care of the sick in the next one hundred years. This is the power of Röntgen's legacy, which we remember in 1995.

As we write it is uncertain if this publication will result in a profit. Any profits that do result will be given to the foundations of the associations whose members purchase the book.

Given more time and resources some of the regional gaps in this volume might have been filled. They exist not because we failed to try to have them remedied.

Brian Lentle
John Aldrich

Milestones in Radiology

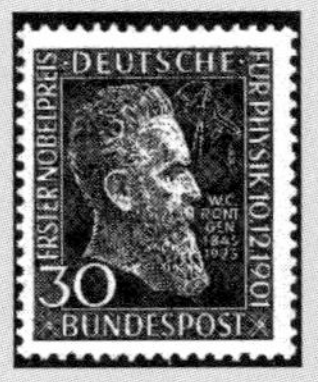

Professor Röntgen discovers x-rays in Germany

First clinical radiograph in Canada

Alexander Graham Bell experiments with x-rays in Baddeck, Nova Scotia

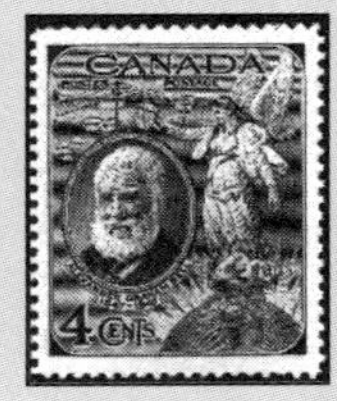

Ernest Rutherford begins a series of publications on atomic structure

First biological tracer work by George Hevesy

Les Rayons X published in Montréal

First plastic x-ray film

Coolidge tube developed

Walter Dandy develops pneumo-encephalography

Egas Moniz develops angiography in Portugal

First Canadian radiological technologist organization formed (Manitoba)

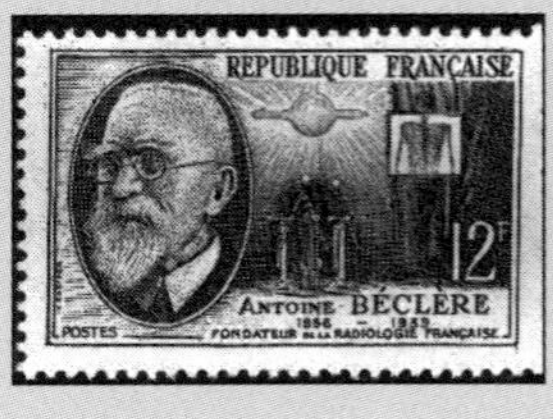

Catheterization done for first time by Forssmain in Germany

The first usable contrast medium

Canadian Association of Radiologists formed

First automatic film processor

1895 | 1900 | 1905 | 1910 | 1915 | 1920 | 1925 | 1930 | 1935 | 1940 | 1945

First image intensifier

First scintillation scanner developed by Benedict Cassen

First clinical ultrasound of soft tissue

Gamma camera invented by Hal Anger

First axial tomographic brain scan (PET) David Kuhl

First Tc-99m made

Houndsfield and Cormack develop computed tomography

Phenomenon of NMR reported by Block and Purcell

Rare earth screens available

First clinical MRI scans produced

First clinical echoplanar imaging

Interventional MRI developed

DICOM Standard

1950 1955 1960 1965 1970 1975 1980 1985 1990 1995 2000

Canadian Association of Radiologists' Journal first published

World's first cobalt-60 unit developed in Saskatoon

First Canadian isotope scanner used

First Canadian medical physicists' organization formed

Remote RF room prototype, Montreal

C-arm angiography developed in Montréal

Canada's first gamma camera developed in Saskatoon

Shoe-fitting fluoroscopes abandoned

First Canadian CT scanner at MNI

Digital subtraction angiography developed in Toronto

First MRT installed in Canada (UBC)

Stereotactic surgical techniques pioneered at MNI

Canada's first high field MRI at MNI

A New Kind of Ray is published

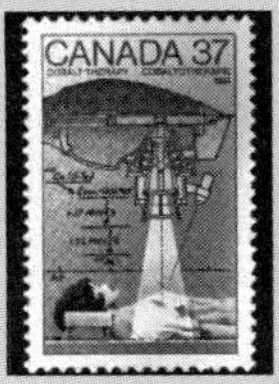

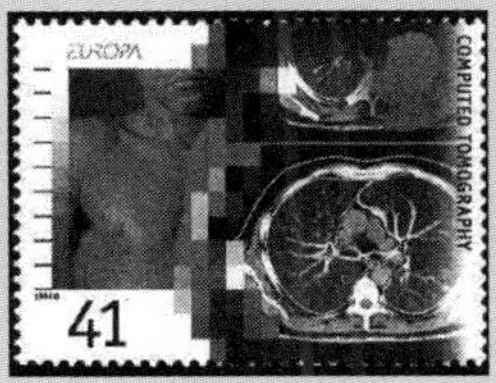

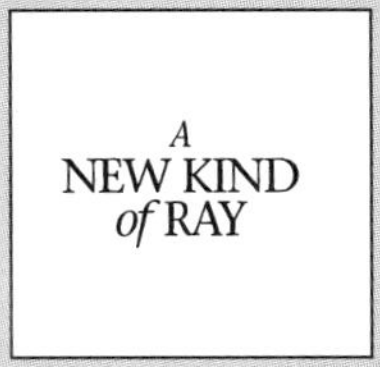

Sponsors

CORPORATE SPONSORS

All of those involved in the radiological sciences in Canada are indebted to the following associations, corporations and societies for their major sponsorship of this volume:

AGFA Canada Inc
ATL Canada Inc
Berlex Canada Inc
Canadian Association of Medical Radiation Technologists
Canadian Association of Radiologists
Canadian Organization of Medical Physicists
Cook (Canada) Inc
  A Cook Group Company
Diasonics Canada Ltd
Dupont Canada Inc Medical Products
Elscint (Canada) Ltd
GE Medical Systems
Kodak Canada Inc Health Sciences Division
Konica Canada Inc Medical Division
Mallinckrodt Medical Inc
Phillips Medical Systems Canada
Picker International Canada Inc
Sanofi Winthrop
Siemens Electric Ltd Medical Systems Division
Therapex Inc
  Division de/of E-Z-EM Canada Inc
Toshiba of Canada Ltd
  Medical Systems Division
3 M Canada Inc
  Medical Imaging Systems Division
Vancouver Hospital and Health Sciences Centre Foundation
Varian Canada Inc
X-Ray Centennial Foundation of Canada Inc

INDIVIDUAL SPONSORS

The following individuals and organizations have also generously sponsored this publication:

Dr Raymond Archambault
Dr Adel Assaf
Associated Radiologists of Saskatoon
Dr RJ Aucoin
Dr E Michel Azouz

Dr Céline Carole Bard
Dr G Barton
Dr CG Beauregard
Dr Gérard Bélanger
Dr Adrien Bernard
Dr Denys Bertrand
Dr Christian Blais
Dr AJ Bliek
Dr A Boubalos
Dr Gordon Bray
Dr Spencer Bridger
Dr William G Brown
Dr Ronald Burr

Dr AJ Campbell
Employees of the Canadian Association of Radiologists
  Suzanne Charette
  Françoise Doyen Caden
  Muriel Gillespie
  Louise Joly
  Bich Vu
Dr Gordon E Catton
Dr John A Chadwick
Dr Jean Chalaoui
Dr Rosemary Jane Chambers
Clinique Radiologie Audet Enr
Dr Sonia Cloutier
Dr A Colantonio
Dr James R Coughlin
Dr Donald Frank Crang
Mr Larry Curtis

Dr Monique Desaulniers
Dr G Desmond
Dr James E Dickie
Dr Conway J Don
Mr William Doern
Dr Ian Doris
Dr Gilles Dubuc

Dr Hugh Edgar

Dr Raffaele Filice
Dr P Fong
Dr J Ford

Dr David B Fraser
Dr WR Fumerton

Dr David Garrow
Dr John D Gibson
Dr George Goodman
Dr GL Goth
Dr DJ Grant
Dr David G Gray
Dr Karen Gulenchyn

Dr Susan Hacking
Sister Noreen Hammill
Dr Ian Hammond
Dr Clayton Hann
Dr T Hanna
Dr ER Harrigan
Dr Sylvie Harvey
Dr Derek Harwood-Nash
Dr Mary-Jane Hendel
Dr Donald Henderson
Dr Erland E Henderson
Mr Robin Hesler
Dr Barry B Hobbs
Dr Brian Holmes
Dr C Stuart Houston
Ms Rita Hudec
Dr Linda C Hutton
Dr Brahm B Hyams
Dr David M Hynes

Dr David H James
Dr Jean-Pierre Jean

Dr Benoit Langevin
Dr Richard Lauzon
Dr Claude Léger
Dr JA Lewin
Dr David Li
Dr Walter M Little
Dr John A Liver
Dr Grant Llewellyn
Dr Andrea Lum

Dr Douglas MacEwan
Dr LR MacFadyen

Dr C Lamont MacMillan
Dr Nestor E Maslo
Dr John T Mason
Dr William F Mason
Dr John Alexander Matheson
Mr Arbo A Mattila
Dr Karl Matzinger
Dr Beverley McKee
Dr Brian McPhilipps
Dr HE Meema
Dr Ian BD Middlemass
Dr S Miller
Dr Steven F Millward
Dr Michael Mindel
Dr Hugh F Morrish
Dr AEW Morton

Newfoundland Association of Medical Radiation Technologists
Dr Donald E Newman
Dr LG Stephens Newsham

Octostop Inc
Dr Gregory Olscamp
Ottawa General Radiology Associates

Dr Edward G Parkinson
Dr Norman Patt
Dr DB Pengelly
Dr Lyette Perrault

Dr AM Quarrington

Dr John W Radomsky
Dr Richard N Rankin
Dr ER Reddy
Dr Martin H Reed
Dr AJ Richards

Dr Louise Samson
Dr Emilio Sanchez
Dr Alastair Scarth
Dr Charles H Shaul
Dr DL Shea
Dr John Stapleton
Dr Giles W Stevenson

Dr William B Stewart
Dr Harald O Stolberg
Dr Ian Suchet
Dr John B (Ian) Sutherland
Dr S Sutherland
Dr Jacques Sylvestre

Dr Donald H Taves
Dr Graham Thompson
Dr Lynette Thurber
Dr Raymond Torbiak
Dr Martin Tropper
Dr J Marc Turcotte

Dr William C Vezina
Vancouver General Radiology Associates
- Dr Nestor Müller
- Dr Jocelyne S Lapointe
- Dr Ann R (Jean) Buckley
- Dr Nigel Clark
- Dr Douglas Connell
- Dr Helen Emmons
- Dr J Stephen Fache
- Dr Douglas Graeb
- Dr Dennis Janzen
- Dr Tom Marotta
- Dr John Mayo
- Dr D Christopher Morris
- Dr Robert Nugent
- Dr V Allan Rowley
- Dr Ian Weir
- Dr Charles V Zwirewich

Dr Warren A Wass
Dr Edward Whelan
Mr G Archie Wilkinson
Mr Jim Williams
Dr Stephanie R Wilson
Dr Stanley Windle
Dr Terry L Woods

Dr Michael L Yuen

Dr Arthur Zalev

IN MEMORIAM

Donations in support of this publication have been received in memory of the following persons:

Mr William Brodie
- *In Memoriam*
- Mr John C Brodie

Ms Suzanne Charette
- *In Memoriam*
- Mrs Cécile Hainault Charette

Dr John Flatman
- *In Memoriam*
- Mr Robert (Bob) Flatman
- *In Memoriam*
- Dr Theodore (Ted) Kozlik

Dr Peter Munk
- *In Memoriam*
- Mrs Margaret Lhotak Munk

Dr Charles H Shaul
- *In Memoriam*
- Dr Douglas Vernon McFarlane

Dr Michael L Yuen
- *In Memoriam*
- Dr Peter W Cockshott

Dr PB Gordon,
Dr WJ Knickerbocker,
Dr LJ Warren
- *In Memoriam*
- Francis Albert Olacke

Contents

The annexes and references accompanying each chapter are reproduced in Part Ten

Part Five: People 231

Penetrating Radiation and Imaging and Treating Disease

The Electromagnetic Spectrum

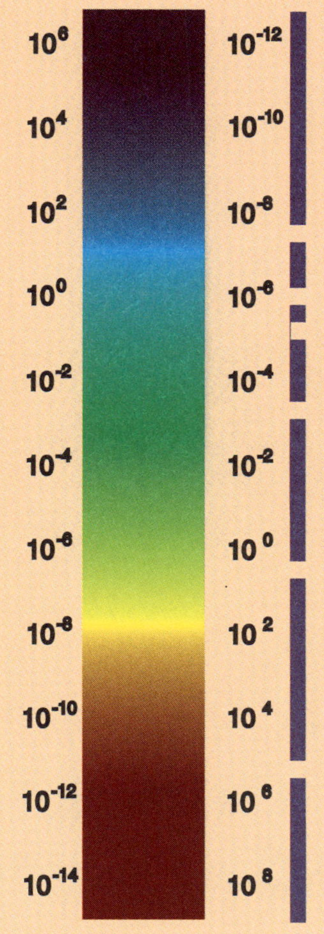

	Diagnosis	Treatment
X-rays and Gamma rays	Positron emission tomography Radionuclide imaging X-ray imaging	Linear accelerators Co–60 treatment Orthovoltage x-ray therapy Superficial x-ray therapy
Ultra violet		UVB (Psoriasis)
Visible	Vision Microscopy Diaphanography	Photodynamic therapy
Infra red	Thermography Non invasive infra-red scanning	
Micro-waves	Microwave imaging Microwave tomography	
Radio waves	Magnetic resonance imaging Magnetic resonance spectroscopy	Radiofrequency tissue destruction Diathermy
Electric current	Magnetic source imaging Electrical impedence tomography	Electrocautery Diathermy
Sound Waves	Ultrasonography	Tissue ablation Lithotripsy Diathermy
Particles +++	Heavy ion radiography	Radiation therapy
+ positrons	Positron emission tomography	
- electrons (electric current)	Electron microscopy Magnetic source imaging Electrical impedance tomography	Radiation therapy

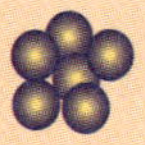

Verlé Harrop

An autobiographical note

REMOTE SENSING 10
Changing States:
Higher Space–Time
Dimensions 147x137cm
Textiles, acrylic, floppy disk,
wire
1989

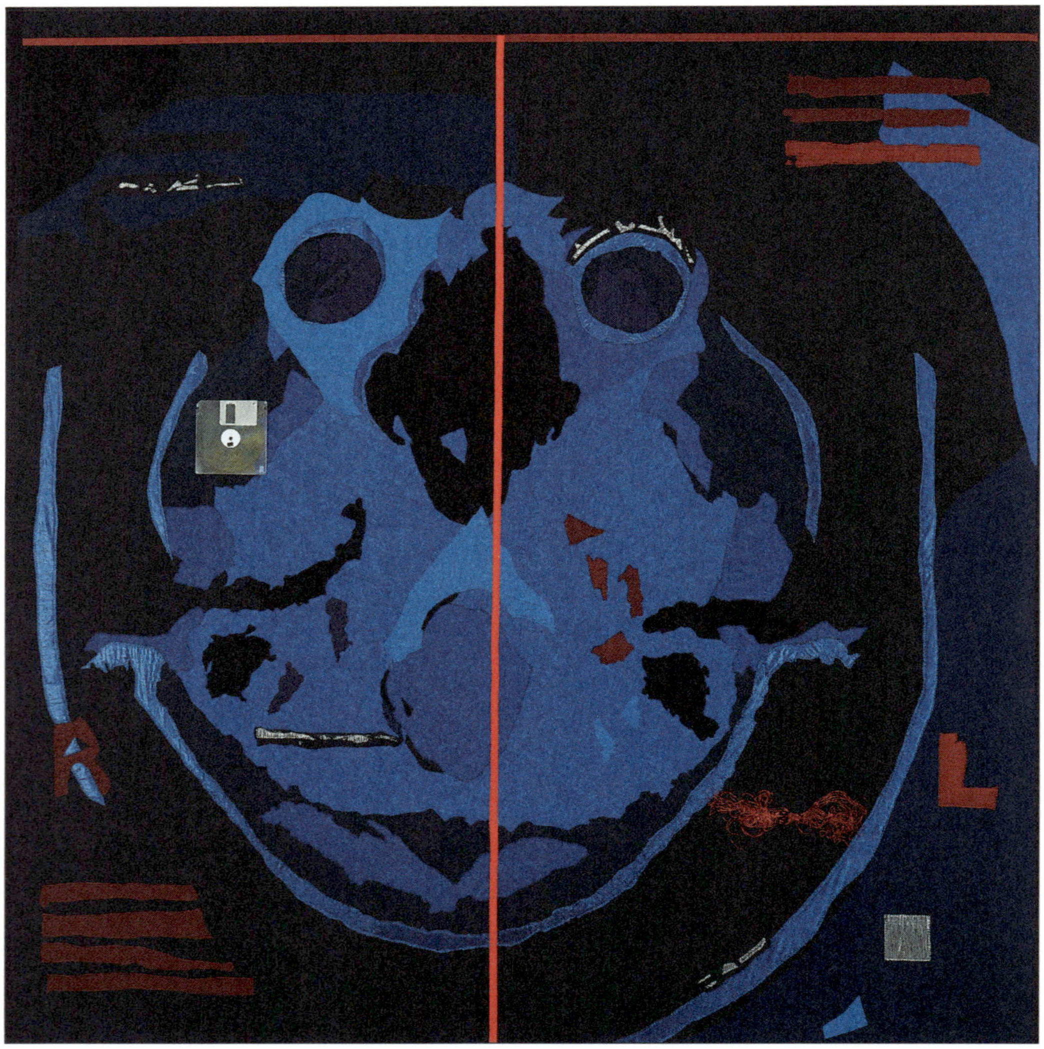

Verlé grew up on a farm, attended a one-room schoolhouse and spent most of her childhood on a bike exploring the rigid grid-work of roads, fences and fields of southern Ontario. Just as her farmer-parents wrestled with the earth, so Verlé has explored similar themes in her artistic work—the simultaneous mapping of internal and external landscapes and the juxtaposition of linear and organic, pre-scriptive and holistic images. Her fascination with the rapid societal changes, in the context of the natural sciences and technology, has led her to contrast these themes in a medical technological context. The works shown in this book reflect her recent interest in the juxtaposition of medical and other images.

Verlé maintains a studio in Halifax, and as well as being artist-in-residence at the Medical School of Dalhousie University, has an active exhibition schedule. Her work is used on the cover, which features a collage of a magnetic resonance brain image and a map of Canada.

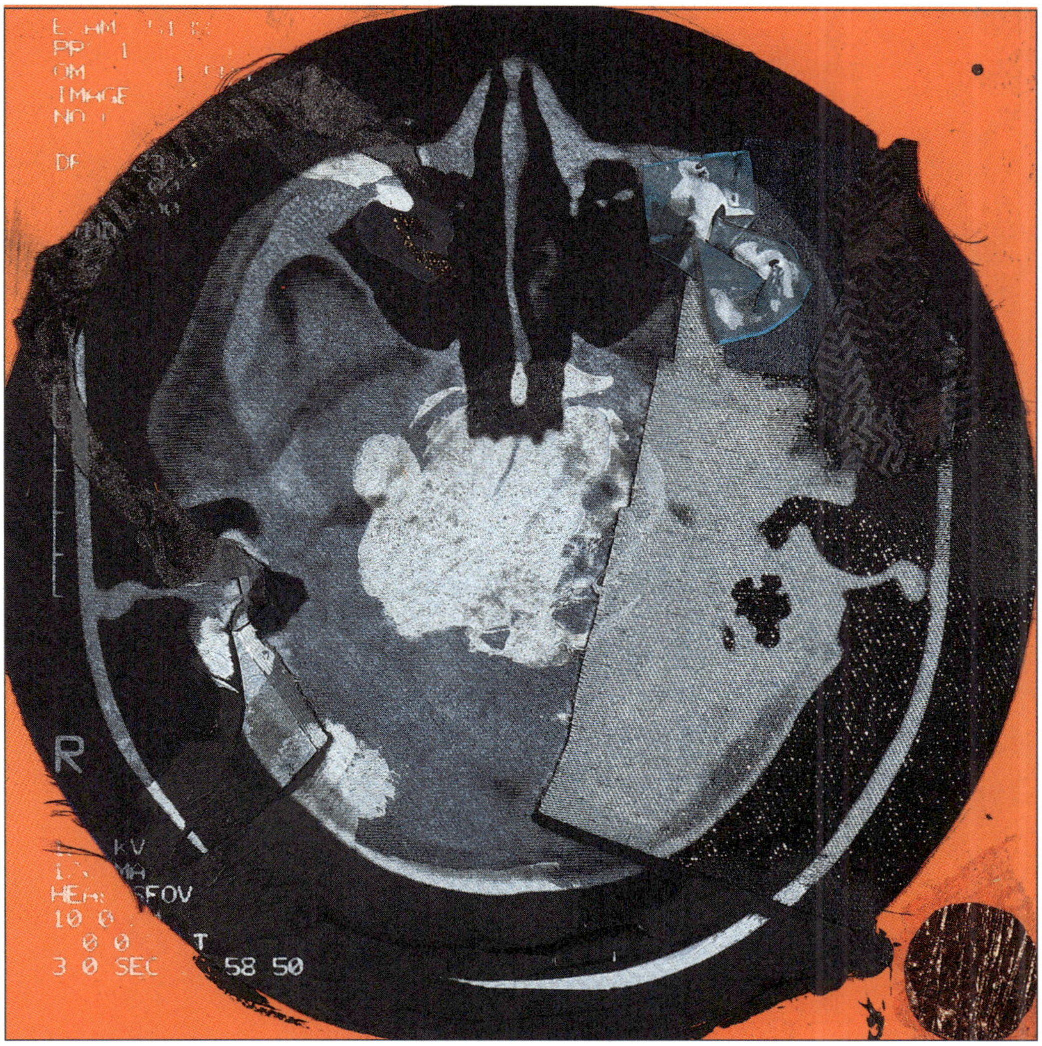

REMOTE SENSING
Tête à Tête 5
30.5x30.5cm
Textiles, acrylic/paper
1993

cover
REMOTE SENSING
Mapping
Linear vs Organic 001624
44.5x37.2cm
Ink/atlas page
1993

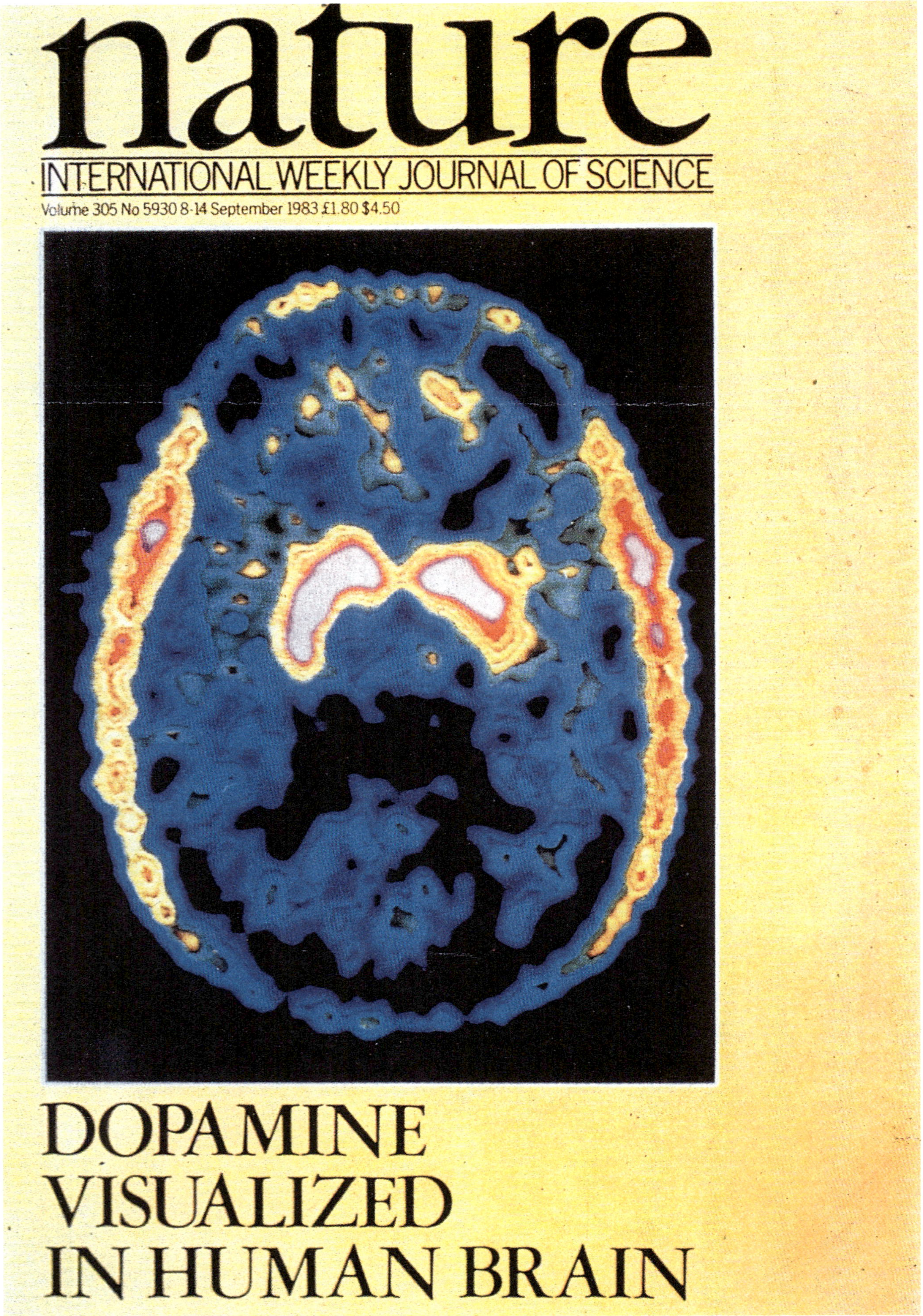

First brain receptor image. Reprinted with permission from *Nature* 1983, 305, Cover. Copyright 1983 MacMillan Magazines Ltd. Image obtained at McMaster University Department of Radiology, Courtesy of Dr. Clande Nahmias. (see page 58)

Contributors

***Douglas N Abrams** PhD*
Dr Abrams is radiopharmacist and Assistant Director of Radiopharmacy at the Health Sciences Centre Winnipeg and an Assistant Professor at the University of Manitoba. He is a former president of the Canadian Association of Radiopharmaceutical Scientists.

***John Aldrich** PhD FCCPM*
Dr Aldrich is Clinical Professor and Head of the Division of Basic Sciences of the Department of Radiology, University of British Columbia and Vancouver Hospital and Health Sciences Centre. Formerly of Dalhousie University, Dr Aldrich has published about the early days of radiology in the Maritimes.

***Laurent Aubé** MD CSPQ*
Dr Aubé est un professeur de radiologie à l'Université de Laval et ancien chef de service en radiologie à l'Hôtel-Dieu de Québec.

***Rosalind Aylmer** BA Dipl Photog*
Ms Aylmer is co-owner and manager of QED Communications Ltd, a Vancouver based firm specializing in the art and technology of communication.

***Louis-Philippe Belisle** MD CSPQ*
Dr Belisle était un radiologiste à l'Hôtel-Dieu de Montréal et un radiologiste consultant à la Ligue Antituberculeuse de Montréal et à l'Hôpital de Bordeaux.

***GF Boult** MD*
Dr Boult was a radiologist at the Health Sciences Centre and in private practice in Winnipeg.

***H Joachim Burhenne** MD FRCPC*
Dr Burhenne is former Professor and Head of the Department of Radiology at the University of British Columbia and the Vancouver Hospital and Health Sciences Centre.

***Patrice Bret** MD CSPQ*
Dr Bret is Professor and Chairman of the Department of Radiology at McGill University and Chief of Radiology at Montréal General Hospital.

***Ross E Brown** MD FRCPC*
Dr Brown is Vice-President, Medicine at St Boniface Hospital in Winnipeg and a former president of the American Institute of Ultrasound in Medicine.

***Ronald C Burr** MD*
Dr Burr is retired, having been Professor and Head of Radiation Oncology at Queen's University. He is a former president of the Canadian Association of Radiologists.

***Montague Cohen** PhD FCCPM*
Dr Montague Cohen was Director of Medical Physics at McGill University from 1975–1991. He is now Professor of Physics (post-retirement) at McGill University, Curator of the Rutherford Museum and President of the X-ray Centennial Foundation of Canada.

***JTH Connor** PhD*
Dr Connor is Executive Director of the Hannah Institute for the History of Medicine.

***Douglas V Cormack** PhD FCCPM*
Dr Cormack is a consultant in the Department of Medical Physics, Tom Baker Cancer Centre, Calgary.

***Trevor Cradduck** PhD FCCPM*
Dr Trevor Cradduck is internationally known for his work in nuclear medicine physics. A former Chairman of Nuclear Medicine at University of Western Ontario and secretary of the Society of Nuclear Medicine he is now Manager of LargeNet in London.

***Sister Marie De Lellis Crowley** SCIC RM RT BSc*
Sister Crowley organised the first meeting of the New Brunswick Society of X-ray Technicians and was the first president of that society. She wrote an otherwise unpublished history of the Canadian Society of Radiological Technicians in 1948 in partial fulfillment of the requirements for a bachelor of science degree at St Louis University.

***William Doern** RT*
Mr Doern is a technologist and former president of the Canadian Society of Radiological Technicians.

***Conway Don** MB FRCPC*
Dr Don is former Professor and Chairman of the Department of Radiology at the University of Ottawa.

***Guy Duckett** MD CSPQ FRCPC*
Dr Duckett est un radiologiste, anciennement Chef du Département de Radiologie à l'Hôpital Jean Talon, Montréal.

***Lewis Edwards** RT*
Mr Edwards is a past President of the Canadian Association of Medical Radiation Technologists.

***Günes Ege** MD FRCPC*
Dr Ege is a radiation oncologist at the Toronto-Bayview Regional Cancer Centre, Toronto, Ontario.

Peter Feddersen
Mr Feddersen is Vice-President and General Manager, Medical Systems Division, Toshiba of Canada Ltd.

***Sylvia Fedoruk** OC SOM MA DSc FCCPM*
Dr Fedoruk is the former Lieutenant

Governor of Saskatchewan and a former Director of Physics Services for the Saskatchewan Cancer Foundation.

William Feindel *OC MD CM DPHIL FRCSC*
Dr William Feindel has been involved since 1956 in many diagnostic advances including the early days of nuclear scanning. As Director of the Montréal Neurological Institute (1972–1984), he established the Brain Imaging Centre, integrating gamma-encephalography, CT, PET, EEG, MRI and MRS.

Peter J Fitzpatrick *MD FRCPC*
Dr Fitzpatrick is Chairman of the Department of Radiation Oncology, Dalhousie University, Halifax, Nova Scotia.

Chen Fong *MD FRCPC*
Dr Fong is Professor and Chairman of the Department of Radiology, Foothills Hospital and the University of Calgary.

David Fraser *MD FRCPC*
Dr Fraser is Professor and Head of the Department of Radiology at Dalhousie University and Chief of Radiology at the Royal Victoria Hospital.

Marie Flore Gagné *AMJ*
Soeur Gagné est une religieuse certifieé en nursing, radiographie, radiothérapie et médecine nucléaire, et qui en plus de travailler au service de radiothérapie de l'Hôtel-Dieu de Québec (1948–1979), y organiza l'Ecole de Radiothérapie (1957) et est l'auteure de "Quarante ans d'histoire des Techniciens en radiologie au Québec 1941–1981."

Colette Gazdic *MRT(R)*
Mrs Gazdic is a retired technologist living in Sudbury. She served on the Ontario Association of Medical Radiation Technologists (OAMRT) Board of Directors from 1982–1986 and was president in 1985. She was OAMRT archivist from 1989 to 1992 and continues to be an executive officer of the OAMRT Northern Section.

James Gillies *MD FRCPC*
Dr Gillies was Head of Radiation Oncology at the Manitoba Cancer Treatment and Research Foundation.

Yves Gingras *PHD*
Dr Gingras est professeur d'histoire et de sociologie des sciences à l'Université du Québec à Montréal (UQAM). Il est l'auteur de plusieurs ouvrages dont le plus récent est *Pour l'avancement des sciences. Histoire de l'ACFAS 1923–1993.* (Boréal, 1994).

George Goodman *MD FRCPC*
Dr Goodman is Professor Emeritus in the Division of Radiation Oncology at the University of British Columbia and a member of the honorary attending medical staff of the British Columbia Cancer Agency and the Vancouver Hospital and Health Sciences Centre.

Clive L Greenstock *PHD*
Dr Greenstock is a research scientist at the Chalk River Laboratories of AECL.

Colin Harrison *MD FRCPC (deceased)*
Dr Harrison was a radiologist in private practice in Vancouver.

Philip Harrison *MD FRCPC*
Dr Harrison is a radiologist at St Paul's Hospital and President of the British Columbia Association of Radiologists.

RW Harrison *MSc*
Mr Harrison is a physicist at the British Columbia Cancer Agency.

Verlé Harrop
Ms Harrop is an artist, currently artist-in-residence in the Faculty of Medicine of Dalhousie University.

Charles RR Hayter *BA MA MD FRCPC*
Dr Hayter is a member of the Division of Radiation Oncology, Department of Oncology, Queen's University, Kingston, Ontario.

Guy Hébert *MD FRCPC*
Dr Hébert est Professeur et Chef Universitaire du Département de Radiologie à l'Université de Montréal.

Stuart Houston *OC SOM MD DLITT FRCPC*
Dr Houston was a former Professor and Head of the Department of Radiology at the University of Saskatchewan and the Royal University Hospital, Saskatoon. He is a past President of the Canadian Society for the History of Medicine and served as editor of the *Canadian Association of Radiologists Journal.* He has numerous publications to his credit in the context of ornithology and Canadian history in addition to those concerning his scientific work.

Rita Hudec *RT*
Ms Hudec is the Controller, Canadian Association of Medical Radiation Technologists.

Stewart M Jackson *MD FRCR FRCPC*
Dr Jackson is a Clinical Professor at the University of British Columbia and Chairman of the Division of Radiation Oncology, British Columbia Cancer Agency.

EE Johnston *MD FRCPC*
Dr Johnston is a retired radiologist and former Chief of Radiology at Victoria Hospital, London.

William A Jones *MD (deceased)*
Dr WA Jones was Professor and Head of the Department of Radiology at Queen's University and the first President of the Canadian Association of Radiologists.

Albert Jutras *OC MD CSPQ (deceased)*
Dr Jutras était Professeur et Chef Universitaire du Département de Radiologie à l'Université de Montréal. et président de l'Association des Radiologistes de Langue Français du Canada.

AS Kirkland *MD (deceased)*
Dr Kirkland was one of the earliest radiologsts in New Brunswick and the first to be educated elsewhere (at McGill). He served a term as president of the New Brunswick Medical Society (1929–1930) and was a president of the Section on Radiology of the Canadian Medical Association in the days before there was a Canadian Association of Radiologists.

RO Kornelson *PHD*
Dr Kornelson is a former Head of the Department of Medical Physics at the British Columbia Cancer Agency.

Gabriel Lam *PHD*
Dr Lam is Head of the Section of Developmental Physics at the British Columbia Cancer Agency, having graduated from the University of Toronto. He is engaged in research concerning mathematical biology and particle therapy.

Jocelyne Lapointe *MD FRCPC*
Dr Lapointe is an Associate Professor in the Department of Radiology at the University of British Columbia and a neuroradiologist at the Vancouver Hospital and Health Sciences Centre.

Étienne LeBel *MD CSPQ*
Dr LeBel est Professeur, département de médecine nucléaire et de radiobiologie, Faculté de Médecine, Université de Sherbrooke et anciennement directeur du centre de recherches cliniques au Centre Hospitalier de l'Université de Sherbrooke.

Brian Lentle *BCH MD DMRD FRCPC*
Dr Lentle is Professor and Head of the Department of Radiology at the University of British Columbia and the Vancouver Hospital and Health Sciences Centre, former Head of the Division of Nuclear Medicine and former editor of the *Canadian Association of Radiologists Journal.*

John K Lipinski *MD FRCPC*
Dr Lipinski is a radiologist in Toronto, Ontario. He has had a long-standing interest in the history of Canadian radiology.

Edward Lyons MD FRCPC
Dr Ted Lyons is Professor and Chairman of the Department of Radiology at the University of Manitoba and Chief of Radiology at the Winnipeg Health Sciences Centre.

Douglas MacEwan MD FRCPC
Dr MacEwan is a former Professor and Head of the Department of Radiology at the University of Manitoba and former president of both the Canadian Association of Radiologists and the Radiological Society of North America (RSNA). He is also a recipient of the gold medal of the RSNA.

Alexander JB McEwan MB FRCPC
Dr McEwan is Professor and Chairman of the Department of Radiology at the University of Alberta and Chief of Radiology at the University of Alberta Hospitals.

Patrick J McManamon MD FRCPC
Dr McManamon is Professor and Head of the Department of Radiology at Memorial University in St John's, Newfoundland.

Robert A McPherson MD CM FACR
Dr McPherson is a former Professor and Chairman of the Department of Radiology at the University of Manitoba.

Frank Manning MD FRCPC
Dr Manning is the Head of the Department of Obstetrics and Gynecology at the University of Manitoba.

Peter Munk MD FRCPC
Dr Munk is an Associate Professor in the Department of Radiology at the University of British Columbia and Director of Interventional Radiology at the Vancouver Clinic of the British Columbia Cancer Agency.

Robert Nolan MD FRCPC
Dr Nolan is Professor and Head of the Department of Radiology at Queen's University and Chief of Radiology at Kingston General Hospital.

Terry Peters PHD FCCPM
Dr Peters is a Professor at McGill University in Montréal in the Deparments of Neurology and Neurosurgery, Radiology, Biomedical Engineering and Medical Physics. He directs a laboratory at the Montréal Neurological Institute dealing with the use of 3-D neurological images in neurology and neurosurgery.

William (Bill) B Parsons MD FRCPC *(deceased)*
Dr Parsons was a radiologist at Red Deer Hospital and the Parsons' Clinic in Red Deer, Alberta.

Roch D DesRochers ING
Roch DesRochers is an engineer with the Commission de la santé et de la sécurité du travail (CSST) du Québec. He was the second president of the Canadian Radiation Protection Association in 1980–1981.

Wallace Roy MD FRCPC
Dr Roy is a retired radiologist living in Ontario and a former President of the Canadian Association of Radiologists.

Edward Shorter PHD
Dr Shorter is Hannah Professor in the History of Medicine in the Faculty of Medicine at the University of Toronto.

Lloyd D Skarsgard PHD
Dr Skarsgard is Head of Biophysics at the British Columbia Cancer Agency and an Associate Professor of Physics at the University of British Columbia.

Giles Stevenson MD FRCPC
Dr Stevenson is Professor and Head of the Department of Radiology at McMaster University.

William Q Stirling RT
Mr Stirling was the first president of the British Columbia organization of radiological technologists.

Douglas L Wilansky MD FRCPC
Dr Wilansky is Chief of Nuclear Medicine at the Etobicoke General Hospital.

Ron Wood RT
Mr Wood is Administrative Director of the Department of Radiology at the Vancouver Hospital and Health Sciences Centre.

Elwood Wylie RT
Mr Elwood Wylie was Manager of the Department of Radiology, Vancouver Hospitals and Health Sciences Centre, from 1967 to 1992.

Carl Zylak MD FRCPC
Dr Zylak is Chief of Radiology, Henry Ford Hospital, Detroit, Michigan and former Professor and Chairman of the Department of Radiology at McMaster University. Dr Zylak is also a former president of both the Canadian Association of Radiologists and the Radiological Society of North America.

Introduction

Brian Lentle

X-rays are a hoax.
— Lord Kelvin

When Wilhelm Röntgen discovered the existence of x-rays in 1895, he created a legacy which is still very much alive. What began as the experiments of a physicist in a laboratory in a small German university town now touches the lives of people worldwide. At present no modern clinic or hospital is complete without a radiological service which uses x-rays to diagnose disease.

The story of the serendipitous discovery of x-rays is almost legendary, but it bears retelling in this volume. Chance alone will rarely account for such a discovery, for scientific discovery requires a mind which both remains open to new ideas and can recognize the importance of new facts when they emerge.[1,2] Although Röntgen was a remarkable man he likely did not foresee just how far his discovery would lead in the next century. That story has not been confined by national boundaries.

The use of x-rays for medical purposes spread internationally with remarkable speed. Only weeks were to elapse before x-rays were being used clinically not only in Canada but worldwide. It is unlikely that anything comparable might happen now given the degree to which discoveries are hedged in by regulations and restrictions.

As physicians turned to physicists for help in using this new diagnostic tool so the applications of x-rays were extended. In time, the clinical specialty of radiology emerged, but the multidisciplinary flavour has fortunately survived. Despite its small population, Canada has played a full part in the early uses of radiation, for example Rutherford's discovery of alpha particles, cobalt-60 treatment for cancer, Alexander Graham Bell's experiments, and one of the very first uses of a radiograph in helping a surgeon to operate successfully. Canadians also have reason to be proud of the contributions made in this land to developments in early radiation treatment machines, treatment planning theory, digital radiography, image transfer, computed tomography systems and nuclear medicine imaging devices. Indeed the number of Canadian innovations arising from radiologists and technologists collaborating with industry is a quite remarkable tribute to those concerned.[3] This book celebrates the many aspects of the use of radiation in medicine.

And in the last quarter of the century which has elapsed since Röntgen's discovery, radiology has taken on some remarkable dimensions. At first, x-rays were mainly used to examine the skeleton since bones are so much more dense than soft tissues. At the same time, air in the lungs provided low-density contrast for the diagnosis of chest disease. Later, contrast materials were introduced to allow examination of blood vessels, kidneys and bowel.

X-rays are but one kind of the penetrating energies which have been used in medical diagnosis. Gamma radiation from injected radioactive tracers is imaged for diagnostic purposes in the specialty of nuclear medicine. Ultrasound energy likewise can map tissues and this lead to the development of the subspecialty of ultrasonology which has a particularly proud record in Canada. More recently radio frequency radiation superimposed upon a magnetic field has led to the development of the new and powerful method of investigating disease called magnetic resonance imaging (MRI).

Above all, the introduction of powerful and rapid computers has radically altered radiology. Such data processing capability has made possible computed tomography (CT), positron emission tomography (PET), single-photon emission tomography (SPECT), digital radiography and MRI. All these methods involve solving large numbers of equations to produce images with a speed that would not be possible without computers. All except digital radiography also provide sectional images. The advantage of these is that bodily structures are not superimposed as they are, for example, on a chest radiograph. The result is that disease is more readily diagnosed.

From its earliest beginnings radiology was concerned with both diagnosis and treatment. Radiation was and is used predominantly to treat cancer. Eventually the amount of information required to be able to practice both aspects of radiology became overwhelming, and radiology divided in Canada into the two sibling specialties of diagnostic radiology and radiation oncology. Parallel to the evolution of radiology, a number of professions playing pivotal roles in the medical radiation sciences has emerged. Indeed, a large hospital department of radiology (or imaging) may be an example of the pluralism that will increasingly characterize health care. Parallel groups of technologists who carry much of the burden of direct patient care work alongside the radiologists, radiation oncologists and nuclear medicine specialists. Physicists, computer scientists and engineers may be employed in contexts such as quality assurance, radiation protection, machine and software development. Radiopharmacists are responsible for making the tracers injected in nuclear medicine. Not least are nurses sharing in the care of the patient in what may be long and complex procedures. The roster is completed by secretaries, receptionists and porters who—to be realistic—make the whole enterprise work.

Because radiation is a two-edged sword having the potential for both good and harm, experts both on the impact of radiation on health and on the regulation of radiation exposure have also emerged.

While the range of energies that might be used to image the body and diagnose its disorders is finite, the future of radiology remains rich in promise. Magnetic resonance is becoming used to examine chemical reactions in the body, such as those which supply the energy we use in living. It is also possible to image the very weak magnetic fields that result from electrical activities in the brain and heart, a phenomenon called biomagnetism, magnetoencephalography (MEG) or magnetic source imaging (MSI). Most of these methods can be expanded and refined by the use of improved contrast agents, and their combined use, which has been called fusion imaging, may yield even larger dividends. Displays which superimpose information about bodily structure and function are proving to be very powerful.

Thus, the legacy of Röntgen is vitally alive. Indeed, it is flourishing in ways he might not have anticipated but would certainly understand and endorse.

At this time of great change and opportunity in radiology there is some scepticism about the role of high-technology tools in medicine. It has even been suggested that such high-technology applications account for a disproportionate fraction of the cost of modern health care. One analysis has identified (a) the apparently insatiable demand by the public for more and better health service and access to the latest technology (the market pull), (b) the thrust of scientific advances and new technology (the market push), and (c) the limits on the public's ability or willingness to pay for the costs associated with an unabated demand for, and use of, new technology. Certainly radiology is "high-tech." However, radiology actually accounts for only a small fraction of the budget for care. Also, methods such as tissue biopsies guided by either ultrasonography, CT or MRI have often replaced exploratory surgery which would cost more and require hospital admission. Thus, radiology may well be part of the solution to the dilemma of the funding of health care in the future. To this extent, technology may be an answer to society's need for an increased ability to treat disease using limited and dwindling resources.

The interaction between radiology and industry is complex. Young has observed that the relationship is unsatisfactory, albeit working to the advantage of the patient.[4] Blume has imagined that the relationship is conspiratorial, while seeming to ignore the physical constraints on what is and is not possible and effective.[5]

The real challenge for radiology in this era is to ensure that the machines do not come between patient and caregivers. There must not only be care of the patient but also caring for the patient, a distinction first made by Francis Peabody.[6]

Radiological research has been criticized for its focus on new machines and new techniques. That, too, is changing as investigators increasingly focus on the assessment of technology. In addition, the newer techniques available to the radiological sciences, particularly magnetic resonance imaging and spectroscopy, and PET, now permit the investigation of disease mechanisms at a molecular level, but in life rather than in the test tube or morgue. In radiation oncology the progression from x-ray (orthovoltage) treatment to the gamma radiation from cobalt-60 and then to the use of linear accelerators and the implantation of radioactive sources has increased the effectiveness of tumor cell killing while reducing damage to normal tissues.

The recent rapid advances in molecular biology have had their impact on nuclear medicine. The use of nuclear medicine for anatomic imaging, as in colloid liver scintigraphy, has declined, to be replaced by, for example, the use of labeled peptides and cytokines, monoclonal antibodies and agents which measure cerebral perfusion. These approaches exploit the sensitivity and tissue specificity of the tracer method and ensure that progress continues while positron emission tomography (PET) is making the transition from research laboratory to clinic.

Although there are unlikely to be vast changes in the nature of the technologies available in a department of radiology and nuclear medicine in future, their use is sure to change. When the second-centennial celebrations of Röntgen's discovery come around, it is likely that imaging disease at an early stage will have become even more pivotal in the prevention of disease and the care of the sick. More and more, the diagnostic and interventional or treatment aspects of the radiological sciences will become inseparable. Ultimately the use of virtual-reality methods will combine medicine and surgery with radiology,[7] enabling the physician to "see through" the patient when planning or performing surgery. Patient care will reach the point at which the boundaries of the radiological sciences with other specialties will blur and radiology will have become intrinsic to the entire art and science of medicine. That juncture will be the ultimate measure of the power of Röntgen's "new kind of ray".

Acknowledgement:
I am grateful to Dr John Aldrich for constructive comment.

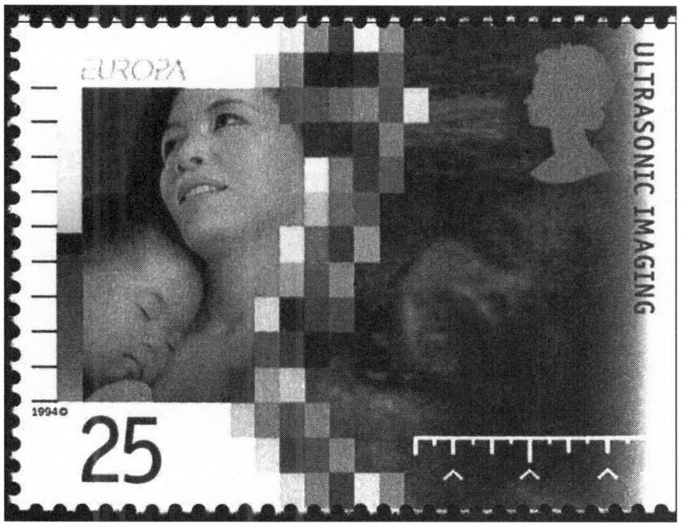
EUROPA
ULTRASONIC IMAGING
1994©
25

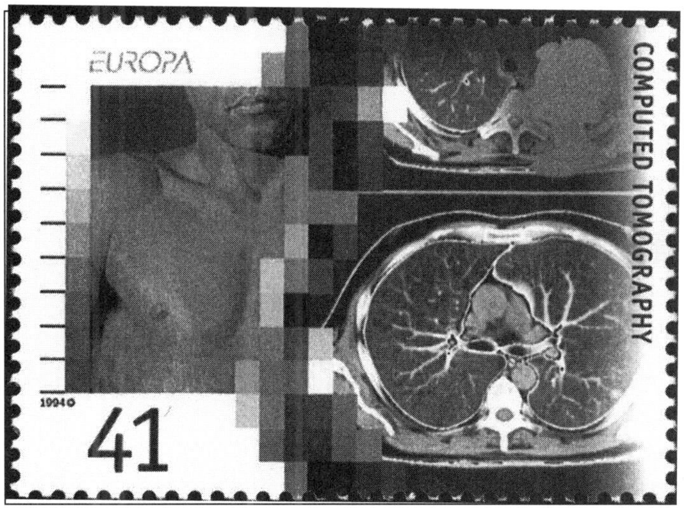
EUROPA
COMPUTED TOMOGRAPHY
1994©
41

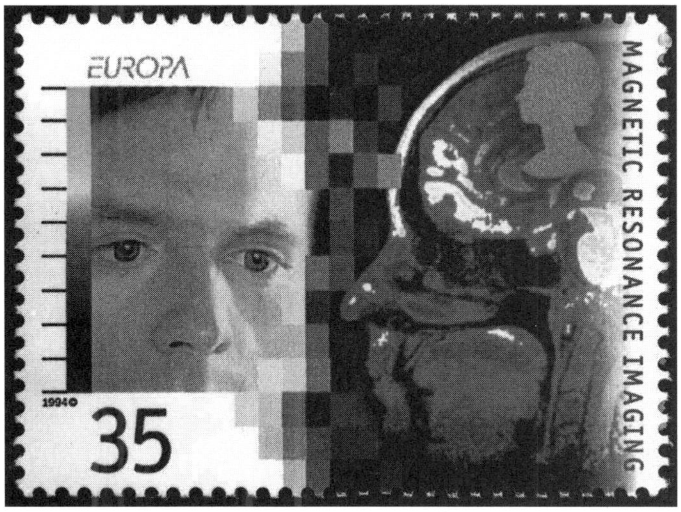
EUROPA
MAGNETIC RESONANCE IMAGING
1994©
35

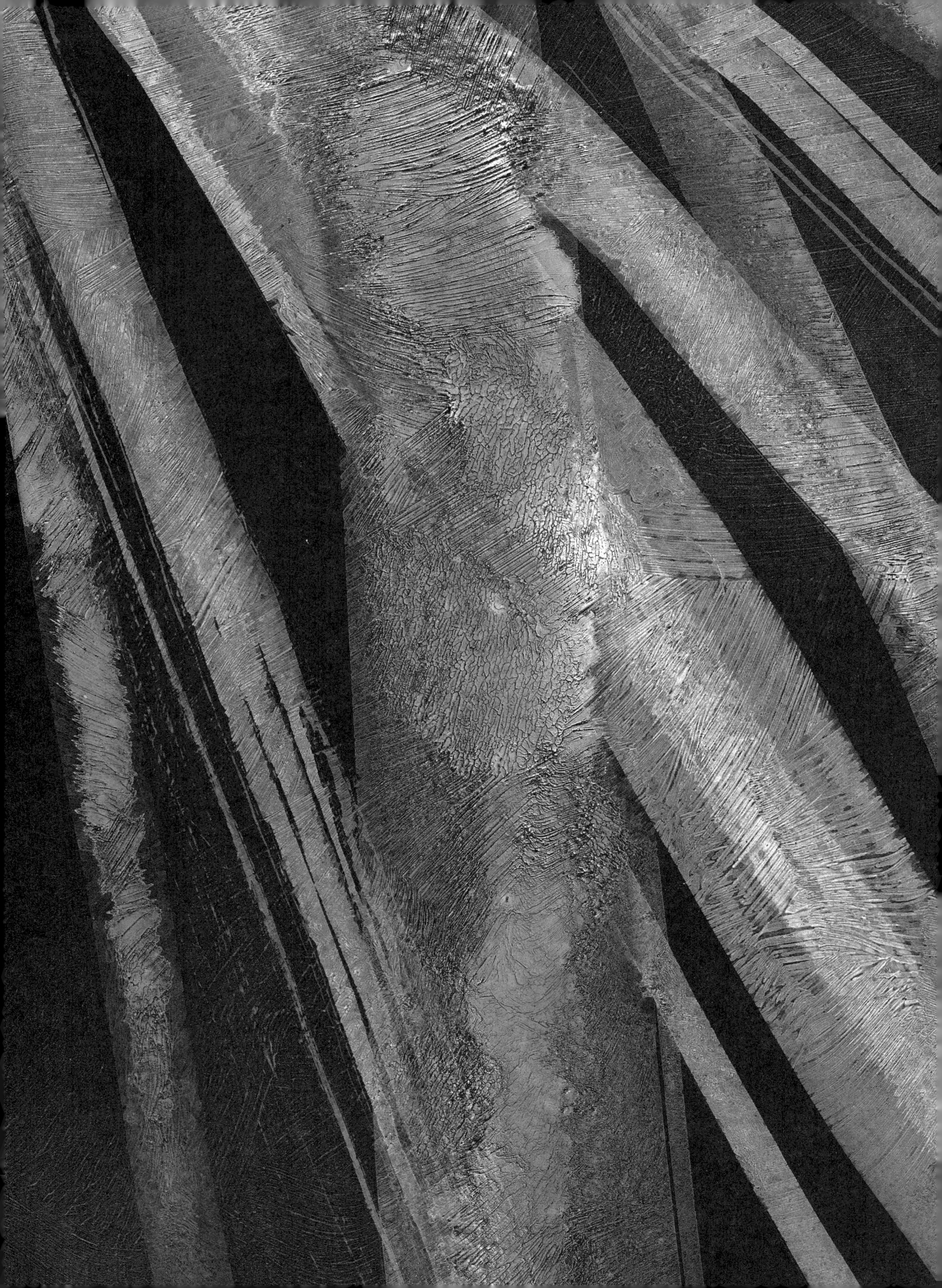

Part One
Origins

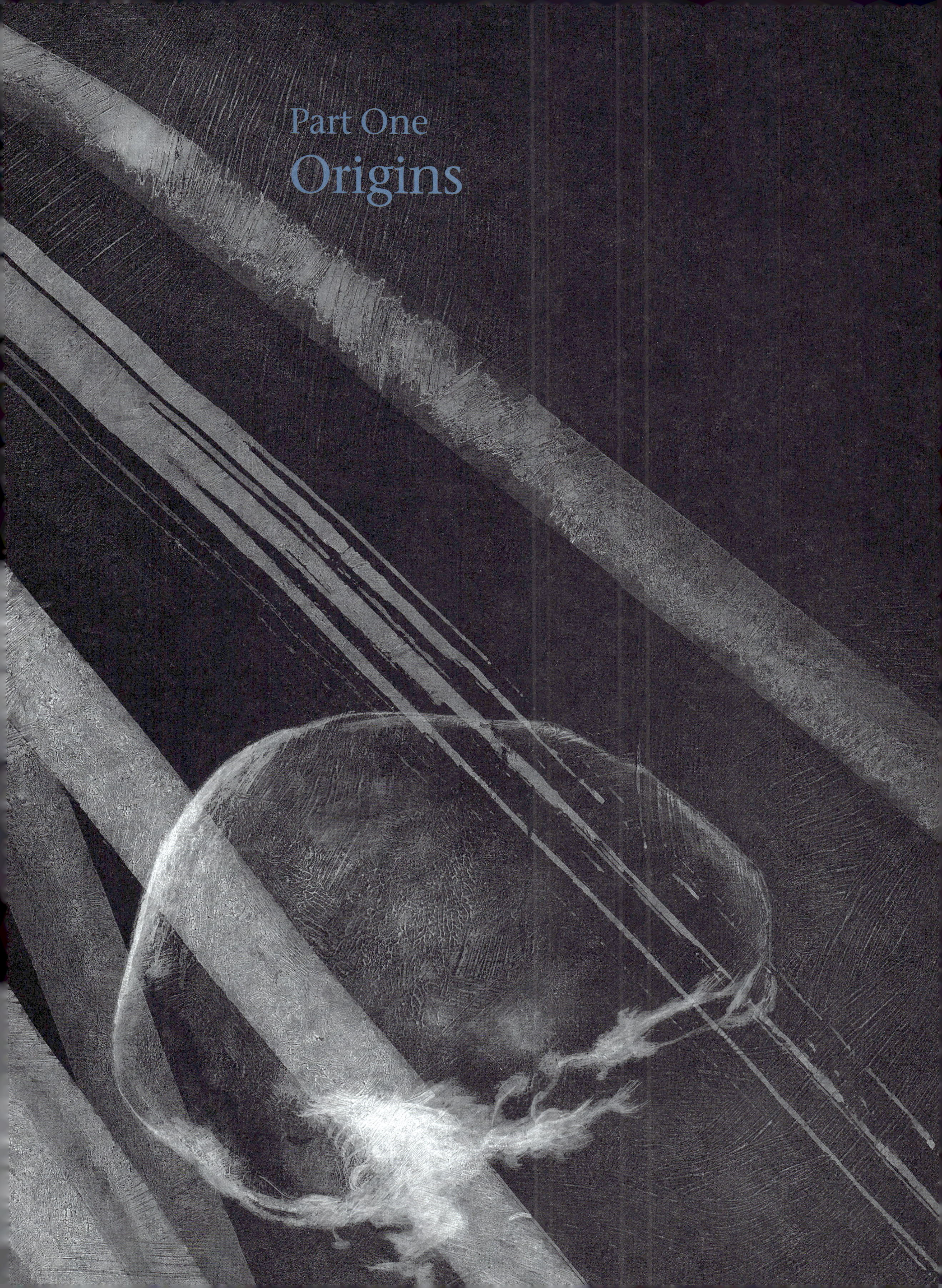

It is difficult even from this historical distance to comprehend the enormity of Röntgen's discovery on that November day in 1895. His work started out in a very ordinary way: he had worked on gases and on the electrical properties of dielectrics and had decided to devote himself to the study of electrical discharges in gases. He built all his own equipment, and he carefully repeated the work which had been performed by previous investigators. It must have taken him months to construct his apparatus: it took more than four days just to evacuate one Crookes' tube!

Many scientists produced x-rays before Röntgen. Many could even show documentary evidence after the event. However, Röntgen alone was able to connect a shimmering light in the corner of his laboratory with an entirely unknown form of radiation. His careful scientific method allowed him to make this momentous discovery.

— John Aldrich

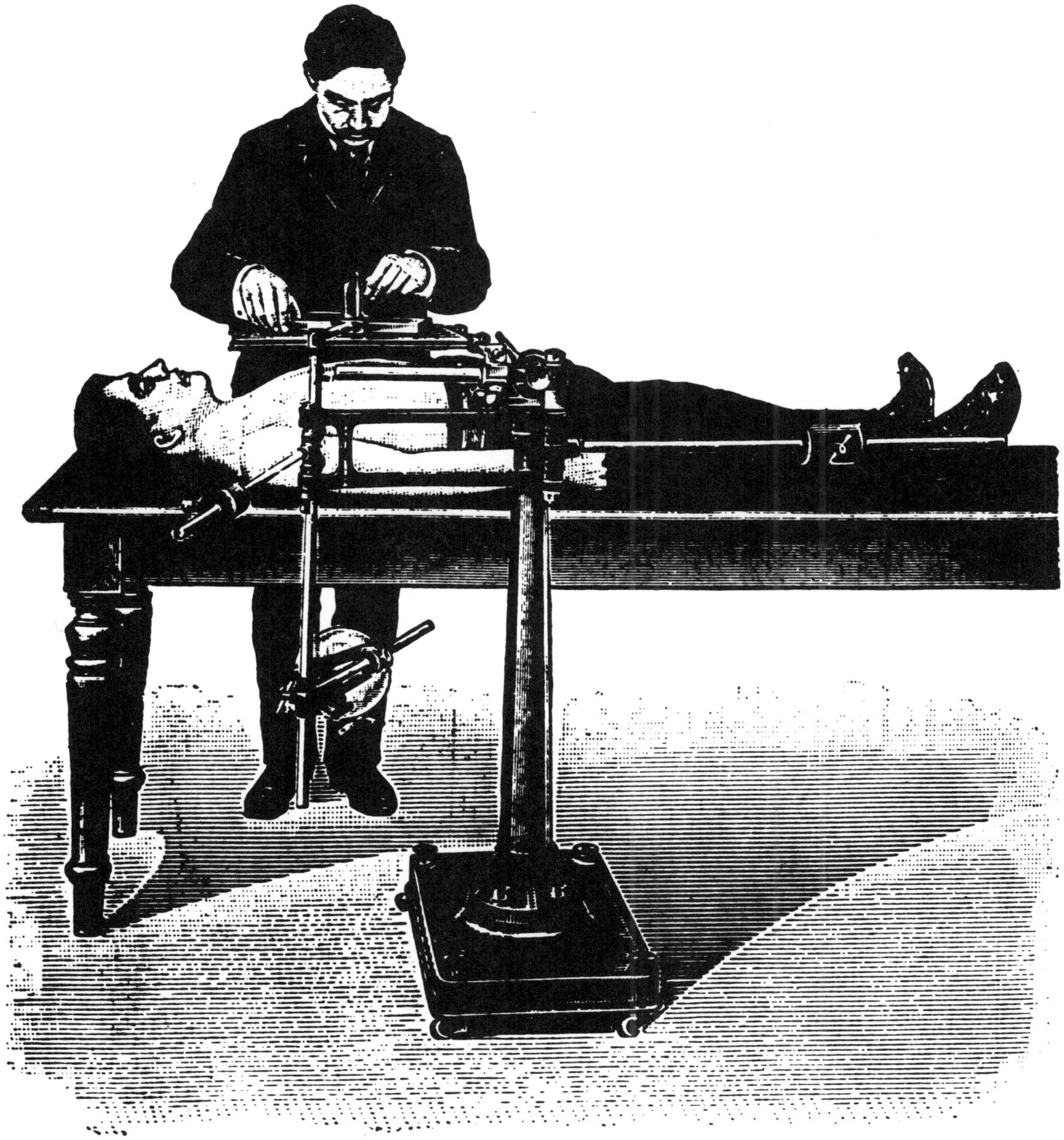

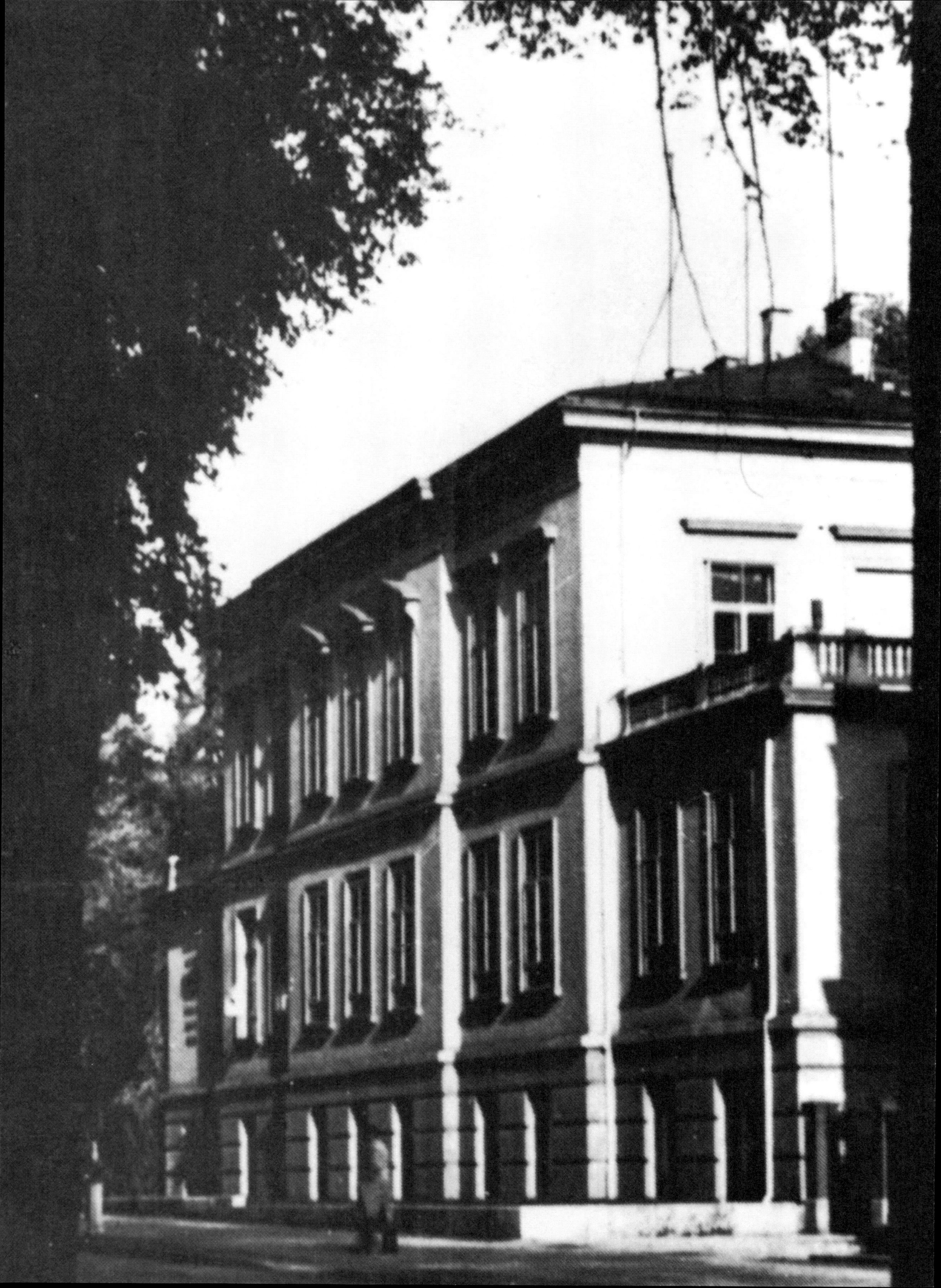

Chapter I • # *Röntgen*

and the Discovery of X-rays

JOHN ALDRICH

INTRODUCTION

In the fields of observation, chance favours only the prepared mind.
— Louis Pasteur

Although the discovery of x-rays is associated with Röntgen, he was certainly not the first person to produce them. During the 18th and 19th centuries there arose an enormous interest in high voltage discharges through gases. As early as 1709 Francis Hauksbee, instrument maker to the Royal Society in London, described colours produced in evacuated vessels containing a few drops of mercury when they were shaken. He could produce the same glow when an evacuated spherical vessel was rotated and charged with static electricity. In 1785 William Morgan experimented to find whether electricity would pass through a perfect vacuum. He formed such a vacuum by boiling the mercury of a Torricellian barometer to expel all the gas. He demonstrated that electricity could not be forced through the vacuum. In the course of one of his experiments the glass tube cracked and very slowly admitted air. Morgan then saw a succession of colours, beginning with yellowish-green and passing through blue and purple to red. He reported these findings to the Royal Society, suggesting that the degree of vacuum could be determined by the colour of the electrical discharge. Quite clearly, both Hauksbee and Morgan had produced x-rays.[1]

In the 1850s Heinrich Geissler made two crucial contributions towards the study of electrical discharges.[2] He was a skilled glass-blower and was able to make the complex shapes which the early experimenters used in these studies. He also designed a new form of mercury vacuum pump which consisted of two glass vessels connected by a long narrow rubber tube. The upper vessel was connected by a stopcock to the vessel to be evacuated. Mercury was added to both

Left
University of Würzburg

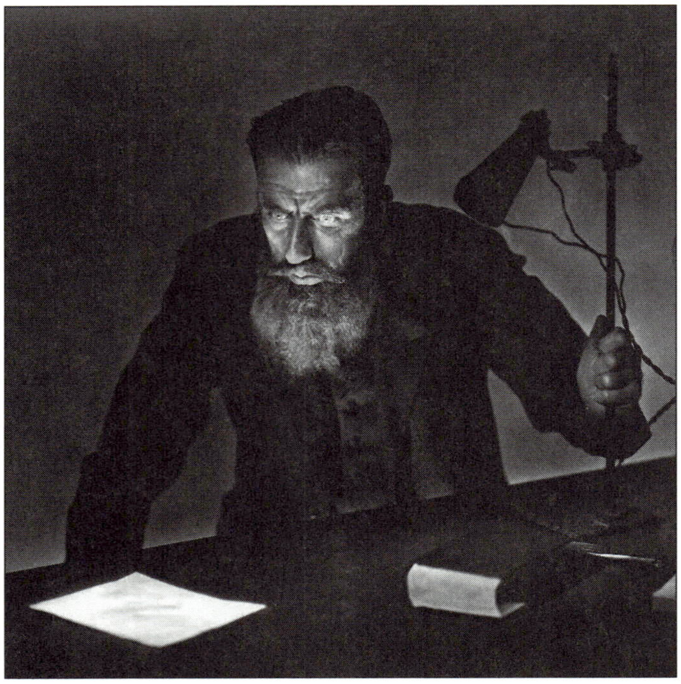

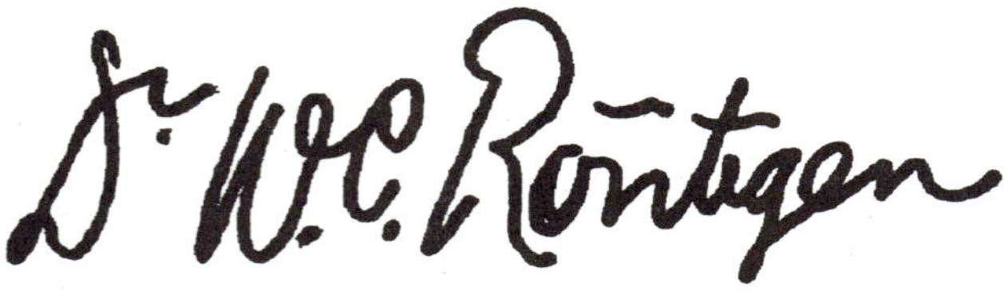

Above
Röntgen's moment of discovery

Right
Röntgen giving a lecture

glass vessels and, by raising and lowering the upper vessel and opening and closing the stopcock, the air could be efficiently removed from the apparatus. The more times the cycle of raising and lowering the mercury was performed the better the vacuum. A vacuum of about 0.05 mm mercury could be achieved. Geissler was able to produce a range of glass vessels with platinum wires sealed in each end, and he was able to evacuate the vessels with his mercury pump. After sending a high voltage from a Ruhmkorff coil, he observed bands of colour in the tubes which varied with the shape of the tubes and arrangement of the electrodes.

Sir William Crookes spent many years in similar investigations, developing a pump for producing even better vacuums, and high vacuum tubes became known as "Crookes' tubes". In the 1870s Crookes demonstrated that when high voltages were passed through evacuated tubes entirely new phenomena were produced. He studied nearly every phase: the production of colours, their stratification, dark spaces, the changes around cathode and anode, and the cathode ray. He showed that the luminous colours radiated in straight lines if the vacuum were sufficiently high, cast shadows of objects placed within the tubes, and could even melt refractory metals such as platinum. Within the tubes diamonds, rubies and various chemical compounds glowed with striking brilliancy. Crookes' work was considered a perfect example of pure science safely remote from possible utility. Nevertheless, Crookes had used a vacuum of one millionth of an atmosphere, which is within the limits of making x-ray production possible. He had noted the greenish-yellow colour of the gas so familiar to workers with early x-ray tubes, and he had studied the spectrum of the light. Unknowingly, he was generating x-rays in more than sufficient quantity for practical diagnostic work.

WILHELM CONRAD RÖNTGEN

Wilhelm Conrad Röntgen was born in the town of Lennep on March 27 1845, the only child of Friedrich and Charlotte Röntgen.[3] When he was three, the Röntgens moved to Apeldoorn in Holland, where Charlotte's parents had made their home. As the son of a fairly wealthy, if conservative, textile merchant, Wilhelm had a pleasant upbringing and came to appreciate culture and good living. At first he attended state schools, and then a private boarding school. At seventeen he attended a technical school in Utrecht and took all the usual courses in mathematics, chemistry and physics. Because of a prank by a fellow student, Wilhelm was expelled from the technical school, and his father spent many months trying to obtain permission for Wilhelm to take a private examination that would allow him to enter university. After a year's preparation he did not pass the examination but registered at the University of Utrecht in January 1865 with permission to audit courses as a student of philosophy. However, he soon learned that it was possible to enter the Zurich Technical School by taking an entrance test. As it turned out, he was accepted into this school based solely on his school record, and for three years he applied himself to study. His marks when he took his final exams in 1868 were excellent.

After graduating from the school in engineering Röntgen stayed on in Zurich to take a few more mathematics courses and August Kundt's course on the theory of light. In Kundt's laboratory he made his first experiments and started to realize that physics was a subject of interest to him. After a year of study with Kundt, Röntgen submitted his thesis, *Studies on Gases*, for which he was awarded his doctorate in philosophy in 1869. Röntgen became Kundt's assistant and in 1870 followed Kundt when he took up a new position in Würzburg. His ties to Zurich were to continue, however, for in January 1872 he returned to that city to marry Anna Bertha Ludwig. Her father Johann was the proprietor of a cafe that Röntgen had frequented as a student. Johann had been forced to flee from Germany because of his revolutionary activities as a student. He had continued his scholarly activities to some extent with private tutoring and translating and often livened discussions in the cafe with his wit and conversation.

Shortly after the wedding, Röntgen and Kundt took up new appointments at the University of Strasbourg. Apart from a year at Hohenheim in Württemberg, Röntgen spent seven years in Strasbourg and worked in several areas, including thermodynamics, solar energy, solid state properties and electrical discharges. This work led to many publications and an offer of a post at the University of Giessen in 1879, which he accepted. He continued his work for a further eight years at Giessen, and he considered his time there to be some of the happiest years of his life. He lectured to a large circle of students and colleagues, and he could indulge his love for hikes in the mountains.

Röntgen's reputation as a skilled investigator continued to bring offers of positions from several universities.[4] Eventually, in 1888, he accepted the Chair of Physics at the Königliche University of Würzburg in the town where he and his bride had made their first home. His teaching schedule was as full as ever, and he developed a certain reputation: He lectured in a black cut-away coat and allowed his moustache and beard to grow freely, acquiring a patriarchal appearance that matched his demeanor. His

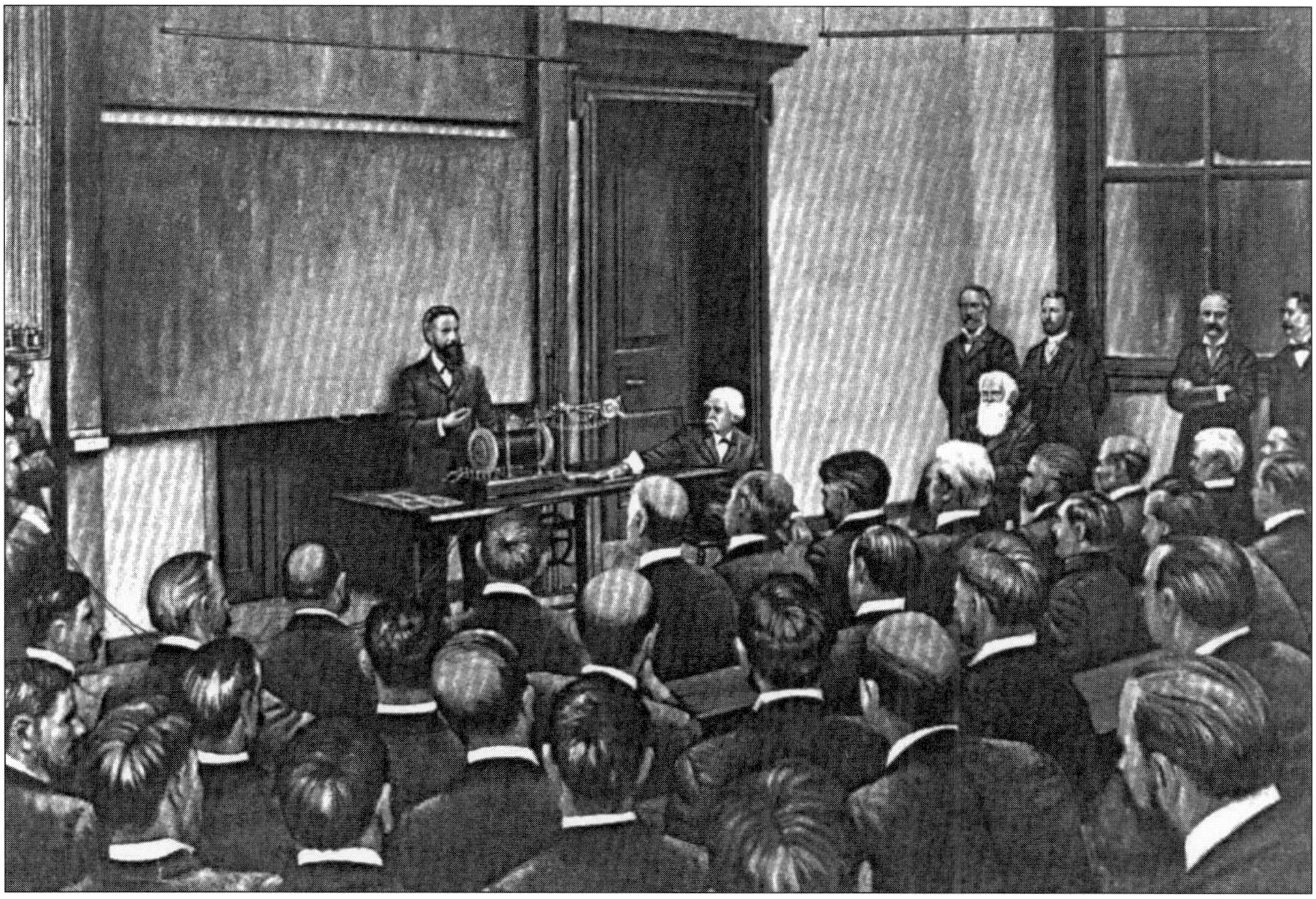

lectures were meticulously prepared but monotonously delivered in a fast, deep voice which was difficult to follow. The examinations were comprehensive, difficult and dreaded ("Don't pamper the students; let each find his own way out of difficulty" was his motto[3]). Despite his classroom commitments, he continued both research and publication.

THE DISCOVERY

Soon Röntgen's attention turned to cathode rays. Lenard had extended the work of Crookes on cathode rays by constructing a discharge tube with a thin aluminum window opposite the cathode. By this means he could observe the cathode rays *outside* the discharge tube. He showed that cathode rays produced fluorescence of certain salts, fogged photographic plates, and were easily absorbed in a few centimetres of air. As was common practice then, Röntgen decided to repeat Lenard's experiments, and he acquired a Lenard tube, fluorescent salts, and photographic plates. He covered the Lenard tube with closely fitting cardboard and tin foil as an electro-static shield to protect the thin window. Thus, just as Lenard had done, he could observe—without interference from the glow within the tube—the fluorescence of the platinocyanide screen held close to the end window. Röntgen had to pay special attention to this process because of his poor eyesight.

On Friday, November 8, 1895, Röntgen was continuing these experiments *but this time with a high vacuum Crookes' tube* covered with a tight fitting cardboard cover.[3] To ascertain that the jacket was light-proof, he connected the electrodes to an induction coil and passed a high voltage through the tube. In the darkness, he noticed a shimmering light that came from a point about a metre away from the tube. With the aid of a match he identified the object—the platinocyanide coated fluorescent screen. Obviously, something had excited the fluorescence across a much greater distance than was possible for cathode rays.

Röntgen became absorbed in his work and devoted all his attention to the study of this new phenomenon, eating his meals in the laboratory, sometimes even sleeping there. He spoke to no one about his work, and his assistants found him irritable and less approachable than usual. For weeks and weeks he repeated the experiments to satisfy himself that what he was seeing was in fact correct. Finally, his wife demanded to know what had so drastically changed his character over the previous few weeks. Röntgen eventually took his wife to the laboratory where he explained his experiments and took the first radiograph of her hand.

On December 28, 1895, Röntgen delivered to the secretary of Würzburg Physical and Medical Society a handwritten paper entitled "On a New Kind of Ray." In this report Röntgen described his experiment with the energized Crookes' tube in a darkened room and how a screen of platinocyanide would glow if placed near the tube. He reported that a bound book of a thousand pages offered little resistance to the rays and, similarly, that two packs of playing cards, several layers of tin foil and a pine board three centimetres thick were all easily penetrated. Glass alone seemed unusual; although transparent to visible light, flint glass stopped the new rays remarkably well because of the lead content. He described, too, the eerie sight of the bones of the hand surrounded by the partially transparent flesh. He tried to formulate a theory to account for the transparencies of different substances to the new rays, and he concluded that the transparency varied inversely with the atomic weight of the material, uranium being the most opaque, lithium the least.

In a footnote he explained that to differentiate these new rays from other rays he would call them x-rays.[3]

Röntgen attempted to study refraction and reflection of x-rays but with inconclusive results. He showed that, as with visible light, the intensity of the x-rays was inversely proportional to the square of the distance from the source of the rays. He described the effect of the x-rays on photographic plates, which enabled him to more easily quantify the effects of x-rays, but which also made him aware that photographic film should be kept away from the x-ray equipment! It was clear to Röntgen that the x-rays were different from the cathode rays described by Lenard (it was not until two years later that JJ Thomson confirmed that cathode rays were in fact electrons[2]). The x-rays were far more penetrating and were not deflected by magnetic fields. Finally, Röntgen described several shadow-pictures which he had taken, including a hand, a compass and some weights in a box. One radiograph showed the shadows produced when an x-ray picture was taken through a door. He had had to have the door dismantled in order to explain the unusual lines on the radiograph, which were caused by the lead paint covering.

On New Year's day Röntgen sent printed copies of his article and some of his radiographs to a few colleagues. One of these leaked the news to the *Vienna Free Press* which carried it as front page news on January 5, 1896. The news rapidly spread worldwide.

Röntgen was astonished by the public and scientific interest in his rather straightforward paper. The university and the Röntgen residence became the focus of world attention from the press and the curious. Letters of praise and condemnation came in from all parts of the world. Scientists sent examples of their equipment to Röntgen for his approval. "As soon as the paper was published our domestic peace was gone," Frau Röntgen complained in a letter to a friend. X-ray pictures were even stolen from the laboratory, and postcards bearing Röntgen's signature never reached their destination.

Early in 1896 Röntgen was summoned to appear at the court of Emperor Wilhelm II to demonstrate his discovery. He set up his apparatus and was able to demonstrate how the x-rays penetrated solid objects. In order not to strain his x-ray tube he did not make any radiographs of human anatomy but showed the pictures he had taken in his laboratory. Röntgen was decorated by the Emperor with the Prussian Order of the Crown.

At the insistence of his scientific colleagues at the university, Röntgen gave one of his few scientific lectures to the Würzburg Physical-Medical Society on January 23. Not surprisingly, everyone, including his scientific colleagues, officials of both the university and town, and his students and friends, wanted to attend the lecture. The auditorium was full long before the lecture, and Röntgen arrived to warm applause. He described his experiments and gave due credit to those, such as Lenard and Hertz, who had paved the way for his discovery. He demonstrated the properties of x-rays, their ability to penetrate various objects, and he showed several pictures he had taken with x-rays.

Röntgen then asked Professor von Kölliker, the famous anatomist of the university, if he could make an x-ray picture of his hand. Von Kölliker eagerly agreed and, when the film was finally developed, there was tremendous applause from the gathered assembly. Von Kölliker gave an impassioned speech in which he thanked Röntgen and said that he felt that this was the most significant lecture he had ever attended. In tribute to Röntgen's discovery he proposed that henceforth the x-rays be known as "Röntgen's rays," and the crowd again expressed its approval.

On March 9 Röntgen published his second paper. Here, continuing from his first paper, he cautioned investigators about accepting the results of x-ray investigations without the proper precautions. He described a large zinc box in which he could conduct his experiments; the box was needed to overcome some of the confounding factors associated with x-ray work. The wall opposite the door was covered in lead except for a small opening covered in aluminum. X-rays from a tube outside the box could pass through the aluminum window so that experiments could be conducted free of perturbation inside. He described the ability of x-rays to discharge electrostatic charges on insulators and conductors.

In his third paper (March 10, 1896) Röntgen discussed in more detail the scattering of x-rays in air and the dependence of x-ray intensity on various factors, including

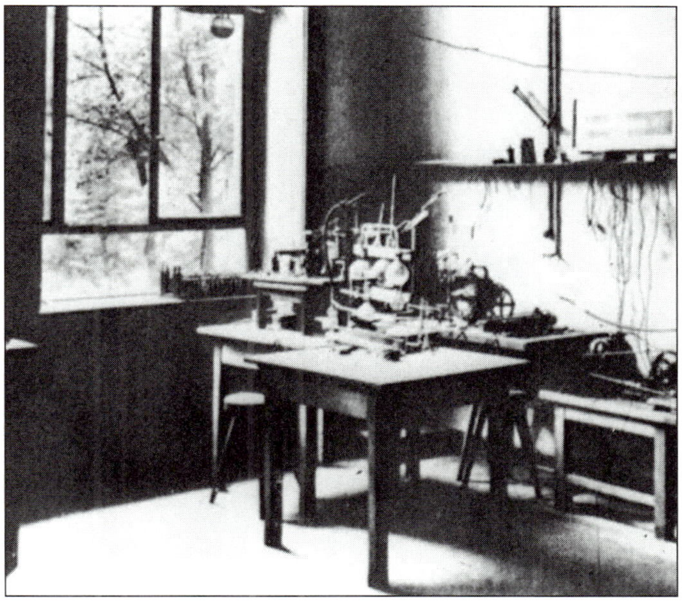

Röntgen's laboratory at the Königliche University, Würzburg

current and the effect of the angle of the target to the cathode ray stream. He also described his attempts to produce a greater intensity of x-rays from his tubes and the type of rays produced by 'soft' (low vacuum) and 'hard' tubes. He correctly surmised that the harder tubes produced more penetrating rays.

Röntgen moved to Munich in 1900 and continued his research on the physical properties of crystals. Numerous awards, medals, and honorary memberships of learned societies were bestowed on him. Perhaps the greatest honour was the 1901 Nobel Prize for Physics, the first ever to be awarded, and Röntgen attended in person to receive the prize. He donated the prize money to the University of Würzburg to be used for research.

After moving to Munich, Frau Röntgen was subject to bouts of chronic pain attributed to renal colic, which severely limited her mobility. She died in 1919 during an attack of the illness. Röntgen himself retired from his university post in 1920, but two rooms were set aside in the laboratory for his continued use. Finally on February 10, 1923, Wilhelm Conrad Röntgen died in Munich at the age of 77. The world lost a great physicist and scholar, and a man of integrity who never doubted the value of his science. His name and his work will endure.

Acknowledgements:
The illustration of Röntgen lecturing at Würtzburg is reproduced by kind permission of Parke-Davis Corporation. The painting of Röntgen's discovery is reproduced by kind permission of General Electric Corporation. All other illustrations are by permission of the Röntgen-Kuratorium, Würtzburg.

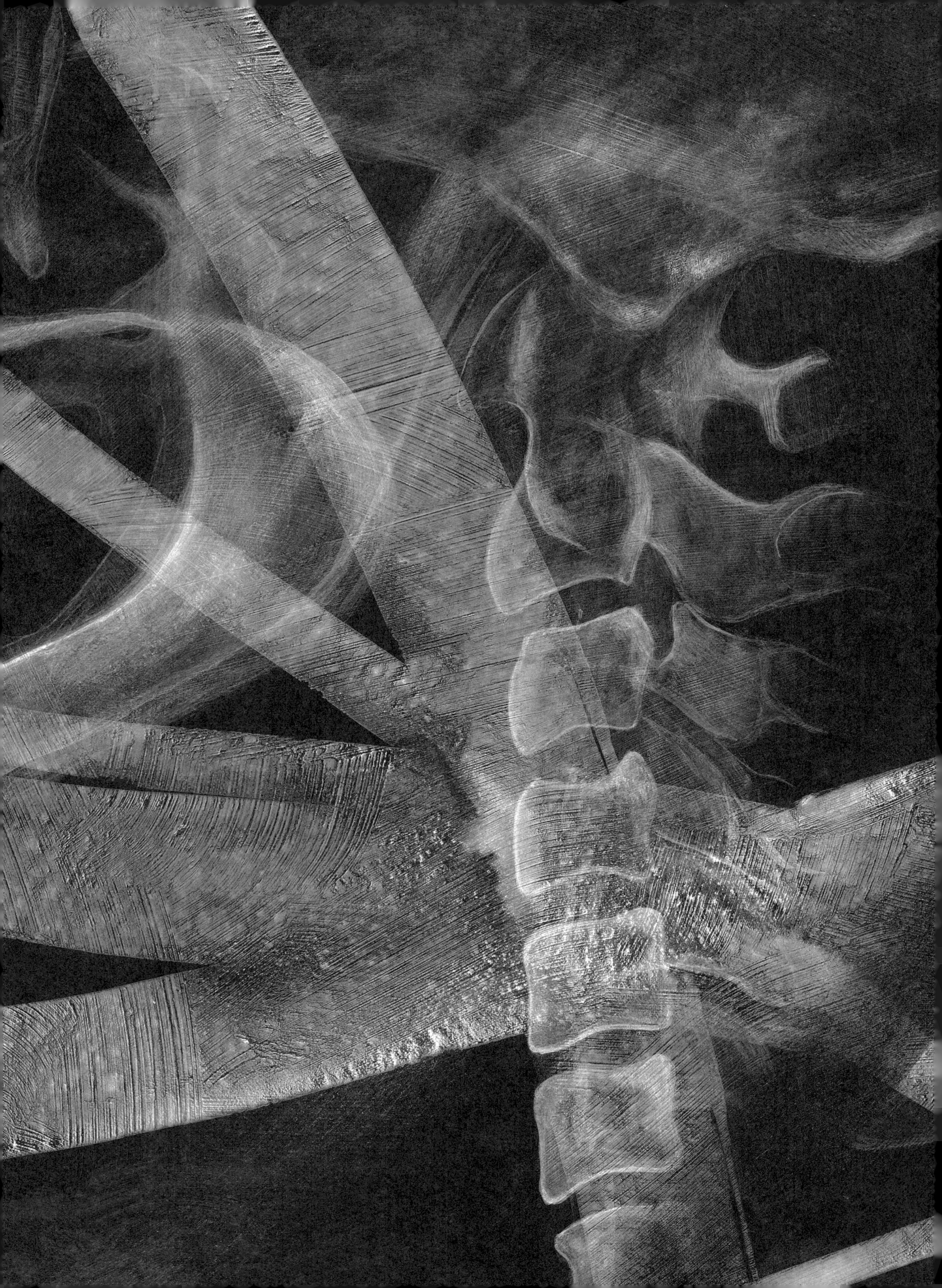

Part Two

The Pioneers

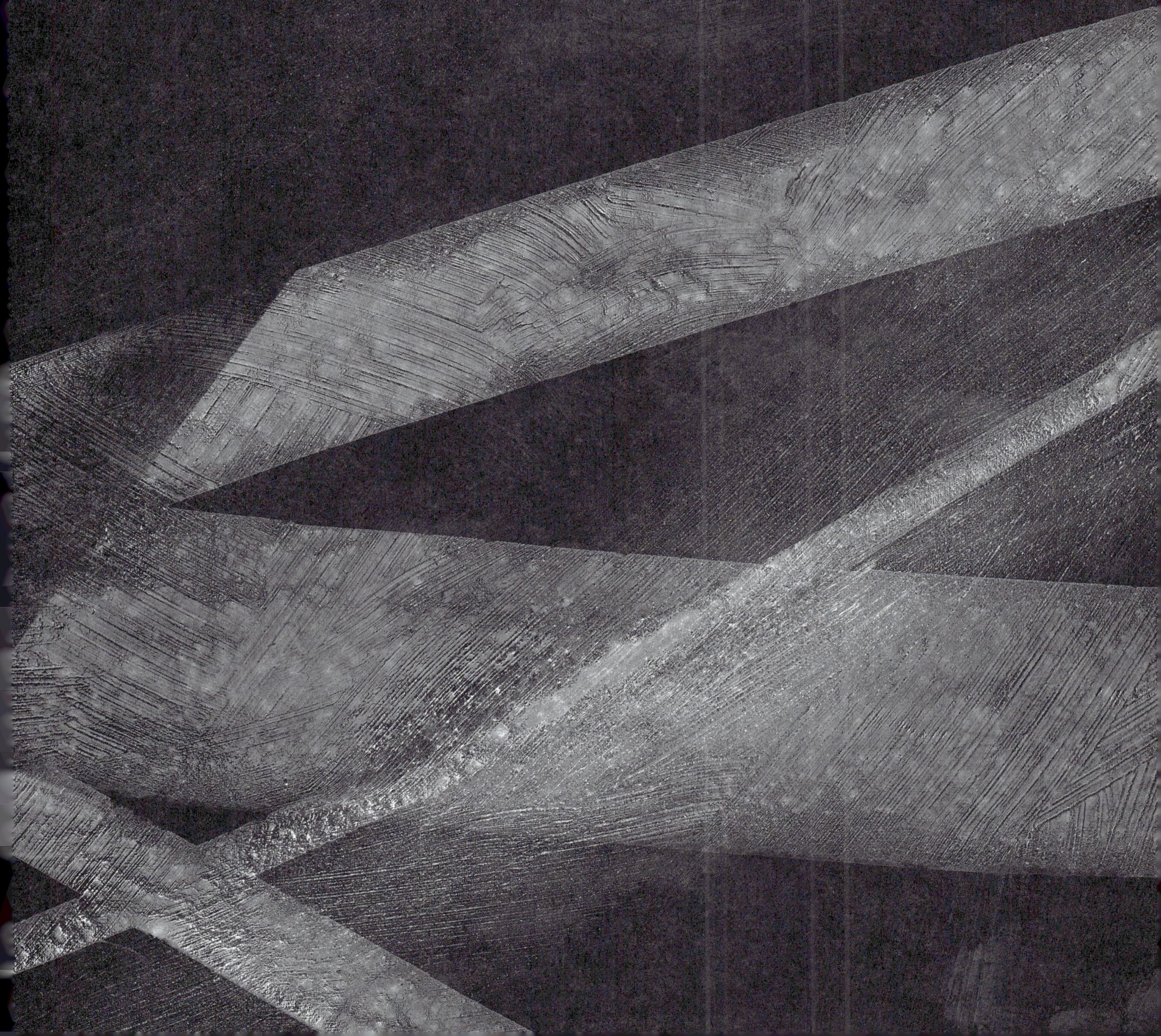

The equipment required to produce x-rays was widely available in university physics laboratories by the end of last century. Within months of Röntgen's discovery x-rays were being produced all over the world. Dr John Cox, professor of physics at McGill University, was one of the first to be involved in the clinical use of x-rays. Later he also helped foster the research of Rutherford.

The early tubes were very difficult to use because they were not completely evacuated. A hand radiograph might take a minute, a chest radiograph thirty minutes.

Alexander Graham Bell knew no bounds to his inventive genius. As soon as x-rays were discovered and he had read about them in the journals, he was thinking of new uses for them. It is not surprising, then, that he was using x-rays in Nova Scotia within six months of their discovery.

— John Aldrich

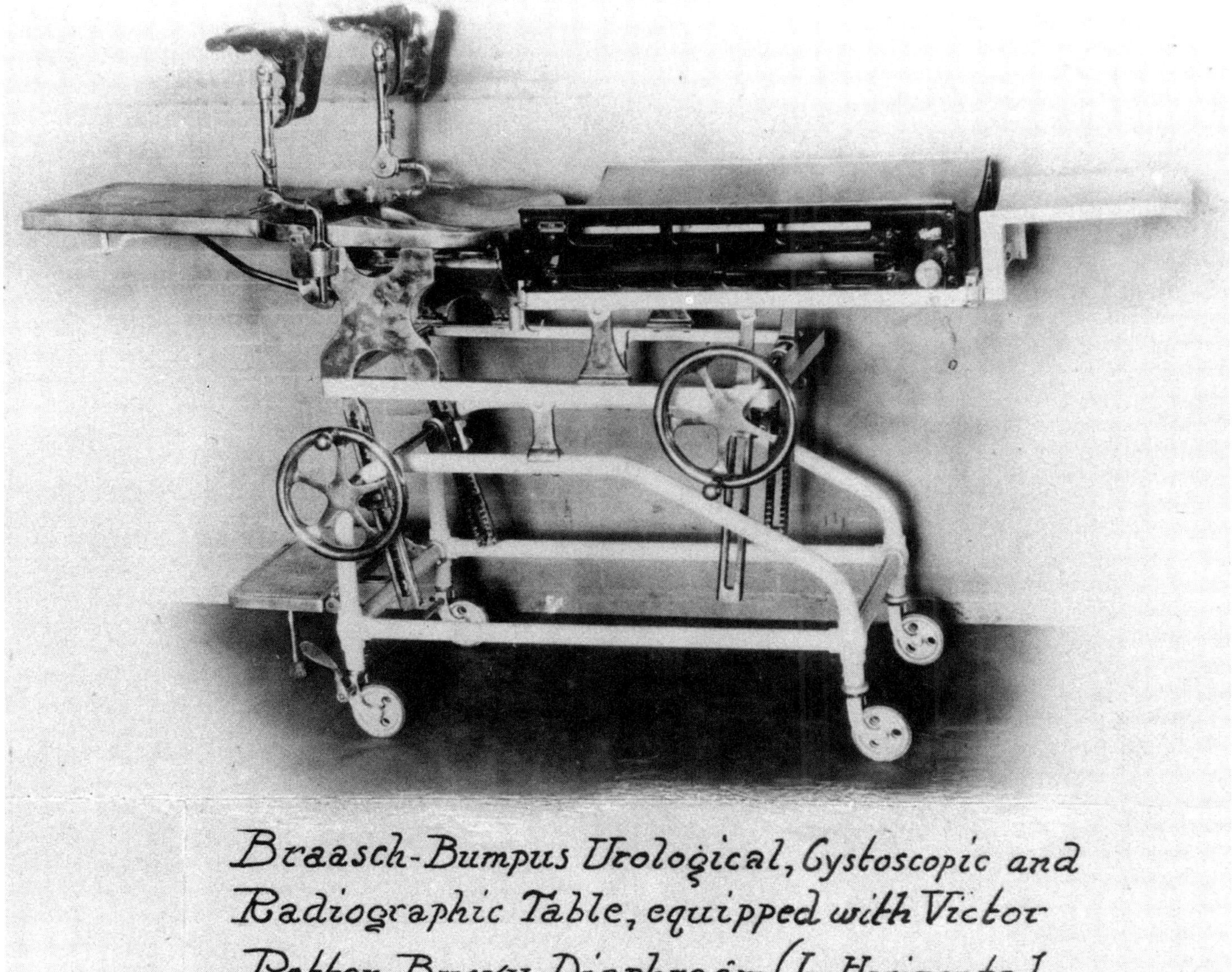

From an equipment catalogue, 1920's

Chapter I • *Gas Tubes*

John Aldrich

It is often thought that early x-ray tubes consisted of a heated coil, like that of an electric light bulb, from which electrons were accelerated towards a heavy tungsten anode, where the x-rays were produced. However, this was not at all the way in which x-ray tubes operated before 1913, when William Coolidge invented a new type of tube from which modern types have developed. In fact, the period from 1896 until 1913 was the so-called "gas tube years."[1] X-ray tubes then consisted basically of a glass tube, evacuated to about a millionth of an atmosphere, with a positive and negative electrode. When a high voltage discharge passed through the tube, many molecules were ionized and the positive ions driven towards the cathode. Positive-ion bombardment of the cathode liberated electrons. These electrons or cathode rays were accelerated in the direction of the anode and produced x-rays with whatever material they collided with, such as the glass of the tube, the anode, or any other target placed in the tube.[2]

Quite clearly, a small amount of gas in the tube was essential for the operation of this type of tube. When the high tension was placed across these tubes and x-rays were produced, there was a tendency for the tube to become more and more evacuated. The early workers had a very difficult time judging the hardness of the vacuum in the tube so that they could, if necessary, intervene. They judged the vacuum by noting the colour of the discharge and by recognizing the sound the discharge made. In order to increase the amount of gas in the tube to a reasonable level, the tube was warmed by, for example, the flame of a small spirit lamp. This procedure was very hazardous

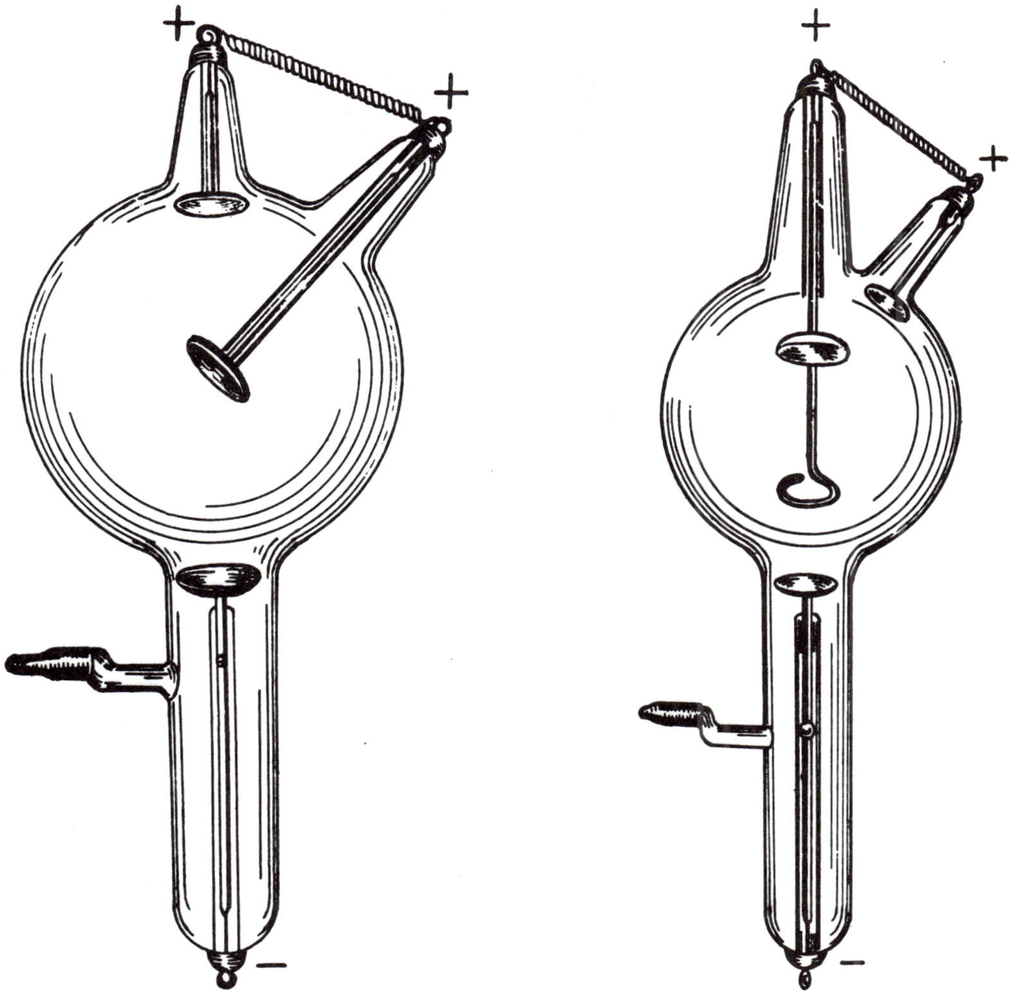

because lowering the vacuum too much or melting the glass would cause the tube to explode inwards (a result especially disliked by child patients). In making an exposure of, say, half an hour the operator had to turn off the current, warm the tube and turn on the current again perhaps fifteen or twenty times.[3]

Gas tubes from about 1900

The vacuum was not the only problem in the operation of the gas tubes. The only way of judging the voltage across the tube was by gauging the length of spark produced. The length of spark in inches multiplied by ten plus ten was a rough indication of the kVp (the peak voltage across the x-ray tube). The thickness of the spark gave some idea of the possible output of the tube. Of course, there were no measurements of the actual radiation output of the tubes, and it was not realized until later that a whole spectrum of x-rays was produced by an x-ray tube and that filters have a profound effect on the properties of an x-ray beam.

THE

MONTREAL MEDICAL JOURNAL.

VOL. XXIV. MARCH, 1896. No. 9.

Original Communications.

THE NEW PHOTOGRAPHY WITH REPORT OF A CASE IN WHICH A BULLET WAS PHOTOGRAPHED IN THE LEG.[1]

By J. Cox, M.A.
Wm. C. McDonald Professor of Physics, McGill University, Montreal.
AND
Robt. C. Kirkpatrick, B.A., M.D.,
Demonstrator of Surgery, McGill University; Surgeon to the Montreal General Hospital.

Everyone is familiar with the phenomena produced by discharging an induction coil through an ordinary Geissler tube. The vacuum of such a tube corresponds to a pressure of about one-thousandth of an atmosphere, or something less than one millimetre of mercury. On closer inspection the negative electrode, or Kathode, is seen to be covered with a velvety glow. Next comes a short dark space from which a faint violet cone spreads along the tube; the rest, and by far the larger part of the tube, is filled with a cloudy light whose colour depends on the gas within the tube. This light is generally arranged in regular patches or striæ and extends right up to the anode or positive pole.

Some twenty years ago Crookes showed to the British Association a number of tubes in which the exhaustion was carried to the millionth of an atmosphere. In these tubes the phenomena, as had been previously observed by Hittorf, are entirely different. As the vacuum increases the dark space spreads from the Kathode till it fills the whole tube, and the faint violet cone of rays from the Kathode excites brilliant fluorescence in the walls of the tube or any mineral or screen placed to receive them. Crookes exhibited experiments to

[1] Demonstrated before the Montreal Medico-Chirurgical Society, Feb. 7, 1896.

Chapter II • *Canada's First Clinical X-Ray*

Montague Cohen

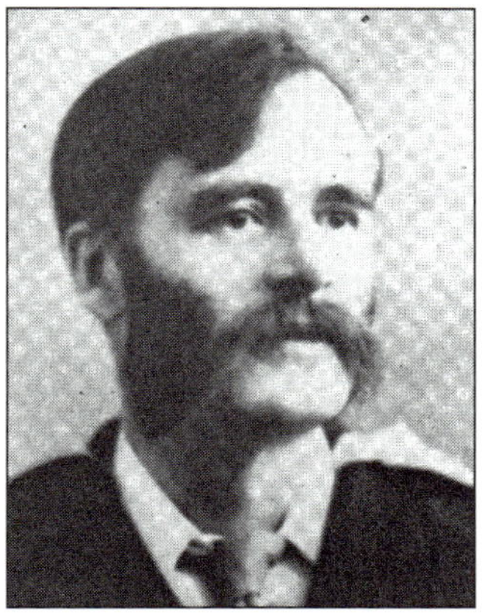

Professor John Cox

The news of Röntgen's discovery of x-rays disseminated rapidly in Europe and the United Kingdom in the first week of January 1896. Reprints of Röntgen's original paper soon became available. However, the early reports reaching North America by cable were lacking in details about the apparatus used for the production of the rays, and it was almost the end of January before this information reached scientists in the United States and Canada. Fortunately, the apparatus needed was readily available in physical laboratories, and experiments could begin almost immediately.

The first verified use of x-rays in North America—there were several unverified prior claims—occurred on January 27, 1896. On that day Arthur Williams Wright, professor of experimental physics at Yale University, obtained an x-ray photograph (with a 15-minute exposure) of some small objects including a pair of scissors and a 25-cent piece.[1] A week later, on February 3, the first authenticated *diagnostic* radiograph in North America was made at Dartmouth College, Hanover, New Hampshire. Edwin B Frost, a professor of astronomy, and CF Emerson, a professor of physics, had begun experimenting with x-rays in the physics laboratory on February 1. Two days later, Frost's brother, a physician, brought a young patient with a broken forearm to the laboratory. A 20-minute exposure was made and, according to the report published on February 14, 1896, "the plate on development showed the fracture of the ulna very distinctly."[2] The article, however, was concerned mainly with the physical investigations of the new radiation made by Emerson and Frost and did not include a reproduction of the clinical radiograph.

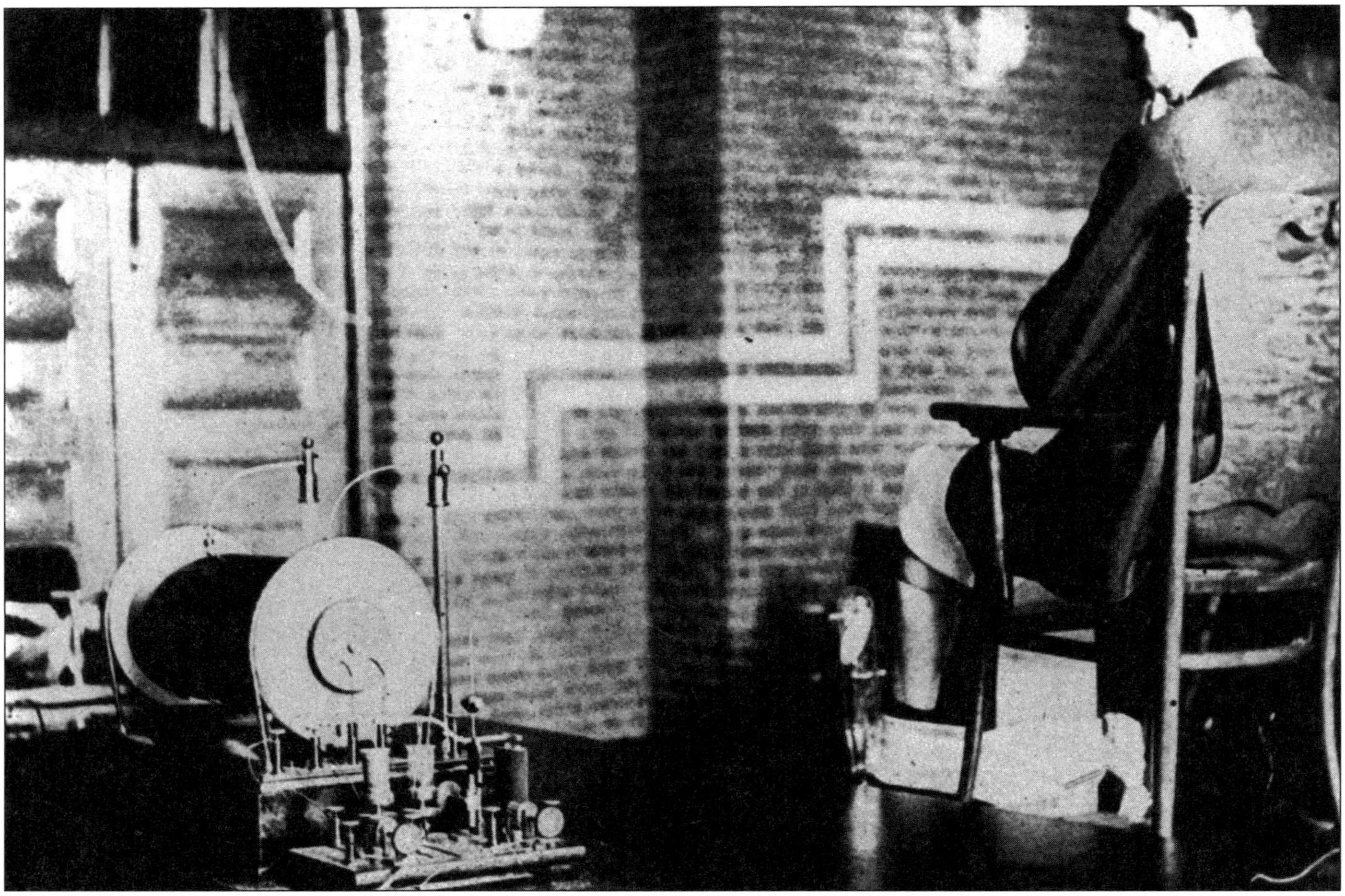

Canada's first diagnostic radiograph was made just four days after the one in Dartmouth. Professor John Cox, Director of the Macdonald Physics Laboratory of McGill University in Montréal, assembled the apparatus to produce x-rays on February 3 and soon obtained excellent pictures of the hands of his assistants. Two days later, a Montréal physician sent Cox a patient with a hip injury, but Cox was unable to obtain a picture even with an exposure of one hour.

On February 7 Dr Robert Kirkpatrick, a surgeon at the Montréal General Hospital, brought another patient to Cox's laboratory. Tolsen Cunning, a young man, had been shot in the leg during a street brawl on Christmas Day, 1895. The doctors at the hospital were unable to locate the bullet by probing, and the wound healed with the bullet *in situ*. However, in early February the leg began to trouble Tolsen again, and Dr Kirkpatrick decided to try the new Röntgen photography. A 45 minute exposure resulted in a plate clearly showing the bullet lying against the outer edge of the tibia. A print made from the underexposed plate and subsequently published was much less clear. The young man re-entered the hospital the same day, and the bullet was surgically removed with the aid of the radiograph.

As it happened, a meeting of the Montréal Medico-Chirurgical Society was scheduled for the same evening, February 7th. Cox and Kirkpatrick were invited to speak, and they showed the plate of Tolsen's leg, as well as those of the hands taken earlier. The lecture was published in the March 1896 issue of the *Montréal Medical Journal*[3].

A little later, Tolsen Cunning sued the man who had shot him, and the x-ray plate was accepted as evidence in the case. It seems, therefore, that the x-ray photograph made by Cox on February 7, 1896 was (a) the first clinical radiograph in North America to be used as an adjunct to surgery, and (b) the first possibly in the world to be accepted as evidence in a court of law. Unfortunately, the original x-ray plate is no longer extant.

Cox and his colleague Hugh Callendar, the Macdonald Professor of Experimental Physics at McGill, continued to experiment with x-rays, at least for a short period. Their joint paper on "Some Experiments on the X-Rays" was read at a meeting of the Royal Society of Canada on May 28, 1896[4]. They revealed that, out of a collection of more than fifty Crookes' tubes acquired by the Macdonald Physics Laboratory in 1894, only one (a "phosphorescent lamp tube of Puluj") was found to retain a sufficiently perfect vacuum during the long exposures required for the x-ray photographs demonstrated on February 7.

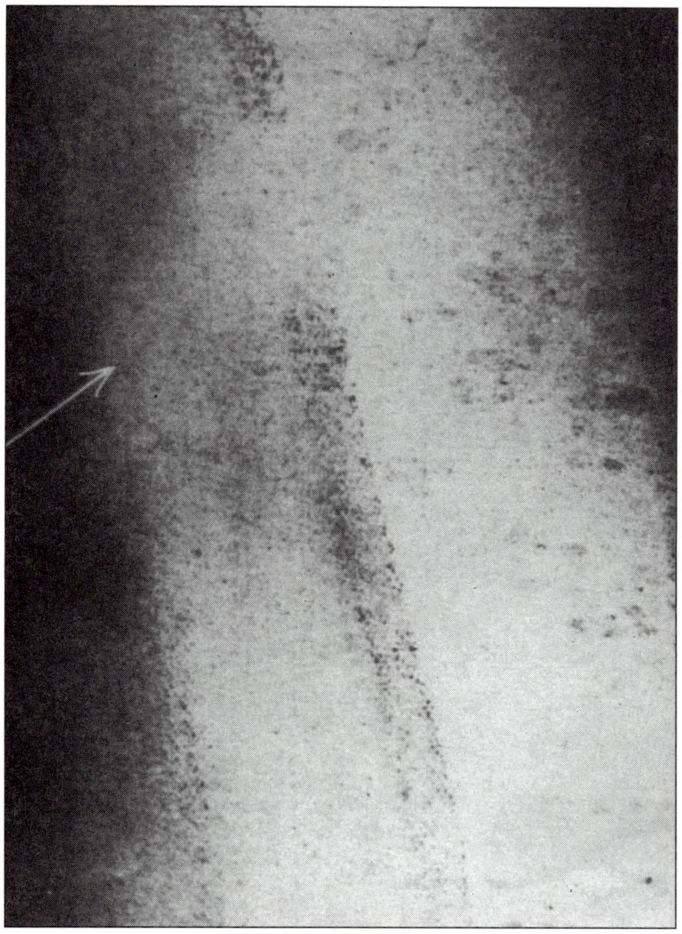

Far left
Apparatus used by Cox for taking an x-ray photograph of a patient's leg (Ref 3)

Left
Print of x-ray photograph of patient's leg with bullet lying against the outer edge of the tibia (Ref 3)

Subsequently Callendar devised and constructed over 30 tubes of different patterns. These tubes were used for taking "a number of anatomical and other photographs, including several surgical cases...and most of the experiments of Röntgen and other observers were repeated and verified." He found that the most satisfactory type of tube was the "focus tube" in which the cathode rays were concentrated by means of a concave electrode on a plate of platinum.[5] A tube of this type was used for a number of trials of "anatomical photography," including the location of a bullet in the brain of a 12-year-old child, a broken hip joint, a drainage tube in the lung, a fracture of the skull and a pus cavity in the lung. The intensity of the radiation emitted by a "focus tube" was so much greater than that of the original Crookes' tubes that exposures of ten to fifteen minutes were sufficient to give usable pictures even of the trunk.

Among the physical experiments described by Cox and Callendar were the following: (a) attempts to deflect the x-rays in a magnetic field (an apparent effect here could be attributed to deflection of the cathode rays within the tube and hence a shift in the position of the focus); (b) action of x-rays on a selenium photo-electric cell (no action was discernible); (c) absorption of x-rays by liquids ("we found the opacity of water to be much greater than we had expected"); and (d) measurement of the velocity of the x-rays. The method here was to pass the rays between the teeth of two rapidly revolving wheels fixed a metre apart on a rigid axis. Three variations of this method were tried, leading to the conclusion that "the lower limit of the velocity...is in all probability not less than 200 kilometres per second." (The actual value is 300,000 km/sec.)

Unfortunately it seems that neither Cox nor Callendar followed up these early experiments on x-rays. Cox was not an experimental physicist, and he presumably either lost interest or became too immersed in his teaching and administrative duties. Callendar returned to his main subject—the measurement of heat—and left McGill less than two years later.

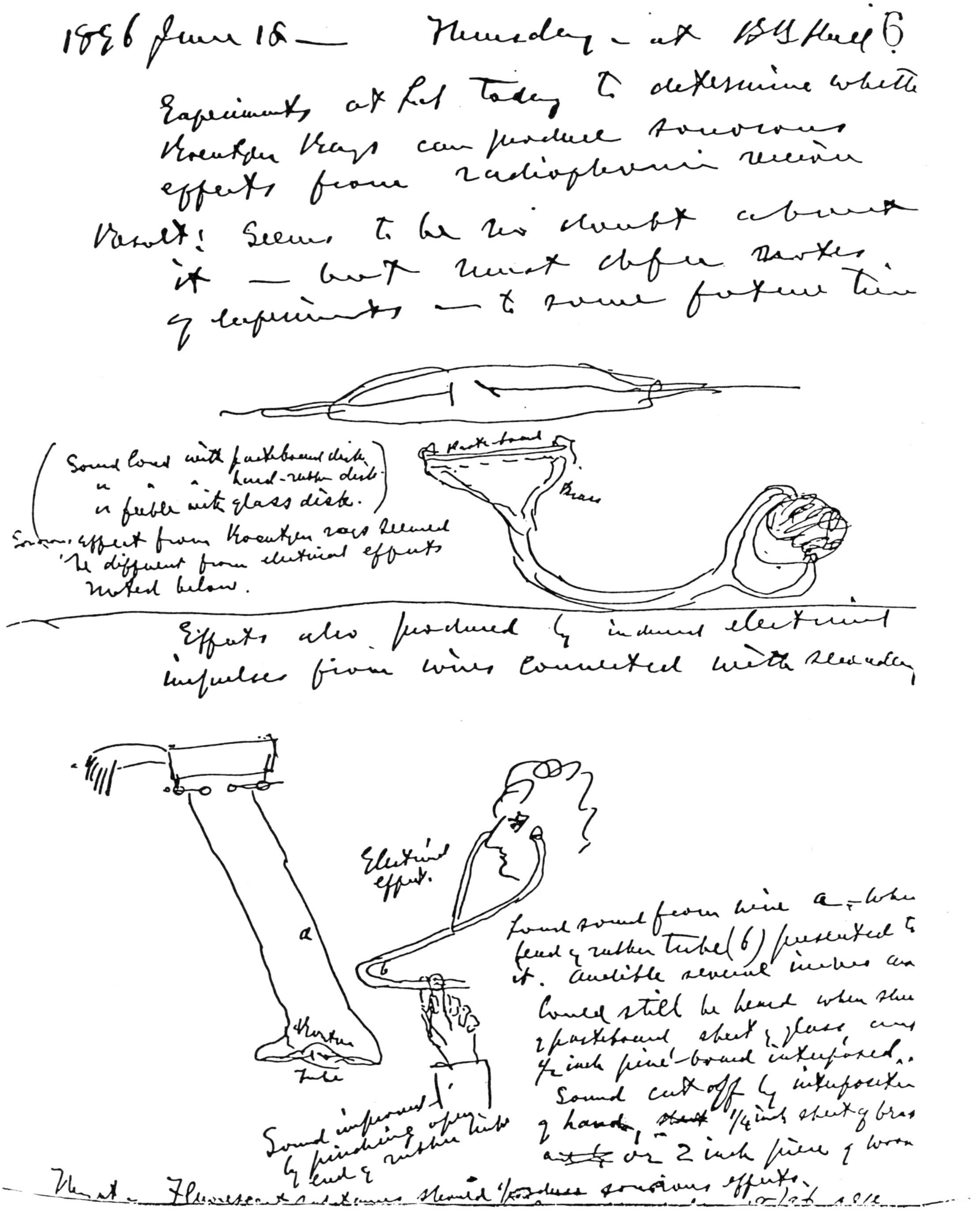
1896 June 18 — Thursday — at B.G. Hall 6

Experiments at Lab today to determine whether Roentgen Rays can produce sonorous effects from radiophonic receiver

Result! Seems to be no doubt about it — but must defer details of experiments — to some future time

Effects also produced by induced electrical impulses from wires connected with secondary

Found sound from wire a — when fed by rubber tube (b) presented to it. Audible several inches and could still be heard when sheet of pasteboard sheet of glass and 1/4 inch pine-board interposed. Sound cut off by interposition of hand, ~~sheet~~ 1/4 inch sheet of brass ~~at~~ or 2 inch piece of wood

Sound improved by pinching open end of rubber tube

Next — Fluorescent substances should produce sonorous effects.

Chapter III • # *Alexander Graham Bell*

John Aldrich

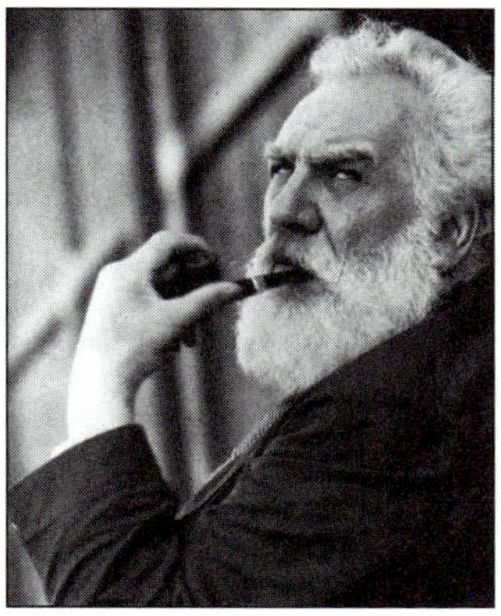

Alexander Graham Bell in a reflective mood in 1896

Alexander Graham Bell was born in Edinburgh in 1847. Both his paternal grandfather and his father were professors of elocution, and both men had studied the anatomy and physiology of speech in a scientific manner in order to help their patients. Bell's father developed a method for visualizing the organ positions necessary to produce phonetic sounds, and Alexander became thoroughly familiar with his methods. Bell studied anatomy and physiology at University College London and often attended medical rounds at the nearby University College Hospital. The Bell family moved to Canada in 1870 largely for health reasons. The Bells had already lost two sons to tuberculosis, and Alexander had shown early signs of the disease. However, after a summer in Brantford, Ontario, Alexander had recovered, and he soon moved to teach at the Boston School for Deaf Mutes.

Over the next few years he spent much time continuing to develop the multiple telegraph and telephone for which he eventually obtained patents. He married one of his deaf students, Mabel Hubbard, whose father, Gardiner Hubbard, became one of his main financial backers. The couple moved to Washington, close to Mabel's parents, but this had one serious drawback: the oppressive summers, which made Bell headachy and miserable. Consequently, each summer Bell and his family left the city for the coolness of the coast of Massachusetts or the mountains of Maryland. In 1885 Bell, his father and the Hubbards planned a trip to Newfoundland, where the elder Bell had spent some time, and to Nova Scotia, so that Gardiner could visit a mining interest in Glace Bay, Cape Breton.

Left
A page from Bell's notebook: the effect of x-rays on the telephone

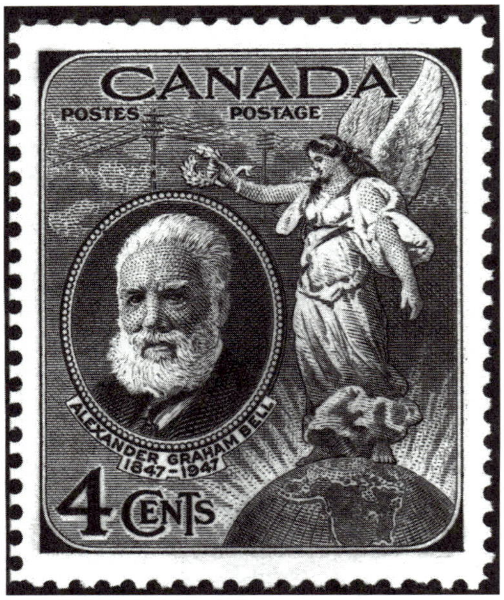

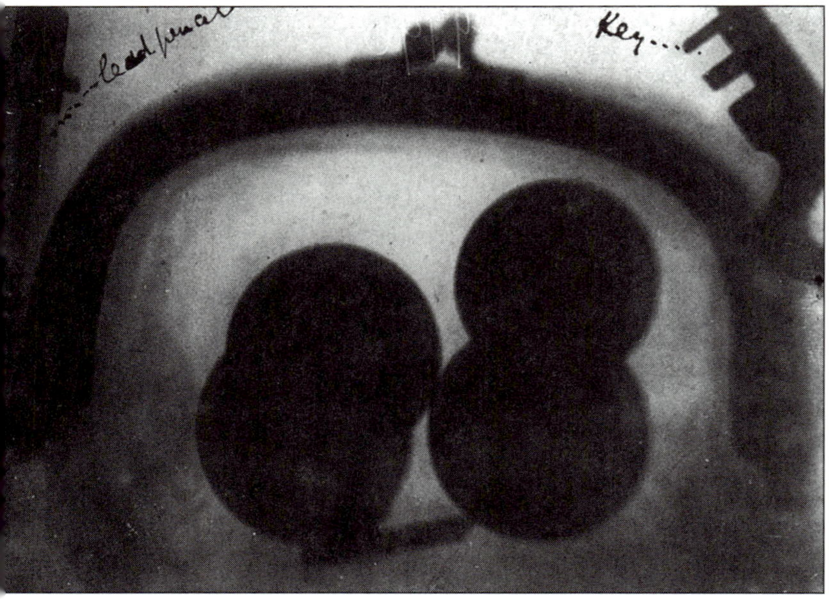

The group passed through Baddeck en route, and the Bells immediately fell in love with its hills and lochs and even its names; the area reminded Alex so much of his native Scotland. For the next thirty-six years, the Bells spent the summers from May until November or December in Baddeck. They completed a thirteen-room house there, *Beinn Bhreagh,* in 1893.[1]

Alexander Graham Bell has been described as a "generalist," and an examination of his notebooks reveals a tremendous range of interests. He had daydreamed for some time about "seeing with electricity," a parallel to his work in developing the telephone, and perhaps this is why he became interested in x-rays. Certainly he was an avid reader of journals, and from the middle of February 1896 his notebooks are full of references to the descriptions of x-rays then appearing in the scientific literature together with his ideas and theories about the origins and uses of the new rays.

On April 13 he purchased a Crookes' tube and other equipment for x-ray work from Queen and Company of Philadelphia. (This company later became famous for the Queen's Self-Regulating Tube, in which a protuberance containing potassium carbonate was heated by sparking when the vacuum became harder, thus maintaining the required gas in the tube.) Bell set this equipment aside to be worked upon when he moved to Baddeck for the summer in May. The x-ray tube and induction coil he used are on display at the Bell Museum in Baddeck. Just six months after the discovery of x-rays he wrote:

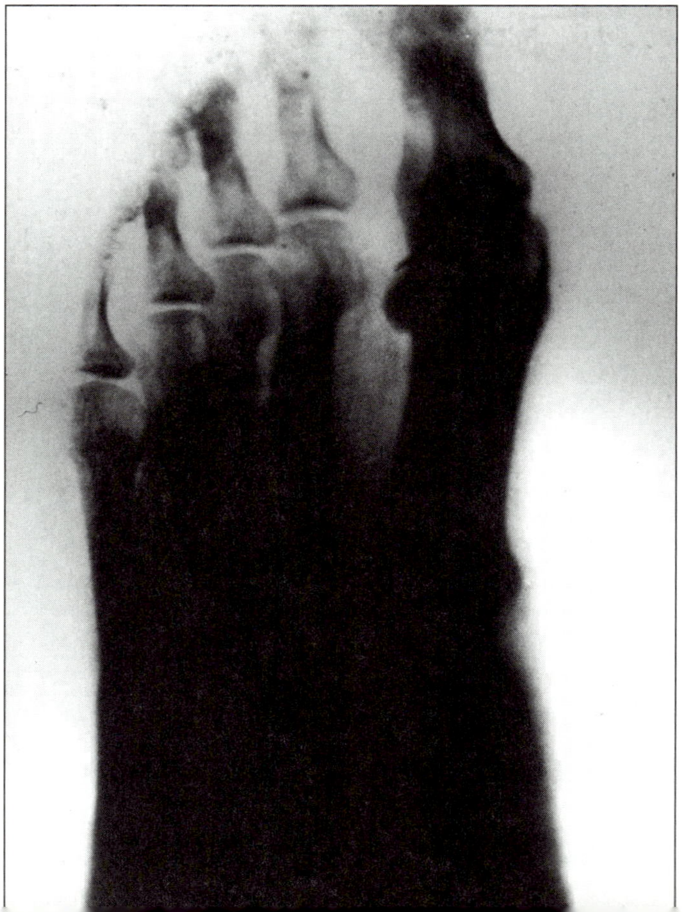

Top
Canadian postage stamp

Above
"Mr. Ellis' purse with coins" taken June 10, 1896

Right
Radiograph of the foot of Donald MacDonald showing a needle embedded in the joint of the big toe

Stereoscopic Radiograph. Try to produce a stereoscopic picture. Two radiographs of the same object placed side by side at the same time. Now combine stereoscopically! Good idea. Skeleton in three dimensions! Viscera etc. in place etc etc.[2]

The earliest known of his radiographs, "Mr. Ellis' purse with coins" was taken on June 10, 1896, during his early x-ray experiments with his assistant William Ellis. A few days later Bell was wondering whether x-rays would produce sounds in his telephone,[3] and indeed he found that they did. Perhaps this was the first recorded attempt at teleradiology!

Bell took several clinical radiographs over the next couple of years—usually for local physicians—similar to the one illustrated taken in October, 1897, of a needle in Donald MacDonald's foot. How his mind leapt from subject to subject is demonstrated in a page of his notebook for June 25, 1898.[4] Here he described four radiographs, discussed the problem of counter-rotating propellers, and gave a design of a child's pull toy with flapping wings, a whirling tail and a passenger taking off his hat!

Bell, who had x-ray equipment both in Baddeck and Washington, was obviously regarded as an authority on x-rays. In 1898 he gave a talk in Washington on x-rays and was proposing to write a paper on the subject. His breadth of vision seems to have overruled any prejudice he might have. He had already invented a surgical probe, based upon the principle of the telephone, for detecting metal objects in a patient (he had personally but unsuccessfully used the probe in an attempt to locate the assassin's bullet in President Garfield), but he was still very open to the possibilities of x-rays, which, of course, eventually made his probe obsolete.

Bell has also been regarded as one of the first to suggest the use of radium for the treatment of deep-seated cancers. In 1903 he wrote to his physician Dr ZT Sowerby:[5]

I understand from you that the Röntgen x-rays, and the rays emitted by Radium, have been found to have a marked curative effect upon external cancers, but that the effects upon deep-seated cancers have not thus far proved satisfactory. It has occurred to me that one reason for the unsatisfactory nature of these latter experiments arises from the fact that the rays have been applied externally, thus having to pass through healthy tissues of various depths to reach the cancerous matter. The Crookes' tube from which the Röntgen rays are emitted is, of course too bulky to be inserted into the middle of a mass of cancer; but there is no reason why a tiny fragment of Radium sealed up in a fine glass tube should not be inserted into the very heart of the cancer, thus acting directly upon the diseased material. Would it not be worth making experiments upon this line?

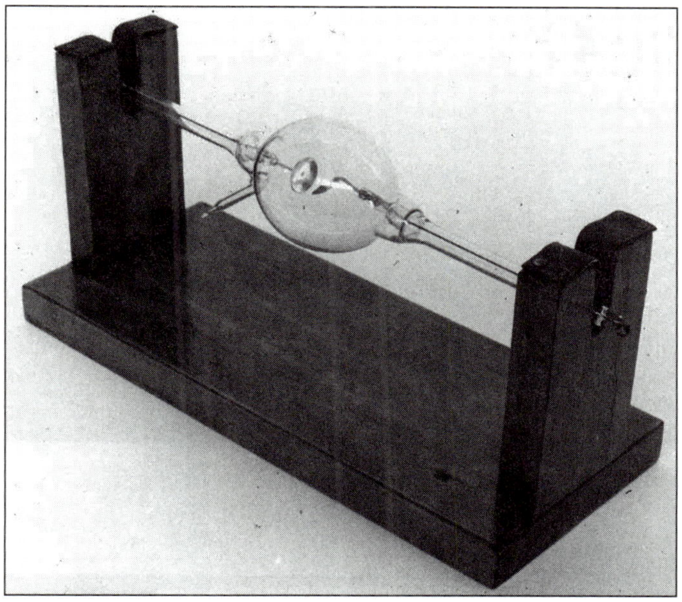

One of the x-ray tubes used by Bell at Baddeck, probably purchased from Queen and Company of Philadelphia in April 1896

This was certainly a letter in which one of the earliest suggestions about the use of radium in cancer therapy was made.

Perhaps because Bell invented the telephone so early in his career, he could turn his creative genius to other problems of the day. His interests covered a vast area from medicine to aeronautics, marine engineering to genetics. He performed much of his work at his quiet retreat in Baddeck. There his airplane Silver Dart made the first flight in the British Empire in 1909, and his hydrofoil HD-4 achieved the remarkable speed of 110 kilometres per hour in 1919.

Bell spent every summer in Baddeck for the last 37 years of his life until his death there at the age of 75. He saw great changes in society over his lifetime and many of these changes were due to technological developments Bell himself had initiated.

Acknowledgement:

Special thanks to the Bell Museum in Baddeck, Nova Scotia for access to its archives and permission to publish the photographs of Bell and his work.

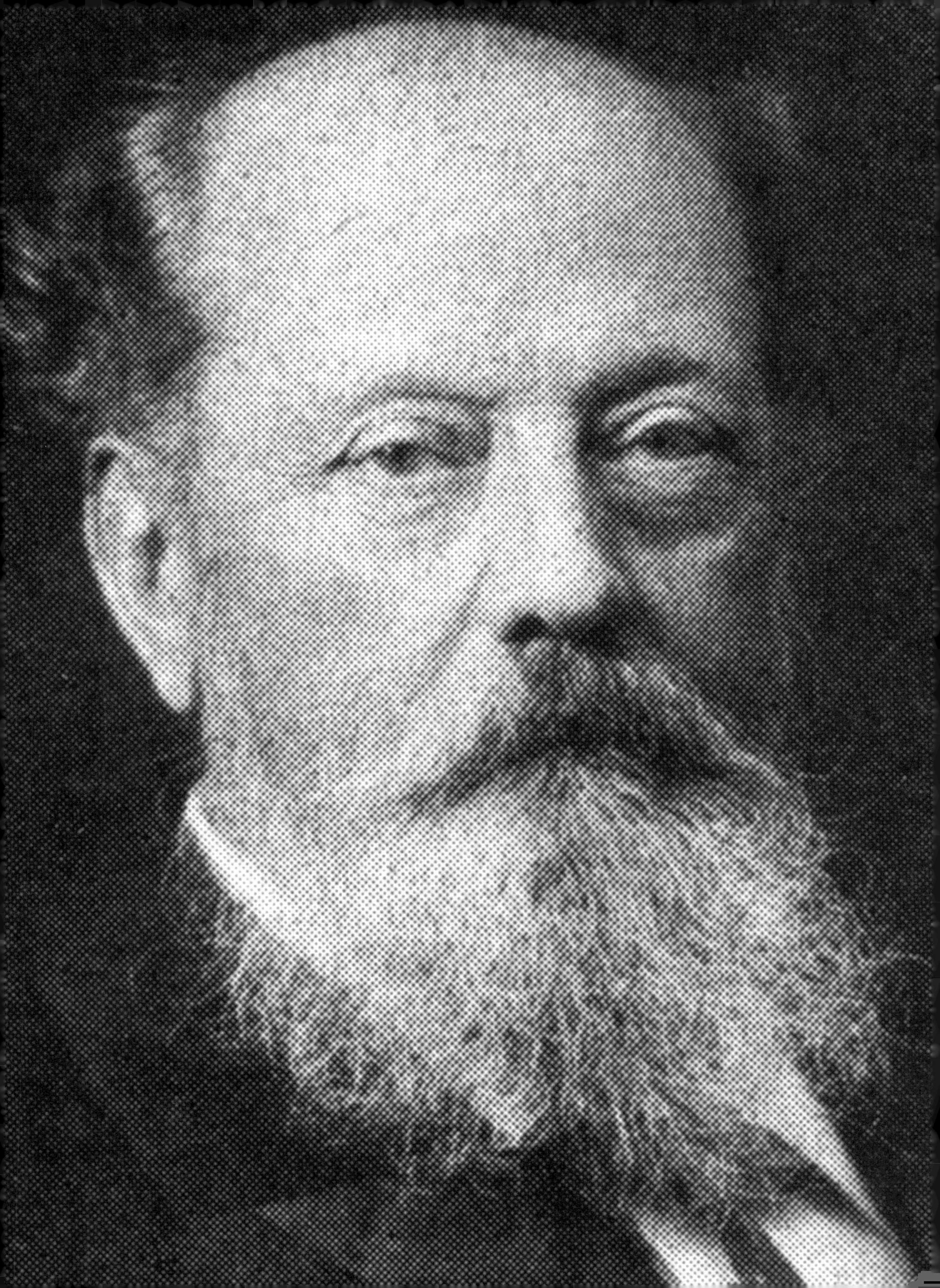

Chapter IV • Some Observations on

Early Diagnostic Radiology

in Canada

J Kenneth Lipinski

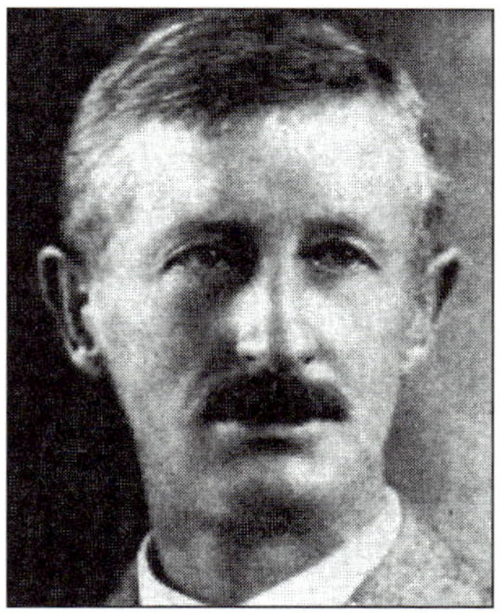

Dr Alexander Howard Pirie

The 20th century has been filled with breakthroughs that have altered diagnostic and therapeutic approaches in medicine. Of particular significance in radiology has been the development of computer-assisted tomography and computer-digitized angiography. The importance of these innovations is best appreciated in the context of the early history of radiology.

Conrad Röntgen announced the discovery of the new rays in late 1895 and within a few months newspapers around the world had front page headlines and illustrations of the new photography. X-rays, and electricity itself, were held in awe by the public at the turn of the century.

The medical profession was quick to see applications for these rays in examining body tissues and within six months of their discovery began to publish clinical reports. In one of the first, from Montréal Professors John Cox and RC Kirkpatrick at McGill University, reported localizing a foreign body in the leg of a victim of a gun blast.[1] While it was obvious that x-rays were here to stay, their significance was not then fully appreciated.

Physicians were accustomed to using new instruments, but previous inventions had been logical extensions of the human senses. The ophthalmoscope and microscope were extensions of the eye. The stethoscope was an extension of the ear. The analysis of body fluids had always been a routine part of practice, even of the primitives; the only difference was sophistication of technique.

X-rays, however, offered a way of visualizing body tissues that had not been theorized and had no relationship to other diagnostic

Left
Professor Gilbert Girdwood

techniques used in clinical medicine. It was in this context that the Röntgen pioneers experimented with equipment, areas of the body to be examined, and the development of methods of visualizing the anatomy.

Canada had its pioneers, based mainly in Montréal. The most prominent early figure was Professor Gilbert P Girdwood, who was to become known as the grandfather of radiology in Canada.

Girdwood was born in England in 1832. He was admitted to the Royal College of Surgeons in 1854 after completing his training at University College and St George's School of Medicine, London. He decided on a military career which was to bring him to Canada in 1862 as surgeon to the 1st Battalion of the Grenadier Guards during the Trent Affair. He returned to Britain but later relinquished his post to return to Canada and the 3rd Regiment of the Victoria Rifles, again as surgeon.

His interests also included physics and chemistry, particularly as related to forensic medicine, and in London he had helped develop a sensitive test for strychnine poisoning. This expertise made him a frequent witness for the prosecution in legal cases. In 1869 he became associated with McGill University as a lecturer, later advancing to professor of chemistry in the faculty of medicine. His teaching continued until he retired in 1911 at the age of 79.

Girdwood's interest in radiology started in 1896 with a small unit he had constructed. He started taking skiagraphs at the Montréal General and Royal Victoria hospitals, and in 1901 his involvement with the latter institution was formalized when he was appointed head of the Medical-Electrical Department. The 1902 annual report of that hospital documented over 500 skiagraphs for the year, 400 of these taken of the bones and joints and more than 100 of the chest.

Girdwood was also interested in the use of stereo techniques for viewing the tissue planes and documented many of these cases in his publications. In the same year he also served as president of the American Roentgen Ray Society.

Girdwood retired in 1911, leaving a developed department that was making use of all the latest applications of x-rays.

It was this early start that gave the Royal Victoria Hospital its international reputation in radiology and enabled it to attract Dr Alexander Howard Pirie who would continue this activity.

Pirie was born in Dundee, Scotland, in 1875, the son of a physician. He was educated at the universities of St Andrew's and Edinburgh and immediately took up the study of radiology when he graduated in 1896. This early

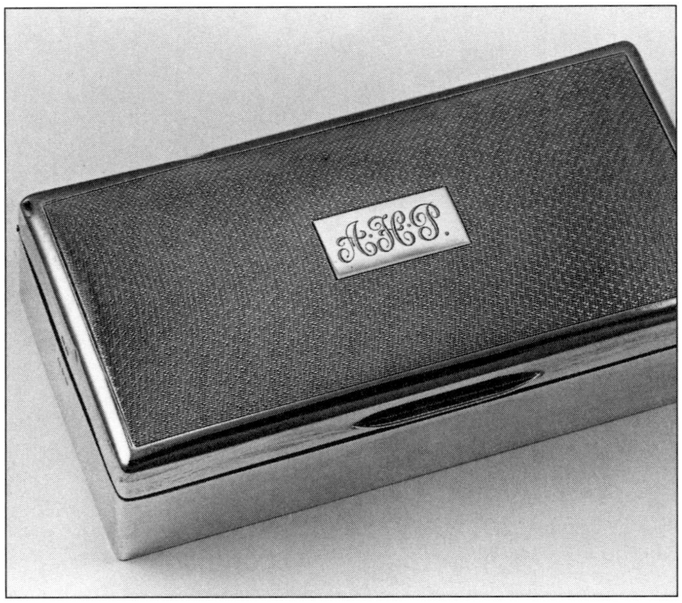

interest was a result of his brother George's similar interest.

Prior to 1911, Howard Pirie held hospital appointments at St Bartholomew's and University College hospitals, London, and maintained a private radiology practice at Harley Street. He was a frequent discussant in the *British Medical Journal* and also published in the specialty publications. In 1911 he was invited by the governors of the Royal Victoria Hospital in Montréal to replace Professor Girdwood as the head of the Medical-Electrical and X-ray Department. Pirie had been a visitor to Canada so was likely aware of living conditions in Québec. As well, Royal Victoria Hospital looked very much like a Scottish hospital. Soon after settling in Montréal, the war in Europe was to take him and a number of other McGill physicians overseas. He was in charge of several radiology facilities as well as the training of a number of new radiologists. He continued to publish articles during the war, particularly on the methods of localization of foreign bodies, which was of great help to surgeons.

In 1915 Pirie was awarded honorary membership in the Röntgen Ray Society of London. This acknowledgment of his contribution to the development of the medical uses of x-rays was significant in that only a few other scientists had been so honoured, including Sir William Crookes, Sir Oliver Lodge, Sir Ernest Rutherford, Professors Holznecht and Leduc, and, naturally, Conrad Röntgen.

After the war Pirie returned to his duties in Montréal. He retired in 1938. Under his direction the department was equal to any in the United States or Europe, and many of its trainees became important figures in Canadian radiology.

Similar developments had also occurred in French Canadian hospitals. Monseigneur JCK LaFlamme, professor

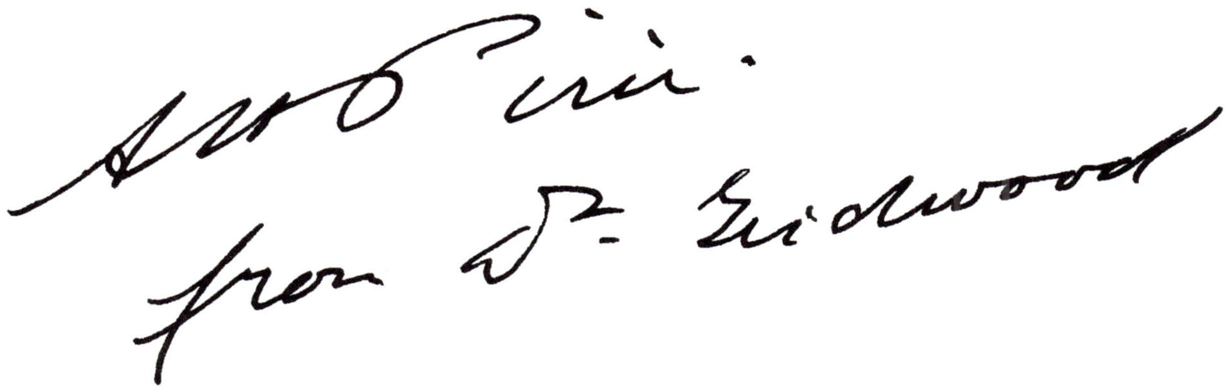

of natural sciences at the Université Laval de Montréal, was duplicating Röntgen's experiments shortly after the discoverer's announcement. At the time of the announcement in Europe, several French-Canadian doctors were studying in Germany and France. With their return to Québec they brought the techniques into use. These men included Charles De Blois, Charles Verge and Henri Lasnier. Lasnier was a diagnostician in Montréal for a long time. His work included the publication of the first radiology journal in Canada, *les Rayons-X*, in 1910.

Probably the most well known of these early radiologists was Léo Pariseau. He obtained his medical degree from the Université Laval de Montréal in 1904 and became head at l'Hôpital Notre-Dame de Montréal from 1906-1909. Prior to the war he spent time as the medical health officer in Sherbrooke and simultaneously radiologist to St Vincent's Hospital. During the war he served as radiologist to l'Hôpital Laval de St-Cloud and from 1919 as director of electroradiology at Hôtel-Dieu de Montréal, a position which he held until his death in 1938.

Pariseau was a well-rounded academic and lectured and published not only in medicine but also in history, ethics, sociology and bibliology [sic]. His extensive library was bequeathed to the Université de Montréal. He was also instrumental in forming the Société Canadienne Française d'Électro-Radiology in 1924.

Acknowledgements:
This article is reprinted from the *Canadian Medical Association Journal* (1983; 129: 766–768) with the kind permission of both the *Journal* and the author.

Left
A silver box given to Dr Pirie as a leaving gift

Above
Signature of Dr Girdwood

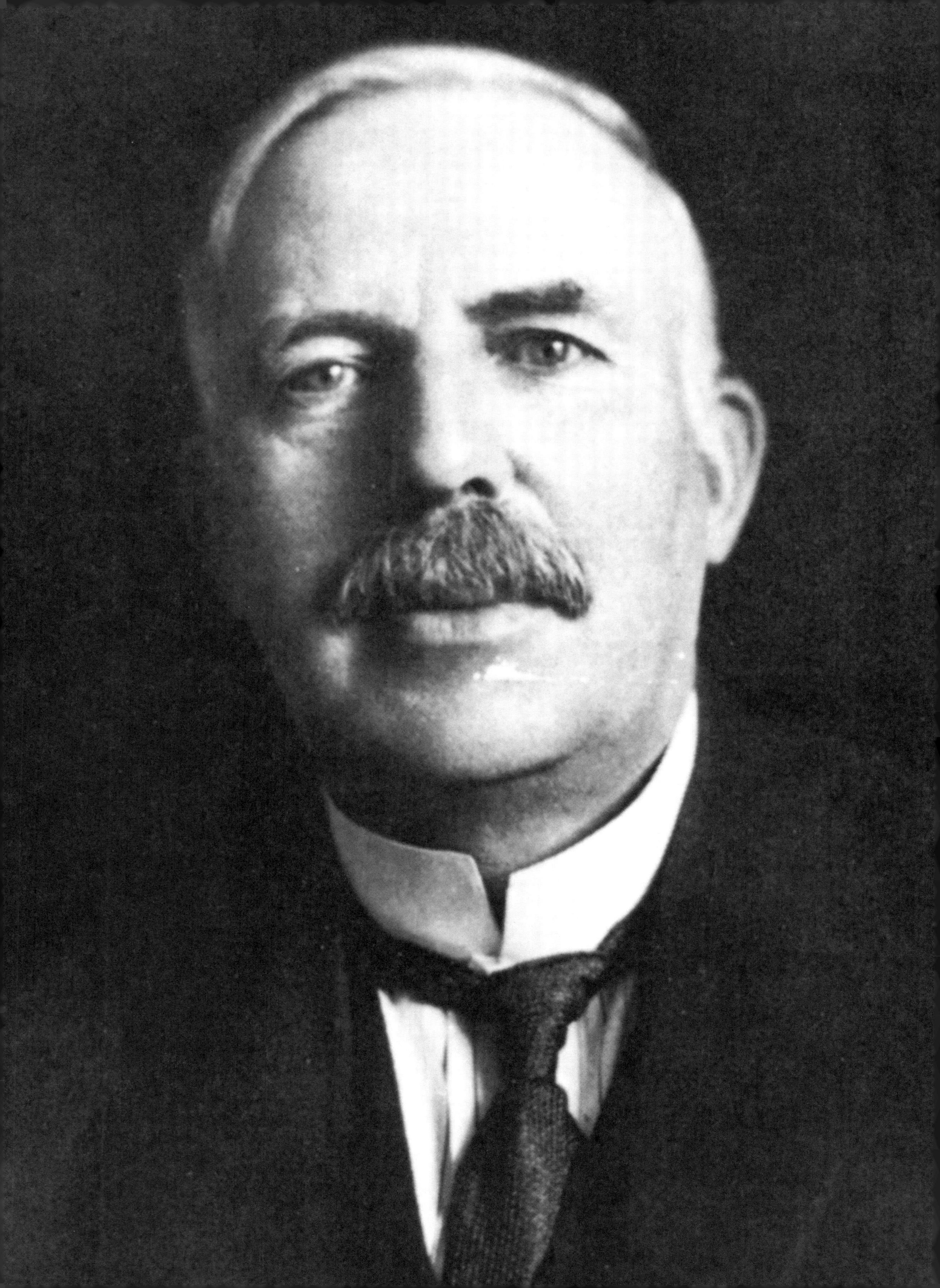

Chapter V •

Ernest Rutherford

at McGill University

MONTAGUE COHEN

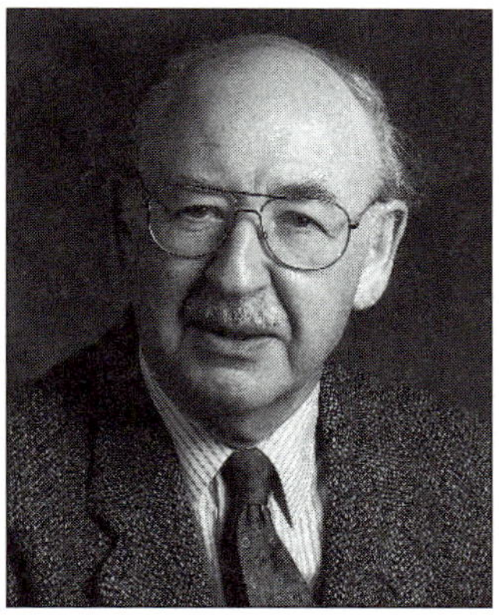

Professor Montague Cohen

Ernest Rutherford was born on August 30, 1871 in a rural community near Nelson on the South Island of New Zealand. He was the fourth of the twelve children of James and Martha Rutherford, who had emigrated to New Zealand from Scotland and England respectively. Ernest attended local schools and Nelson College, a secondary school from which he graduated in 1889 with honours in all subjects.

A scholarship took Rutherford to Canterbury College in Christchurch, the principal city of the South Island; here he obtained the Bachelor and Master of Arts degrees in 1892 and 1893 respectively, with first class honours in mathematics and physical science. He remained in Christchurch for two further years in order to obtain a Bachelor of Science qualification, which at that time was a research degree. Rutherford's laboratory in the basement of Canterbury College, where he worked in cramped conditions with largely home-made apparatus, is preserved as a museum.

Rutherford's research at Canterbury College was in the field of magnetism. His earliest papers, published in 1894 and 1895 in the *Transactions of the New Zealand Institute*, were titled "Magnetization of iron by high-frequency discharges" and "Magnetic viscosity."

In 1895 Rutherford received an 1851 Exhibition Science Scholarship tenable in the United Kingdom. Only one such award was available that year to New Zealand applicants, and Rutherford was actually the runner-up. However, the winner, JC Maclaurin (a chemist) declined the award for personal reasons—he was about to be married—and the scholarship fell to Rutherford. It was the only

Left
Baron Rutherford of Nelson (courtesy of the National Portrait Gallery, London)

time in his career that luck played a decisive role. Years later, when his colleague (and subsequent biographer) Arthur Stewart Eve playfully accused Rutherford of "always riding on the crest of the wave," he replied, "Well, I created the wave, didn't I?"

RESEARCH IN CAMBRIDGE

Rutherford chose to take up his scholarship at the Cavendish Laboratory in Cambridge, under the direction of one of the most distinguished British scientists, Sir Joseph John ("JJ") Thomson. Rutherford was the first non-Cambridge graduate to take advantage of a new rule which permitted non-Cambridge graduates to undertake graduate research at the University. Using apparatus brought from New Zealand Rutherford continued his investigations on magnetism, especially the application of magnetic phenomena for the detection of Hertzian (radio) waves. His home-made detector received radio signals from half a mile away, a better distance than Marconi could achieve at the time. Rutherford's first publication in the *Transactions of the Royal Society*, in June 1896, was "A magnetic detector of electrical waves and some of its applications." However, in April 1896 he switched his main interest from the long to the short wavelength end of the electromagnetic spectrum. This change came about at the suggestion—or rather, invitation—of "JJ."

JJ Thomson had already carried out extensive work on the conduction of electricity in gases at low pressure, the phenomena of the discharge tube which, in November 1895, led to Röntgen's discovery of x-rays. The publication of Röntgen's *Preliminary Communication* in January 1896 (English translations appeared in *Nature* on January 23 and in *The Electrician* on January 24) immediately led to a flurry of activity by scientists anxious to investigate the new phenomenon. Here was a means whereby air could be rendered conducting even at atmospheric pressure! Thomson was already impressed by Rutherford's research ability and invited the young graduate to join him in an investigation of the conducting power of gases exposed to Röntgen rays. The first paper on this topic, by Thomson and Rutherford, was published in the *Philosophical Magazine* in November 1896. This publication was followed, in 1897 and 1898, by three papers by Rutherford alone in which he investigated the phenomena in more detail, including the relationship between the rate of leak in a gas (i.e., the ionization current) and the intensity of the radiation; he also studied the velocity and rate of recombination of the ions produced by the radiation.

Rutherford's sixth and last paper in his Cambridge period[1] was published in *Philosophical Magazine* in January 1899, by which time he was already in Montréal. The paper discussing work carried out in the Cavendish Laboratory was in many ways the most significant for Rutherford's subsequent career, since it marked a move from x-rays into the new phenomenon of radioactivity (which had been discovered by Henri Becquerel in March 1896 and subsequently investigated by Marie and Pierre Curie in Paris). In his research Rutherford spread uranium metal or compounds in powdered form over the centre of a horizontal zinc plate which formed the lower electrode of a parallel-plate ionization chamber. The uranium radiation caused a leak between the two electrodes, which was measured by the rate of movement of a quadrant electrometer connected to the upper plate. Rutherford placed successive layers of aluminum foil (thickness 0.005 mm) over the uranium compound and determined the rate of leak for each additional layer. He observed that the rate of leak (i.e., the intensity of the radiation) diminished according to the ordinary (exponential) absorption law for the first three layers but, after the fourth thickness, the intensity fell only slightly when another eight layers were added. Rutherford concluded:

> *These experiments show that the uranium radiation is complex, and that there are present at least two distinct types of radiation—one that is very readily absorbed, which will be termed for convenience the α-radiation, and one of a more penetrative character, which will be termed the β-radiation.*

The discovery of a third, even more penetrating, component of the radiation is usually attributed to Villard in 1900,[34] but Wilson, in his exhaustive biography of Rutherford,[35] argues strongly that Rutherford himself was the discoverer, although he did not apply the term "gamma rays" until 1904.

In the work cited above in which Rutherford first named the α and β components of uranium radiation, he also investigated the radiation emitted by thorium compounds, the radioactivity of which had been discovered by Gerhard Schmidt in Erlangen in April 1898.[36] (Unlike uranium and radium, high-purity thorium compounds were readily available and were used in much of Rutherford's early work.) Rutherford noted that the thorium radiation differed in penetrating power from that of uranium, and that "thorium nitrate when first exposed to the air on a platinum plate was not a steady source of radiation, and for a time the rate of leak varied very capriciously, being sometimes five times as great as at others." This was clearly Rutherford's first encounter with "emanation," which was subsequently to play a major role in the unfolding of the radioactivity story.

THE MOVE TO MONTRÉAL

In 1898 Rutherford left Cambridge to take up an appointment as Macdonald Professor of Experimental Physics at McGill University in Montréal. The vacancy arose because the previous incumbent, Hugh L Callendar (himself a Cambridge graduate), was appointed to a chair at University College, London. The director of the McGill physics laboratory, Professor John Cox, and the principal of the university, William Peterson, travelled to Cambridge to seek a replacement. It seems that at first Rutherford was hesitant to offer himself as a candidate but soon decided to apply, and in due course he received the appointment, an outcome which must be attributed to his own canvassing as well as to Thomson's strong recommendation.[37]

At first sight it is strange that Rutherford wished to move from Cambridge to Montréal. At that time the centre of scientific research was firmly in Europe, including the United Kingdom. Canada was not a major player on the scientific stage and even the United States was not yet a scientific power, although it was already demonstrating its facility in applying science to practical ends, for example in electrical technology. A young scientist established in the Cavendish Laboratory would have been well advised to stay put rather than move across the Atlantic.

Nevertheless, several arguments favoured the move. First, McGill offered Rutherford a full professorship at the early age of 26. (He was just 27 when he took up the appointment in September 1898.) It was doubtful if he could have attained that status in England in less than five years, more probably ten. Second, the salary offered, £500 a year ($2500), was considerably higher than he could expect in England, and Rutherford needed the money, especially since he was engaged to be married. (It was not until May 1900 that Rutherford had saved enough to return to New Zealand to marry and bring his bride Mary Newton, daughter of his landlady at Christchurch, to Canada.) In the event, third, the physics laboratory at McGill was housed in a new building (opened in 1893), built and equipped by tobacco millionaire Sir William Macdonald and reputed to be one of the finest science buildings in the world, perhaps even *the* finest. Next, the post at McGill was essentially a *research* rather than a teaching professorship, which was what Rutherford wanted. Finally, and perhaps most important of all, Rutherford was a young man of immense self-confidence—often hidden behind an outward show of diffidence—who felt that he could surmount the problems imposed by a voluntary "exile" on the other side of the Atlantic. He was right. However, he never expected his move to Canada to be permanent, and almost certainly his stay of nine years was longer than he originally intended.

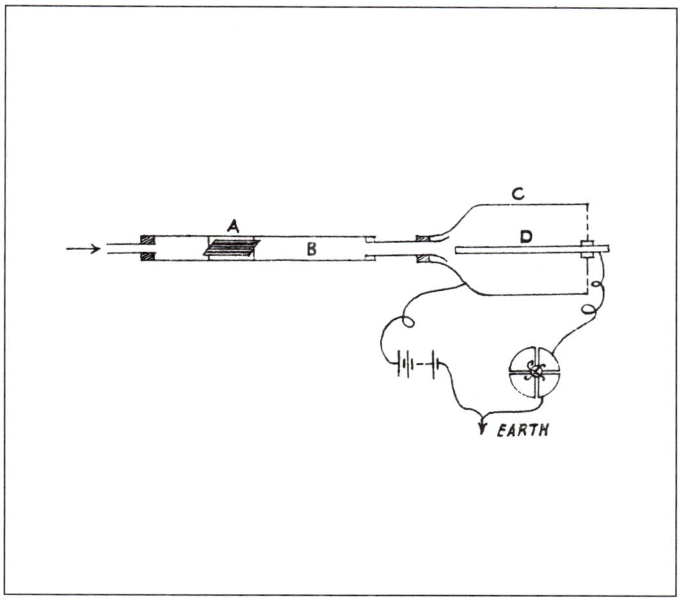

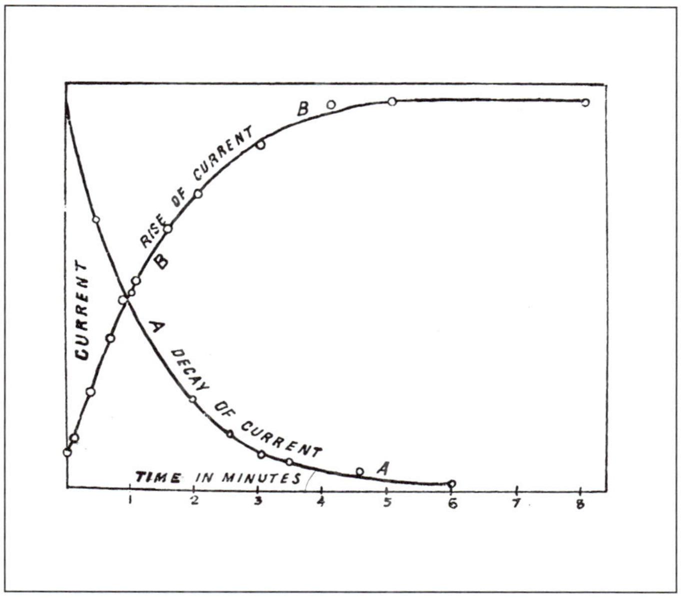

Top
Apparatus for determining the rate of decay of thorium emanation.
A: thorium oxide enclosed in two thicknesses of paper, which absorbed the α-rays emitted by the thorium but allowed the emanation to pass through.
B: metal tube, through which passed a slow current of air.
C: cylindrical ionization chamber with small holes in end plate for passage of air.
D: central electrode connected to quadrant electrometer
(Rutherford, ref 3)

Above
Curve A: Decrease in current in ionization chamber of Fig. 1 when the flow of air was stopped.
Curve B: Rise in current in an ionization chamber due to gradual build-up of emanation from a thorium source.
A steady state is reached when the production of new emanation by the thorium balances the decay of the existing emanation
(Rutherford, ref 3)

The Physics Department (or "laboratory") at McGill University comprised two professors (Cox and Rutherford), three demonstrators and a small number of graduate students. The teaching of physics at the undergraduate level was mainly directed to students of other disciplines, such as engineering, mining, chemistry, medicine and the liberal arts, since very few young Canadian men—and even fewer young women—elected to become professional physicists. The senior professor, Cox, was an excellent teacher but not a good researcher: so he reduced Rutherford's teaching load to a minimum, enabling him to devote a high proportion of his time to research.

EMANATION AND EXCITED RADIOACTIVITY

Rutherford's first research at McGill was nominally a continuation of his last investigation in Cambridge, i.e., measurement of the ionization of air induced by radiations emitted by compounds of uranium and thorium. However, he made an important, and decisive, shift in emphasis: he was no longer interested primarily in the mechanism of ionization and the nature of the "leak" across the electrodes of the parallel-plate chamber. Instead, he treated the rate of leak as a tool for the study of the radiations emitted by radioactive substances and hence for the elucidation of the nature of radioactivity itself.

Rutherford's first published paper in Canada, read before the Royal Society of Canada in May 1899, compared the radiation emitted by thorium and uranium.[2] He confirmed his previous observation that thorium radiation was more penetrating. Furthermore, the same kinds of radiation were emitted by thorium oxide, sulphate and nitrate: radioactivity was apparently an *atomic* phenomenon. The "capricious" behaviour previously observed in thorium nitrate was found also, to an even greater extent, in the oxide:

> *It was found that if the substance was enclosed in a lead box with a door, the rate of leak [of the electrometer] was much slower with the door open than closed. The addition of a slight draught of air caused by opening or shutting the door of the room diminished the rate of leak still more.*

This paper was quickly followed by another on the same theme, submitted in September 1899 and published in January 1900.[3] In this paper he emphasized the significance of the capricious behavior of the thorium compound in the presence of draughts of air. Rutherford explained the observed rate of leak of the ionization chamber by the supposition that:

> *in addition to the ordinary radiation [emitted by the thorium compound] a large number of radioactive particles are given out from the mass of the active substance. This 'emanation' can pass through considerable thicknesses of paper.... The explanation of the action of slight currents of air is clear on the 'emanation' theory...extremely minute motions of air, if continuous, remove many of the radioactive centres from between the plates.*

This is the first mention of "emanation," a name coined by Rutherford to avoid the use of terms such as "gas" or "vapour" which would define the (as yet unknown) nature of the "radioactive centres." Emanation [thoron and radon] was destined to play a central role in elucidating the nature of radioactivity. In an ingenious experiment Rutherford separated the emanation from the thorium compound and showed that its radioactivity diminished rapidly, with a half-life of about a minute, while the activity of new emanation from the "de-emanated" thorium builds up at an equal but inverse rate. The paper ends on a remarkable note: the positive ions produced in a gas by the emanation are able to induce radioactivity in all substances on which they fall. (The term "excited radioactivity" was first used in a follow-up paper[4] published in February 1900.) This power to emit radiation lasts for several days, with a half-life of about 11 hours, and the radiation is more penetrating than that emitted by thorium or uranium. Rutherford concludes that "the emanation from thorium compounds thus has properties which the thorium itself does not possess." Here was the genesis of the theory of atomic transmutation, but over two more years of further research, and a historical partnership with a brilliant young chemist, were needed before the theory could be formally presented to the scientific world.

Up to this point Rutherford had observed the property of induced radioactivity only with thorium compounds. However, in November 1899 Pierre and Marie Curie announced the discovery of radioactivity induced by radium and polonium,[38] using sources of much greater activity and purity than were available to Rutherford at the time. Rutherford acknowledged this discovery in a postscript to his February 1900 paper,[4] but added that he had already disproved (at least in the case of thorium) the explanation suggested by the Curies; that induced radioactivity is a kind of phosphorescence excited by the primary radiation.

Rutherford's next advance in the emanation/excited radioactivity story occurred over a year later, by which time he had acquired a reasonably strong and pure source of radium. (Meanwhile, he had travelled to New Zealand to get married and had investigated various aspects of the ionization of gases, as will be discussed later.) Rutherford showed that, when a radium source was heated below red heat, its emanating power increased over 10,000 times, but this power was largely destroyed at higher temperatures. The emanation, obtained by passing a slow current of air over heated radium, preserved its radioactivity and exciting power for weeks when kept in a closed metal container.[5] The longer life of radium emanation, as compared with thorium emanation, rendered the former suitable for the next investigation: to elucidate the nature of the emanation by measuring its molecular (or atomic) weight.

The amount of emanation available was far too small for a direct measurement of molecular weight by standard chemical techniques. Instead Rutherford chose an indirect method, based on the rate of diffusion of a gas in air, which was known to be a function of molecular weight. In this investigation he was assisted by Harriet Brooks, a young graduate student who showed every promise of becoming "Canada's Marie Curie" but unfortunately never attained that status before she gave up science altogether in 1907 when she married.[39]

Rutherford and Brooks passed air containing radium emanation into one half of a long cylindrical ionization chamber divided into two parts by a metal slide. When the ionization current (as measured by an electrometer) became steady, the input of emanation was stopped, the chamber sealed and the dividing slide removed. The ionization in the other half-chamber, resulting from the gradual diffusion of emanation, was measured with a second electrometer. In this way the rate of diffusion, and hence the molecular weight, of the emanation could be calculated.[6] However, the experiment was subject to considerable uncertainty and the estimated molecular weight—between 40 and 100—was far too low. Rutherford concluded that the emanation could not be radium in vapour form, since Mme Curie had shown that the atomic weight of radium was greater than that of barium, i.e., 137 or more.[40] This conclusion was, of course, unjustified at the time, since the real atomic weight of radium emanation (radon) is 222, very close to that of radium (226). However, in the circumstances this valuable piece of evidence supported the transmutation theory beginning to take shape in Rutherford's mind. Further progress now depended on the possibility of completely separating the original radioactive substance (thorium or radium) from both the emanation and the excited radioactivity, and proving that each component was chemically distinct. This task required the collaboration of a skilled chemist, and, fortunately, one presented himself at the right moment.

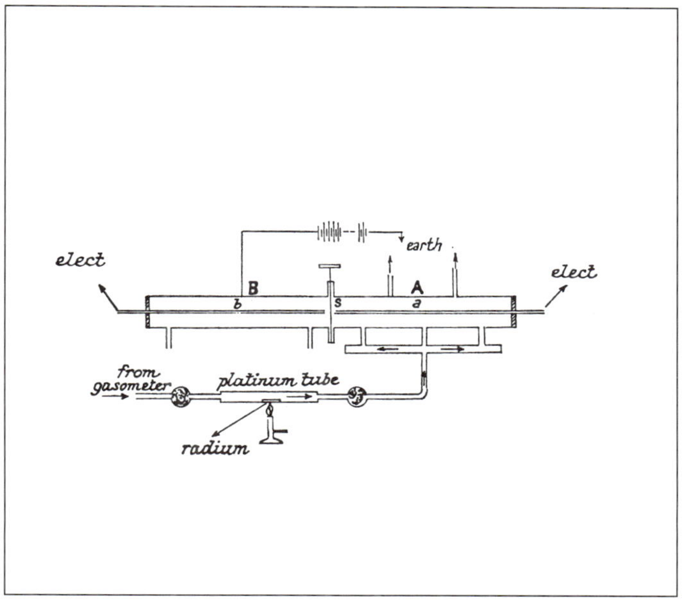

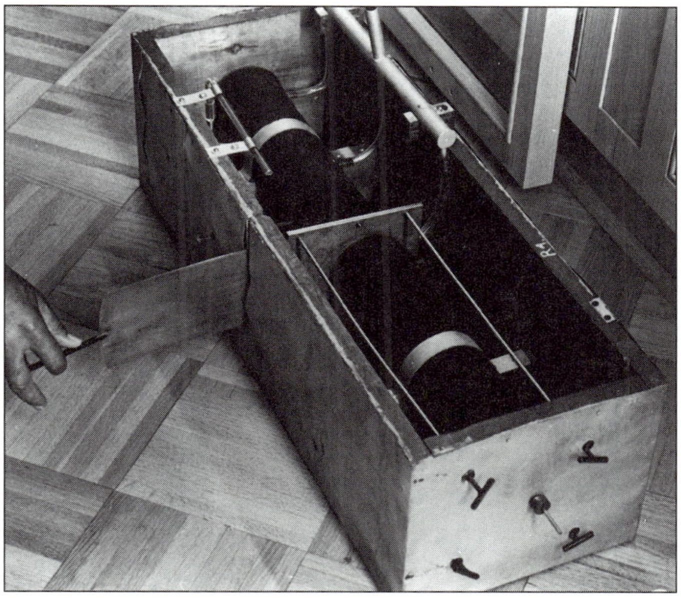

Top
Apparatus for determining the molecular weight of radium emanation by measuring its rate of diffusion; see text for explanation (Rutherford and Brooks, ref 6)

Above
Photograph of apparatus in Fig 3. The cylindrical ionization chambers were covered with felt and enclosed in a box filled with cotton wool in order to maintain a steady temperature (Rutherford Museum, McGill University)

THE RUTHERFORD–SODDY COLLABORATION

Frederick Soddy (1877–1956) was a young English chemist,

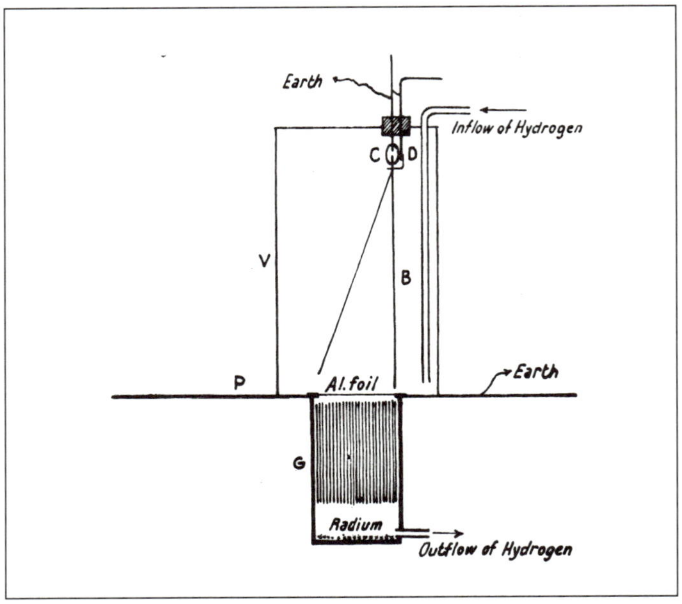

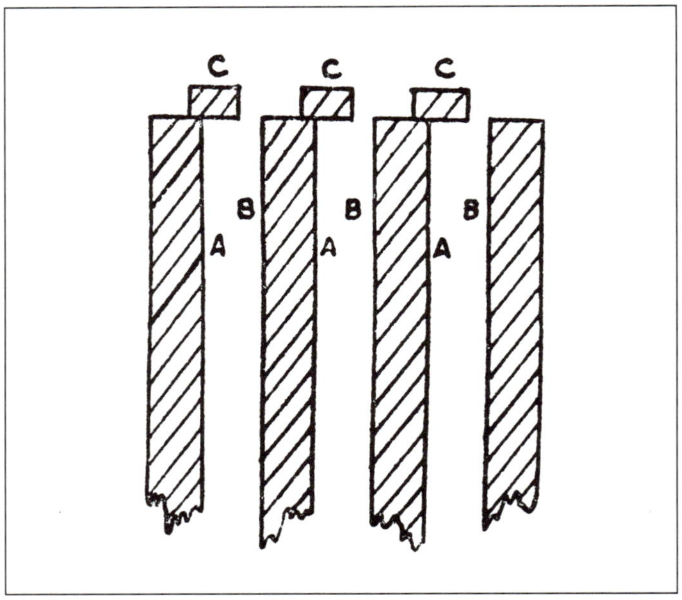

Top
Apparatus for observing the deviation of α-rays in a magnetic field. The α-rays from a thin layer of radium passed between the parallel brass plates G into the vessel V containing a gold-leaf electroscope, B. The plates G were located between the poles of an electromagnet.

Above
Modification of parallel plates by half covering the openings (Rutherford, ref 11)

an Oxford graduate, who had come to Canada in the spring of 1900 in the hope of obtaining the vacant chair of chemistry in Toronto, only to find that the post had already been filled. He then accepted a post at a much lower level, that of demonstrator in chemistry, at McGill. Soddy's first direct encounter with Rutherford was in March 1901, when he stoutly defended the non-divisibility of the chemical atom in a debate organized by the McGill Physical Society on "The existence of bodies smaller than the atom." In spite of the considerable heat generated by this debate, Soddy left the door open to collaboration with Rutherford; the opportunity came in the autumn of 1901.

The Rutherford-Soddy collaboration at McGill University lasted only 18 months (October 1901 to March 1903) but was one of the most important, and fruitful, in the history of science. Soddy carried out the chemical procedures in the Chemistry Building while the physical measurements were made by Rutherford, and to some extent also by Soddy, in the Physics Building. While standard chemical techniques, such as heat, solvents, precipitation and filtration, could be used to *separate* the elements in a given compound or mixture, the actual amounts of the radioactive substances were far too small to be measured on a balance or even spectroscopically. Instead, the presence or absence of radioactivity (as measured by an ionization chamber) plus the characteristics of the radioactivity—that is its rate of change with time and the penetrating power of the radiation—were used as an index of the sample under investigation and to distinguish one element from another: all together an early example of a radioactive tracer technique.

Between January 1902 and May 1903 Rutherford and Soddy published nine joint papers, totalling about 160 printed pages. The most important of these were "The Radioactivity of Thorium Compounds," published in two parts in the *Transactions of the Chemical Society*,[7] and "The Cause and Nature of Radioactivity," also in two parts and published in *Philosophical Magazine*.[8] The latter paper was essentially an updated version of the first but intended for a wider audience.

A complete account of the Rutherford-Soddy collaboration requires a book in itself: indeed, such a book has been written: *The Self-Splitting Atom* by Thaddeus Trenn.[54] Perhaps the best summary of the advances achieved by their partnership was that written by Rutherford himself, in a letter of reference for Soddy dated January 1904 (Soddy had left McGill in March 1903) and quoted by Muriel Howorth in her biography of Soddy:[41]

> *...In my opinion, the most important advances made in these researches were:*

1. The separation from thorium of the radioactive substance thorium X and its connection with the radioactivity of thorium.
2. Proof that the emanations behave as chemically inert gases and are produced by radium and thorium at a constant rate under all conditions.
3. Discovery of the condensation of the radioactive emanations and an accurate determination of their condensation points.
4. Proof that radioactivity is in all cases due to the continuous and spontaneous productions of new kinds of active matter.
5. Development of the disintegration theory to explore the phenomenon of radioactivity; evidence of the large amount of energy associated with radioactive changes and the suggestion that helium was produced from radioactive bodies.

The first item in the list was particularly significant: the addition of ammonium hydroxide to a solution of thorium nitrate gave rise to a soluble filtrate of ammonium nitrate which in principle should have been non-radioactive since it contained no thorium. In practice, however, the filtrate gave rise to 75 per cent of the α-rays, all the β-rays and all the emanating power. On the other hand, the insoluble precipitate should have contained all the thorium (as hydroxide) but in fact it produced only 25 per cent of the α-rays and had no emanating power. Clearly, an unknown radioactive substance, with chemical properties different from that of thorium, was present in the filtrate. This was presumably the "active constituent" of thorium, thorium X, the existence of which had been discovered the previous year by Baskerville.[42] However, some residual activity clearly remained in the thorium precipitate, and repeated chemical separation failed to deactivate the thorium completely. Furthermore, the residual activity actually increased with time, while that of the soluble filtrate containing thorium X decreased with time, both in geometrical progression, i.e., exponentially. Meanwhile, in December 1901 Becquerel reported a similar situation with uranium and "uranium X."[43]

Evidence of the chemical properties, or rather the *absence* of chemical properties, of the gaseous emanation, was reported in Part II of the paper *Cause and nature of radioactivity*.[13] Emanation, carried in a current of air, hydrogen or carbon dioxide, was passed through red-hot platinum, magnesium powder, zinc dust and other reagents. In each case the emanation emerged unchanged. The paper notes that "...the only known gases capable of passing in unchanged amount through all the reagents employed are the recently discovered members of the argon family." Towards the end of 1902 the Macdonald Physics Building acquired a liquid-air machine, and it was then possible to demonstrate that the emanation was indeed a gas with a fixed condensation point: i.e., –120° C for thorium emanation and –150° C for radium emanation. Furthermore the emanation lost its activity at the same rate at the temperature of liquid air as at room temperature. This and other results showed "that the rate of decay is unaffected by any physical or chemical agency."[9]

The transformation theory of radioactivity underwent a number of changes in a short period. The notion that radioactivity involved the transformation of the atoms of a chemical element had taken root in Rutherford's mind even before the partnership with Soddy began. (The term "transmutation" was avoided because chemists associated it with discredited medieval alchemy.) At first, the transformation of the atom and the emission of radiation were considered to be separate processes, and this made sense because the only material particles emitted were thought to be the β-rays, whose mass was a tiny fraction of that of the lightest atom, hydrogen. The α-rays were considered to be non-particulate—similar to soft x-rays—because attempts to deviate the rays in a magnetic or electric field had yielded negative results. The penetrating γ-rays were also non-deviable. However, by mid-1902 the transformation theory required a re-examination of the nature of the "easily absorbed rays from radium." In a paper on the transmission of excited radioactivity, submitted in July 1902 and published in January 1903[10], Rutherford summarized the evidence that α-rays were actually heavy charged particles, an idea previously suggested by Strutt and by Crookes. However, to demonstrate deviation of the particles required (a) a very strong magnetic and/or electric field, (b) a powerful source of α-rays, and (c) a very sensitive detector. Towards the end of 1902 Rutherford was able to fulfill all three conditions with a powerful electromagnet borrowed from the Electrical Engineering Department (maximum field strength 8370 cgs units, i.e., 0.84 tesla), a strong source of radium, and a gold-leaf electroscope, which was much more sensitive than a quadrant electrometer.

Between the poles of the electromagnet Rutherford placed a set of 25 parallel metal plates of length 3.7 cm and average spacing 0.4 mm. The radium source was below the plates, while the electroscope was above, separated by a very thin aluminum window. The electroscope and the plates were flushed with a stream of hydrogen, which carried away the radium emanation and, at the same time, increased the ionization in the electroscope due to the α-rays. With the magnetic field at its maximum strength the reading of the electroscope—i.e., the rate of fall of the gold leaf—was reduced to 11% of its value in the absence of the field, indicating that 89% of the α-rays had been deviated into the parallel plates. In a further experiment the exit slits between the plates were half covered by brass strips, and the *direction* of the deviation was ascertained. This experiment showed that the α-particles were positively charged, and calculations gave approximate values of their velocity (2.5 x 10^9 cm/sec) and the ratio of their charge to mass (*e/m* = 6 x 10^3 cgs units).[11] This value of *e/m* was about half that obtained for hydrogen in the electrolysis of water. Assuming, therefore, that the charges (α and H+) were equal, it appeared that α-rays were rapidly moving particles with a mass about twice that of hydrogen.

The "conversion" of the α-rays from non-material to material entities had a major impact on the transformation theory of radioactivity. In their final joint paper, "Radioactive Change," published in May 1903, Rutherford and Soddy reviewed the evidence for the mechanism of radioactivity and concluded:

> *Hence it is not possible to regard radioactivity as a consequence of changes that have already taken place. The rays emitted must be an accompaniment of the change of the radiating system into the one next produced.*[12]

In this paper Rutherford and Soddy introduced the term "radioactive constant" for λ, the proportion of the whole mass of a given radioactive element which changes in unit time. However, Trenn has pointed out[44] that Rutherford and Soddy construed λ to mean not all the atoms of a radioactive material but the fraction undergoing radioactive change. The final step was taken in September 1905 by a Viennese physicist, Egan von Schweidler, in a paper presented at the First International Congress of Radioactivity and Ionization, held in Liège, Belgium. Schwiedler construed the constant t = 1/ λ , i.e., the average life, to mean a property characteristic of *each individual atom* of a given radioactive substance. This development constituted the first step in the emergence of λ as an *atomic constant.*

In March 1903 Soddy left McGill for a post in University College, London under Sir William Ramsey, the chemist who had discovered the inert gases helium, argon, krypton and neon. In the July 16 and August 13 (1903) issues of *Nature*, Ramsey and Soddy reported the presence of helium in the gases obtained from radium bromide, and the production of helium by radium emanation.[45] Up to this time Rutherford and Soddy had speculated that "the presence of helium in minerals and its invariable association with uranium and thorium may...be connected with their radioactivity"[13] and that "possibly helium is an ultimate product of the disintegration of one of the radioactive elements, since it is only found in radioactive minerals."[14] Now it was possible to go a step further. As it happened, Rutherford was in Britain in the summer of 1903 and he immediately commented on the August 13 letter of Ramsey and Soddy. Rutherford's letter, published in the next issue of *Nature* (August 20) states that the available evidence "supports the view that the α-particle is in reality helium."[15] No longer was helium merely an "ultimate product" of radioactivity, but rather an integral part of the disintegration process, identified with the α-particle itself. Rutherford continued to hold this belief although it was not until five years later that he was able to provide a rigorous proof of the identity.[16]

THE RADIOACTIVE SERIES

After Soddy's departure, Rutherford remained at McGill for another four years, an important period of consolidation; he explored (a) the radioactive series, (b) the nature and properties of α-rays, and (c) the energy associated with radioactive transformations and with the production of ions. These topics were, of course, closely linked, but it will be convenient to discuss them separately.

In the spring of 1904 Rutherford gave two important lectures in London, at the Royal Institution, in March, and the Royal Society (the prestigious Bakerian Lecture), in May. Both lectures were published later in the year.[17,18] In the Bakerian lecture, "The succession of changes in radioactive bodies," Rutherford reviewed the evidence for four radioactive series, those of radium, thorium, uranium and actinium, and derived the mathematical theory of successive changes. At this stage the link between uranium and radium was unproven although Rutherford discussed the evidence that uranium is the parent of radium and that radium can also be derived from thorium and actinium. (The concept of *isotopes* had not yet been developed.)

By September 1905 Rutherford had extended the radium series, via emanation, from radium A, B, C and D (now considered the primary constituent in radio-lead) to radium E and, finally, radium F, the active constituent in radio-tellurium and polonium.[19] He suggested that the transformation product of radium F is lead:

> *The view that lead is the final or end-product of the transformation of radium is supported by the fact that lead is always found in the radioactive minerals in about the amount to be theoretically expected from the content of uranium, when the quantity of helium, present in the mineral, is used to compute its probable age. A similar suggestion has recently been advanced by Boltwood [Phil Mag, April 1905, p. 613].*

THE NATURE OF THE α-PARTICLE

A key factor in the elucidation of the radioactive series was the assumption that α-rays are charged atoms of helium, since the loss of five helium atoms in successive transformations would account for the difference in the atomic weights of radium and lead. Indeed, Rutherford speculated that "many of the so-called chemical elements may prove to be compounds of helium, or, in other words, that the helium atom is probably one of the secondary units with which the heavier atoms are built up."[20]

The experiments published two years earlier[11] had clearly demonstrated that α-rays were deviable and, therefore, particulate in nature but had not provided conclusive proof that they were emitted with a positive charge: the charge could have been acquired after emission. Nor had their identity with helium been rigorously proven. Rutherford returned to this problem in 1904 and, during his last years at McGill, devoted a substantial proportion of his research to the α-particle: of his 19 papers published in 1905 and 1906, nine were directly concerned with this problem.

Experiments with α-particles were complicated by the presence of β-rays and by the fact that the alphas emitted by the various members of a radioactive series differ in their initial velocities, as indicated by their ability to penetrate layers of aluminum foil. These problems could be avoided (or, at least, minimized) by using radium at its minimum activity, i.e., by expelling the emanation from a solution of radium bromide and by deflecting the β-rays (electrons) away from the measuring (ionization) chamber by a strong magnetic field. By reversing the polarity of the electrodes in the chamber, Rutherford could prove that the α-particles were emitted with a positive charge[21] and could deduce the product *ne* of the number of α-particles *n* and their charge *e*. However, the experiment did not yield independent values of *n* and *e*, and further deductions depended on the assumption that each particle carried a single ionic charge. Hence, he calculated that the total number of α-particles expelled per second by 1 g of radium at its minimum activity, i.e., without emanation and subsequent products, is 6.2×10^{10}. If, however, the α-particle carries *two* ionic charges, this number reduces to 3.1×10^{10} α-particles per second. (The value later taken as the basis of the *curie*, the unit of radioactivity, is 3.70×10^{10}.)

Rutherford's "definitive" investigation of the α-particle is considered to be that published as two papers (the second with Otto Hahn) in October 1906.[22,23] These papers set out to answer a number of questions, including the identity of the α-particle from different radioactive products; the variation, if any, of *e/m* as the particle passes through matter; the connection between the velocity of the particle and its range of ionization in air; and the connection, if any, between the α-particle and the helium atom. In these experiments five different sources of α-rays were used: (1) a wire exposed to radium emanation acted primarily either as radium C or radium A, depending on the length of exposure to the emanation and the subsequent time in the measuring apparatus (short time, radium A, long time, radium C.); (2) the "radium F" source was a bismuth rod coated with "radio-tellurium;" (3) the actinium α-ray source was a copper plate exposed to actinium emanation; (4 and 5) the thorium B and C source (they could not be separated) was a wire exposed to thorium emanation.

The α-particles emerging from the source passed through a thin mica window into an evacuated cylinder and hence between two parallel brass plates 4 cm high and 0.21 mm apart. The emergent pencil of rays struck a small photographic plate some distance from the exit slit, producing—after a long exposure, or a series of short exposures with a succession of radium A sources—an image of the slit. The image split into two when a deflecting voltage was applied across the parallel plates, and the polarity reversed halfway through the exposure. The separation of the two images increased with voltage and distance between the exit slit and the photographic plate. With a voltage of 508.6 V and a distance of 10.0 cm, a separation (taken from the outer edges of the images) of 3.10 mm was obtained.

These experiments demonstrated that, within the experimental error, the value of *e/m* of α-particles from all five sources is identical although the velocity of expulsion is different for each. (Furthermore, *e/m* remains unchanged as the particle passes through matter.) Rutherford discusses three possibilities: (1) that the α-particle is a *molecule* of hydrogen carrying the ionic charge of hydrogen, or (2) that it is a helium atom carrying *twice* the ionic charge of hydrogen, or (3) that it is *one-half* of the helium atom carrying a single ionic charge. He concludes—the detailed arguments are omitted here—that the second solution is the most probable although (as previously indicated) he still has no irrefutable proof.

Rutherford also investigated the retardation of the α-particle in passing through matter.[24] The apparatus was somewhat different from that described above: here an evacuated brass cylinder contained the α-source, a single slit and a photographic plate; the distances between these items could be altered at will. The whole apparatus was placed in a strong (and reversible) magnetic field so that the velocity of the α-particles emerging from layers of absorbing material placed over the source, could be estimated from the separation of the two images.

Rutherford had previously noted "evidence of a distinct

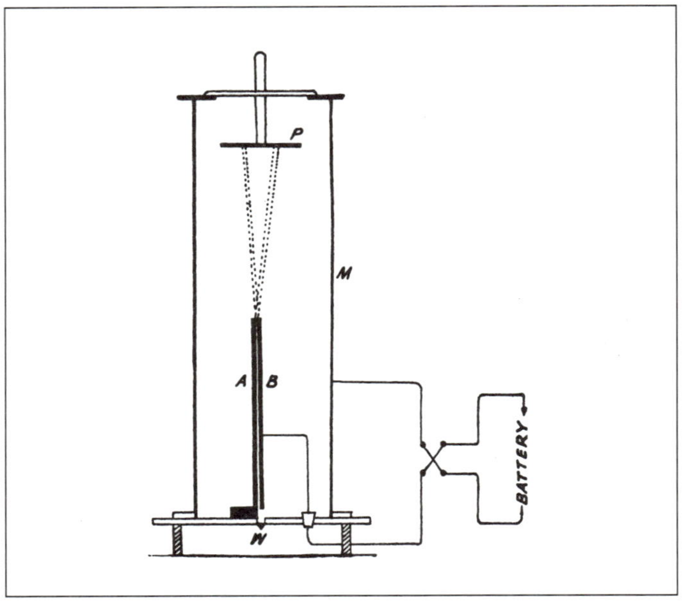

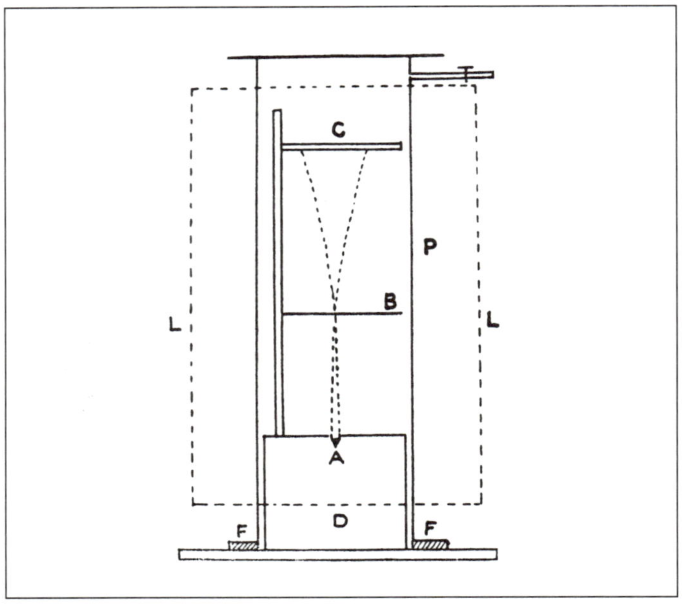

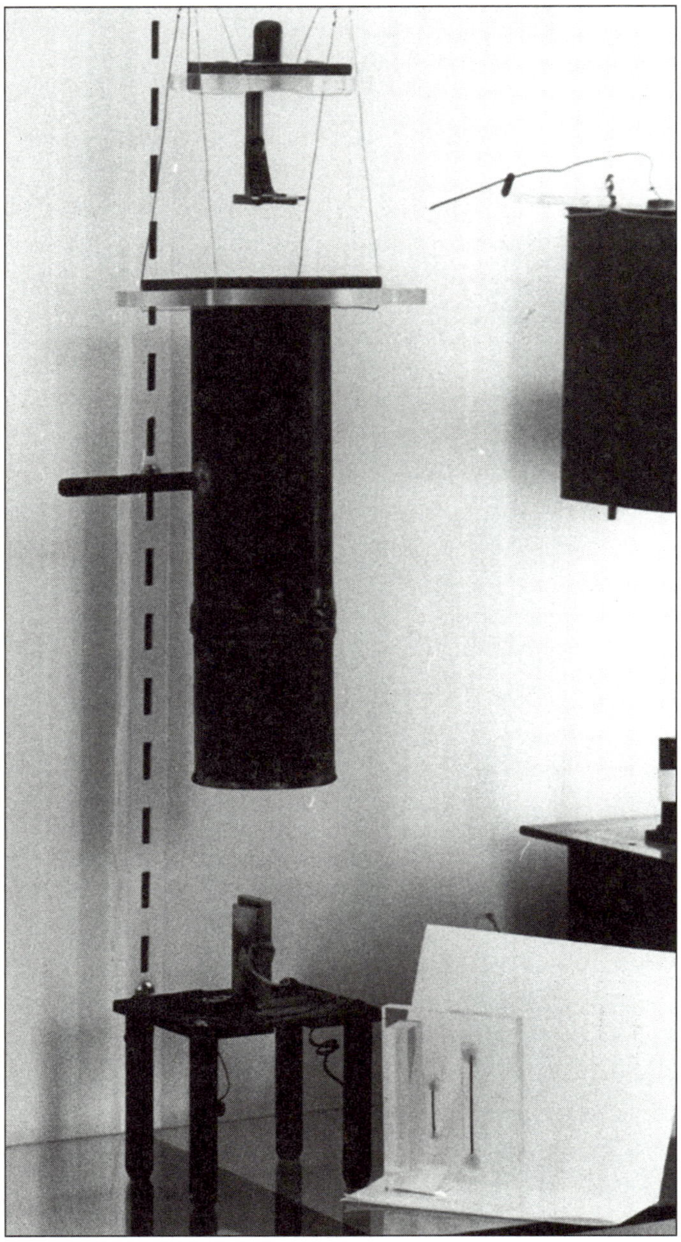

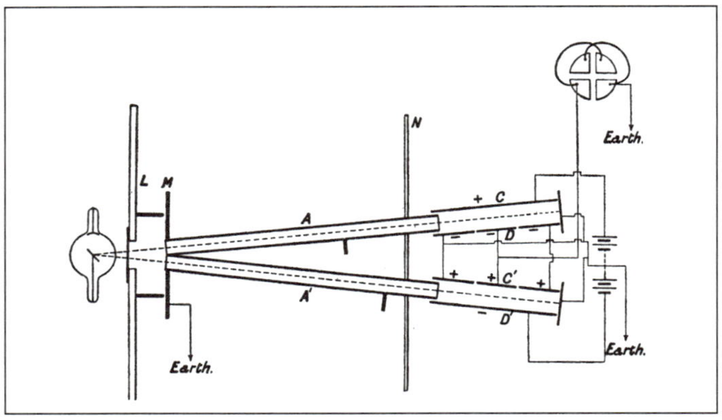

Upper left
Apparatus for determining the ratio of charge to mass of α-particles by deflection in an electric field. W: wire source of α-particles. A,B: parallel metal plates, connected to a reversible voltage. P: photographic plate. M: evacuated vessel (Rutherford, ref 22)

Lower left
Photograph of apparatus (in "exploded" format) in upper left (Rutherford Museum, McGill University)

Top
Apparatus for measuring the retardation of α-particles, from different sources, in matter. A: wire source of alphas. B: movable frame with slit. C: movable holder for photographic plate. P: evacuated brass tube with flange FF ground to form airtight joint with base plate. LL: extent of applied magnetic field (Rutherford, ref 24)

Above
Apparatus for measuring the absorption of x-rays in air. AA′: sealed brass tubes, 118 cm long, 3.4 cm dia, with side tubes for evacuation or increasing air pressure; CD, C′D′, identical parallel-plate ionization chambers. The earthed outer plates formed guard rings, the inner plates C^1 and D were connected together and to the quadrant electrometer so as to register the difference between the two ionization currents; L, M, N: lead screens to eliminate stray radiation (Rutherford and McClung, ref 26)

scattering of the rays from radium C in their passage through air." He now extended this observation by placing a thin sheet of mica, equivalent in stopping power to 3.5 cm of air, over one-half of the slit. The result was a well-defined image on the photographic plate of the uncovered half-slit and a diffuse image of the mica-covered portion. These images resulted with or without the magnetic field, so the effect could not be ascribed to "contaminating" electrons. From the width of the diffuse image Rutherford estimated that some of the particles had been deflected by about 2°. He concludes:

> *The scattering of the α-particles increases, as we should expect, with the decrease of velocity of the α-particle...it can easily be calculated that the change of direction of 2°...of some of the α-particles in passing through the thickness of mica (0.003 cm) would require over that distance an average transverse electric field of about 100 million volts per cm. Such a result brings out clearly the fact that the atoms of matter must be the seat of very intense electrical forces...*

Rutherford did not follow up this observation immediately; in fact, it was not until 1908, by which time he had left McGill for Manchester, that he suggested to Hans Geiger, a young German scientist in Manchester on a John Harling Fellowship, that he carry out a full investigation of the scattering of α-particles in foils of different metals. In part of this investigation Geiger was joined by a graduate student, Ernest Marsden. Their study produced the unexpected result that a few alphas—about 1 in 8000—were scattered by a thin gold foil through 90° or more, a phenomenon described as "diffuse reflection."[46] Rutherford's explanation of α-scattering—the nuclear model of the atom—followed in 1911.[25] Thus the immediate "parent" of the nuclear atom was the scattering investigation in Manchester, but its genesis was the observation of a diffuse image in Montréal.

THE ENERGY OF RADIOACTIVE TRANSFORMATIONS

The third major subject of Rutherford's "post-Soddy" research at McGill concerned the energy associated with radioactive transformations. He had begun this study even before the start of his collaboration with Soddy: in 1900 he carried out a major investigation of the energy of x- (Röntgen) and Becquerel rays, with the assistance of one of the demonstrators in physics, RK McClung. Their joint paper was published in 1901.[26] The energy of the x-rays was determined by partially absorbing the radiation in a grid comprising 3 m of narrow platinum strip wound on a mica frame and measuring the change in resistance arising from the (very small) increase in temperature. The energy of the rays, thus determined, was then used to find the energy required to produce a single ion in gases exposed to x-rays. This, in turn, required a measurement of the ionization current produced by the rays under saturation conditions, i.e., no recombination, together with a measurement of the fraction of the radiation absorbed in a given volume of the gas. The latter was measured by an ingenious arrangement of two identical and quasi-parallel brass tubes, 118 cm long, through which a divided x-ray beam passed before reaching identical ionization chambers. With one tube evacuated and the other filled with air or other gas under known pressure, the difference between the currents measured in the two chambers allowed the absorption coefficient of the gas to be calculated.

These experiments led to a value of W—the average energy required to produce a single ion in air at atmospheric pressure and temperature—of 1.90 x 10^{-10} ergs, equivalent to about 120 electron-volts, several times today's accepted value of 34 eV. Nevertheless, in view of the many difficulties encountered in these investigations (for example, the x-ray source was unstable and the beam inhomogeneous), the result was very commendable.

Rutherford and McClung, in the work just cited,[26] used their value of W to determine the energy emitted per second by a thin layer of uranium oxide or thorium oxide. For this purpose the radioactive layer was placed on a small central area of the lower plate of a parallel-plate ionization chamber, and the resulting ionization current was measured. Hence, it was deduced that 1 g of uranium oxide radiated energy into the air at the rate of 10^{-9} calories per second, with a somewhat greater value for thorium oxide. Radium was known to be at least 100,000 times more active than uranium and was therefore emitting energy at an apparently constant rate of at least 3000 calories per gram per year. (This value was actually far too low. In 1903 Pierre Curie and André Laborde deduced a value of about 100 calories *per hour* for the heat output of 1 g of radium.[47]) Rutherford rejected the theory that radioactive substances acted as transformers of "outside" (atmospheric?) energy. He speculated that their energy was derived internally from a closer aggregation or regrouping of the components of the atom or molecule, which JJ Thomson had suggested was comprised of a large number of positively and negatively charged electrons.

Soon after Soddy's departure from McGill in 1903, Rutherford returned to the problem of the rate of heat emission by a radium source. The value of 100 calories per hour per gram of radium cited above had just been published, and Rutherford and Soddy had recently shown that the radiation from a radium source in equilibrium comprised three components: (1) a "non-separable" radiation that remained when the emanation was driven off by heating the source, entirely α-rays and comprising 25 per cent of the total radiation; (2) the radiation from the emanation occluded in the radium, also entirely α-, about 18 per cent of the total; (3) "excited radiation," comprising α-, β- and γ- rays, arising from the decay products of emanation deposited within the source, about 57 per cent of the total. The purpose of the new investigation was to measure the rate of heat emission by the three components and, if possible, to correlate heat and radioactivity in each component.

In this investigation Rutherford was assisted by Howard Barnes, an assistant professor of physics who had earlier collaborated with Rutherford's predecessor, Callendar, in precision calorimetry. Barnes had, *inter alia* , measured the specific heat of water with great precision over a wide range of temperature.

The method adopted by Rutherford and Barnes was based on a simple differential air calorimeter comprising two identical spherical flasks connected by a manometer which registered differences in pressure.[27] The whole assembly was immersed in a constant-temperature water bath. A central glass tube in each flask allowed a radioactive source to be introduced into one or other flask: either radium bromide from which the emanation had been expelled, or pure emanation. The manometer responded to the expansion of air (in the source-containing flask) arising from the heat emitted by the radioactive source, and the displacement of liquid (xylene) in the manometer could be calibrated by substituting a small resistance coil heated by a known electric current. Measurements were taken at intervals with both the "de-emanated" radium and the emanation source for several days after the initial separation of the emanation. The results indicated a reasonably good correlation between the rate of heat emission and the emission of α-rays: the variation in time of the heat emission of each of the radioactive products is the same as the time variation of the activity (bearing in mind that, at this stage, the full radioactive series from radium to lead was not yet known). The assumption that the energy contributed by β-, x—and γ-rays was only a small fraction of that associated with α-rays seemed to be borne out.

Not all the readers of the Rutherford/Barnes paper were convinced however. Louis Paschen, a highly respected professor of physics at Tübingen in Germany, had carried out his own measurements with an ice calorimeter and had concluded that the γ-rays emitted by radium carried at least as much energy as the alphas. Rutherford and Barnes,

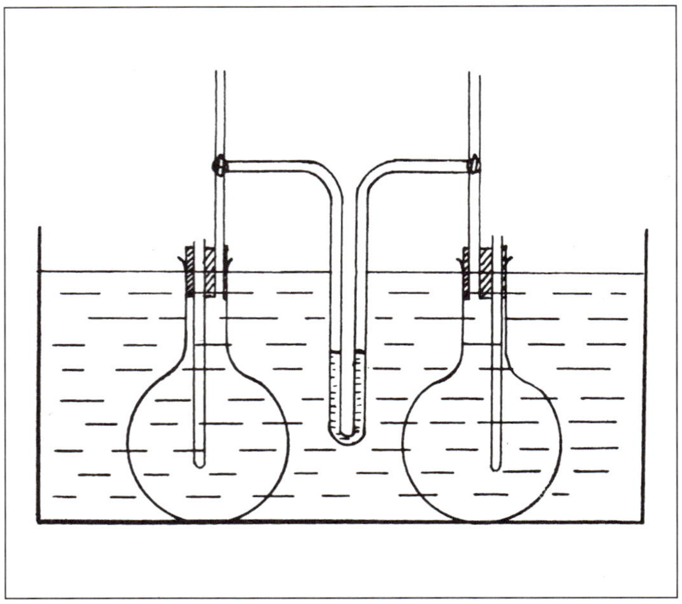

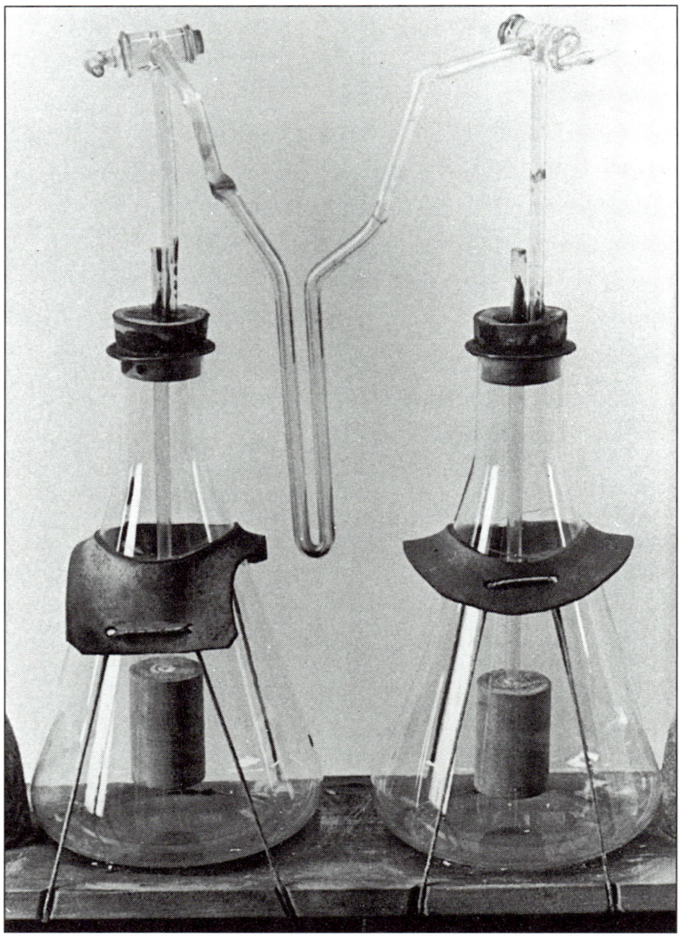

Top

Differential air calorimeter. Two 1-litre flasks were immersed in a constant-temperature water bath. A source of radium or emanation was lowered into the inner tube of one flask and the expansion of the air registered by the manometer. The manometer was calibrated by replacing the source by a wire of known resistance carrying a known current (Rutherford and Barnes, ref 27) in turn, were unconvinced by Paschen's results but, nevertheless, devised another experiment to verify their original assumption. This time they enclosed the inner tube of each flask in a lead cylinder of sufficient size to absorb most of the gammas and betas, as well as the alphas, emitted by the source.[28] The result was virtually the same as before, confirming the assumption that most of the energy emitted in radioactive changes is carried by the α-particles. (Meanwhile, Paschen had carried out further investigations which disproved his earlier conclusions on the energy of the gammas.)

The work of Rutherford and Barnes, together with that of their European contemporaries, on the heat emission by radium had some unexpected repercussions. At the time a fierce controversy raged as to the age of the earth. On the basis of the known temperature gradient in the earth's crust (1° F increase for every 50 feet of descent), and assuming that the whole earth had originally been a molten sphere, Lord Kelvin had calculated that the earth could not be more than 100 million years old—probably less—a duration quite insufficient to account for geological and biological evolution. However, it was known that everything—earth, rocks, water and air—contains a small amount of radioactive material, of the order of one or two parts per million. Rutherford showed that the heat supplied by this tiny amount of radioactivity, if uniformly distributed in the form of uranium (strongly suspected, but not yet proven, to be the parent of radium), with a half-life of hundreds of millions of years, was sufficient to extend the origin of the earth back several billion years. Rutherford argued this case in a "popular" article in *Harper's Magazine*.[29]

RETURN TO ENGLAND

In the summer of 1907 Rutherford left McGill and Canada to return to England as Langworthy Professor of Physics at Manchester University. The following year he was awarded a Nobel Prize (in chemistry, not physics!) for his work in Montréal on radioactivity. Meanwhile, he had received many honours, including the Fellowship of the Royal Society in 1903, the Rumford Medal of the Society in 1905 and honorary doctorates from several universities. In addition to the Bakerian Lecture to the Royal Society already mentioned, Rutherford lectured to the Franklin Institute in Philadelphia in April 1905 and gave the prestigious Silliman Lectures at Yale, also in 1905.

During his nine-year stay at McGill, Rutherford published 70 scientific papers and articles, of which 47 were authored by himself alone and 23 co-authored by a single collaborator.[30] Of these 70 papers at least 30 can be described as "major" works by virtue of their length, content and scientific insight. The McGill papers occupy over 700 pages of Volume I of the *Collected Papers of Lord Rutherford of Nelson*,[31] and constitute the largest of the five components of Rutherford's scientific career, i.e., Canterbury, Cambridge, Montreal, Manchester and Cambridge again. (It should, however, be borne in mind that Rutherford had no administrative or external responsibilities at McGill, not the case in his later posts; in addition, World War I effectively removed several years from his Manchester research.)

Apart from his original research papers, Rutherford's career at McGill was marked by the publication of his book, *Radio-activity*. The first edition was published in 1904 and comprised 399 pages.[32] The rapid growth of the subject is indicated by the expansion of the book to 580 pages in the second edition, published only a year later. Rutherford's third book, published in 1906, contained an updated version of the eleven Silliman lectures delivered at Yale the previous year.[33]

In addition to the 70 papers authored or co-authored by Rutherford during his McGill career, 58 papers were published in this period by members of his "team" on various topics within the general field of radioactivity and ionizing radiation. (Rutherford would never add his own name to a paper unless he had made a major contribution to the research beyond suggesting the topic and discussing the progress of the work.) Most of these papers were published in the second half of Rutherford's tenure, by which time his reputation was sufficient to attract research workers from outside Canada, including Stewart Eve from England, Fanny Cook Gales from the United States, Tadeusz Godlewski from Poland and Otto Hahn and Max Levin from Germany. Many topics not investigated by Rutherford himself, including the nature and properties of the gamma rays, secondary radiation and the radioactivity of the atmosphere. However, as Pyenson has pointed out,[48] Rutherford did not succeed in establishing a European-style "school of physics" in Montréal which survived his own departure. Nevertheless, Rutherford's influence on physics in North America as a whole was profound, and many of the younger scientists who worked with Rutherford at McGill went on to become professors elsewhere in

Left
Modified differential air calorimeter, with lead cylinder surrounding the radium source to absorb the β- and γ-rays as well as the α-particles. The lead weights on the baseplate kept the flasks submerged in a constant-temperature water bath (not shown) (Rutherford and Barnes, ref 28) (Rutherford Museum, McGill University).

Canada or in the United States. Wilson has also argued[49] that the later success of Canadian nuclear research at Chalk River can be attributed, at least in part, to the foundations laid by Rutherford in Montréal at the beginning of the century.

Many pieces of apparatus used by Rutherford in his research in Montréal have been preserved and are on display in the Rutherford Museum of McGill University.[50]

It is, of course, futile to pretend that any branch of science owes its development to a single researcher, however talented. Rutherford was well aware of this and, in letters to his mother and fiancée, often stressed the importance of "keeping ahead of the race." Nevertheless, it is widely recognized that of all the individual contributions to the science of radioactivity—and hence to the structure of the atom—that of Rutherford was supreme. He not only elucidated the *facts* of atomic transformation and the spontaneous emission of radiation but put forward *explanations* that (allowing for subsequent additions and modifications) have stood the test of time. Not without cause is Ernest Rutherford often described as "The Father of the Atomic Age."

"Some of their colleagues gravely expressed the fear that radical ideas about spontaneous transmutation of matter might bring discredit to McGill, and Rutherford was advised to delay publication and proceed more cautiously. However, the senior professor, Cox, quietly gave support to Rutherford and prophesied that the development of radioactivity would bring renown to McGill, and went on to say that Rutherford's experimental work would one day be rated as the greatest since that of Faraday."[1]

"So much has been written of Rutherford as a man that I can add nothing: it was said of him that he never made an enemy and never lost a friend; Sir James Jeans said that those who were honoured by his friendship knew that his greatness as a scientist was matched by his greatness as a man."[1]

1. Allibone TE. *Rutherford, the father of nuclear energy.* Manchester:Manchester University Press, 1973. [The Rutherford Lecture, 1972, delivered at the Polytechnic of Central London.]

Right
X-ray appparatus from the early 1900s

PLATE I.

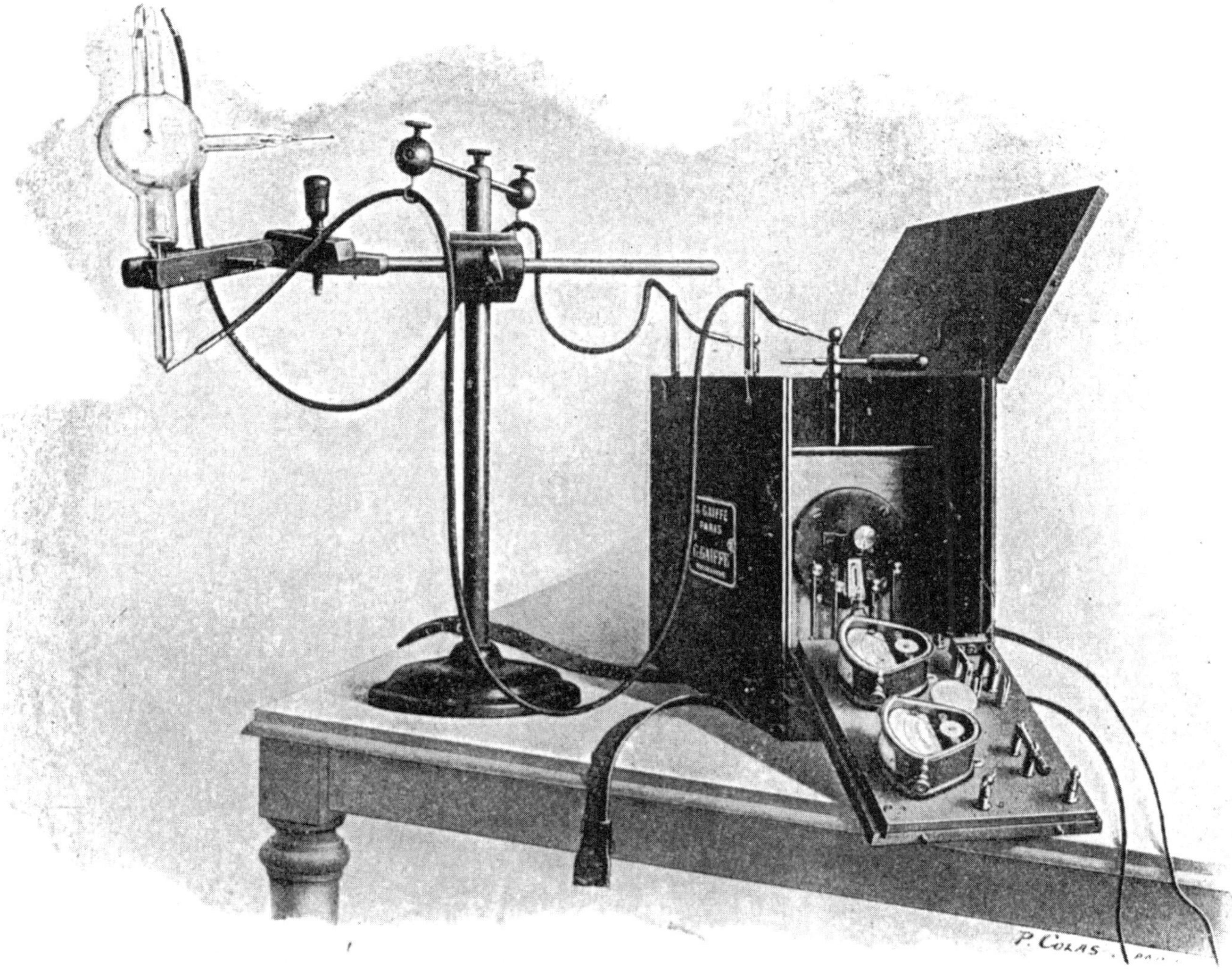

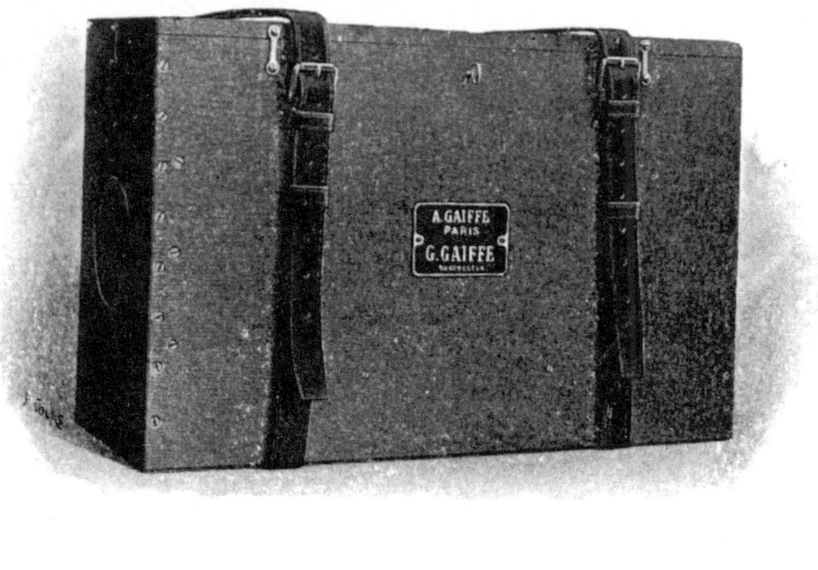

PORTABLE COIL (OPEN AND SHUT).

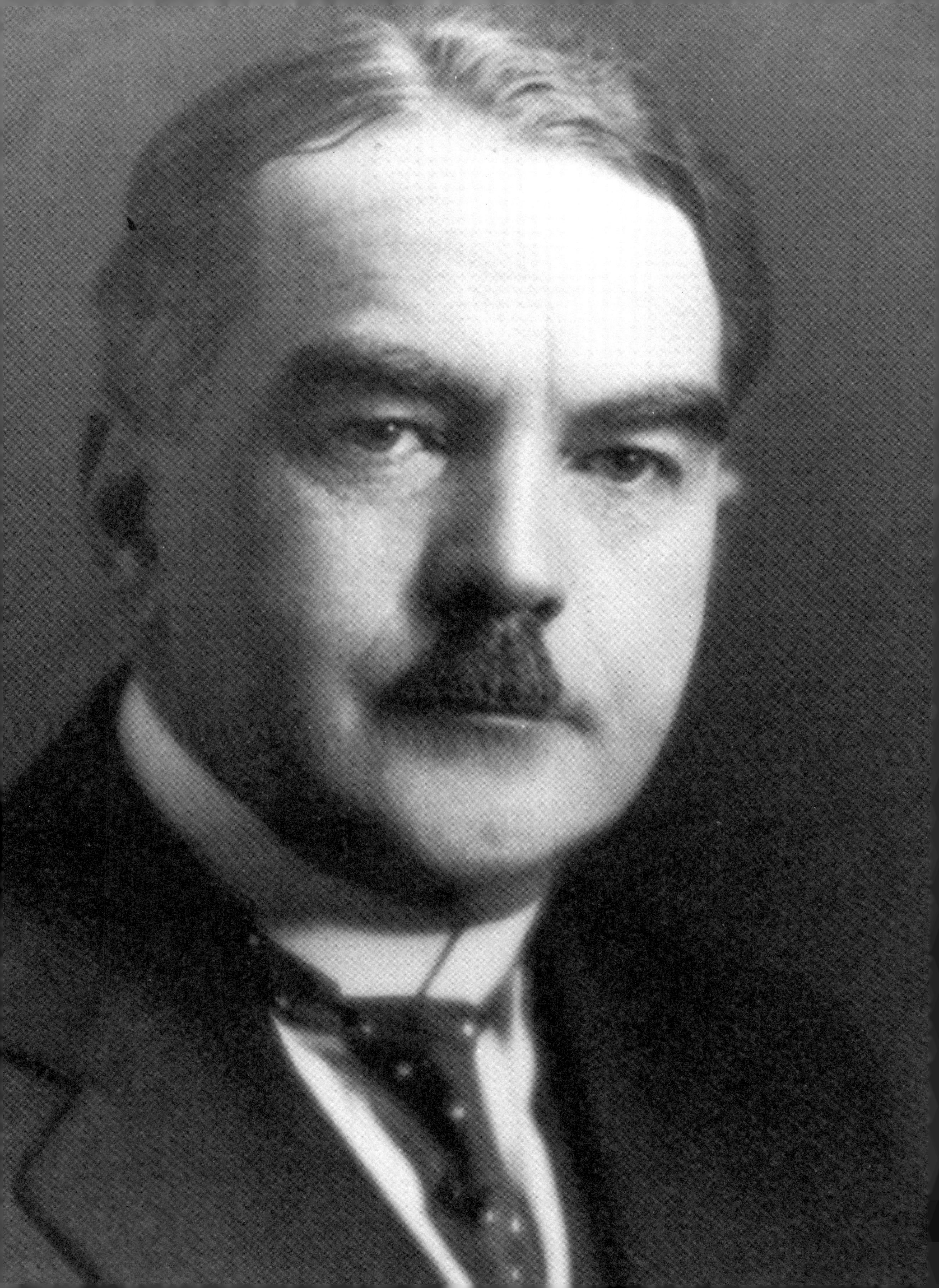

Chapter VI •

Rays of Hope:

The Establishment of Radiation Oncology in Canada 1895–1976

Charles RR Hayter, Günes N Ege, and Peter J Fitzpatrick

PREAMBLE

In 1902 Dr Abraham Groves of Fergus, Ontario was faced with a vexing clinical problem. He had seen a 59-year-old woman with a cancer of the uterus. Over a two-year period the patient had lost weight, become weak and had been bleeding profusely. The disease was too advanced for surgery, and there seemed no hope other than the liberal use of morphine. However, Groves was not willing to let the patient go home and die in pain. Always of an adventurous and pioneering spirit—he had performed the first appendectomy in North America—he had recently acquired an x-ray machine and became interested in the treatment of cancer with x-rays. He decided to treat his patient with radiation and was amazed to note a beneficial effect:

> *Treatment was commenced, lasting on an average 15 minutes per diem, and on the fourteenth day there was no apparent result excepting a partial relief of pain, but after this, the odour decreased with lessened discharge, the ulcerated surface showed healthy signs, granulation occurring, and on the thirtieth day from the commencement of the treatment, there was only a small surface not completely healed, no odour, discharge or hemorrhage, and complete absence from pain. Patient then left the hospital, and ten days afterward I examined her and found the remaining surface had healed and her general health improved in every way. Two months afterwards I found her in perfect health, with absolutely no return of symptoms. I think this may be confidently claimed as a cure.*[1]

Thus began the art and science of applying radiation in the treatment of cancer in Canada.

Left
Dr Gordon Richards

INTRODUCTION

One in three Canadians will develop cancer during his or her lifetime. In men, the commonest cancers arise from the lung, prostate and large bowel; in women, from the breast, lung, large bowel and uterus. About 50 per cent of cancer patients receive radiation therapy at some point during the course of their illness. Radiation therapy may be given for cure or, when cure is not possible, to relieve symptoms such as pain or bleeding. When given for cure, radiation therapy has the advantage that it preserves the function and the normal anatomical contour of body tissues. For example, treatment of cancer of the larynx by radiation therapy allows preservation of the voice, and treatment of breast cancer by removal of the tumour followed by radiation permits retention of the breast.

Radiation oncology is the medical specialty that encompasses the care and treatment of cancer patients with an emphasis on the use of ionizing radiation. Radiation oncologists are medical specialists who, after graduation from medical school, receive a four to five year period of specialized training in the treatment of cancer. Once qualified, most radiation oncologists work in provincial cancer treatment centres, where they see patients in consultation, decide if radiation therapy is appropriate and prescribe and supervise courses of radiation. Radiation oncologists also follow patients closely after treatment and help in their continuing care.

Although the term "radiation oncology" was not formally adopted until 1976, radiation therapy of cancer has a long history in Canada. This chapter will outline the establishment, development and achievements of radiation therapy in Canada from the turn of the century to the 1970s.

1895–1902: THE BEGINNINGS

Within a year after Röntgen's discovery of the x-ray, physicians found that the new rays had the power not only to illuminate the inside of the body but also to destroy diseased tissue. Cancers seemed particularly susceptible to the influence of the rays. Skin cancers melted away, and bulky internal tumours were reduced, relieving pain. Invisible, impalpable and odourless, the rays seemed nothing less than magical. For the first time, doctors had a treatment for cancer that did not involve cutting and removal of tissue.

By the turn of the century, several Canadian physicians reported their experience in the radiation treatment of cancer. Dr Abraham Groves' observations have been noted above; another influential practitioner was Dr James Third of Kingston[2], who reported in 1902 on the successful use

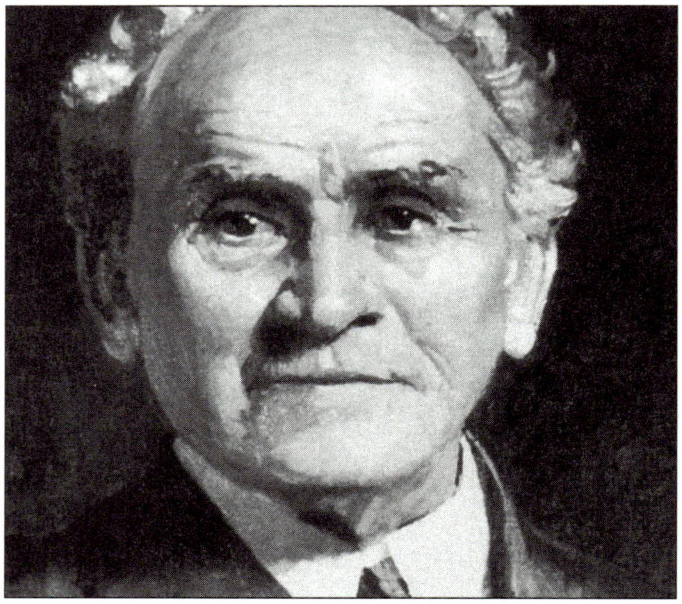

Above
Dr Abraham Groves

Right
Diagram demonsrating early superficial radiotherapy, early 1900s

of radiation to treat chest wall recurrences of breast cancer. In the same year, radiation therapy achieved national recognition when an entire session at the Canadian Medical Association's annual meeting in Montréal was devoted to the topic. Among the speakers was Dr AR Robinson of New York, who asserted that the x-ray would do away with the scalpel.

During this early period the technical aspects of therapy were crude. The source of x-rays was simply placed over the part of the body to be treated, which might be defined by sheet lead. Treatment was carried out daily until a desired therapeutic effect was reached or the skin reaction prevented further exposure.

Despite the primitive nature of early treatment, the results were promising. Doctors such as FW Hett of Berlin (now Kitchener), Ontario recognized the special features of radiation therapy. Writing in the *Dominion Medical Monthly*, Hett listed the advantages of x-ray treatment:[3]

1) *it is painless;*
2) *it leaves small scars, thus doing away with disfigurement;*
3) *it destroys diseased tissue but not the normal;*
4) *it relieves pain;*
5) *it removes odour;*
6) *it removes the dread of an operation.*

1902–1920: THE ERA OF "COTTAGE RADIOTHERAPY"

After the turn of the century, x-ray machines and radium became widely available to medical practitioners. The early decades of this century were the era of "cottage radio-

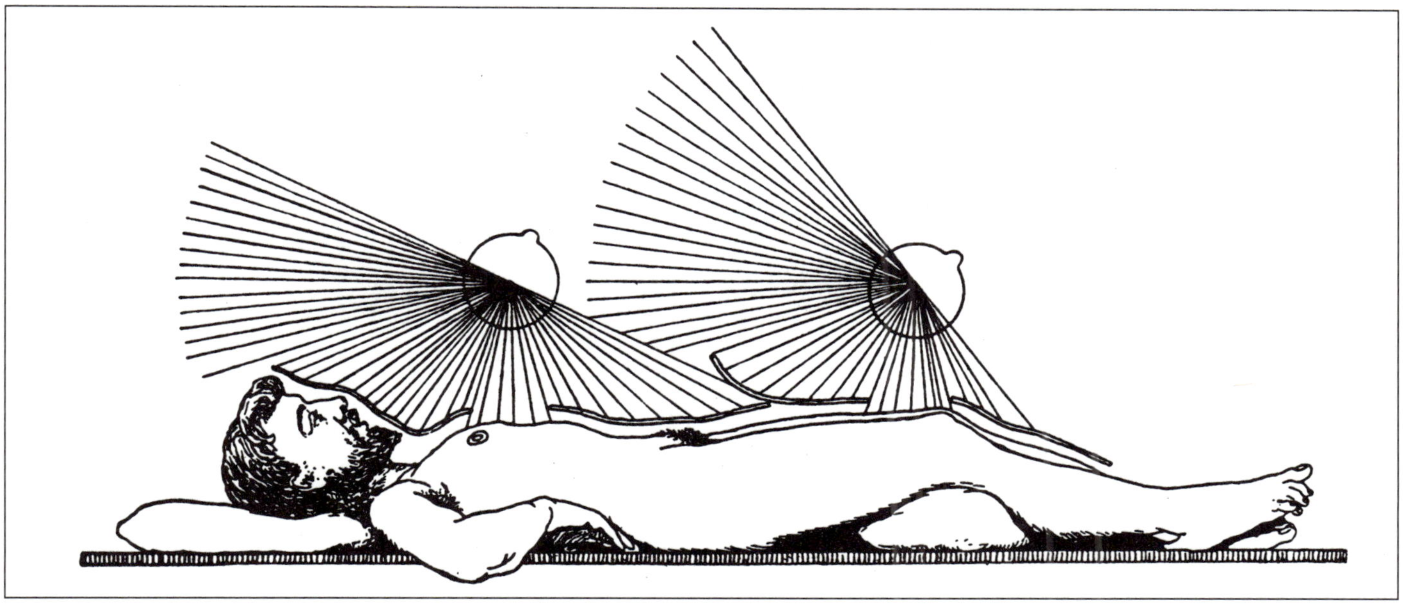

therapy," when treatment was carried on in hospitals, doctors' offices and, in the case of radium, sometimes in patients' homes. The treatment was supervised and given by general practitioners and surgeons.

A glimpse into x-ray therapy in the early part of this century is given by a letter now in the Archives of Ontario written in March 1932 by Mrs James Price Kennedy of Wingham, Ontario to Dr JWS McCullough, the chief inspector of health for Ontario. Mrs Kennedy, a trained nurse, reported that around 1900 she had given x-ray treatment under the supervision of her husband, a country doctor. Dr Kennedy had owned the first x-ray machine in the region and "proved thirty or more years ago that cancer treated by x-ray after operation is curable or rather can be cured". On the strength of her experience, Mrs Kennedy, now a widow with time on her hands, was seeking a position with the newly established cancer treatment clinics in Ontario. She received a polite refusal from Dr McCullough.

In addition to x-ray machines, radium became available in the early years of the century. Radium was first introduced in Canada in 1909 by Dr WH Aitken of Toronto, the first president of the American Radium Society. Like x-ray apparatus, radium became available to the general practitioner, although at enormous cost. In 1922, for example, Dr William F Roberts of Saint John, New Brunswick (later the first minister of health in the British Empire) purchased 60 mg of radium for private use at a cost of six thousand dollars. Dr Roberts used the radium in his physical therapy clinic in Saint John. One current resident of Saint John recalls that his mother was treated at home for breast cancer by Dr Roberts' nurse, who brought the radium to the house in a brown paper parcel and laid it on the tumour for half an hour twice a day[4].

By 1920 the situation in radiation therapy in Canada was near chaos. General practitioners and surgeons owned x-ray equipment and radium and gave treatment for all kinds of conditions, ranging from cancer to tonsillitis to psoriasis to cataracts. Although radiation treatment showed great promise, the results of treatment had not been analyzed properly, and there were no standards for technique or dosage. Serious concerns arose about its safety in the hands of unskilled individuals. In 1928 Dr TL Gray raised his concern in the *Canadian Medical Association Journal* when he wrote that promising reports about x-rays "act as a stimulus to men who simply possess an x-ray outfit to treat promiscuously almost every type of disease known, with results that are either negative or harmful... we also know that disastrous results have followed months and even years after treatment has been discontinued."[5]

1920–1946: SPECIALIZATION AND CENTRALIZATION

As a result of the concern of physicians, the public and government, pressure increased to ensure that radiation therapy to be carried out only by fully trained and qualified specialists in special treatment centres. The era from 1920 to 1946 saw the establishment of cancer treatment organizations and clinics in most of the provinces in Canada and the recognition of radiology as a separate specialty of medicine. Both of these developments are intertwined with the life and career of Gordon Richards, a man rightly called the father of Canadian radiotherapy.

THE CONTRIBUTIONS OF GORDON RICHARDS

Gordon Earle Richards was born in 1885 (the same year as the Northwest Rebellion) in the town of Lyn in eastern

Ontario. In 1908 he graduated in medicine from the University of Toronto and subsequently served as the medical officer of a mining camp in British Columbia. While in the west, his interest in x-rays was awakened by Dr CW Prowd of Vancouver. From 1914 to 1917 Richards served as a radiologist in the Royal Army Medical Corps. Even in this early period he showed a talent for innovation and published a method of making miniature prints of x-ray plates which could be used on the field of battle. On his discharge from the army he was appointed the first radiologist at the Toronto General Hospital. During the early part of his career he practiced both diagnostic and therapeutic radiology, but he soon focused on radiation therapy. As Dr WG Cosbie has said, "Once his feet were set in the way he should go, all his great energy and unflagging industry were concentrated in developing radiotherapy as a means of treating cancer."

In 1937 Richards founded the Canadian Association of Radiologists, and in 1945 he was appointed the first managing director of the Ontario Cancer and Treatment Research Foundation. He died in 1949 of aplastic anemia thought to have been induced by his lifetime exposure to ionizing radiation. His character was summed up by Dr William A Jones, who said, "he was a man to admire for his tremendous capacity for work and detail, his thoroughness and scientific intensity, and with it all, a warm kindness for his patients and a tolerant attitude to his medical confrères."

Richards made many contributions to the development of radiology and radiation oncology in Canada. First, he believed that radiation therapy should only be practiced by skilled and experienced individuals. His attitude is summarized in the following quotation:

> *It is vitally important that the profession should understand that the possession of an x-ray machine means neither more nor less than the possession of a piano, and that satisfactory results in the one case and music in the other are entirely dependent upon the skill, training and experience of the person operating it.*[7]

Largely through his efforts, radiology was recognized as a specialty in 1937 by the Royal College of Physicians and Surgeons of Canada. Richards chaired the first Royal College specialty committee in radiology.

Second, Richards had a large influence on the centralization of radiotherapy services in his own province, Ontario. In 1929 and 1930 Manitoba and Saskatchewan became the first provinces in Canada to recognize the need for special funding and support for the treatment of cancer. In response, the Ontario government established a royal commission to study the use of x-rays and radium

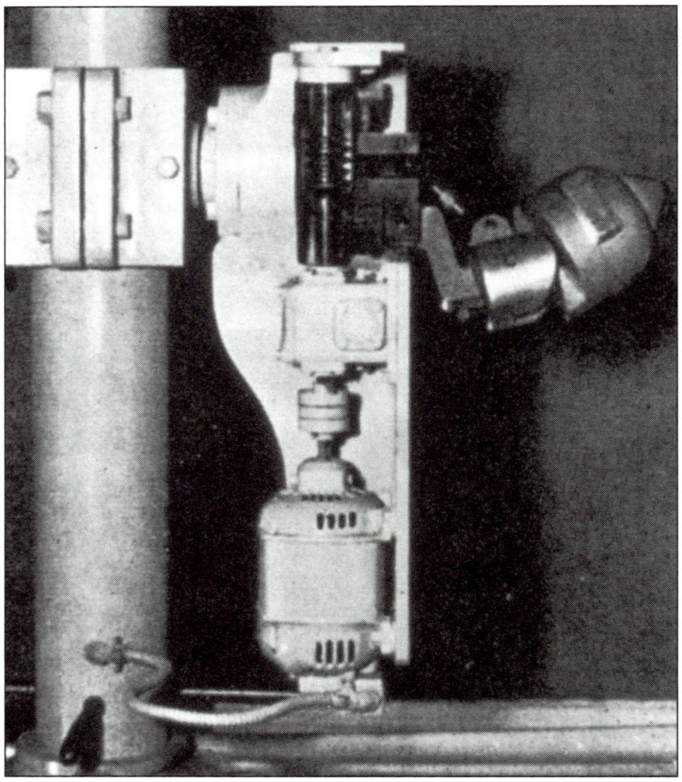

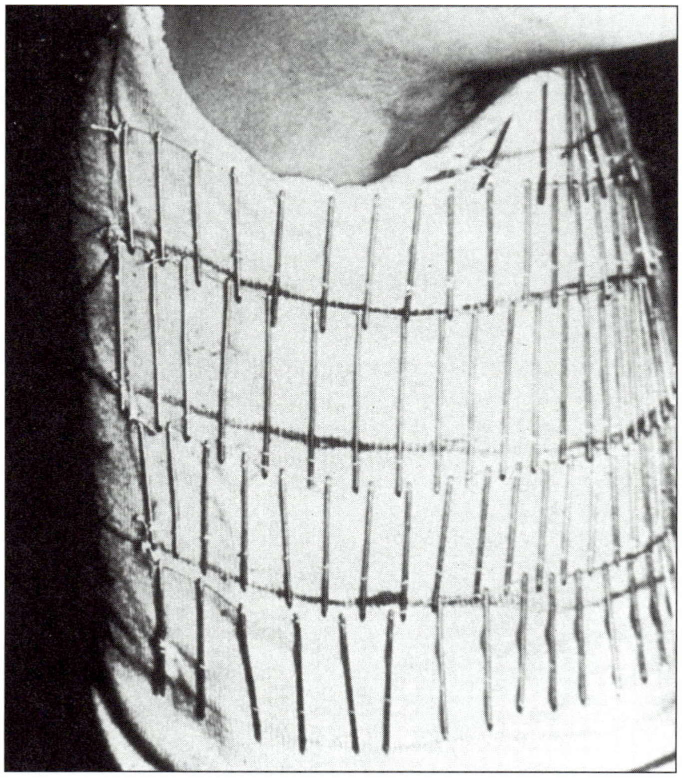

Top
Radium 'bomb'

Above
Radium jacket

in the treatment of the sick. The commission was chaired by Reverend Henry John Cody, president of the University of Toronto; its report, published in 1932, is a magnificent summary of the state of knowledge of cancer and its treatment in the early decades of this century. Although Richards did not sit on the commission, he prepared several briefs and authored most of its key ideas regarding radiation therapy. The report recommended establishing specific treatment centres in larger cities and led to the centralization of cancer services in Ontario and other provinces.

Richards collaborated with physicists, engineers and technicians to apply physical principles to clinical problems. With Picker Engineering, he developed a 400-kilovolt unit with two tubes arranged so that four patients could be treated at one time. The exposure of each of the four ports could be controlled independently. In 1935 he devised a rotational radium "bomb," used for external beam therapy of patients with head, neck or breast cancer. Perhaps his most ingenious contribution was the radium jacket, used for treatment of extensive chest wall recurrences of breast cancer. About a hundred 3 mg radium needles were sewn into pockets in a specially designed felt jacket.

Richards' permanent legacy was his analysis of the outcomes of radiation therapy. Although European investigators had published papers on the results of treatment, before Richards' time there had been no careful analysis of treatment in Canada. He introduced the principle of close follow-up of patients; as a result, he reported in 1936 in the *Canadian Medical Association Journal* the results of treatment of extensive series of patients with tonsillar, tongue, lip, oral cavity and cervix cancer. He reported, for example, a five-year crude survival rate of almost thirty per cent in cervix cancer.[8] These articles established the effectiveness of radiotherapy beyond doubt in Canadian medical literature.

One other significant contribution was Richards' interest in post-graduate training. In 1923 he set up the first training program in radiology at the Toronto General Hospital. Among his students were Dr Clifford Ash, who became the first director of the Ontario Cancer Institute,

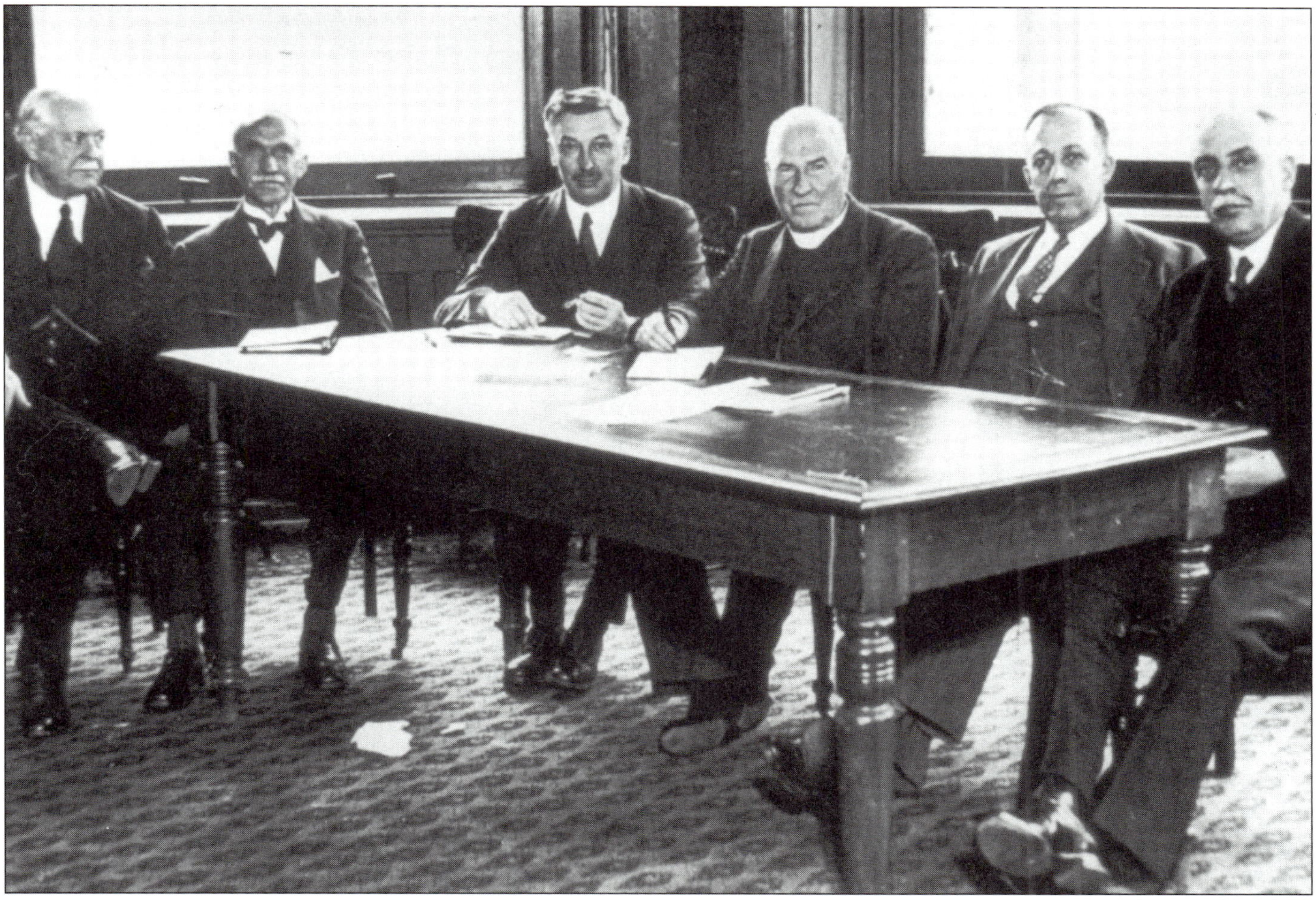

Royal Commission on the Use of Radium and X-Rays, Ontario 1931

Dr Allan Blair who became the director of cancer services in Saskatchewan, and Dr Vera Peters.

THE 1950S AND 1960S: THE FOUNDATIONS OF MODERN PRACTICE

By the end of Richards' lifetime, radiation therapy in Canada was on a firm footing. The new specialty began in earnest when the Royal College of Physicians and Surgeons of Canada carried out the first certification examinations in therapeutic radiology in 1946. By this time cancer treatment centres had been established in all provinces. Dr Allen Blair of Saskatchewan surveyed cancer services in Canada for the National Cancer Institute of Canada in 1947 and found fifty-five x-ray treatment centres and thirty-three radium treatment centres across the country.[9]

Therapeutic radiologists entered the 1950s on a surge of optimism generated by their new-found recognition, the government support of cancer centres, developments in technology which allowed safer and better treatment, and the results of treatment. As the only specialists devoted full-time to the care of patients with cancer, they often found themselves in important administrative positions. For example, Dr John Caskey, a radiation oncologist trained in Edinburgh, headed cancer services in New Brunswick from 1951 to 1977. When he arrived from Scotland, he was appalled to find four radiotherapy centres in a province of only six hundred thousand people and during his career he managed to centralize services in Saint John.

As the number of clinics and cancer incidence increased, the demand for therapeutic radiologists outstripped the supply, and in the 1950s and 1960s Canada imported many radiation oncologists from other countries, notably Britain.[4]

THE DEVELOPMENT OF TECHNOLOGY

Canada has made a substantial contribution to the technical foundations of the discipline of radiation oncology as we know it today. The major limitation of low-kilovoltage x-ray machines available in the early part of the century was the deleterious effect of low energy x-rays on normal skin and subcutaneous tissues before adequate doses could be delivered to underlying tumours. The need for higher energy x-ray machines which could deliver more radiation to tumours with less damage to intervening tissues was obvious. X-ray machines with energies of up to 400 kV were built, but the insulation required was very cumbersome.

Therapy units containing radium sources were designed but only achieved depth doses of the same order as 140-kV x-rays. Larger radium sources were not feasible because of the high cost of radium and because much of the radiation was absorbed by the radium itself.

Through the initiatives of Dr Harold Johns the first 25-MeV medical betatron was installed at the University of Saskatchewan in 1948, enabling the first concerted clinical investigation of multimegavoltage as a therapeutic tool. Depth-dose distributions show clearly the physical advantages of 22-MeV over 200-kV radiation. Both its skin-sparing effect and its high output made the betatron a practical tool for the treatment of deep-seated tumours.[11]

Around the same time it was recognized at Chalk River that artificial radioisotopes could revolutionize the treatment of cancer and that cobalt-60 could replace the radium bomb. In due course it became obvious that cobalt-60 would offer a more economical means of cancer therapy than the betatron which was very expensive to run.

Before 1928 radiation dosimetry was very crudely estimated by hair loss and skin erythema. In that year the röntgen (R) was accepted internationally as the unit of measure of ionization in air. The röntgen was superseded in 1956 by the rad (radiation absorbed dose).

In the 1950s computers in the form of analogue devices were developed to relieve the tedium of dosage calculation in radiation treatment planning as well as to improve accuracy. By 1955 automatic computing machinery produced radiation dose distributions and radiation beam characteristics. The next generation computer, the Programmed Console was designed with an adaptation for graphical input and output. Subsequently, Atomic Energy of Canada Ltd (AECL) has played an important part in the development of computer software for radiotherapy treatment planning.[12]

THE CONTRIBUTIONS OF THE PRINCESS MARGARET HOSPITAL

The Princess Margaret Hospital (PMH) in Toronto is a world-renowned radiation oncology centre. When it opened in 1958, the new hospital housed inpatient wards for the non-surgical treatment of cancer, outpatient facilities for treatment by radiotherapy and chemotherapy, and outpatient clinics for assessment and follow-up of patients. The top three floors of the seven-storey building were devoted to offices and laboratories for Ontario Cancer Institute (OCI) research scientists in medical biophysics and aspects of biological research. The proximity of cancer clinicians and scientists in one building allowed the cross-fertilization of ideas and projects and led to many original discoveries and concepts.

The hospital employed full-time medical staff in radiation and medical oncology, pathology and diagnostic radiology. Dr Clifford Ash, a trainee of Dr Gordon Richards,

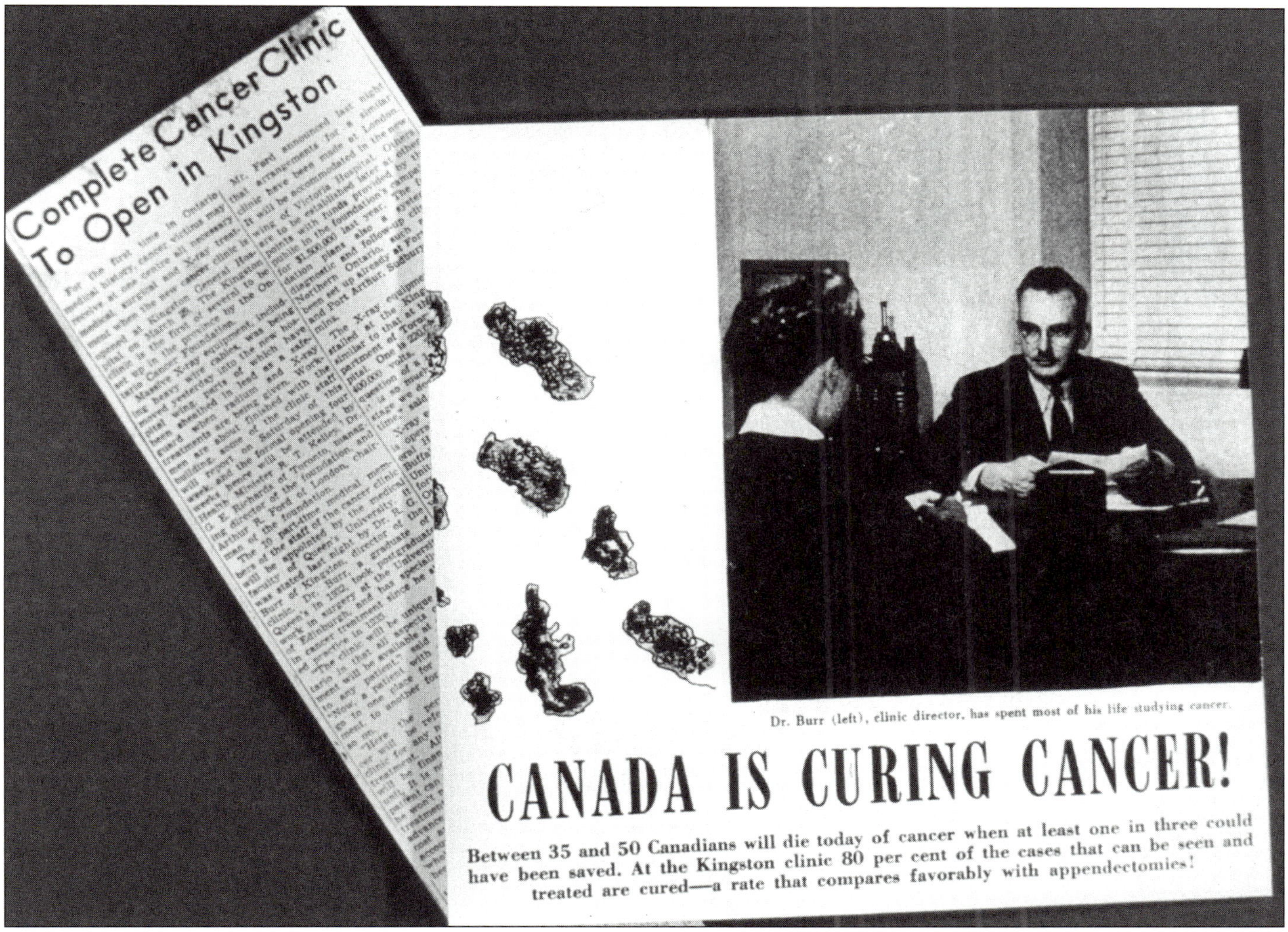

Complete Cancer Clinic To Open in Kingston

Dr. Burr (left), clinic director, has spent most of his life studying cancer.

CANADA IS CURING CANCER!

Between 35 and 50 Canadians will die today of cancer when at least one in three could have been saved. At the Kingston clinic 80 per cent of the cases that can be seen and treated are cured—a rate that compares favorably with appendectomies!

Newspaper article from the 1960s

was the first director of the new OCI/PMH complex. He gave the 1961 Janeway Lecture of the American Radium Society on Oral Cancer. Even at that time, he noted that the rapid increase in medical knowledge and the complexities of management of malignant disease would necessitate close cooperation between the various specialty groups. Consultants in other specialties, particularly the surgical disciplines, attended the clinics of the radiation and medical oncologists, eventually leading to the establishment of specific tumour-site groups, which collected data on both common and rare tumours. Subsequent analysis and reporting of large series of patients with different cancers helped to establish the reputation of the PMH/OCI as an international cancer centre. However, it was the conclusions reached from questions asked in prospective clinical trials that were to establish the PMH/OCI as a cancer research centre of excellence.

The knowledge gained through both success and failure in basic science and clinical care and the contributions they made to the understanding of cancer are outside the scope of this brief review. Information of the work of the PMH/OCI clinical and research activities can be found in the annual reports, together with references to specific work undertaken, presented and published. The following items provide some indication of the importance of careful record keeping and what can be achieved when physicians and scientists from different backgrounds collaborate to deal with specific issues.

In 1951 another of Richards' trainees, Dr Vera Peters, reported on work on Hodgkin's Disease[13] started by Richards. She showed for the first time that the disease was curable with radiation therapy. This certainty led to the first prospective randomized clinical trial on Hodgkin's Disease, which confirmed patterns of spread and defined optimum radiation fields and dose. This knowledge, together with advances in chemotherapy, means that the majority of patients with Hodgkin's Disease can now be cured. In 1975 Dr. Peters showed that localized breast cancer can be managed as effectively by lumpectomy plus radiation as by radical mastectomy.[14] Today, this conservative, less-mutilating treatment is standard management for many women with early breast cancer and provides a

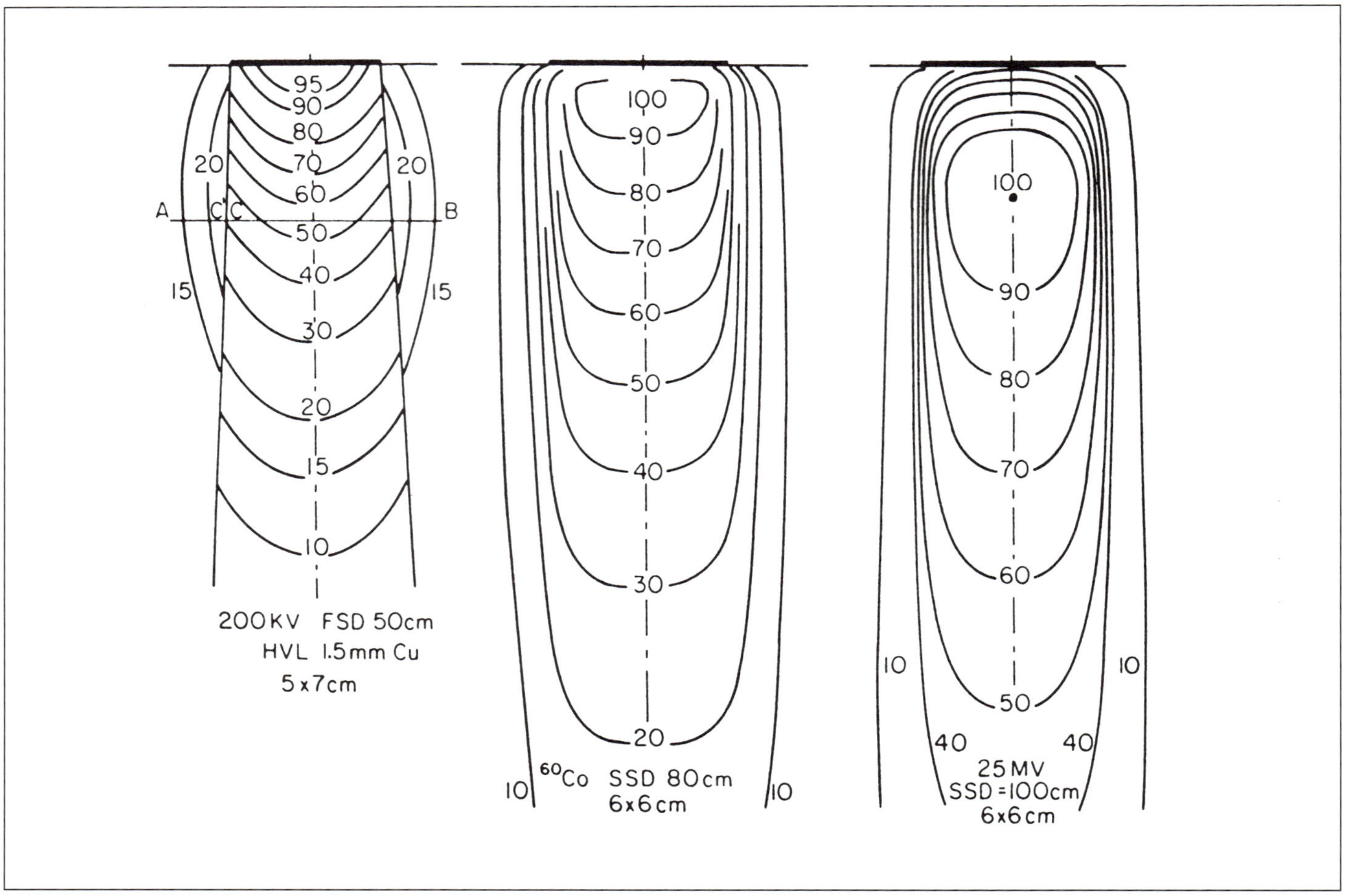

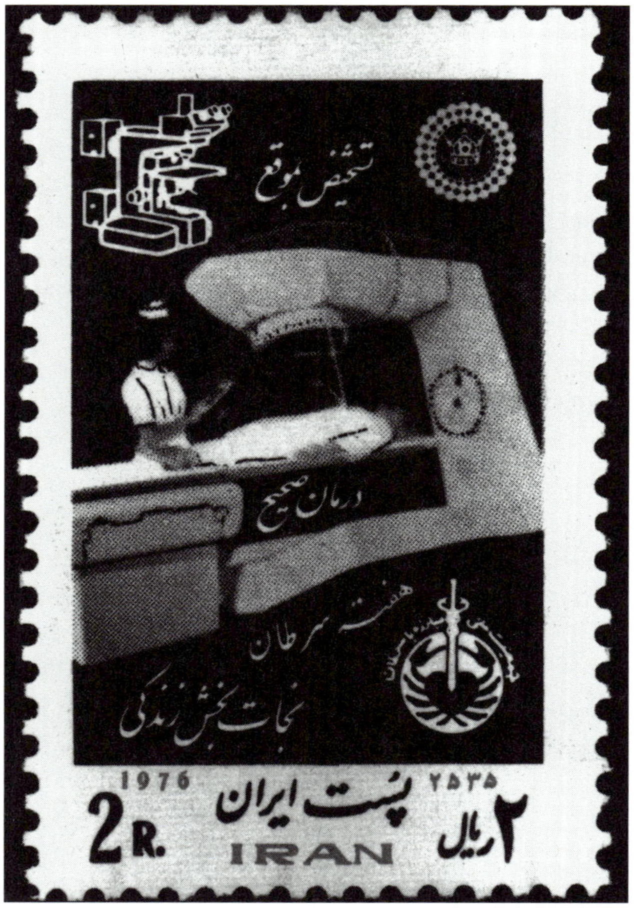

Above

Diagram from text by Dr Harold Johns demonstrating depth-dose curves.

Left

Stamp illustrating Cobalt-60 therapy machine, Iran 1976

much better quality of life.

In head and neck oncology the close cooperation between the university departments of otolaryngology and radiation oncology in the treatment of cancer of the larynx led to the policy of radical radiotherapy, with surgery reserved for salvage if the tumour was not controlled. For many years surgical excision had been the most certain way of controlling cancer of the larynx. A careful review carried out by Dr Douglas Bryce, professor of otolaryngology, and Dr Bill Rider identified two groups of patients whose treatments had produced the same results even though one group had received radical radiotherapy alone while the other group received radical radiotherapy followed by surgery. The advantage of radiotherapy alone was that the voice was preserved, and the quality of life significantly improved. This practice was extended to other tumour sites in the head and neck. From these experiences developed the philosophy of radical radiotherapy followed by observation, with salvage surgery performed only if the disease was not controlled.

Dr Rider also made significant contributions to the management of rectal cancer and noted that adenocarcinomas were much slower to respond to radiotherapy than squamous cell cancers. If the latter responded successfully to treatment, the majority disappeared in four to six weeks, whereas adenocarcinomas often only started to regress at three months. Sometimes regression would continue for over twelve months.

Dr Vera Peters

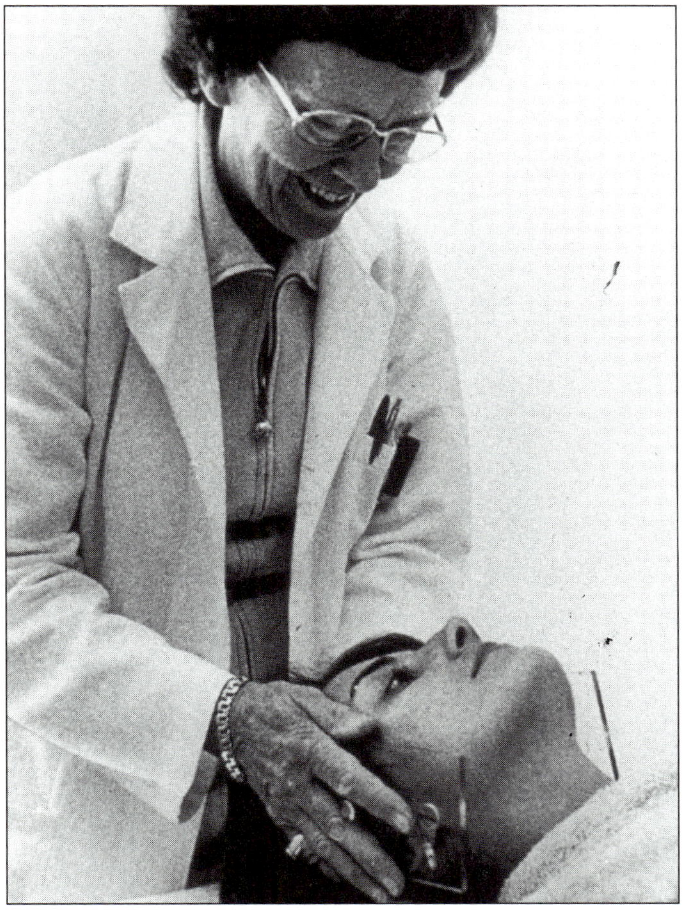

Dr Rider developed wide field radiation in an attempt to use radiotherapy as a systemic treatment for cancer. Total body irradiation found a place in the management of bone marrow transplants; half-body radiotherapy was used to palliate patients with multiple metastases. At the other end of the scale, radioactive plaques and small radiation beam techniques were developed to treat small tumours at the back of the eye while preserving the organ and vision.

Today, portal imaging and beam's-eye-view planning are state-of-the-art radiation technology. Over 30 years ago this technology was available at the PMH when a diagnostic unit was incorporated with a cobalt-60 source on a supervoltage machine called the X-otron. Its development resulted from a collaboration between the departments of medical physics and radiotherapy, but the concept is only just becoming state-of-the-art.

In the 1960s it was recognized that patients with carcinoma of the cervix treated on the betatron fared better than those on a cobalt-60 machine. Previously, patients had been treated on the first available machine. A review showed that cure rates improved and complications were fewer because of the better radiation distribution on the betatron. This betatron development was the combined work of the departments of clinical physics and radiotherapy; Dr Bill Allt played a major part in the analysis of the material.

In the 1960s fewer than 70 radiation oncologists were working in Canada. Many came from the United Kingdom, where Canadian-born radiation oncologists also received much of their training. The radiation oncology residency program under the direction of Dr John Simpson grew gradually, and today, most of the residents are Canadian born and trained.

The honours awarded to staff are numerous and are listed in the annual reports of the OCI/PMH. Of special significance, three staff researchers, Drs Peters, Rider and Johns, received the Astro Gold Medal, the highest award in radiation oncology in North America. No other hospital or institute has ever had three staff members earn this award. Drs Peters and Johns were also honoured as recipients of the Order of Canada.

1976: THE COMPLEAT ONCOLOGIST

Despite the accomplishments outlined above, by the early 1970s radiation oncology faced many struggles. It remained a small specialty, and its members often felt overwhelmed by the large size of its sister discipline, diagnostic radiology. In addition, the specialty often had to face an image problem. The trends to specialization and centralization had the disadvantage of making radiation therapy seem remote, isolated and esoteric. Other specialists often regarded radiation therapists as mere technicians. In response to these problems, in 1976 Dr George Goodman of Vancouver recommended that the name of the specialty change from "therapeutic radiology" to "radiation oncology," a term that reflected the broad interests of radiation oncologists in the general welfare of cancer patients. This emphasis on the clinical aspects of the specialty was reinforced by Dr Raymond Bush in 1982 when he created the concept of the "compleat oncologist." He defined the compleat oncologist as a clinician with competence in all three aspects of clinical practice: evaluation, treatment and long term care of patients with malignancy.[15]

The final stage in the evolution of radiation oncology in Canada was the creation of an independent specialty society, the Canadian Association of Radiation Oncologists (CARO). The story of its development is told in the accompanying papers by Drs Goodman and Jackson.[16,17]

Acknowledgements:
This chapter is based partly on material gathered for the joint CARO/Hannah Institute exhibit, "Controlling Cancer: The First Century of Radiation Oncology in Canada" which is travelling to medical schools across Canada between 1994 and 1997. The authors are grateful to Barbara Clow PhD, Jim Connor PhD, Felicity Pope, Gordon Catton MD, Alan Connor and Sheila Snelgrove for research assistance and support. Thanks to Sherry Mott for preparation of the manuscript.

Tube-holder and support for photographic plates

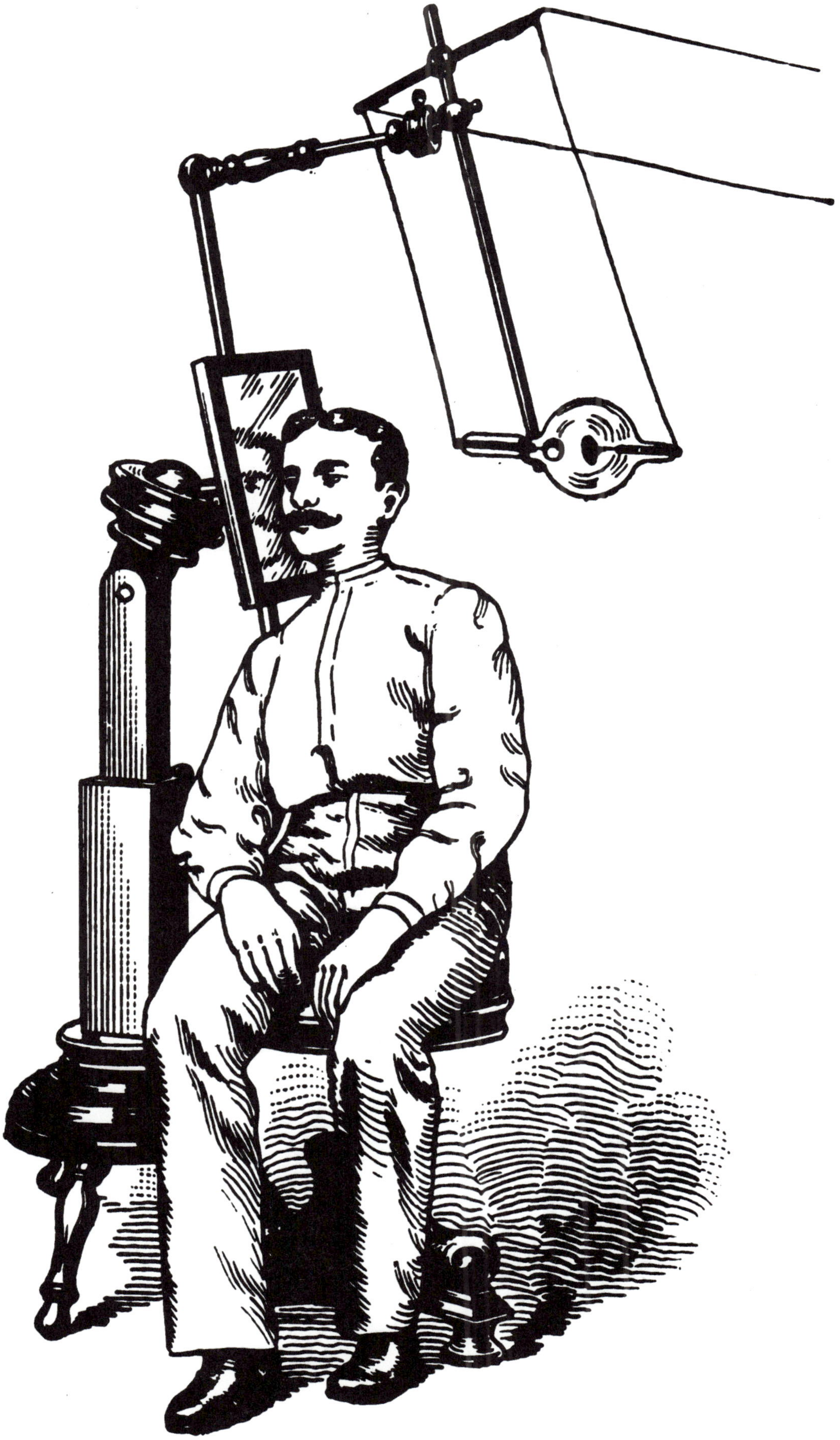

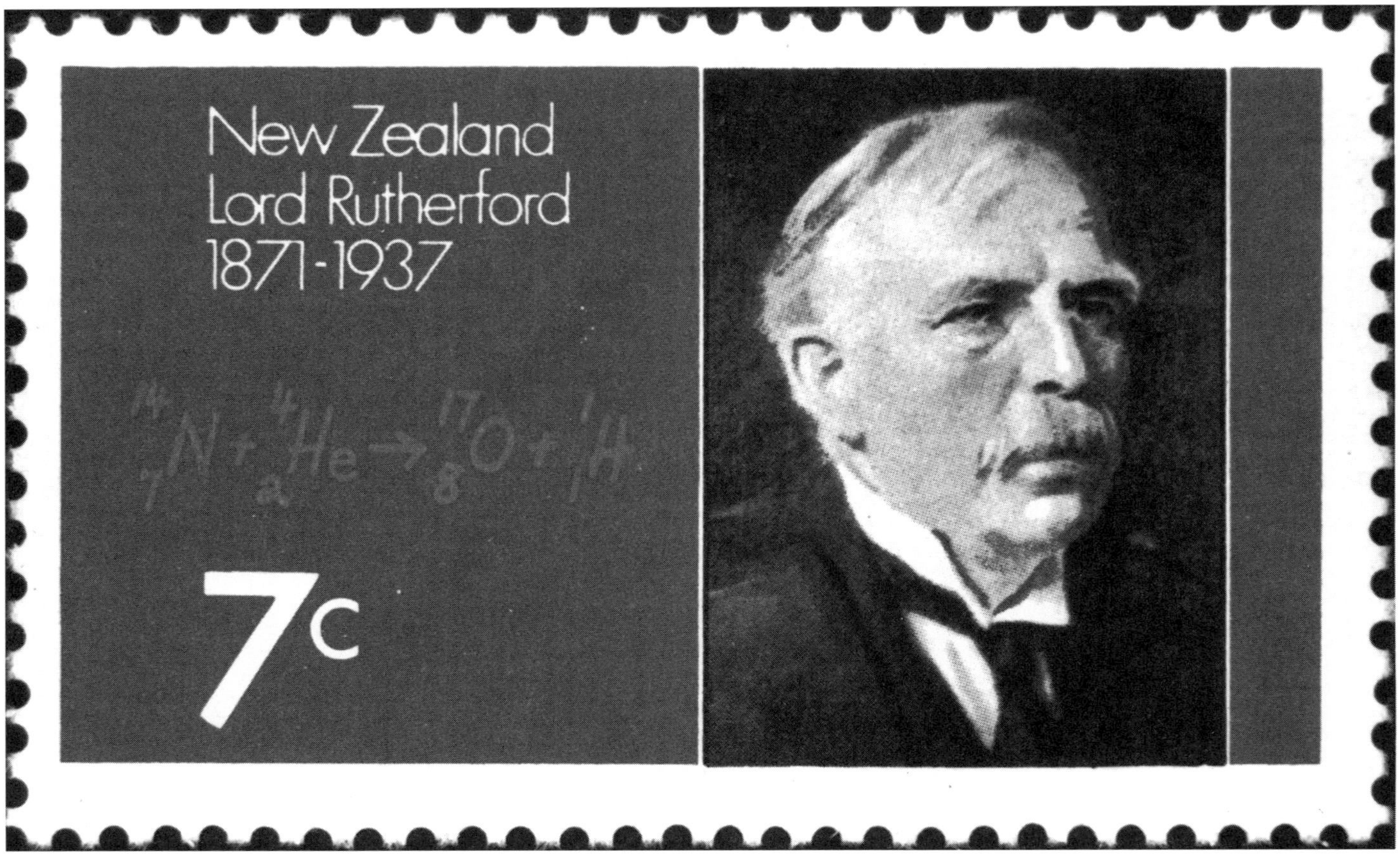
New Zealand
Lord Rutherford
1871-1937
7c

Chapter VII • *The Rutherford Legacy:*

Nuclear Medicine in Canada

BRIAN LENTLE

The very name of this, one of the youngest of the specialties, speaks of the twentieth century. Thus the early days of nuclear medicine are well documented[1,2] and do not reach back into a distant or mythic past, except that the specialty springs from the age-old concern of medicine for the human condition.

No single event, such as Röntgen's discovery of x-rays, can be seen as the birth of nuclear medicine. Donizetti has suggested that Rutherford's theory of the atom ultimately resulted in the specialty of nuclear medicine.[3] Certainly Becquerel's discovery of radioactivity was important.[4] However, the germinal idea, to which the development of nuclear medicine is most often attributed, is the tracer principle of Georg de Hevesy.[5] Working with a radioisotope of lead, and in plants, he proposed that a biological process might be followed by substituting a small amount of a radioactive atom for some of the more usual stable atoms of the same element.[6] A suitable radioactive atom, being detectable as such, would then serve as a marker of the biological process as a whole without perturbing it.

In medicine, iodine-131 was used initially to contribute to a greater understanding of thyroid physiology and disease. However, the impetus to an increase in the scale and scope of the applications of radioactive tracers in medicine was the development of nuclear technology during the Second World War. In particular, in reaction to those consequences which were terrible beyond telling, the atoms-for-peace initiatives (the first conference was held in Geneva in 1955) of the post-war period provided some of the radionuclides and, in embryo, the machines which were to serve as the infrastructure for the specialty.

In particular Anger's invention of the gamma or scintillation camera in 1951, replacing the rectilinear scanner developed by Cassen in 1949, provided a singular impetus in the development of the specialty.[7]
A number of far-sighted physicians in Canada, notably Étienne LeBel and Leonard Rosenthall in Montréal, realized that a gamma camera might enable them to image in a dynamic sense the distribution of radiotracers in patients. These images and the quantitative data they provided were seen as a way of achieving greater insight into disease and pathophysiological processes. As Judson has written in "The Search for Solutions": "[S]cience however pure is incurably dependent on techniques, methods, instruments: a large part of science is technology."[8]

Nuclear medicine is defined as the use of unsealed sources of radiation to diagnose and treat disease. This distinguishes it from other methods used to image disease and from radiation oncology. In these other specialties sealed sources of radiation are used: either machines or encapsulated radionuclides emitting radiation. However, nuclear medicine services usually work closely with other medical radiation sciences and share with them in the make-up of university departments of radiology or radiological sciences. Such departments are sometimes also called "imaging" departments although purists complain both that this is inaccurate and that imaging is not a noun.

While it may be invidious to single out individuals, the development of nuclear medicine in Canada has in no small way owed much to people such as Ms Brenda Clark and Trevor Cradduck. Ms Clark began the educational program for technologists at the British Columbia Institute of Technology. Dr Cradduck, a physicist, served as Secretary of the Society of Nuclear Medicine and became the first non-physician head of a university division of nuclear medicine at the University of Western Ontario. A little known story of what might have been concerns Dr William Paul, now Professor Emeritus of Biochemistry at the University of Toronto. Dr Paul had had education in physics and in 1949 he built a rectilinear scanner and used I-131 serum albumin to image brain tumors. He had previously used As-74 to diagnose brain lesions; this isotope of arsenic decays by positron (ß+) emission, which process was to become central to the technique of positron emission tomogaphy (PET). Dr Paul subsequently attempted to adapt early image intensifiers to detect gamma radiation (1954–1964), work that was only overtaken by the creation of the gamma camera by Hal O Anger in the United States.[8]

A particularly distinguished physicist in medical radiation science has been Ms Sylvia Fedoruk, later the Lieutenant Governor of Saskatchewan, who worked in radiation oncology and nuclear medicine in Saskatoon. Dr Cradduck, as a graduate student there, built the first Canadian "home-grown" gamma camera in 1963.

Dr Sylvia Fedoruk recollected these events in 1989, speaking to the annual meeting of the Canadian Nuclear Association:

> *[A] camera...was developed in Saskatoon by TD Cradduck as a PhD project and used an 11 inch by 0.5 inch thick crystal and 19 photomultiplier tubes. The camera enabled us to study resolution and sensitivity of scintillation cameras and reports of our work received international attention. It also enabled us to learn at first hand the horrors that can occur when a sodium iodide crystal is exposed to a sudden change in temperature during our cold Saskatchewan winters. Today equipment in Saskatoon is located in imaging rooms that have no windows which can be left open during the night.*
>
> *Dr WB (Bill) Reid a dear friend and colleague...as a graduate student along with Dr W Feindel and Dr HE Johns developed a unique brain scanning device. It was a departure from the rectilinear [scanning] approach and had two detectors that scanned the contour of the head in search of brain tumours. The head was scanned in nine arcs...*
>
> *There were only three of these units built and these were used successfully for about 15 years in Saskatoon, the Montreal Neurological Institute and the Princess Margaret Hospital in Toronto. This machine was ahead of its time and never received much international attention. I often wonder what might have happened if microprocessor technology had been available in 1956 when the unit was first put into use. Today the microprocessor is a vital component in camera imaging...*[9]

The first positron emission tomographic detector in Canada was built by Claude Nahmias at McMaster University where a program directed by the late Dr Steve Garnett went on to make important contributions to receptor site imaging in the brain. This group obtained the first images of receptor sites in the basal ganglia of the brain.

There are now PET research programs at the Montréal Neurological Institute and the University of British Columbia (supported in part by the Tri-University Meson Facility or TRIUMF on the UBC campus). A further program has been created more recently at the Clarke Institute in Toronto.

The gamma camera with its ability to image rapidly changing distributions of radiotracer has brought the *in vivo* applications of nuclear medicine to their present maturity and future promise.

Many centres in Canada have served to teach not only Canadian graduates but visitors who, for a week, a month, a year or longer, sought to expand their clinical or scientific horizons. Drs Leonard Rosenthall, Étienne LeBel, Raymonde Chartrand, David Gilday, Al Driedger and others have served as ambassadors of Canadian nuclear medicine in teaching and consulting internationally. Dr Gilday, the chief of nuclear medicine at the Toronto Sick Children's Hospital has been a leader and pioneer in computer applications in nuclear medicine and internationally in the emergence of the discipline of pediatric nuclear medicine (a fact recognized among other ways in an honorary doctorate from the University of Mainz in Germany).

For a small group of clinicians, basic and clinical scientists, the record of nuclear medicine in Canada has been one of promise.

Ultimately, the power of the tracer concept will define the future of nuclear medicine. However, the anomalous position of nuclear medicine in health care in Canada in being regulated federally whereas health care in general is a provincial matter constitutes an anomaly. In the 1990s successive attempts to ensure cost recovery for regulatory activities, first by the Atomic Energy Control Board and then by the Health Protection Branch of Health Canada, have threatened the cost-effectiveness of nuclear medicine. The measures proposed have gone beyond simple cost recovery, and they have become a potential indirect taxation and a unilateral means of altering the balance of federal and provincial health care funding. Such issues are likely to be a microcosm of those to be addressed by the health care industry in the foreseeable future.

Acknowledgements:

I am indebted to Jean Lentle for preparing the manuscript. This text has been slightly modified and enlarged from its earlier publication.[10] It is used with the permission of the Royal College of Physicians and Surgeons.

Chapter VIII • # La Médecine Nucléaire au Québec

Étienne LeBel

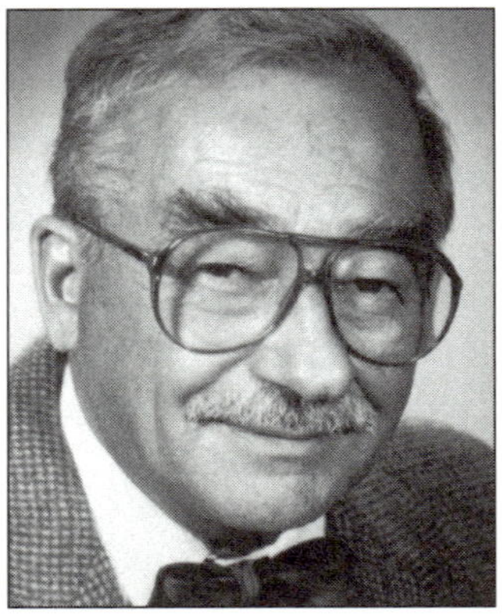

Dr Etienne LeBel

L'évolution de la médecine nucléaire au Québec a été très différente du reste du Canada, non pas à cause du fait français mais à cause d'un contexte social, économique et politique particulier, au début des années 1960. Appelée par l'Histoire la Révolution tranquille, cette période favorisa l'innovation.

Le groupe médical québécois responsable de l'utilisation des radio-isotopes s'est détaché précocement de la tendance générale qui existait à cette époque au Canada pour former un mouvement devant amener la création de la spécialité de médecine nucléaire. L'Association des radiologistes du Québec créa un comité des radio-isotopes présidé tour à tour par les Drs Jacques Lamoureux et Étienne LeBel. En 1967, ce comité déposa un rapport favorisant la création de cette spécialité, qui fut froidement reçu initialement.

Après plusieurs hésitations, le rapport fut soumis au Collège des médecins et chirurgiens de la province de Québec, qui étudia à son tour la possibilité de créer la spécialité de médecine nucléaire au Québec. Le rapport étant accepté, le Collège des médecins et chirurgiens du Québec créa en 1969, une première mondiale, la spécialité de médecine nucléaire, spécialité à part entière exigeant une formation de 4 années de résidence sanctionnée par un examen. Suite à cette création, le collège agréa trois programmes d'enseignement post-doctoral en médecine nucléaire, une autre première, aux universités de Montréal, McGill et Sherbrooke. Quinze médecins radiologistes, internistes et autres ayant une formation adéquate reçurent un certificat de spécialiste. Les autres durent se soumettre à un examen. Les pionniers de cette époque furent les Drs

Jacques Lamoureux, Étienne LeBel, Jacques Plamondon, René Robillard, et Léonard Rosenthal.

La même année, la faculté de médecine de l'Université de Sherbrooke créait sous l'influence du Dr Étienne LeBel, le premier département universitaire de médecine nucléaire et de radiobiologie avec l'objectif d'améliorer la pratique clinique, la recherche et l'en-seignement, département qu'il dirigea jusqu'en 1985. Ce département offre aujourd'hui en plus d'un programme de formation en médecine nucléaire un programme de doctorat en radiobiologie, grâce à une équipe de recherche nationalement reconnue en sciences des radiations, (groupe du Conseil des recherches médicales du Canada), unique au pays dans ce domaine.

Avec l'avènement de cette nouvelle spécialité, le Ministère de l'Education autorisa la création de 4 programmes de formation en Techniques de médecine nucléaire au Québec, qui par la suite fut réduit à un seul à Montréal, recevant 59 étudiants(es) en 1990.

La médecine nucléaire connut donc un essor assez important et l'ensemble des membres de cette spécialité, convaincu des rôles qu'il avait à jouer dans la distribution des services de santé, décida, dans un deuxième temps, de créer l'Association des médecins spécialistes de médecine nucléaire du Québec. Cette association fut donc créée en 1975 et le Dr Étienne LeBel en fut le premier président. Cette association devint membre à part entière de la Fédération des médecins spécialistes du Québec.

Lorsque le Collège royal des médecins et chirurgiens du Canada décida de créer en 1976 la spécialité de médecine nucléaire, les médecins québécois ne purent que se réjouir de cette décision. Pour beaucoup d'entre eux, cette décision arrivait vraiment très tard et eut peu d'impact au Québec.

De 1976 à nos jours, la médecine nucléaire au niveau provincial a connu un développement cyclique avec des hauts et des bas. Du point de vue international dans le monde de la francophonie, elle s'est taillé une place de chef de file. Le Québec a été l'hôte en 1978 du XIXe Colloque de médecine nucléaire de langue française, tenu pour la première fois hors de l'Europe, et en 1990 l'hôte du XXIXe Colloque, une manifestation qui regroupe tous les scientifiques et cliniciens de langue française du monde entier. Ces deux manifestations internationales ont été organisées par l'Association des médecins spécialistes de médecine nucléaire du Québec, présidées en 1978 par le Dr Étienne LeBel et en 1990 par le Dr Jean Léveillé. Il ne faudrait pas oublier le 5e Congrès mondial de biologie et de médecine nucléaire, tenu à Montréal en août 1990, qui fut, grâce à l'Association canadienne de médecine nucléaire et de ses membres, dont fait partie un bon nombre de Québécois, un succès sans précédent, laissant aux invités un souvenir mémorable.

Grâce aux efforts de l'Association des médecins spécialistes de médecine nucléaire du Québec, la population québécoise a accès à cette discipline dans plus de 50 services assurés par 66 spécialistes certifiés. Des services cliniques bien équipés permettent de former une vingtaine de jeunes médecins.

A travers ce bilan très positif, comparé au reste de l'Amérique du Nord, il demeure quand même des lacunes très importantes. On note au point de vue professionnel, l'absence de radiopharmaciens dans les grands services universitaires, et au point de vue matériel, l'absence presque totale de cyclotrons et d'unités de positrons autour desquels on peut regrouper les chercheurs. Seul l'Institut neurologique de Montréal bénéficie de ces resources.

Après plus de 20 ans, la médecine nucléaire québécoise a dépassé l'adolescence. Son évolution aura sûrement marqué le reste du Canada.

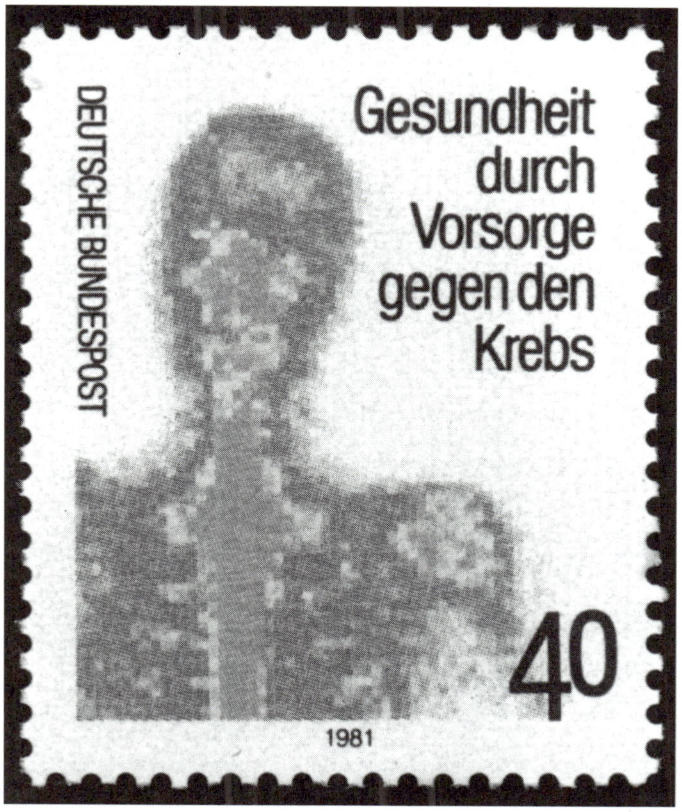

A German stamp illustrating a technetium-99m phosphate bone scan.

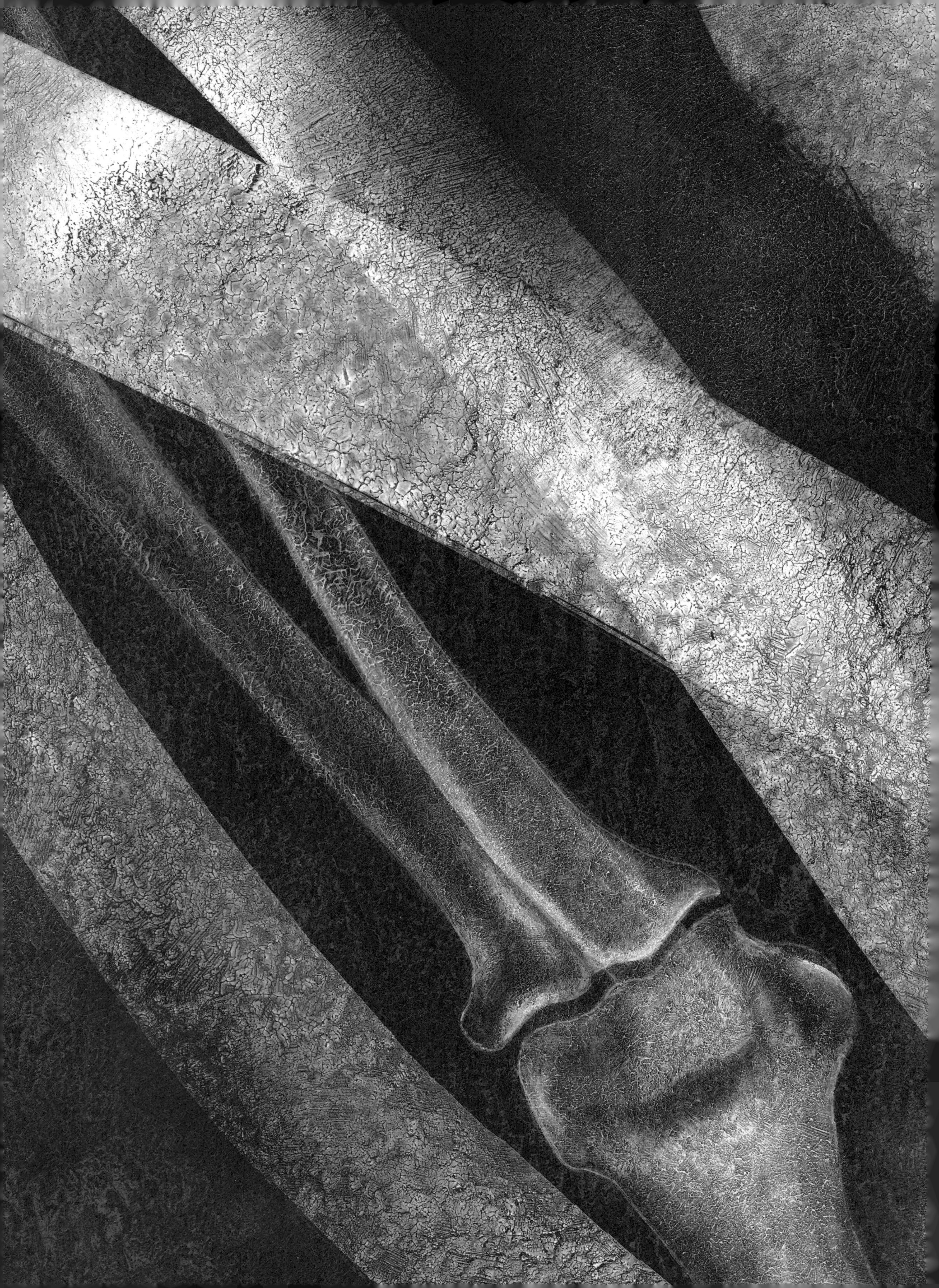

Part Three

Progress by Province

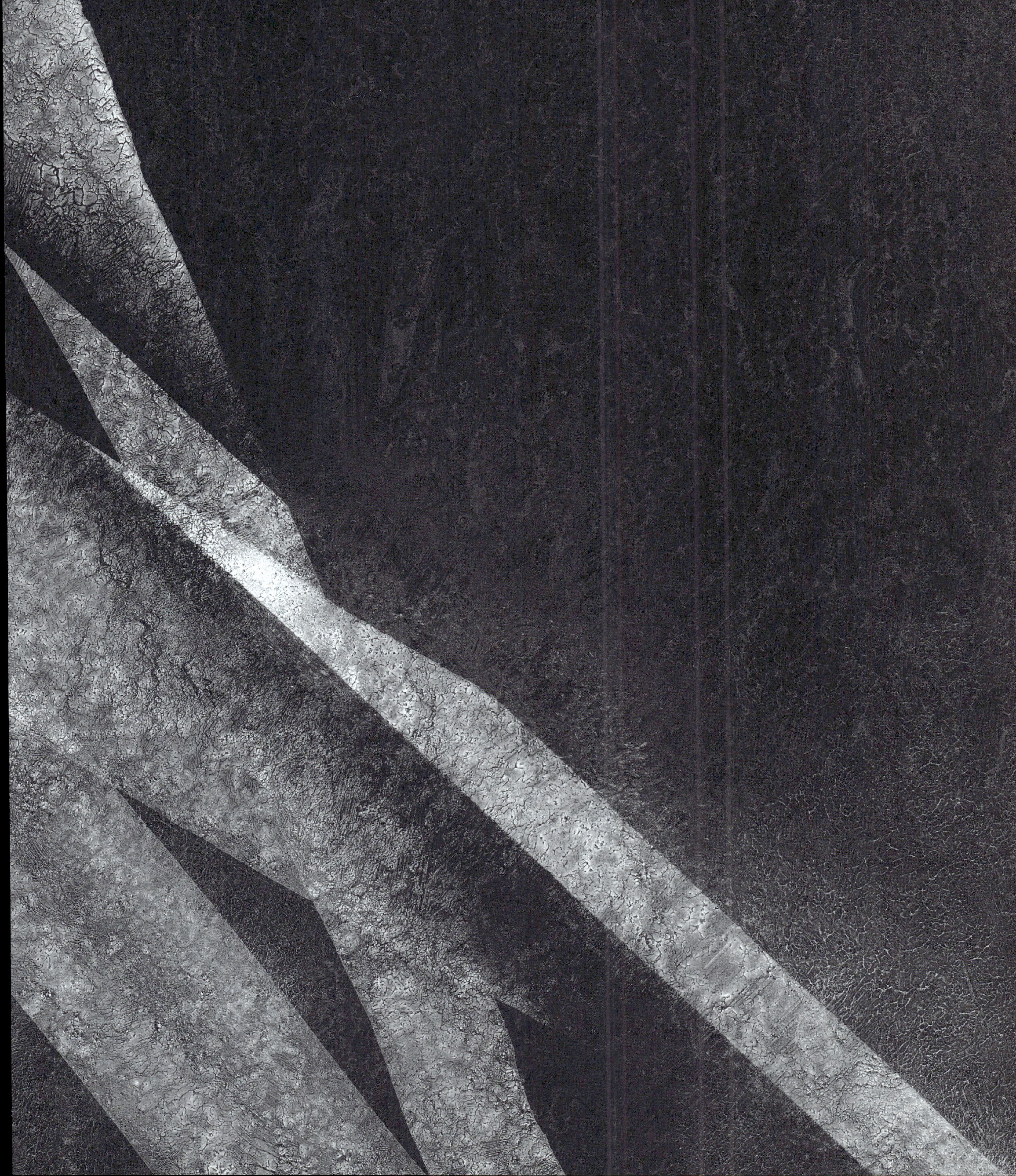

[I]f some countries have too much history, we have too much geography.
— William Lyon Mackenzie King

X-rays were introduced into medical practice across Canada and worldwide with a speed which is unthinkable in modern times. We now recognize more fully the need to assess a technology as it moves from being a tool under investigation to one in clinical use. Indeed, it is now considered proper to ask about not only the efficacy of a new technology but also about its cost effectiveness.

After Röntgen's first scientific report *Die Presse*, Vienna's leading daily paper published news of his discovery on Sunday January 5, 1896. This happened because the editor happened to have a son who was a physicist and who had seen some of Röntgen's x-ray photographs at a dinner party given by Franz Exner, then the professor of physics in Vienna. He had been sent Röntgen's paper to review.[1] This report in Die Presse was followed only a day later by news of this "sensational discovery" in the *Daily Chronicle* of London, England. It is likely that this report was derivative as both mis-spelled Röntgen's name as "Routgen."[1] The news reached the Toronto newspapers first in Canada on January 30, 1896.

Röntgen's discovery was not made because he had access to any unique technology. The tools he used could be found then in any reputable university physics laboratory around the world. Indeed, several scientists subsequently realized to their chagrin that inexplicably fogged film in their laboratory or an unrecognized, fleeting observation of fluorescence might have alerted them to the existence of these "new rays." In reality, Röntgen first made the connection which eluded others and proceeded to establish much of what, even now, we know about x-rays. To describe that discovery as serendipitous does nothing to detract from the genius of Röntgen.[2,3]

Since the tools to generate x-rays were at hand worldwide, there rapidly resulted, in many centres, collaborations between physicists and physicians to use this new diagnostic method. Such collaborations still characterize much superior radiological practice and research. Thus, radiography became the harbinger of "high-tech" medicine. Inevitably, the infrastructure provided by industry was important to the growth and development of radiology, as documented somewhat idiosyncratically by Blume,[3] who believes the evolution of radiology to be in some ways a conspiracy between radiologists and industry. His view ignores the reality of the physical universe, which ultimately constrains what is and is not possible in imaging disease.

X-rays excited not only physicians and other scientists; the media response in that era indicates that x-rays were not only of immense interest to the general public but that they also took on metaphorical dimensions. Certainly, the public rapidly made the connection between seeing through tissues and the potential role of x-rays in medicine. Indeed in that Victorian context there was an interest in seeing not just through tissues but also through clothing. That interest can only be described, from the cartoons that come down to us, as largely prurient.

— Brian Lentle

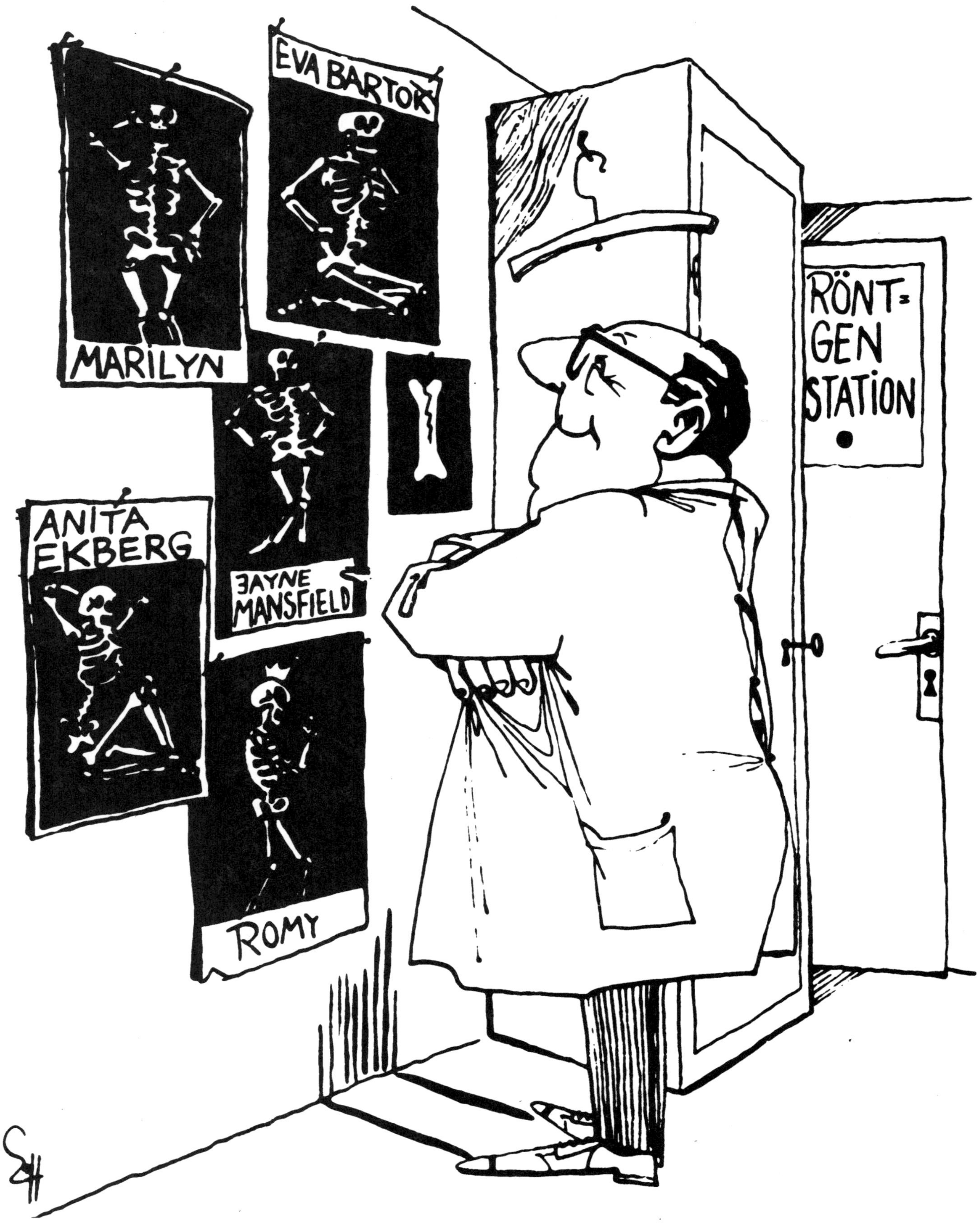
MARILYN
EVA BARTOK
JAYNE MANSFIELD
ANITA EKBERG
ROMY
RÖNT-GEN STATION

Chapter I • Public Perception:

X-rays as Metaphor

Brian Lentle

Where there is much light,
there is also much shadow...
—WC Röntgen
(April 1922)

To read nearly a century later the media responses to the discovery of x-rays makes it clear that Röntgen's work had ramifications beyond the obvious clinical ones. The scientific interest in x-rays was matched or exceeded by the fascination they held for the public. To understand this interest we must leave behind the prejudices of the late 20th century and reflect on the society into which x-rays were announced. Radio had just been invented by Marconi and, with electricity and other modern inventions, seemed to indicate a boundless future of technological promise.

In Britain and Canada, Queen Victoria was in the late years of her reign (1860–1907). It was the high noon of imperialism, and the idea of empire was everywhere prevalent. In Canada the Queen's influence is evident in clues as diverse as the names of an anglophone national holiday and of the capital of British Columbia. Meanwhile, Elgar and Mahler were providing very different but convergent musical visions at the close of the Romantic Period, but with a hint of the neuroticism later to characterize some 20th century music. However, such rumblings had yet to invade the Victorian sense of order, as illusory as it was.

Joseph Conrad had by 1895 only published three books, beginning with *Almayer's Folly,* and his major works lay ahead. These were to include a bleak, ironic and damaging view of imperialism in the novella *Heart of Darkness,* published in a book entitled *Youth.*[1] The Victorian notion of empire was inseparable from, and indeed built upon, a racist view of the world. In turn, Victorian society was deeply class conscious.[2] This latter sense spilled over into Canada.

Left
From the Montréal _Monitor_ published by Philips on the occasion of the 10th International Congress of Radiology, Montréal, August 1962

Tannahill has noted that the peculiar mixture of sexual repression, perversion and commercial sex that we associate with the Victorian era was in no way confined to Britain but was worldwide.[3]

Scientifically the world seemed a tidy place in the early 1890s. Atoms were perceived as tiny and indestructible spheres and the insights of modern physics were only to begin with the discovery of x-rays. A professor of physics of that era is even reputed to have told his students not to become physicists since physics was "over." That scientific sense of an imposed order unrelated to reality perhaps matched the moral environment.

It was into such a world that the discovery of x-rays was announced and rapidly disseminated by newspapers, themselves a relatively new manifestation of technological promise. The different aspects of the public perceptions surrounding the discovery of x-rays can be categorized as follows:

(a) an immediate insight by the public into the potential for x-rays to change the practice of medicine;
(b) an acceptance of x-rays as another aspect of technological mastery which was expected to relieve the human condition. (It was only later that discoveries in physics were to threaten the Victorian sense of solidity and order);
(c) a prurient interest in the fact that these new rays might be used to see through materials, particularly clothing.

Another social consequence of Röntgen's discovery was that hospitals needed to deal with a new influence: that of coping with and funding high-technology medicine, of which the use of x-rays in caring for the sick was the first instance. This aspect of Röntgen's discovery is analyzed here by Connor.[4] In addition there was a uniquely Canadian dimension to the societal response to x-rays, as pointed out by Gingras.[5]

To Victorian sensibilities the ability of x-rays to "see through" the voluminous and confining clothing of that era seems to have been important. That society, certainly in its upper classes, set great store on decency and propriety. X-rays as a means of invading privacy were the subject of many cartoons and much comment in the popular press, as illustrated in this volume and described here by Connor.[4] If the apparel of a well-to-do Victorian, which seems to us today to have been used to deny the reality of flesh and blood, could be made transparent by the use of x-rays, this may have been the first intimation of what we now consider to be the sexual revolution of the 20th century. Thus the established social order and public morality was under technological "threat." Certainly, the great public interest in x-rays in the early years of this century appears to have been not a little prurient. Jack made the following observation but appears to have been less persuaded that the public interest derived from Victorian sexual repression:

> *The public, though, were quick enough to seize on what they thought were certain other possibilities. They had read in the newspapers that [x]-rays could penetrate clothing. Thinking that the invisible ray would reveal the human form in all its naked inglory, that the device was a kind of electronic peeping tom, they raised an outcry against this invasion of Victorian decency. According to Harvey Graham, 'A London firm rose to the occasion, and made a small fortune from the sale of [x]-ray proof underwear,' and in New York there was an attempt to legislate against the use of x-rays in opera glasses.*[6]

Thus, this aspect of the "new kind of ray" was also not lost on entrepreneurs. They were quick to offer for sale underclothing which supposedly afforded protection for affluent and delicate Victorian womanhood against this radiological invasion of privacy.

Moreover, the early interest of certain physicians in using x-rays may have owed something not only to the fact that this was the first time much of the inside of the body was accessible without major surgery, but also that physical examination was impeded by prudery in the Victorian era. Examinations of women—and in that sexist era almost all physicians were men—were then done "under a sheet in a darkened room."[7] As Tannahill notes, these concessions to feminine modesty might lead to a modern physician losing his licence to practice.[7] Nevertheless, these cultural factors may have influenced the reception of the discovery of x-rays by physicians and the public alike, over and above the compelling nature of the technology itself.

Historical accounts such as those in this volume inevitably focus on the far-sighted physicians who were quick to perceive the potential power of x-rays in clinical practice. However, most were not able to make such a rapid connection. Jack contrasts the speedy public interest, albeit somewhat prurient, with the conservative response by the majority of physicians:

> *As has happened so often in the past, the medical profession was slow to grasp the revolutionary advances in diagnosis that the [x]-ray made possible.*[6]

There was, therefore, a selection process at work to ensure that early radiologists were often those physicians with an interest in innovation and with a futuristic bent.

The discovery of x-rays, perhaps with the discovery of radium by the Curies, was in many respects the first of the

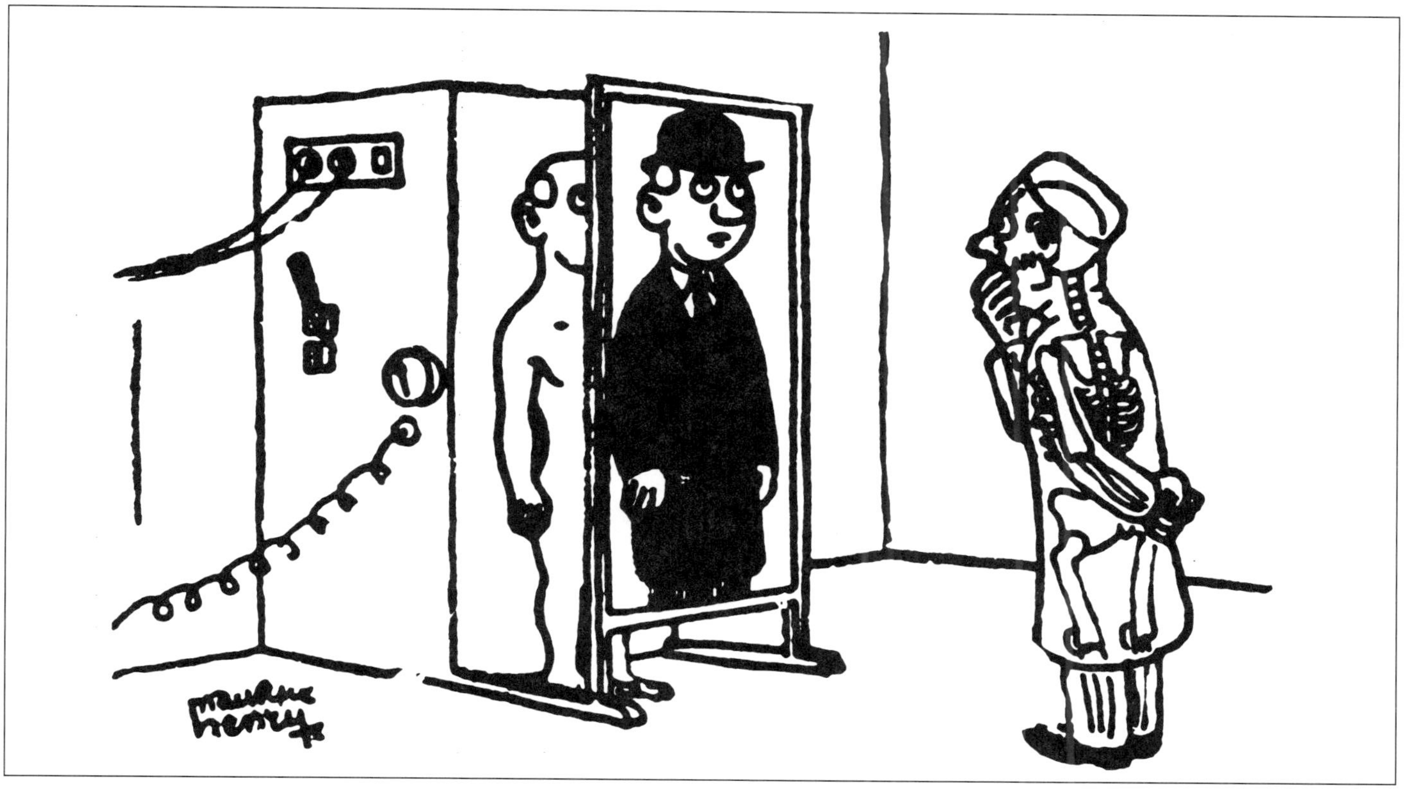

great insights of late 19th and early 20th century physics which together radically changed our world view. At the same time these were, perhaps, the last to be readily understood in the popular imagination. X-rays, if not tangible, could at least be seen by virtue of their effects on photographic film.

Radioactivity, Einstein's theory of relativity, quantum mechanics, the uncertainty principle, the "big bang" and the many-worlds theory—among later insights—were not only increasingly obscure but counterintuitive. On the publication of Einstein's theory it was reputedly said (about a decade after Röntgen's discovery) that "only two people understand relativity, God and Einstein, and God isn't too sure about it." This same sense gave rise to the (appropriately) anonymous American limerick current in the Twenties:[8]

I don't like the family Stein!
There is Gert, there is Ep, there is Ein,
Gert's writings are punk,
Ep's statues are junk,
Nor can anyone understand Ein.

Moreover, science and technology were then still perceived as embodying endless promise for the future. Electricity, radio and telephones were already changing forever people's expectatations, as well as their perception of the world and their place in it. It was to be nearly a century later that the Challenger disaster, Bhopal, Chernobyl and the ozone hole, among many comparable events and findings, made people realize the limits to technology as the potential solution to any problem. In addition there developed a scepticism about the Madison Avenue hype that came to surround technological enterprises. As Richard Feynman was to write in reporting the enquiry into the Challenger disaster, "For a successful technology, reality must take precedence over public relations, for Nature cannot be fooled."[9]

In the years following the discovery of x-rays the optimism that characterised the public response to them came to be replaced by doubt and scepticism about subsequent developments in physics. Einstein's space–time continuum was not only deeply counter-intuitive, but it changed the place which reflective people saw for themselves in the universe. Indeed, Baumer quotes Eddington in proposing that Rutherford's Canadian work had been even more subversive in changing the world view:

If anything, the concept of matter was more thoroughly "bolshevized" than were the concepts of space and time. This, at any rate, was what Sir Arthur Eddington thought as, in the Gifford Lectures of 1927, he surveyed the wreckage of classical physics. Lord Rutherford, he said, not Einstein, was "the real villain of the piece." Eddington's specific reference was to Rutherford's work on the structure of the atom, but he was also thinking generally of the whole new conception of "the atom of action.[10]

When we compare the universe as it is now supposed to be with the universe as we had ordinarily preconceived it, the most arresting change is not the rearrangement of space and time by Einstein but the dissolution of all that we regard as most solid into tiny specks floating in void.[11]

But x-rays were born into a world uninfected with such scepticism. Moreover, their immediate relevance to the human condition was readily grasped. Physicians were able to "see" bones and hence more readily diagnose and set fractures, for example. Thus, the acquisition of radiological equipment by hospitals became a status symbol in the hierarchy of institutions. This aspect of the radiological revolution is analyzed here by Connor.[4] It was to be the financial pressures of the end of the 20th century that finally prompted nearby hospitals to rationalize or merge their services rather than compete. Before that reorganization, competition and the aggressive promotion of image were the rule despite the lack, in Canada, of any fiscal incentive for providing service to more people. For hospitals, image was often indissolubly and not unreasonably linked to what was the latest and best of its radiological and other technological equipment.

The usefulness of x-rays as a metaphor has not entirely ceased. As recently as October 1994 *The Globe and Mail* used as its aphorism for the day the following instruction: "If you really want to get in touch with your inner self, have an x-ray."[12]

A uniquely Canadian aspect to the introduction of x-rays into the public conciousness derives from the insidious implications of empire and class, as well as the historic tensions between the English and French peoples who came to populate this land alongside its first nations. This theme is developed by Gingras.[5] The first experiments with x-rays took place in the province of Québec, and specifically Montréal, and their use took on particular social overtones there well before the quiet revolution.[13] Gingras suggests that the introduction of x-rays into Québec mirrored that province's social structure. He contrasts the experimental approach at the anglophone McGill University, where Cox was available and where Rutherford was to work, with the approach in francophone Canada. The French-speaking universities in Québec had a strong tradition of pedagogy but at that time little tradition of knowledge generation and research. Gingras makes the elegant distinction, *en français*, between knowledge *production* and knowledge *reproduction*. If that social distinction was true at the turn of the century it was to be rapidly reversed by the innovations pioneered by the Québec school of radiologists, chiefly at l'Hôtel-Dieu and l'Hôpital Jean Talon. Included in that school were such innovators as its leader Dr Albert Jutras, along with Dr Paul Roy and Dr Guy Duckett among others.[14]

The use of x-rays in medicine has also come to be symbolic, and much of that symbolism must have to do with the perceived power of technology. It is surprising how often physicians who have no idea how an x-ray film or scan is produced and who may be uncertain about which way up it should be viewed, will choose to be photographed against the dramatic back-drop of back-lit scans or radiographs.

The term x-ray is often used by physicians and patients alike to mean the films or radiographs produced by an x-ray exposure. It is usual to refer to a "chest x-ray," but almost never to a chest radiograph which is the pedantically correct description. Patients themselves may then have an ambiguous relationship with this radiograph and may ask "What is the matter with the x-ray?" or "What does the x-ray show?" instead of "What is the matter with me?" Perhaps this is a way of distancing oneself from potential bad news—it is the x-ray which is abnormal not the person. Using humour to heighten this ambiguity Joey Bishop observed in jest: "My doctor is wonderful. Once in 1955, when I couldn't afford an operation, he touched up the x-rays."[15]

X-rays may be intrinsically invisible. Nevertheless, their introduction seems to have provided as penetrating a commentary on the social fabric of *fin de siècle* Canada as their clinical use offered a penetrating view of the skeleton.

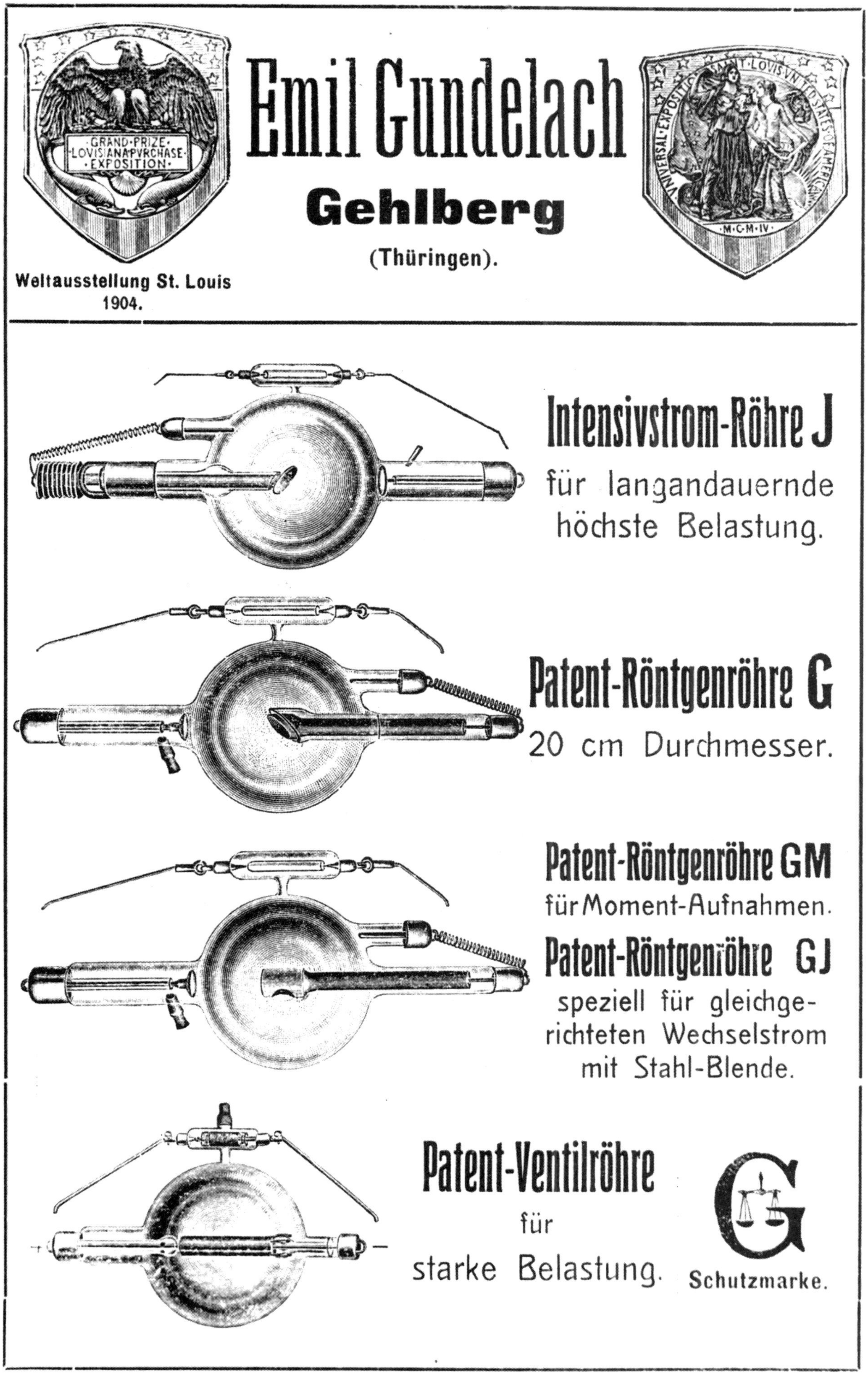
GRAND·PRIZE·
LOVISIANA·PVRCHASE·
·EXPOSITION·
Emil Gundelach
Gehlberg
(Thüringen).
Weltausstellung St. Louis
1904.
M·C·M·IV
Intensivstrom-Röhre J
für langandauernde
höchste Belastung.
Patent-Röntgenröhre G
20 cm Durchmesser.
Patent-Röntgenröhre GM
für Moment-Aufnahmen.
Patent-Röntgenröhre GJ
speziell für gleichge-
richteten Wechselstrom
mit Stahl-Blende.
Patent-Ventilröhre
für
starke Belastung.
G
Schutzmarke.

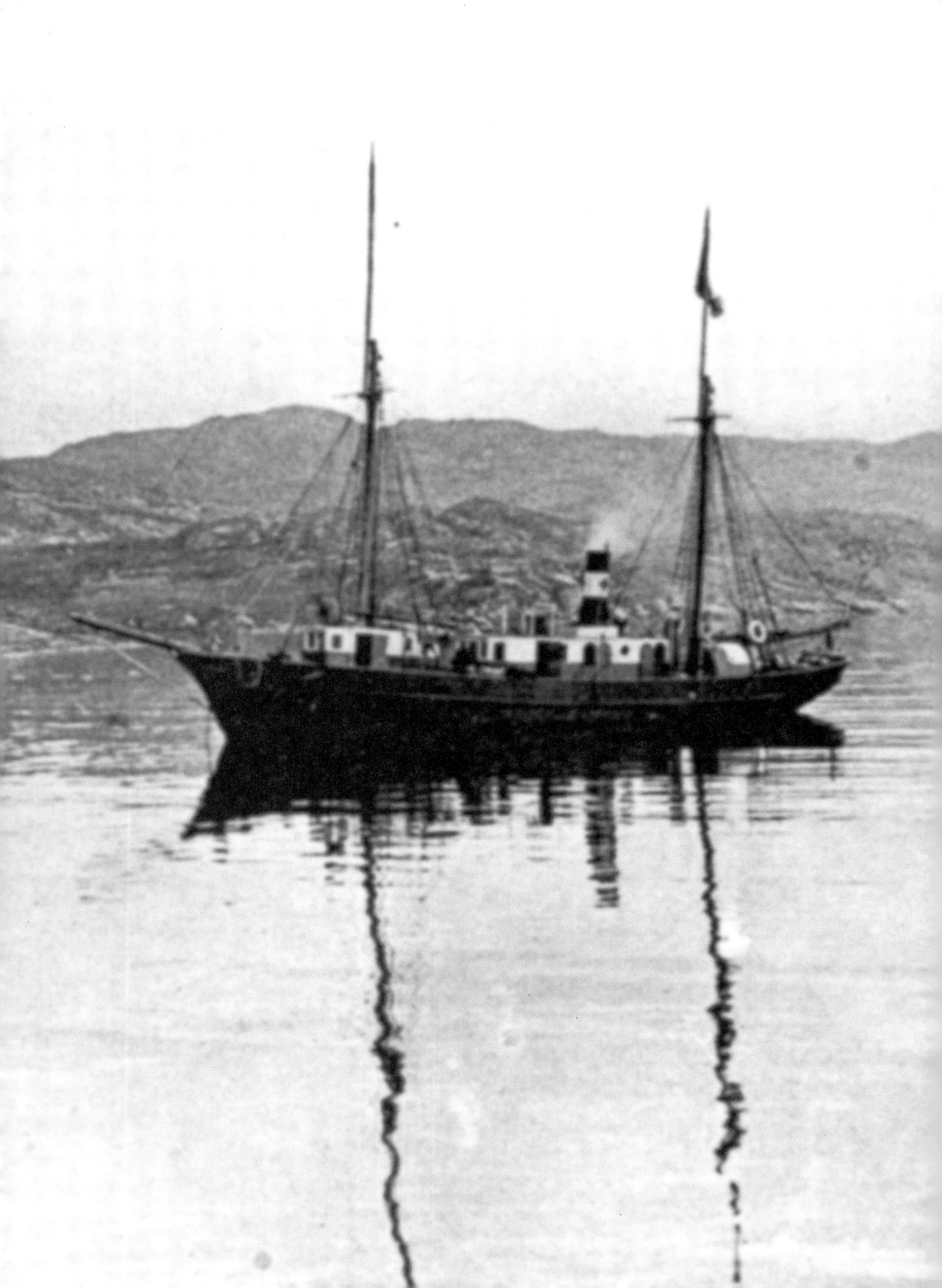

Chapter II • Radiology in Newfoundland

Patrick J McManamon

The story of the introduction of the medical use of x-rays into Newfoundland long antedates the entry of the province into the Canadian confederation.

The first x-ray machine to be used clinically in Newfoundland was at the St John's General Hospital, then located on Forest Road. The first radiograph was made in 1909 by a technologist by the name of Daisy Long.

During the development of the clinical use of x-rays, the machines were used not only for diagnosis but in the treatment of sciatica, lupus and skin cancer.

When Wilfred Grenfell (later Sir Wilfred) arrived in Newfoundland in 1892, he perceived a great need for a mission ship to travel the coasts of Newfoundland and Labrador.[1] This ship would be used to treat the many people scattered along the coastal settlements and, in particular, fishermen at sea. In that era there were few roads to link widely separated outports. Grenfell finally convinced the people of the Labrador Mission to build a vessel. The *SS Strathcona* arrived at Battle Harbour in 1899 fully equipped with an on-board hospital which included an x-ray facility. The total cost of building the *Strathcona* was £3000. (Newfoundland was not to become a province of Canada until 1948, hence the citation in British currency.) The chief patron was Lord Strathcona, after whom the vessel was named.

The base hospital of the Labrador Mission was at St Anthony in Labrador, where it has been succeeded by the Grenfell Regional Health Services. This hospital received delivery of its own x-ray

Left
SS.Strathcona (Grenfell Mission).

machine in 1912. It was installed by the Marconi operator from the *Strathcona.*

After 1912 x-ray equipment was installed in more and more hospitals throughout the province.

With the establishment of a medical school at Memorial University in St John's in 1967, the faculty of medicine began and an educational head, Dr CJ Hodson, was appointed in 1968. Dr Hodson was recruited from Great Britain, where he had already made a number of major contributions to his specialty, particularly in the radiological diagnosis and natural history of renal infections.[2] He was succeeded by Dr EA MacLaughlin in 1977. Dr Patrick McManamon was then appointed in 1989 and continues to hold the reins.

Right
Sir Wilfred Grenfell

Below
Canadian commemorative stamp

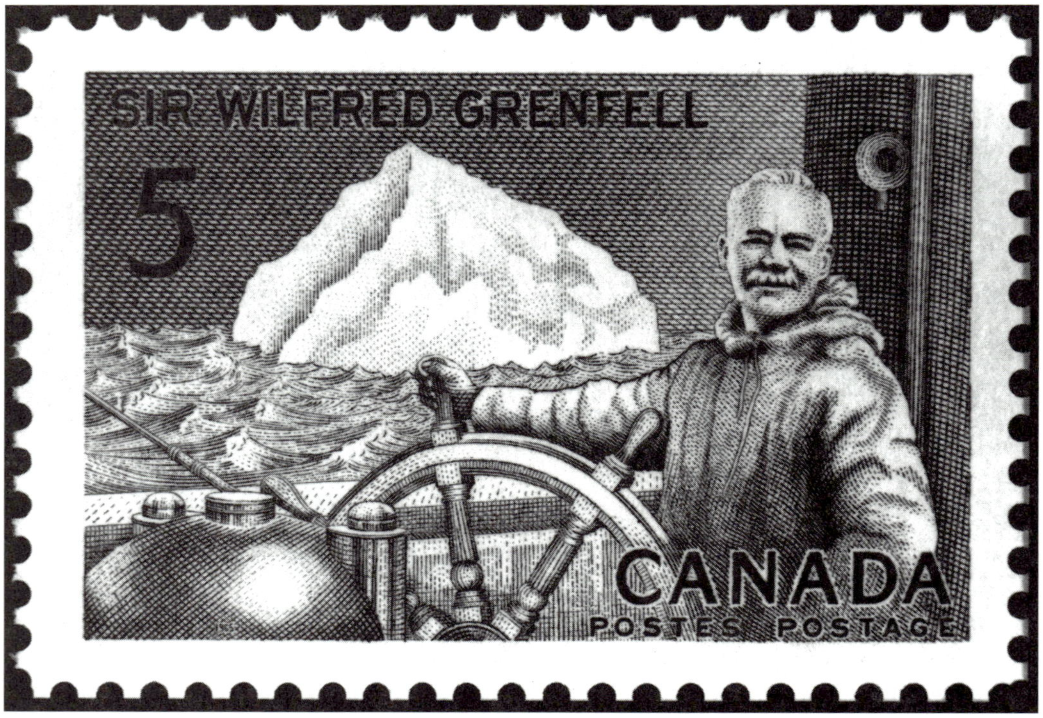

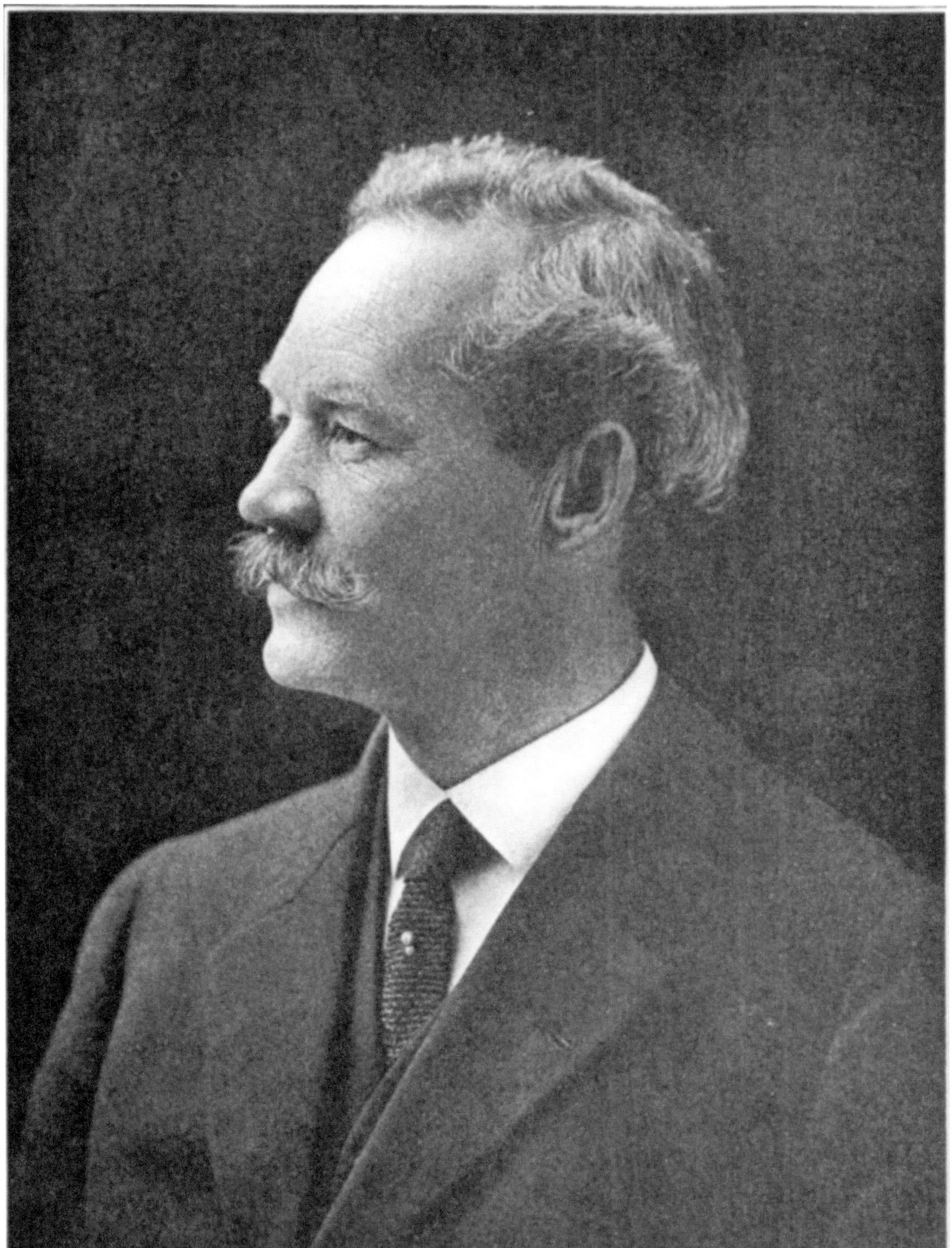

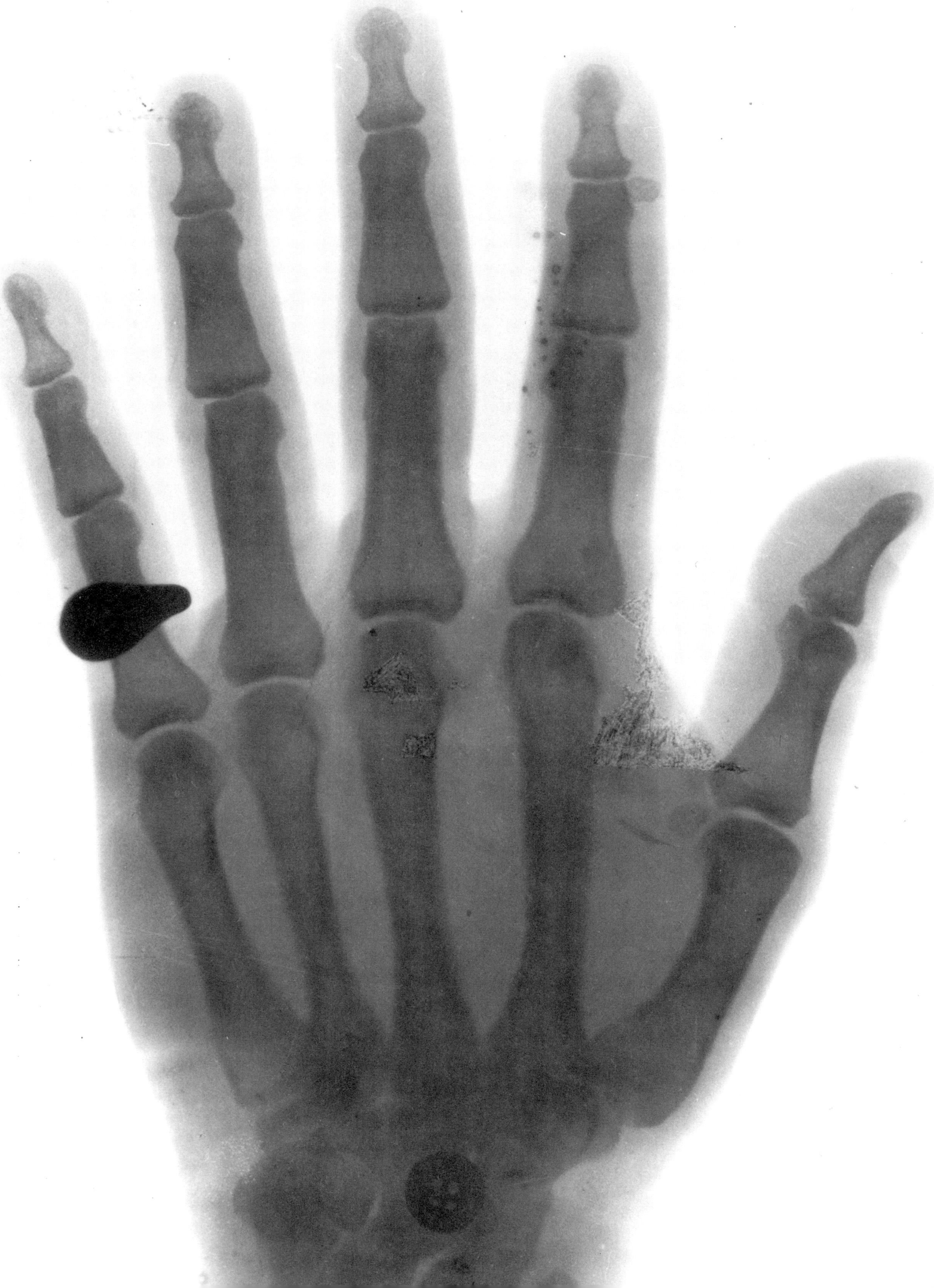

Chapter III • *History of the Use of*

X-rays in Nova Scotia

John Aldrich

X-RAYS IN HALIFAX

At the turn of the century, close ties existed between the medical communities in the Maritimes and in Britain. Meetings of the Maritime Medical Association as well as meetings of the Maritime's branch of the British Medical Association took place. Not surprisingly, then, we find in the March issue of the *Maritime Medical News* for 1896[1] a reprint from the *British Medical Journal* of Röntgen's discovery of x-rays. Clearly, the physicians in the area would have known about x-rays from this article and others which they would have read in other journals. Ties also existed between the Maritimes and the McGill Medical School. In fact, in each monthly issue of the *Maritime Medical News* there was an advertisement for the McGill School, where Professor Cox[2] had used x-rays in clinical diagnosis in February 1896. The official histories of the time attribute the installation of the first x-ray equipment in Nova Scotia to Dr Weaver, at the Victoria General Hospital in the fall of 1903.[3] Was it likely, this author wondered, that physicians in the area would really have waited seven years before availing themselves of such a valuable tool?

That x-rays were being used in Halifax before 1903 is recorded in the minutes of the meetings of the Nova Scotia Branch of the British Medical Society and reported in the *Maritime Medical News*. On November 5, 1897, Dr Edward Farrell, a prominent surgeon of the city, reported a case involving a needle in a lady's wrist which "could not be detected by probing but was located by means of the x-rays and successfully removed."[4] On April 19, 1900, Dr Edward D Farrell, son of the above Dr Edward Farrell (and the sixth Dr Edward Farrell in the family) "related the history of a boy who had been wounded

Left
An early radiograph taken by A Robie Cogswell probably of his own left hand

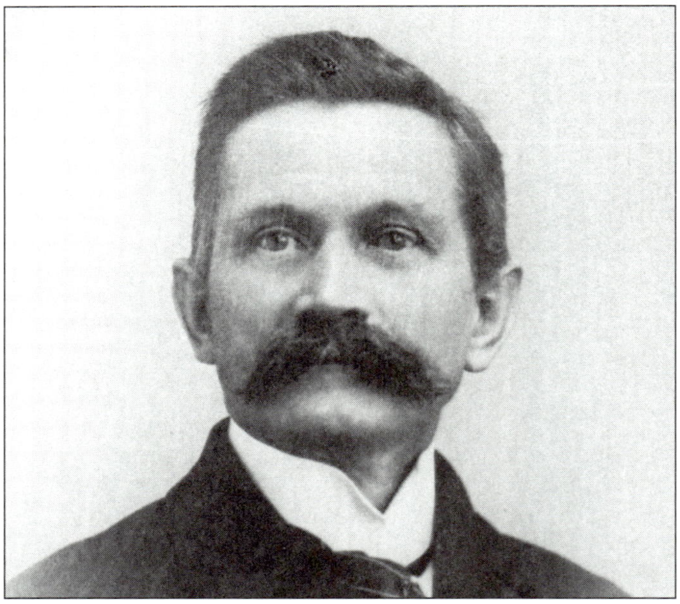

in the leg by a bullet, and showed an excellent radiograph of the case, by which means the bullet had been located."[5] Perhaps the most interesting report is by Dr Edward D Farrell, who on September 29, 1900 went to see a patient who, while painting, had fallen 25 feet to the ground.[6] He had a marked prominence between the fourth and fifth cervical vertebrae with complete loss of motion and sensation of the lower two-thirds of the trunk. Dr Farrell continues: "on the same night I again saw him accompanied by my father (Dr Edward Farrell) and Mr Cogswell of the Electric Studio, Barrington Street for the purpose of making a radiograph but found that Mr Cogswell's apparatus was not sufficiently powerful to outline clearly the spinal column."

Mr A Robie Cogswell, a professional photographer based in Halifax, was known especially for his interest in unusual photographic techniques, such as multiple exposures and collage. It is not surprising that he would have been interested in "the photography of the invisible," as radiography was often referred to in these early days, and he would, of course, have had all the equipment and expertise necessary for the developing and printing of glass photographic plates. Only one radiograph taken by Cogswell exists probably a radiograph of the left hand of Cogswell himself. Although x-rays seem to have been available to the physician in his private office, patients in hospital appear to have been less fortunate. In the surgical records of the Victoria General Hospital, for example, no mention of x-rays occurs before 1903 even for the most complicated fracture.

HERBERT D WEAVER

Herbert Weaver was born in Altrincham, Cheshire, England and came to Canada as a boy.[7] His family took up residence in Woodstock, Ontario. In 1897 he graduated from Trinity University, Toronto, in medicine. He practiced in Albert, New Brunswick for a while, came to Halifax in the fall of 1898[8] and became a lecturer in histology at Halifax Medical College in 1899. In the summer of 1901 he took a special course on "electricity" in Toronto and then fitted out his office at 41 Spring Garden Road with new equipment, including "a ten plate static machine with x-ray attachments, Crookes' tubes, etc."[9] It was reported that Dr Weaver was then able to "carry out x-ray work for diagnostic purposes promptly; and from what we have seen satisfactorily; and also any electrical treatment that may be suggested by the attending physician."

Two types of high voltage generators had been in use for electrotherapy for some years, the electrostatic generator and the induction coil, used also as high voltage sources for x-ray tubes. Both had their problems. The induction coil needed an "interrupter" to produce the alternating current from batteries, but interrupters were generally unreliable. The static machine was somewhat simpler to use and could be powered by an electric motor or by hand but was prone to failure due to humidity which, in the coastal province of Nova Scotia, may have been a frequent problem. However, by November 1901 Weaver appears to have become the local x-ray expert, discussing fluoroscopic techniques at a meeting of the Nova Scotia branch of the British Medical Association.[10] In the fall of 1903, Dr Weaver joined the staff at the Victoria General Hospital as head of the Electrotherapeutic Department and arranged the purchase of x-ray equipment for the hospital, a system apparently similar to that in his private office. He was obviously highly regarded, because he was asked in 1904 to give a talk—"Some Experiences with the X-ray Therapeutically"—at the annual meeting of the Nova Scotia Medical Society.

At this same meeting an invited speaker, Dr EA Codman from Boston, Massachusetts, spoke on "The use of the x-ray in the Surgery of the Diseases of Bones."[11] Dr Codman, a staunch proponent of the use of x-rays, was concerned that they be used correctly. In 1902, for example, he conscientiously reviewed all the papers on x-ray injuries that he could find[12] and unearthed fewer than two hundred cases. At that time a widespread impression held that injuries from x-rays had been more numerous, but Dr Codman explained that individual cases were being reported repeatedly in one publication after another. It seemed also that such injuries were becoming rarer as the years progressed. Of the 88 x-ray injuries which

Doctor Codman could definitely date from published accounts, 55 had occurred in 1896, but only one had been reported in 1901. This decline, of course, might have been due to the fact that x-ray injuries were no longer news and therefore went unreported. However, Dr Codman preferred to believe that the record was actually improving. He reasoned that the reported cases were less attributable to the hazards of radiation than to the wanton folly of those who had abused their equipment. As an example, Dr Codman cited a physician who bought an x-ray machine from Otis Clapp & Son of Boston early in 1899. Soon after installing the machine, he tested it by exposing himself to the rays for 45 minutes with the tube only five inches from his groin. A forty-five minute exposure at 5 inches would have been risky even in 1896.

With the far more powerful equipment that became available later, prolonged exposure was extremely dangerous and would certainly have been malpractice if attempted on a patient. "A most uncomfortable burn followed." Dr Codman reported, "necessitating a severe operation producing disability for one and a half years." The physician thereupon sued the Clapp firm for $20 000.00 in damages, alleging that the company had guaranteed that its apparatus would not burn. Many of the country's foremost authorities testified on behalf of the manu-facturer, including Dr Codman, and yet the physician was awarded substantial damages of $6750.00 in 1901. Soon afterwards the first tragic deaths attributed to x-rays started to occur and the deleterious effects of x-rays became apparent. At the 1904 meeting of the Nova Scotia Medical Society Dr Weaver proposed a vote of thanks to Dr Codman for his talk.

Left
Edward Farrell MD

Right
Herbert Weaver MD

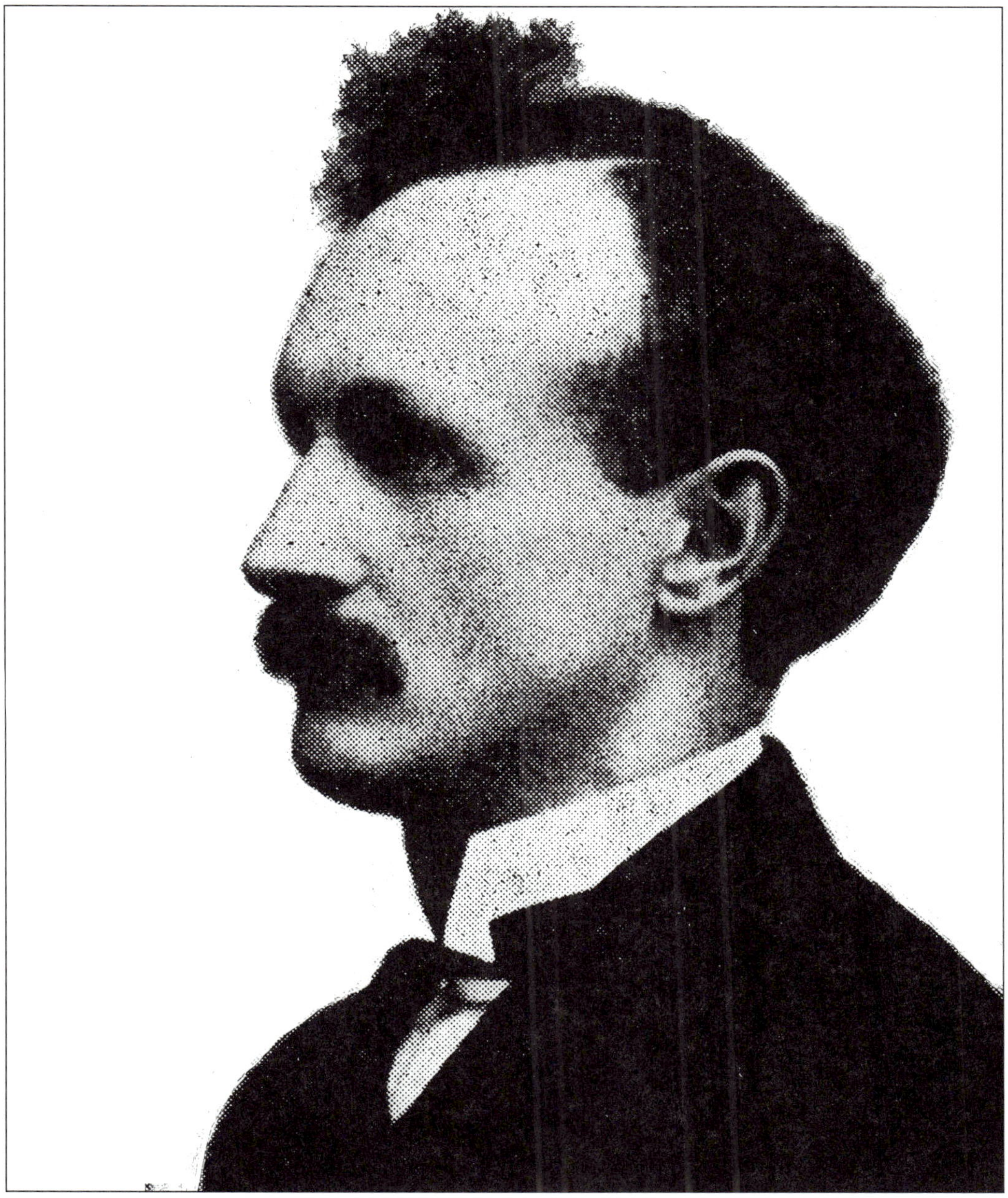

While in Halifax, Dr Weaver became keenly interested in his medical students, especially Miss Alice Thomas, whom he eventually married. About the same time Dr Weaver approached the commission regarding remuneration for his work in the Electrotherapeutic Department of the Victoria General Hospital. He was told that all the other members of the staff were giving their services gratis and that he should do likewise. This answer was apparently a real disappointment to the young professor, and by December of 1904 he had resigned from the Victoria General Hospital and left Halifax in favour of Saskatoon, taking his own x-ray machine with him. He came back in June 1906 to marry Miss Thomas and take her to Saskatoon with him.

In Saskatoon Dr Weaver decided not to continue in radiological practice, perhaps partly because he lost his left index finger to x-ray burns; he continued instead in general practice. He did, however, help establish radiology in Saskatoon. Dr Weaver became prominent in Saskatoon life and was especially remembered for his work in horticulture. He was a member of the Saskatoon Parks Board for many years and established one of the first nurseries in northern Saskatchewan where he carried on experimentation for the purpose of introducing trees, shrubs and perennials suited to the climatic conditions of the Prairies.

The electrostatic generator which Dr Weaver first used in Halifax in 1901 and which is now in the museum of the Physics Department of the University of Saskatchewan in Saskatoon was made by the company of Waite and Bartlett of New York. The instruction manual which came with the generator has the following instructions: "When the x-ray tube is properly connected, it will be illuminated with a bright green light showing plainly in one half of the tube. When your tube is properly illuminated, place the object to be x-rayed one inch from the tube and the fluorescent screen against the object on the other side, and you get the desired result."[13]

CHARLES PUTTNER

After Dr Weaver left for Saskatoon, the Electrotherapeutic Department was left in the hands of Charles Puttner. Puttner was something of an institution at the Victoria General Hospital in its early days. In 1867 a year after the Victoria General Hospital opened, Charles Puttner was appointed apothecary and clerk.[14] Puttner, a fully qualified pharmacist, trained in New York, where he was born. His departure from the United States came as the result of the Civil War. Puttner's family was loyal to the Confederacy and they came to Nova Scotia in 1861 on a blockade runner.[15] As well as his duties as the apothecary for the hospital, he performed many other functions. He acted as purchasing agent, buying the food, fuel, equipment, surgical supplies and drugs used in the hospital. In 1897, when Mr W Wallace Kenny became the first non-medical superintendent of the hospital,[16] Charles Puttner became his right-hand man, assistant superintendent.

At that time a large variety of home-made concoctions was made in the pharmacy, and Puttner deserves credit for developing a more palatable form for the dispensing of cod liver oil, often considered a valuable factor in the treatment of pulmonary tuberculosis. To overcome revulsion to this medicine, Puttner decided to emulsify it. So Puttner's Emulsion of Cod Liver Oil was born. He secured the patent and then sold it to the National Drug Company. The following advertisement for this preparation appeared in each edition of the *Maritime Medical News*:

> **OF THE MANY PREPARATIONS**
> *of Cod liver Oil now offered to the Physician*
> **PUTTNER'S EMULSION,**
> *introduced twenty years ago,*
> **IS UNDOUBTEDLY THE BEST**
> *maintaining its superiority over all competitors,*
> **RICH IN OIL**
> *partially predigested by pancreatine,*
> **PALATABLE AND ACCEPTABLE**
> *even to delicate stomachs,*
> **IN LARGE BOTTLES**
> *making it the cheapest to the patient,*
> **ALWAYS FRESH**
> *being made daily in Halifax,*
> **IT DESERVES THE PREFERENCE**
> *of the intelligent prescriber.*

No doubt Puttner would have been intimately involved in setting up the Electrotherapeutic Department in 1903 and no doubt he arranged payment for the first x-ray "plant" which cost $1173.41.[17] By comparison, for the same year the total cost of drugs for the hospital was $3906.11, and the cost of "stimulants" (alcoholic beverages) was $1041.70. Some of the patients or staff must have had rich palates since $22 of this total was for champagne! After morning surgery the doctors congregated in the pharmacy for a refreshing glass of spirits!

Puttner's familiarity with the early uses of the x-ray machine must have put him in good stead for carrying on this work after Weaver left. The work seems to have started off slowly. In 1907, for example, 118 procedures were

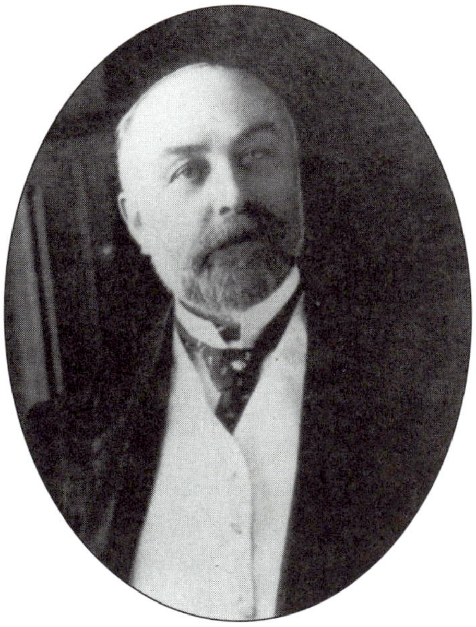

performed using x-rays, while 250 electrotherapy treatments using the static machine and induction coil were still performed. The number of x-ray procedures gradually increased until immediately before World War I 698 procedures were performed. During the war years the number of procedures increased sharply, reaching a maximum of 1540 during 1917. The cost of x-ray supplies follows this gradual rise, from $183.76 in 1907 to $1002.00 in 1917. From 1905 until 1917, Puttner is listed in the hospital staff as pharmacist and electrotherapeutist. In the 1919 Annual Report he is listed as pharmacist and roentgenologist. In the annual reports for the X-ray Department, he called himself the radiographer in 1913, but the radiologist from 1914 to 1917.

Charles Puttner was obviously a major figure in the history of the Victoria General Hospital. In 1905 he was

Above
Charles E Puttner PhM DPharm in 1904.

Below
Static machine used by Weaver in Halifax in 1901, now at the University of Saskatchewan.

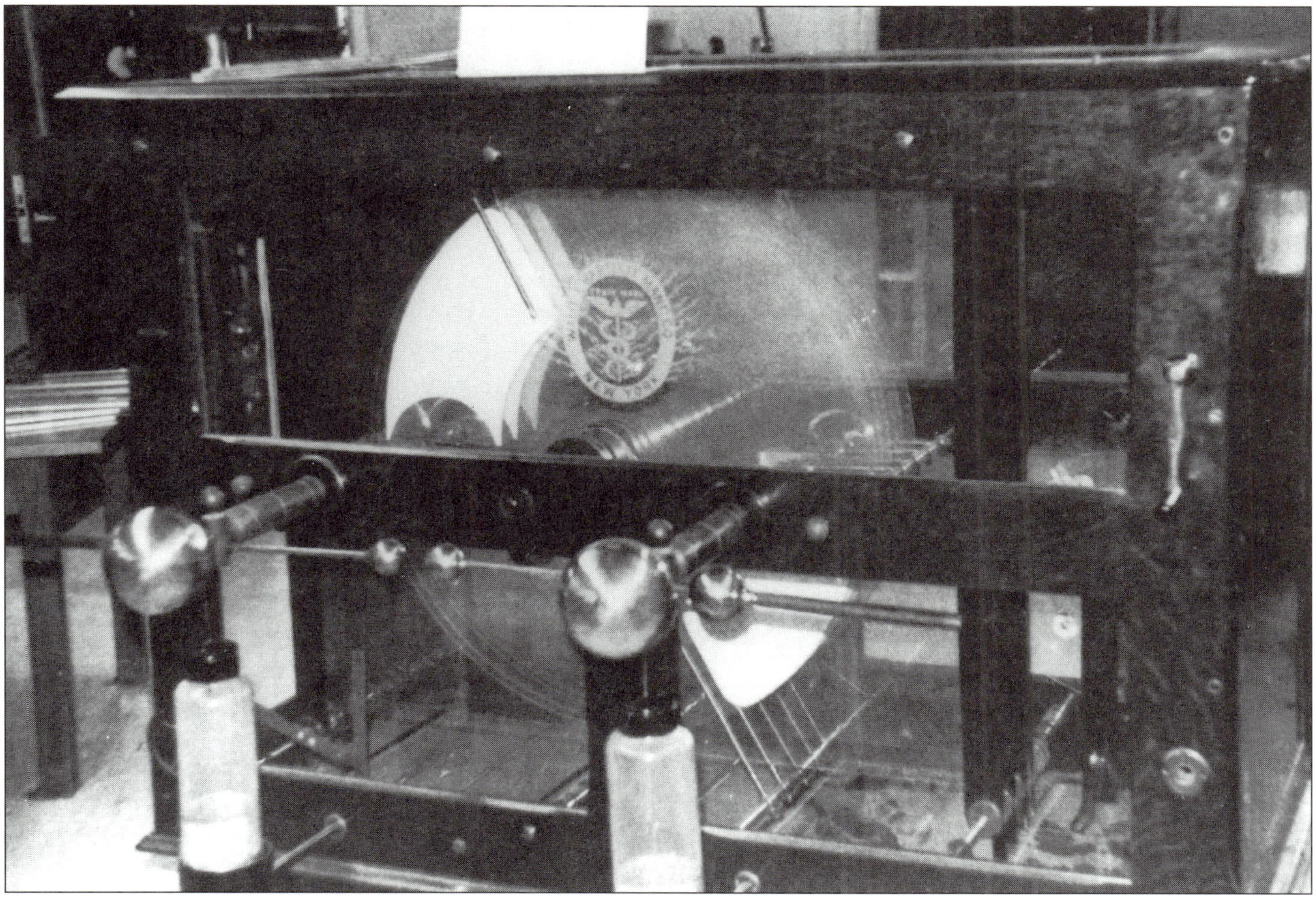

awarded an honorary doctorate by the Halifax Medical College. His degree of Doctor of Pharmacy still hangs near his photograph in the South Wing of the present Victoria building of the hospital. He was on the staff of the hospital for fifty-three continuous years until his death in 1920 (at age 75). Few people would have had the experience that Dr Puttner had in his lifetime and it is even more doubtful that anyone would have been apothecary, clerk, accountant, pharmacist, electrotherapeutist, radiographer, radiologist and roentgenologist in any one lifetime. He also had enough time to be very active in freemasonry and gave a lecture course on "Practical Materia Medica" at the Halifax Medical College for many years.

ERNEST CODMAN

As material for this article was assembled, I realized that most of the x-ray pioneers were to play a part in the aftermath of the Halifax Explosion. One of these was Dr Codman, and some background on his life is necessary to explain his part in the disaster.

Ernest Amory Codman, brought up with exceptional social and educational advantages, attended private school in Boston and subsequently obtaining his MD from Harvard.[18] He started in private practice in December 1895, just as the announcements of Röntgen's discovery were being published. He at once realized the potential importance of x-rays to surgery and collaborated with Professor John Trowbridge of Harvard and Elihu Thomson of the General Electric Company to perform some of the first clinical x-ray experiments in the United States. As early as the summer of 1898 Codman had compiled a complete atlas of 74 x-ray photographs of the human skeleton which was donated to the Countway Library of Medicine at Harvard. Codman devoted much of the next five years to the study of x-rays until he was offered the post of outpatient surgeon at the Massachusetts General Hospital. Although he now became less directly involved with the use of x-rays, he continued his interest in x-rays as applied to surgery, especially to bone and upper abdomen disorders. As an expert in these matters he gave a talk in Halifax in 1904.

The turning point in Codman's career came in 1910 when he was forty years old. By any standards he was a successful man: assistant visiting surgeon at the Massachusetts General Hospital and the author of many important papers on general surgery as well as on x-rays. But new events propelled his career even further. His whole life became consumed by what he called the "End Result Idea." The idea was that "every hospital should follow every patient it treats long enough to determine whether or not the treatment has been successful, and then to inquire, if not, why not?"[19] Although perhaps self-evident nowadays, this idea was not generally accepted for several years and was somewhat unpopular with his peers at the time. Codman also took the tenet to mean that the contribution of each hospital physician should be assessed and that promotion should be based upon a physician's patient successes. He resigned from the Massachusetts General Hospital in protest against promotion by seniority rather than by merit and, shortly after started his own hospital, the Codman Hospital Clinic, where he could test out his principles.

No doubt Codman was a sincere and honest man. Self-assured, he lost no opportunity to promote his ideas. Characteristically, his definitive book, *The Shoulder*,[20] begins with a 36-page autobiographical preface, including a page of minute details about his ancestry, interests, education and income over his lifetime! In this preface he tries to explain the motives for his actions and blames a "pure English Puritan" heritage for unswerving devotion to an ideal, which many times brought him public disgrace and near financial ruin. However, by 1917 many of his ideas were adopted in hospitals and clinics throughout the country. The United States entered the war on April 6, 1917, but Codman remained in Boston, believing that work in his hospital made a major contribution to the war effort. This same Codman also left his mark on radiology with his description of "Codman's Triangle."

DECEMBER 6, 1917

The morning of December 6 was crisp and clear in Halifax, a pleasant, early winter day. Robie Cogswell enjoyed the short walk from his home to his now successful photographic store on Granville Street in the business district of Halifax. Patients in the Victoria General Hospital were also enjoying the morning sunshine, and the wards were settling down to their daily routine. The contrast between the calm in the hospital and the horror about to happen can scarcely be imagined. Suddenly, a few minutes after nine o'clock, a terrifying blast blew in most of the windows of the hospital.[21] Many thought the hospital was being shelled, but the news soon spread that the reason was the collision and subsequent explosion of the Mont Blanc, a ship laden with 2600 tons of high explosives, with a Belgian relief ship, the Imo, in the narrows of Halifax Harbour. The Mont Blanc was bringing explosives to Halifax to be convoyed to the war effort in Europe.[22] The blast from the explosion completely laid waste the northern part of the city, damaging practically every building in the city, killing over 1600 persons, injuring

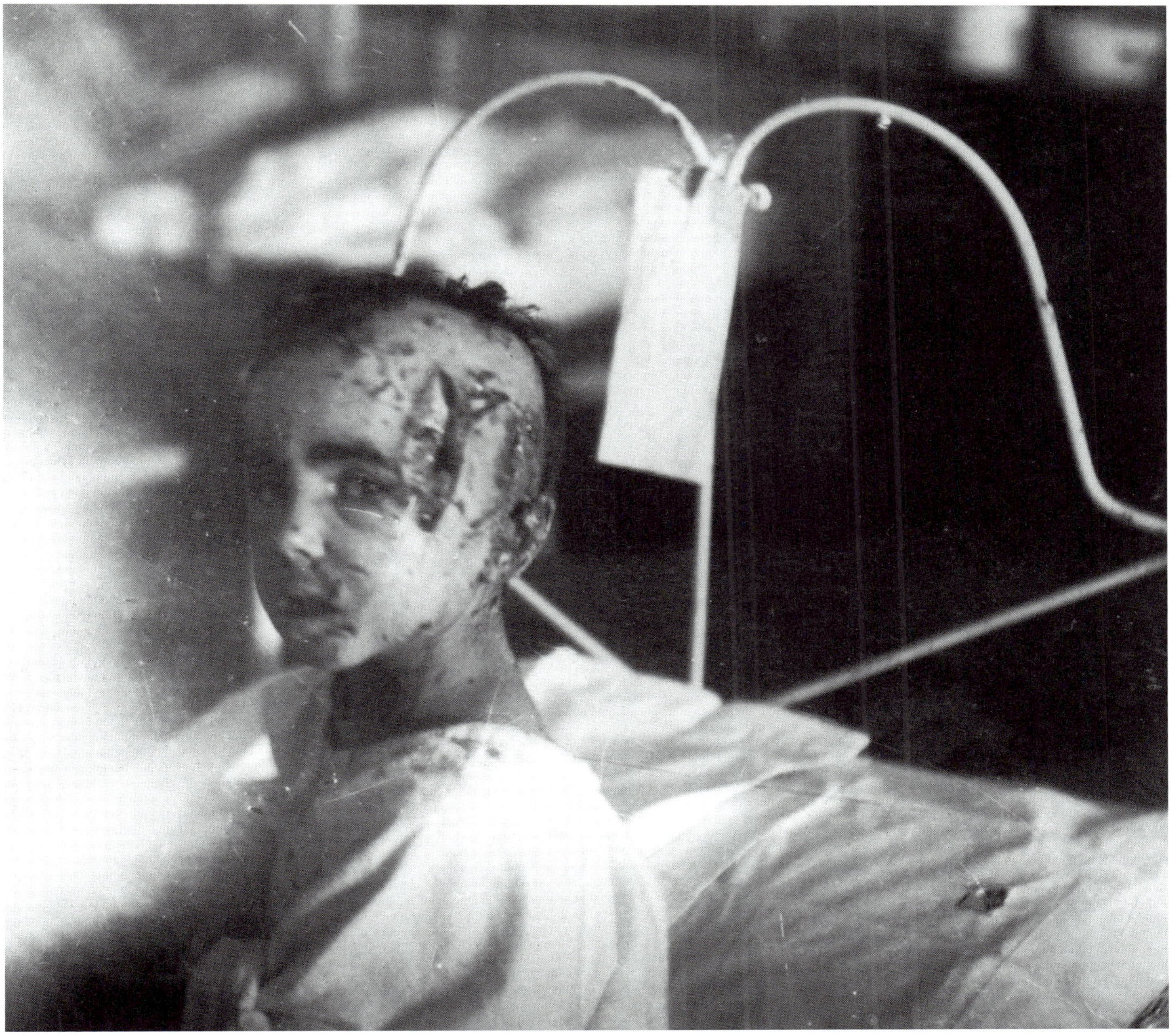

Explosion victim in the Victoria General Hospital Photograph taken by A Robie Cogswell some 9000 and leaving homeless nearly 25 000, many of whom were small children or young people.

The blast was heard as far away as Baddeck, 177 miles distant. Several members of the *Beinn Breagh* household felt the ground shake and heard the windows rattle, and many thought there had been an earthquake. The Halifax business district suffered less than the north end of the city, but damage from flying glass was, nevertheless, substantial. Apart from broken windows, the damage to the Victoria General Hospital was relatively minor, and there were no serious injuries. Soon the enormity of the situation became apparent at the hospital, where every driveway became filled by vehicles of all sorts bearing the injured, dead and dying. The scene was ghastly, even to the trained hospital staff, because the severe mutilations and freely flowing blood from facial injuries caused by flying glass were so widespread.[23]

How could the work of the hospital be administered under such conditions? The superintendent of the hospital was away at a convention in the United States and the burden fell to his deputy, Dr Charles Puttner. He turned no one away. Soon every bed and cot was full, and when no more were available, the wounded and dying were laid gently on the floors of the wards, the halls, the offices and even the cellar. The hospital was also besieged by those seeking information concerning injured or lost friends and relatives. Puttner must have needed all his considerable experience and kindness to handle the situation. To the horrors of the disaster was added another complication brought on by the weather. The two days following the disaster were bitterly cold with high winds and driving snow, two of the worst days of a long winter.

Dr Puttner laboured day and night, stopping only for food, in dealing with the enormous problems of the hospital. Finally, on the third day, Puttner, now 73, collapsed with a heart attack and became a patient himself. He was put in a room with Dr Murdoch Chisholm, the senior surgeon of the hospital. After the explosion Dr Chisholm, at first reported dead, had been found unconscious, bleeding freely from a severed artery. A colleague had realized the extent of the wound, revived him and sent him off to hospital. There, a few days later Chisholm had the unique experience of reading his own obituary in the local paper. On seeing it he quipped, "That man, Chisholm. He was quite a man."[24]

The other hospitals in the city were also filled to capacity and to relieve the tremendous overload some patients were even moved by train to New Glasgow, Truro and Windsor. Offers of money and help came pouring in as soon as the news of the disaster spread.[25] The Alexander Graham Bell household packed up blankets and clothes—including one of Alexander's own winter coats—to be shipped to Halifax. Casey Baldwin, one of Bell's associates, left immediately to help in the relief efforts, and a few days later a dozen of Bell's staff joined Baldwin in the reconstruction work.

Two trainloads of medical staff and supplies left Boston soon after the explosion. The first was organized by the Massachusetts Relief Commission, the second by Dr Codman, who put his complete hospital on a train. He set up an emergency hospital in the Halifax YMCA building with two local doctors. He organized the hospital according to his own original ideas of health management and was pleased to find that his system worked well even in a city destroyed by such a disaster. With a simplicity that won the hearts of all the people, he generously placed his skill and that of his staff at the service of the poorest and humblest of the sufferers.

Why he felt so strongly about the disaster in Halifax is not known. He had been born and had lived all his life in Boston. He did visit both Nova Scotia and New Brunswick four times between 1890 and 1904, probably to hunt and fish (the other consuming passions of his life), and he had made many friends there. It is possible, too, that the ties to his hospital which had prevented him from offering himself for military service troubled his puritan conscience, and the Halifax disaster was a very concrete way in which he could help the war effort. The following year he joined the United States Medical Corps.

The x-ray facilities in Halifax at the time of the Explosion were modest, to say the least, with no significant improvement between 1903 and 1917. With Dr Puttner in poor shape during the aftermath of the crisis, probably no one could carry on the x-ray work in the hospital. Fortunately, the American Red Cross provided a complete x-ray system and operators to carry out this important work for sufferers of the disaster. This modern equipment may have been a revelation to Puttner, for in his 1917 annual report he calls attention to "the urgent necessity of improving our present x-ray plant by the addition of more modern and up-to-date equipment..."

Within five years of the Halifax Explosion, Nova Scotia had lost all of its x-ray pioneers. Bell and Puttner were now dead; Farrell had died earlier, in 1900. Weaver had moved to Saskatoon, Codman returned to his beloved Boston, and Cogswell retired to Florida. A new generation of radiologist was arriving on the scene with new departments and specialized equipment; the discipline was about to enter an expansionary phase in the province.

Acknowledgements:

The author would like to acknowledge the help and encouragement given by many friends and colleagues. Special thanks is due to the staff of the Public Archives of Nova Scotia in Halifax, the Physics Department of the University of Saskatchewan in Saskatoon and the Francis A Countway Library of Medicine at Harvard. Part of this account has been previously published in the *Canadian Medical Association Journal* and the *Canadian Pharmaceutical Journal* and is reproduced here with the permission of the publishers.

Lead radiation safety mask to protect the face and eyes without undue interference with vision and breathing (1920s)

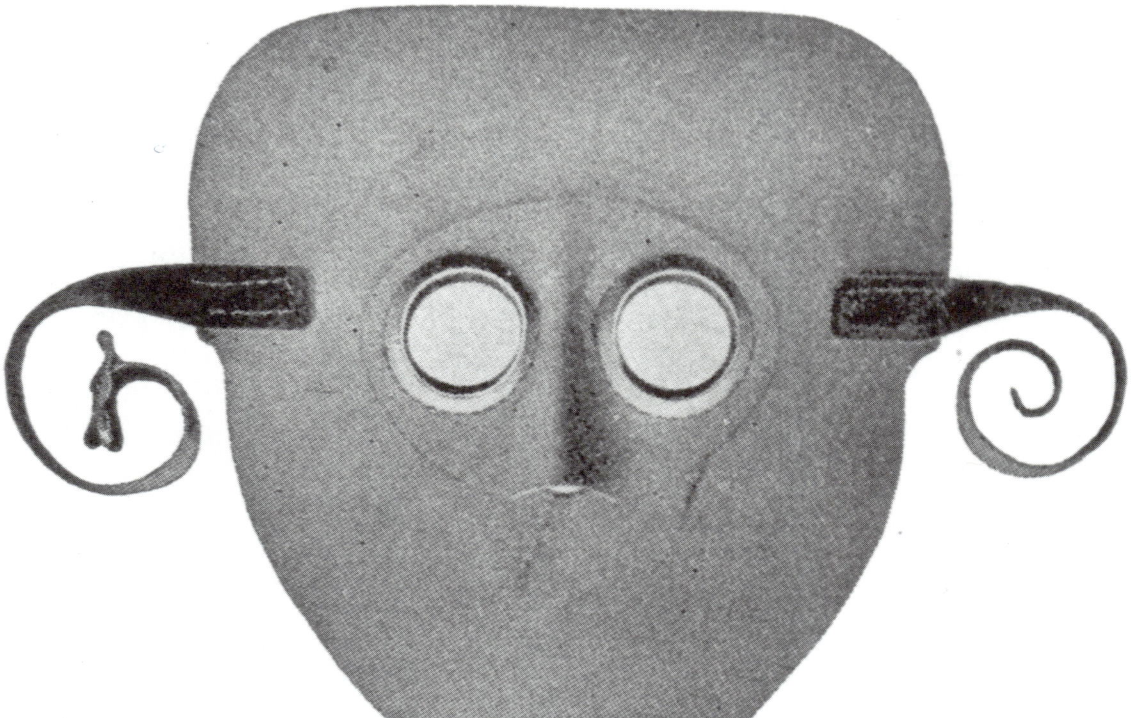

"WHO SAID FRACTURES?"

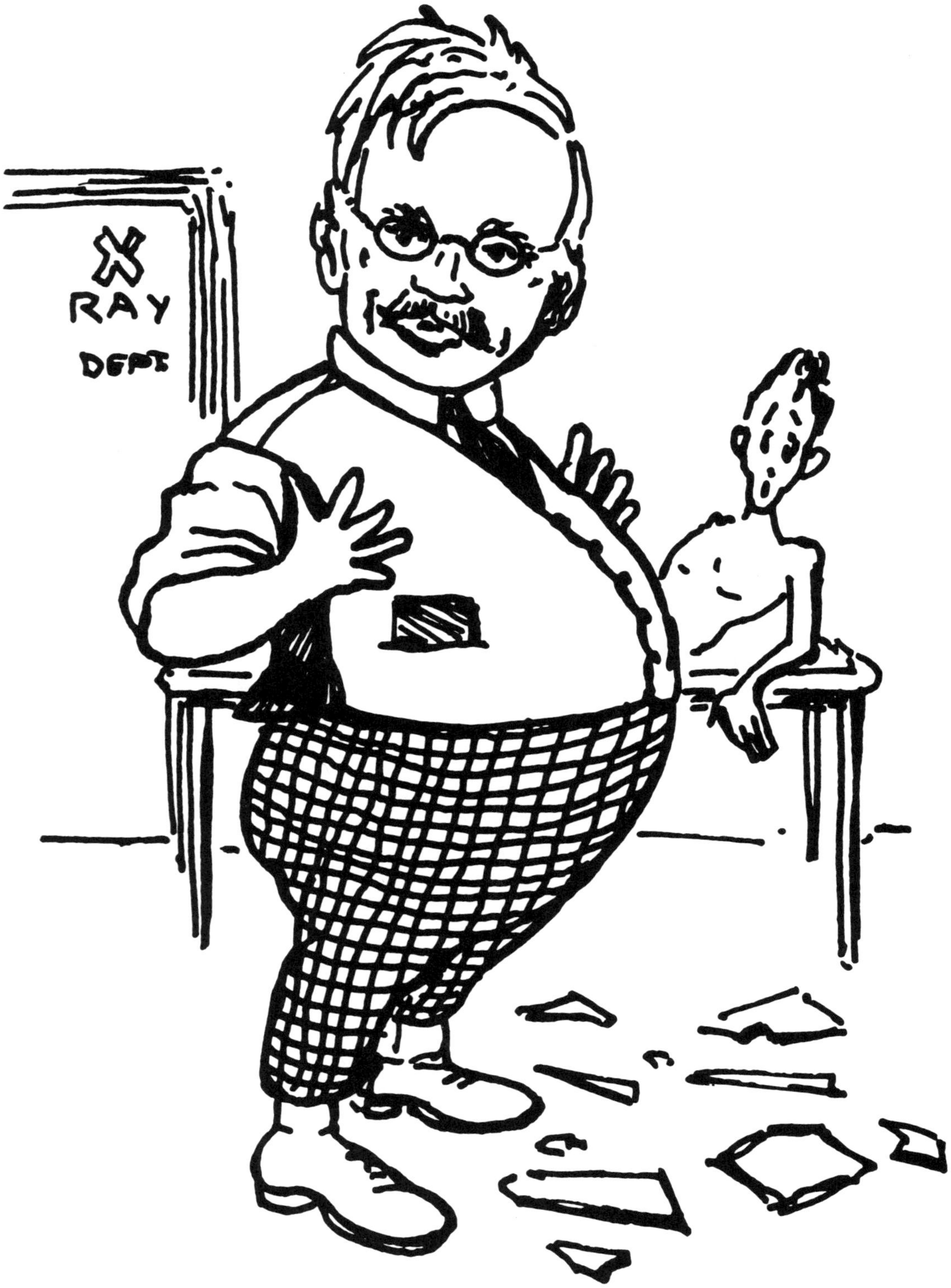

Chapter IV • *Memories of*

Early Radiology in New Brunswick

AS Kirkland

[Dr Kirkland was writing in 1958]

In 1940 "x-ray" was a relatively new word, and x-ray machines were even more of a novelty. X-ray men had appeared about the time of the first machines. Some were physicians, some not. Many of the physicians did much to further the clinical use of these machines. Later, a few physicians began to provide a full-time service in expanding x-ray departments. My teacher, Dr Walter Wilkins of Montréal, was one of these.

Some years ago, I was chosen as the first of "older members" to be honoured by the Saint John Medical Society. I took this opportunity to consider the story of x-rays in New Brunswick. Later, I recorded what I remembered and what has been told to me about radiology in this province. This is that record.

Two sources of accurate information were available. The minutes of the Board of Commissioners of the old Saint John General Public Hospital and the private records of the late Dr G Clowes VanWart of Fredericton, provided through the courtesy of his son, Dr Arthur VanWart.

The first x-ray machine in New Brunswick, bought in 1902 at the cost of $500.00 it was, perhaps, the first such machine in the Maritimes. Installed in the Victoria Public Hospital in Fredericton, it was later placed in the electrical department of the University of New Brunswick and used for teaching purposes.

Left
Cartoon: In the days of glass plates "fracture" might apply to the patient or the film (from the *Canadian X-ray Newsletter*, circa 1945)

The money to buy this machine was raised by public subscription. Several doctors supervised the medical uses of the machine but, from the first, the operator was William S (Doc) Kelly who had been an orderly in the Fredericton Hospital since 1896. He was stone deaf but perceptive. and he possessed great manual dexterity. He continued as x-ray technician until 1937, when Dr Hynes became the first full-time radiologist in Fredericton. "Doc" Kelly was an expert surgical assistant, a skilled cystoscopist and a good laboratory technician.

Early in the life of this machine, Dr VanWart, assisted by "Doc" Kelly, removed a bullet from a patient's skull. During the operation they used a hand fluoroscope with enthusiasm but not too much care: The patient survived, but the left side of his head remained permanently bald.

The next x-ray machine acquired cost $294.00 and was, I believe, second hand, picked up in Boston. After much debate by the hospital commission, a group of three physicians was given charge of the machine. One of the physicians was Dr Stewart Skinner, whose son, Dr Norman Skinner, also became a radiologist.

A number of physicians gave greater or lesser amounts of time and interest to radiology in this old hospital. Worthy of note are Dr GG Corbet, who was later Officer Commanding Number 14 Field Ambulance Overseas in World War I; Dr Henry Heddon, one-time superintendent of the hospital; and Dr John H Allingham, one of New Brunswick's brilliant surgeons, who performed the earliest thoracoplastics in the Maritimes with outstanding success.

During the period 1910–1922 an excellent radiology service was provided in the Saint John Infirmary, later St Joseph's Hospital, by Dr Clement Kelly, who like Dr Allingham was an able surgeon practicing radiology as an adjunct to his surgery.

In 1921 Hon WF Roberts, MD, the first minister of health in the British Empire, and Mr King Kelly were appointed as a search committee of the Board of Commissioners of the Saint John General Hospital to employ a full-time radiologist. This writer, Dr A Stanley Kirkland, was their choice, and he reported for duty on May 1, 1922. He remained as a Director of Radiology until June 1955, when he was appointed Emeritus Director.

In 1922 the radiology equipment comprised:

1	Campbell combination table with fluoroscope and transformer
1	Waite and Bartlett portable x-ray unit
1	soapstone developing and fixing tank
1	dozen plate hangers
2	14 x 17 film hangers

The Department was located on the top floor of the old hospital.

In this (to me) strange Maritime atmosphere the new radiologist quickly and unofficially organized a small diagnostic unit about himself, including the pathologist Dr HL Abrams a graduate of Yale, and three McGill alumni: Dr JH Allingham and Dr CM Kelly, surgeons, and Dr WE Rowley, physician, all of whom have passed to their rewards. These rewards would have to be superlative to equal their abilities, generosity of heart and charity of thought and deed.

The new radiologist was the third full-time specialist in Saint John in 1922; the others were Dr Abramson, pathologist, and Dr L DeV Chipman, eye, ear, nose and throat—and now in 1958, just count them!

In 1924 a new department was opened in the old morgue and other rooms on the first floor of the old building, and next to the telephone switchboard. Switchboard operator Marion Lawlor served without pay as receptionist, financial advisor and public relations officer for the X-ray Department for many years.

The new equipment purchased at the time included an up-to-date Snook transformer and General Electric (GE) Table, a good darkroom which was well equipped and a new Coolidge tube and table for therapy. This table, by the way, was a revamped autopsy table and still in use in 1958.

In 1930 a new hospital was built, including a new x-ray department, much more space and much new equipment: a GE stabilizer valve, rectified transformers, tilt tables, new portables, a deep therapy unit, superficial therapy unit, radiographic cystoscopic tables etc.

In 1947 when the New Brunswick Department of Health took over the responsibility for the care of patients with cancer, further diagnostic and treatment units were made available.

Radium in small amounts was provided in 1936 by the Independent Order of Daughters of the Empire and was increased in amount slowly by private donations. After 1947 the Cancer Control Director of the New Brunswick Department of Health supplied very generous amounts of radium to the Saint John General Hospital, where all radium therapy for the province has since been carried out.

In 1958 a new wing of the Saint John General Hospital is about ready for use, with a splendid radiotherapy department partly sunk into the rock of the hillside; elsewhere, protection is provided by concrete and lead. Here, the cobalt source is available, as well as röntgen therapy units of various voltages, radium storage, mould rooms, an isotope laboratory, and an office and work room for the full-time physicist. This new department is supervised by Dr J A Caskey, Director and Dr Douglas Smith, Assistant Director.

The diagnostic x-ray department will expand into

much larger new space near its old location. Several new machines are being installed to carry out new techniques and to handle the great increase of routine work expected to follow the introduction of welfare medical services sponsored by the federal and provincial governments.

The diagnostic x-ray services were provided by Dr Norman Skinner, Director, and Dr John Stevenson, Assistant Director.

The Saint John General Hospital is qualified in 1958 to give the first two years of instruction in radiology to students preparing for the examinations of the Royal College of Physicians and Surgeons of Canada. This hospital department has come a long way in the years from 1922 to 1958.

The following statistics are samples for 1922 and 1953 while I was the radiologist in charge.

In 1922—Work done in the department:

Fluoroscopics [sic]	161
Radiographs	2049
X-ray treatments	727

In 1953—Diagnostic examinations:

Number of patients	15,594
Radiographs	53,681
Areas examined	17,389
Fluoroscopics	3,241
Miniature chest films	3,401

In 1953—Radiotherapeutic procedures:

New patients	474
Follow-up examinations	1,401
Postal follow-ups	700
X-ray treatments	8,111
Radium treatments	122

The above figures are the bare bones of this story; more important, perhaps, are personal and personnel achievements. The training of technicians began in 1923. The first technician from this hospital registered in the American Society was Miss Ethel Thompson in 1926. Since that time our own registered technicians have staffed our department and may have been employed in various hospitals in the United States and Canada. When the Canadian Society of Radiographers was established, this hospital had more registered technicians than any hospital east of Toronto.

The routine of giving nurses chest radiographs began in our hospital in 1926 with the approval of Miss Margaret Murdock, RN, the head of the Training School of Nurses.

I, the radiologist since 1922, have provided diagnostic and therapeutic services for the city of Saint John and district. I have also served as consultant to the Saint John Tuberculosis Hospital and consultant and chief radiologist to the DSCR [?] and Department of Veterans Affairs in this same district.

To qualify for my first appointment at Saint John I had:

Four years internship at Montréal General Hospital in medicine and surgery.
Three years as an x-ray officer in Britain, France, Belgium and Germany with No 1, CCCS, CAMC.
Three years post-graduate x-ray study at Montréal General Hospital, 1919–1922.

As a Radiologist, I was a member of:

The Canadian Medical Association
The American Roentgen Ray Society
The Radiological Society of North America
The American College of Radiology
The Canadian Association of Radiologists
as well as a diplomate of the American Board of Radiology and a specialist certified in Radiology by the Royal College of Physicians and Surgeons of Canada.

As a physician specializing in radiology I was honoured by my contemporaries by being made:

A Fellow of the Royal College of Physicians and Surgeons of Canada
President of the New Brunswick Medical Society
President of the Medical Council of New Brunswick
President of the Medical Council of Canada
A Member of the Council and a Member of the Executive of the CMA
President of the Section on Radiology of the CMA.
A Charter Member of the Advisory Committee of the NB Cancer Control Program
Official Canadian delegate representing Canada at the Radiological Congress Stockholm in 1929—at which the "röntgen" was accepted as the measurement of x-radiation
A Lt Colonel in the RCAMA commanding the 14th Field Ambulance "Active" and "Reserve" in World War II

From records preserved in the Saint John General Hospital since 1922, superficial x-ray therapy dosage was recorded (for example) thus (I never used pastilles):

5 mA ; 3mm. Aluminium Filter; 8"–10" distance
8" spark gap; aperture and shielding varied for obvious reasons—cones as required.

The conditions treated in 1922–23 are interesting in retrospect: cancer of the breast, post-operatively as well as for palliation without operation; sarcoma of bone and chest etc; warts, acne, carbuncle, furuncle, angina pectoris, pruritus ani, enlarged and diseased tonsils, deafness, whooping cough, enlarged thymus, leukaemia, paronychia, ringworm of nails and scalp, favus, blastomycosis, rodent ulcer, cancer of the lip, Hodgkin's Disease, epidermoid cancer, tuberculus glands, keloid eczema, lupus, haemangioma, melanoma, simple adenitis, simple goitre, cancer of the thyroid, mastitis, diphtheria carriers (tonsils), tinea barbae, cancer of the uterus, psoriasis, asthma, parotid tumour, moles, papilloma, hypertrophy of the prostate gland and menorrhagia.

Much of the above is my own experience because for a long time I was alone in the specialty in New Brunswick. I was fortunate in having x-ray friends in Montréal, Toronto, Detroit, Cleveland, Boston and New York, and I visited all of them at frequent intervals. For many years the Atlantic Coast Meetings of the Radiological Society of North America at Atlantic City in January was a get-together of the greatest value providing an opportunity to hear the best men on the continent and to make new friends who corresponded freely on x-ray problems. The meetings of the New England group of x-ray men was another profitable source of inspiration.

Carl Darnell, physicist for the Victor X-ray Corporation (GE) visited Saint John on occasion and Montréal more frequently, and I learned much from him. Real physics was always beyond me, but Carl wrote out rule-of-thumb instructions which even I could follow, and his "jam sessions" were tops.

Dr Stephen Johnson and Dr Wm Eagar of Halifax were staunch colleagues and personal friends. Dr A H Pirie of Montréal and Dr Case of Battle Creek guided my steps in the American societies, and Dr Gordon Richards was an inspiring friend from the earliest days.

Dr McGuffin of Calgary and Dr Currie McMillan of Winnipeg were long-time friends and correspondents, while Dr Hamish McIntosh and Dr Prowd of Vancouver were friends first and brother radiologists always.

After a while other radiologists entered practice in New Brunswick, and, as time passed, good radiology departments developed in St Joseph's Hospital in Saint John with Dr EA Petrie in charge, Dr Hynes in Fredericton; and Dr Ripley in Moncton, to name but a few. Later, a large number of young, eager and forward-looking certified radiologists began to work in other centres.

As an aging radiologist, scarred by loss of skin from face and fingers, I feel an inward assurance that in my next incarnation, or whatever life follows this one, I have nothing to fear. I have experienced it in this life. If I had it to do all over, I would say, "Remembrance is sufficient of the beauty I have seen."

Acknowledgement:
This account was found in the Canadian Association of Radiologists' archives among material collected by Dr EM Crawford. It has been reproduced with slight editing but no changes of substance.

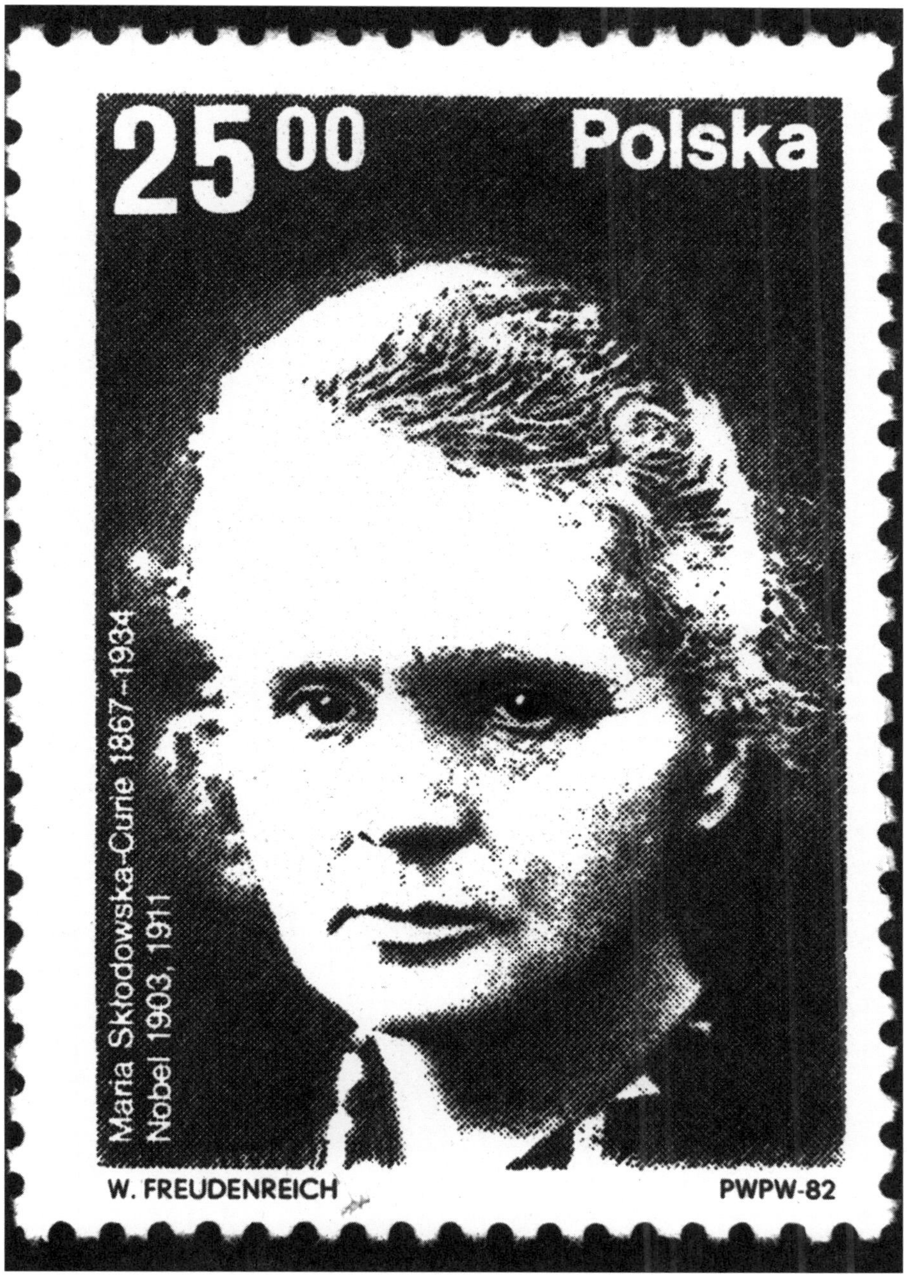
25 00
Polska
Maria Skłodowska-Curie 1867–1934
Nobel 1903, 1911
W. FREUDENREICH
PWPW-82

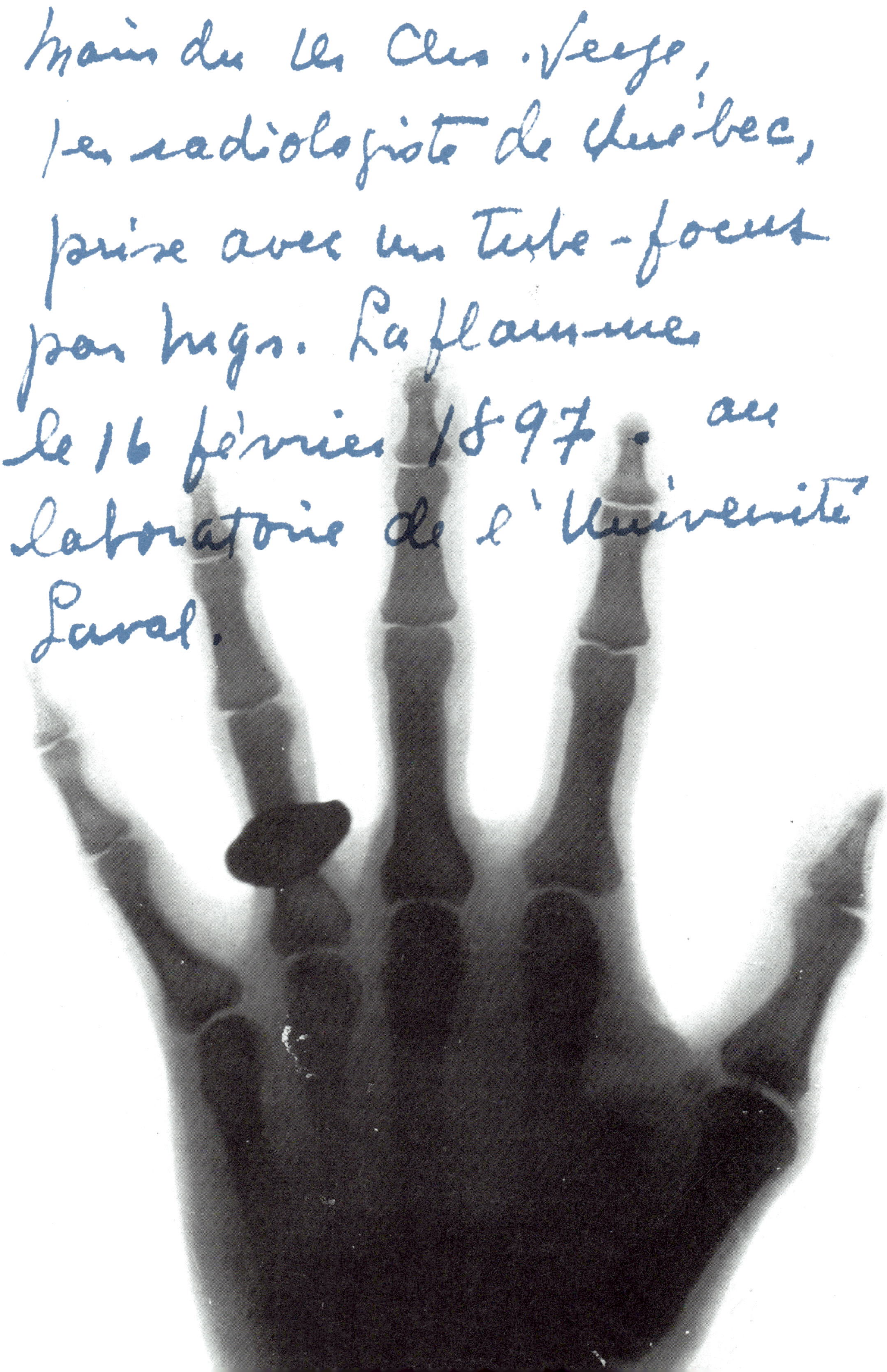
Main du Dr Chs. Verge,
1er radiologiste de Québec,
prise avec un tube-focus
par Mgr. Laflamme
le 16 février 1897. au
laboratoire de l'Université
Laval.

Chapter V • *Histoire de la*

Radiologie au Canada Français

Louis-Philippe Bélisle

Le 6 juin 1958, la Société Canadienne-française d'Électro-Radiologie célébrait par un grand dîner le 30ième anniversaire de sa fondation. A cette occasion, le Dr L-P Bélisle a esquissé brièvement l'histoire des débuts de la Radiologie au Canada français et les circonstances qui ont entouré la fondation de la Société. Celle-ci a rendu, on le sait, d'inappréciables services dans l'élaboration des standards de formation professionnelle des radiologistes, dans le recrutement du personnel compétent pour nos services hospitaliers, etc.

L'Union médicale du Canada félicite chaleureusement la Société, ses membres-fondateurs et tous ses membres actuels. C'est pour rendre hommage à l'oeuvre méritoire de nos radiologistes canadiens-français que nous commençons aujourd'hui la publication de cette "Histoire de la Radiologie au Canada français." écrite par le docteur Bélisle.

NOS PIONNIERS— LES PROFESSEURS DE PHYSIQUES Mgr J-C-K Laflamme (1896–1902)

Main du Dr Charles Verge, 1er radiologiste de Québec, prise avec un tube-focus par Mgr Laflamme le 16 février 1897 au laboratoire de l'Université de Laval

Au moment où William Conrad Röntgen, ayant déjà l'intuition de la géniale découverte dont il allait doter le monde quelques jours plus tard annonçait à sa femme " je ne rentrerai pas ce soir " et s'enfermait dans son laboratoire, six médecins canadiens-français en stage à Paris: Lesage, Rousseau, Lasnier, De Blois, Martel et St-Denis se réunissaient à l'Hôtel des Balcons, rue Casimir-de-la-Vigne pour fêter joyeusement la Noël.

Lesage et Rousseau: deux grands noms de la médecine canadienne-française, deux personnalités attachantes, tous deux futurs doyens de la faculté, l'un à Montréal, l'autre à Québec.

Quant à Lasnier et De Blois, alors attachés à l'hôpital d'Auteuil à titre d'interne bénévole, ils joueront un rôle important dans l'histoire de la radiologie au Canada français. C'est donc à Paris même que ceux qui devaient devenir nos initiateurs en radiologie reçurent le choc de la stupéfiante découverte, en virent les premières applications françaises, sous l'impulsion d'Antoine Béclère, alors que déjà, les dernières semaines de janvier, la traînée de poudre des expérimentateurs se répand comme une fièvre dans le monde entier.

A Paris, une main d'enfant radiographiée par Oudin et Berthélémy confirme devant l'Académie des Sciences le diagnostic de TB osseuse posé par le professeur Lannelongue. Puis, Montpellier, puis le Guy's Hospital de Londres; puis Genève où Dufour exhibe à la Société Médicale ses radiographies de poissons et de grenouilles.

Aux États-Unis, la première radiographie est réalisée le 27 janvier 1896 par le professeur Wright à l'Université de Yale. Au Canada, ce n'est que le 6 février que *La Presse* avec presque un mois de retard sur le *New-York Times* (9 janvier) annonçait la découverte de Röntgen au Canada français.[1]

Mais l'Université McGill n'avait pas perdu de temps et c'est la veille même (5 février) que le professeur John Cox y réussissait la première radiographie canadienne.[2]

A cette époque, l'Université Laval de Québec avait comme professeur de physique un homme de grande intelligence et d'un rare savoir: Monseigneur J-C-K Laflamme, Supérieur du petit Séminaire, deux fois secrétaire de l'Université Laval, professeur de sciences naturelles durant quatre ans. Monseigneur Laflamme se fit chez-nous, malgré l'amorphisme de l'enseignement des sciences de l'époque fin-de-siècle, le fervent apôtre de la physique, de l'électricité, de la géologie, de la botanique, de la météréologie et même de l'astronomie. Il fut le premier à préconiser dans des conférences publiques extrêmement populaires où ses dons d'orateur faisaient un bel effet, l'exploitation de nos ressources hydrauliques et des richesses de notre sous-sol québécois. Ses conférences à Québec et à Louiseville en 1880 et 1888, sur les dépôts de gaz naturel, firent gloser tous les journaux de l'époque. "Toute la province, disait un jour Benjamin Sulte dans un réunion mondaine, connaissait l'existence du gaz naturel; mais il lui manquait *la flamme*." Au cours d'un voyage d'études en Europe en 1881, il est élu membre de la Société Française de Géologie. Il publie, à son tour son excellent Traité de Minéralogie et de Géologie, le premier du genre au Canada français.

En 1891, une mise en congé du Séminaire lui permet de s'adonner à ses travaux préférés. Durant dix années, il parcourra maintes régions québécoises en vue de relevés géologiques: le Saguenay, le Lac St.-Jean, la Beauce, Charlevoix, les vallées du St-Maurice et de la rivière Batiscan.

Il affectionne en particulier la Minéralogie et la Paléontologie; on le voit souvent en compagnie de quelques amis Anglais[4] piolet en main, fouiller les sous-sols des maisons en démolition. Il étudie passionnément les schistes de Cap Diamant et les dépôts aurifères de la Beauce. Il découvre même, au cours de ses périgrinations—fait unique dans notre histoire minière—un gisement d'émeraude au Saguenay.

Il prononce toujours des conférences très écoutées. Il fonde en 1884 le "Club des Naturalistes" et commence à monter patiemment ce qui deviendra, grâce à lui, l'excellent musée actuel de Géologie et de Paléontologie de l'Université Laval. Nommé la même année membre de l'Association Britannique pour l'Avancement des Sciences, il innove dans le milieu québécois en prenant peu après une part active à son Congrès de Montréal.

Un nouveau voyage d'études le ramène en Europe en 1888. A peine de retour, il cherche sur place pour le compte de la Commission Géologique Fédérale dont le président Robert Bell est un de ses fervents amis, l'existence de champs pétrolifères en Anticosti.

Mais voilà, en 1888, ce géoloque impénitent qui devient dans notre province le pionnier génial d'une science assez nouvelle et peu connue: la Météréologie. En 20 ans (de 1888 à 1908) il ne fera pas moins de trois enquêtes sur "les conditions de naissance et la direction des orages dans la région québécoise", croyant avec raison rendre service à l'Agriculture, au Transport et au Tourisme. Mais hélas! la distribution de 1500 questionnaires-réponses aux curés, aux vicaires et autres observateurs bénévoles n'amène qu'une rentrée trop maigre pour pouvoir tirer des conclusions scientifiques....Et c'est avec amertume que Mgr Laflamme doit abandonner la partie.

En 1889, il est nommé membre de la Société Royale et président de la section de Géologie.

En 1891, il participe au Congrès International de Géologie à Washington et devient en même temps membre de la Société Américaine de Géologie. "C'est avec Mgr Laflamme", note avec humour René Bureau,[5] "qu'est né à l'Université Laval cette louable habitude de participer aux Congrès. Avant lui, cette mode n'était pas très en vogue, c'est avec raison qu'on a dit un jour de l'Université Laval "qu'elle n'était pas sorteuse."[6] Nommé Évêque de Chicoutimi en 1892, il refuse; cet homme de science est comme pris de panique devant les responsabilités officielles du devoir pastoral; il croit qu'il peut rendre plus de services dans l'enseignement scientifique. Il écrit à l'abbé Huard, alors résident à Chicoutimi: "Vous n'avez pas des coeurs tellement de pierre qu'il faille le marteau d'un évêque géologue pour les cliver."[7] Il ne devait accepter le titre de

Monsignor que quelques années plus tard.

C'est à cette période que se place l'incident...géologico-comique entre Mgr Laflamme et M Horace Dumais, arpenteur géologue du Lac St-Jean. Frappé par la grandeur des rives de la rivière Saguenay, Arthur Buies avait invoqué l'action d'un cataclysme préhistorique pour en expliquer la formation; Mgr Laflamme à son tour, voyait dans ces bouleversements le résultat de causes géologiques beaucoup plus classiques et refusait de donner dans le romantisme littéraire de Buies. Mais M Dumais avait relevé le gant dans un article extrêmement prolixe publié dans le "Naturaliste Canadien" où il prenait à partie de façon cinglante les prétentions scientifiques de Mgr Laflamme. Une "prise de bec" nouveau genre pour l'époque était en perspective!...Mais Mgr Laflamme fait la sourde oreille; on a beau lui promettre d'élaguer dans le texte de Dumais toute allusion personnelle ou blessante, rien ne le fait se désister de son silence.

Il écrit à l'abbé Huard, alors directeur du "Naturaliste Canadien":

La craque de M. Dumais me fascine; mais elle me fait peur. S'il avait publié un semblant de carte, on y verrait plus clair, mais nous n'avons eu qu'une interminable série de noms, impossibles à retenir, que l'on prononce à la romaine ou à la canadienne. De plus, ce savant parait très batailleur. Il manie la science un peu comme les manchons de la charrue. C'est effrayant. Voilà pourquoi je suis très perplexe.[8]

Je ne sais que vous répondre à propos du travail de M. Dumais. J'ai lu le susdit travail, il y a déjà des mois, de sorte que j'ai un peu perdu de vue comment il est bâti. Le souvenir qui m'en est resté, c'est qu'il y a un bon nombre de pages et qu'il manque un peu de sens au point de vue géologique. Quant à vous dire ce qu'il y aurait à retrancher, j'y renonce. Mes souvenirs sont trop vagues.

Toutefois, je puis bien vous dire une chose, c'est que je serais on ne peut plus marri si vous retranchiez ce qui me regarde. Ce n'est pas malin du tout; il y a sur ce point des choses qui arrivent fort bien tout en n'étant pas de nature à faire fouetter un chat.

Encore une fois, mon impression première a été que cette étude est un peu trop longue, pas assez nerveuse, et comme thèse générale, repose sur une interprétation quelquefois fantaisiste d'observations incomplètes, ne s'appuyant pas sur des connaissances géologiques suffisantes.

Publiez, mais ne retranchez pas ce qui me concerne, c'est ce qu'il y a de plus joli.

Ce qu'il y aurait de mieux, ce serait que l'auteur abrégeât (3 fois). Qu'il cite d'abord ses observations, puis qu'il discute sérieusement à la lumière des lois reconnues en géologie. Son travail y perdra énormément en dimension et y gagnera beaucoup en valeur.

Voilà pour notre gouverne personnelle. Je serais vraiment chagrin si mes paroles empêchaient la publication des pages de Monsieur Dumais. Elles renferment beaucoup de bon (les faits). Il s'agit d'émonder. Mais qu'il laisse bien tout ce qui me regarde, c'est le plus drôle.[9]

Et c'est ainsi qu'on ne sut jamais si la "craque de Dumais" méritait plus de respect que l'hypothèse Laflamme sur le travail classique de l'érosion après le retrait de la mer Champlain! En 1897 M Fitzpatrick informe Mgr Laflamme que M Laurier désire le voir représenter le Canada au Congrès International de Géologie de St-Petersbourg. Il accepte après un moment d'hésitation et part pour la Russie. Puis de passage à Paris, il complète par des achats l'instrumentation scientifique de l'Université Laval. Il ne revient pas assez tôt pour assister à Toronto, au Congrès de l'Association Britannique pour l'Avancement des Sciences; mais une communication de lui y est lue en français. C'est en français d'ailleurs que Mgr Laflamme, patriote convaincu, s'adressait toujours, où que ce soit, dans les congrès scientifiques.

Nommé Chevalier de la Légion d'Honneur en 1898, membre titulaire de la Société Belge d'Astronomie en 1904, il continua à faire connaître, par son enseignement, ses expériences et sa participation scientifique aux congrès, le Canada français aux quatre coins du monde, jusqu'à sa mort survenue en 1910 au Séminaire, près des collections et des musées qu'il avait organisés grâce au patient labeur de ses mains.

J'ai omis volontairement pour y revenir ici, le rôle de pionnier, joué par Mgr Laflamme dans le Québec au moment de la découverte des rayons-X.

Membre de plusieurs sociétés scientifiques, dont la Société Française de Physique, Mgr Laflamme entretenait depuis avril 1891 une correspondance suivie avec son trésorier M Gay. Celui-ci ne paraît pas outre mesure frappé par la découverte du 22 décembre; en effet, sa lettre qui parvient à Mgr Laflamme au début de janvier 1896 ne contient que de banaux souhaits du Nouvel An.

Nous avons vu que Wright à Yale réussissait le 27 janvier sa première radiographie, alors que le même honneur au Canada revient au professeur John Cox de McGill. Passionné d'expériences physiques, Mgr Laflamme aurait pu au même titre que Wright de Yale ou Cox de McGill revendiquer l'honneur d'une première radiographie sur le continent américain. "En effet, raconte le docteur J Edmour Perron, le laboratoire de physique de l'Université Laval est équipé d'un grand nombre de tubes de Crookes, dont les uns sont montés pour l'étude des rayons

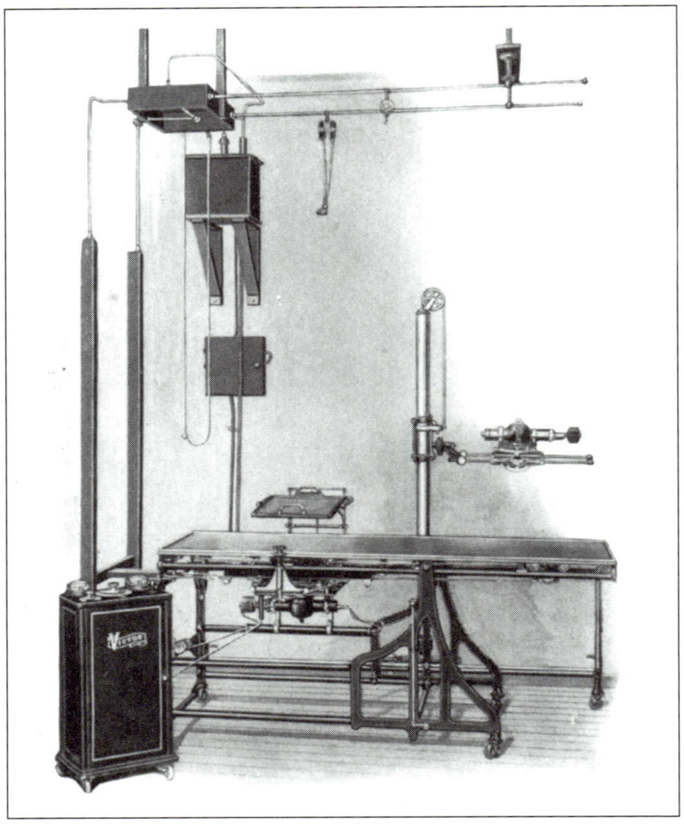

En haut
Equipement complet de diagnostic radiographique et fluoroscopique, avec un tube Coolidge de type "Radiateur"

Droit
Table motorisée de modèl Victor (circa 1920)

cathodiques, et ont été fabriqués par Radiguet et Massiot, de Paris. Le laboratoire possède ces tubes (d'après un catalogue) depuis plusieurs années avant 1896. Il y a en plus trois bobines de Ruhmkorff capables de donner dix, quinze et vingt centimètres d'étincelle, puis un interrupteur Carpentier qui s'adapte à ces bobines."[10]

Mais ce n'est que le 12 février, puis deux jours plus tard que Mgr Laflamme tente sans succès ses premières expériences, avec 20 et 25 minutes de pose. "Le procédé est simple, mais la lumière si faible", note avec scepticisme le chroniqueur du Séminaire. "On se demande comment les choses peuvent se passer comme on dit!"[11]

Le 17 février, lettre de M Gay, la première où il soit fait allusion aux rayons X, encore que celle-ci soit des plus discrète et toute dénuée de commentaires. Il y donne à Mgr Laflamme certaines indications sur la façon de procéder. Un catalogue d'appareillage radiologique Ducretet, étonnamment varié pour l'époque accompagnait cette lettre.[12]

Durant le mois de mars, il tente plusieurs expériences toujours infructueuses. Enfin le 2 avril 1896: "Mgr Laflamme qui avait fait hier des expériences photographiques à la Röntgen a reçu aujourd'hui les clichés de la Maison Livernois. Ils sont admirablement réussis." Et le 5 avril: "Mgr Laflamme a continué aujourd'hui ses expériences avec les rayons X. Il a radiographié la main et le pied d'un enfant. Le petit bonhomme a du poser au-delà d'une demi-heure et a trouvé le temps très long."[13]

Le 18 mai, John Cox de McGill, devenu grand expert, remercie Mgr Laflamme pour son envoi de radiographies. Le monde entier, depuis quelques mois étudiait avec fièvre les implications de la découverte nouvelle.

Le 16 mars, à l'Académie de Médecine de Paris, Pinard exhibait la radiographie d'un utérus gravide extirpé en 1894 et conservé dans l'alcool. Les observations se multipliaient: on annonçait maintenant la possibilité d'observer au fluoroscope[14] le crâne, le coeur, l'aorte, les poumons, etc...

Le Kinescope, frère de lait des rayons Röntgen, fait aussi ses premiers pas; et c'est dans la ferveur générale que le premier cinéma "Lumière" ouvre ses portes au 96 de la rue St-Laurent. Déjà la jurisprudence s'élabore sur des données médico-légales nouvelles fournies par la jeune radiologie. Dès le 10 février, un individu du nom de Cunning, blessé d'une balle à l'épaule est radiographié par Cox qui localise la balle, permet son extraction, exhibe ses radiographies en cour où elles produisent, on s'en doute bien, un effet dramatique et les verse au dossier comme pièce à conviction avec l'assentiment du juge.[15] Quelques mois plus tard d'autres radiographies d'une épaule prises par Cox apportaient un témoignage concluant dans une cause demeurée célèbre.[16] Un accident de voiture survenu à l'automne 1896 dans le midi de la France causa une fracture de la clavicule. Une radiographie ayant démontré l'existence d'une consolidation vicieuse, des dommages-intérêts de 1500 francs furent accordés par le tribunal civil de Marseille.

Que de chemin parcouru déjà, depuis 1862, alors que Nélaton fouillait de ses sondes aveugles à la recherche d'une balle, la blessure ouverte du pied de Garibaldi! Ici dans la province, le monde médical commence à s'émouvoir. Et cependant, le 6 octobre, à l'hôpital Notre-Dame de Montréal dans son allocution d'ouverture des cours de clinique médicale, le docteur E-P Benoît ne fait aucune allusion à la découverte stupéfiante qui avait déjà commencé de révolutionner le monde scientifique.

Mais c'est plutôt le public non médical que les rayons röntgen jettent dans un état voisin de la panique. Il éprouve l'appréhension bien légitime qu'au train où vont les choses, rien de plus intime de l'être, dans son corps ou sa pensée ne pourrait résister à sa pénétration—*nil in ultum remanebit*—Et les rebatteurs de journaux populaires et les exploiteurs ès publicité d'entrer dans la danse. Il faut lire ces coupures de réclame charlatanesque que le regretté docteur Edmour Perron s'est amusé à colliger dans les journaux de l'époque. Il y eut, entre autres dans la Presse[17] cette annonce d'un tissu supposé imperméable aux rayons X: "Attention, Mesdames, à ces porteurs de rayons X dont la réputation infâme se répand de plus en plus, et qui porteurs d'un instrument qui leur permet de vous "ombrographier" vont apercevoir votre photographie intime, l'argent que vous portez et vos bijoux. Le textile Buckskin, imperméable à la pluie, aux vents et aux rayons X constitue la protection assurée contre ce malappris à vingt-cinq sous la verge".

La litanie des commentaires benêts sur les pouvoirs sans limites des nouveaux rayons allait de la révélation du contenu du portefeuille au dosage de pureté du charbon à chauffage. Certains hommes de sciences, aussi, donnaient dans l'euphorie générale. Thomas Edison lui-même, perdant toute retenue, ne désespérait pas de photographier la pensée. Durant toute l'année 1896, partout à Montréal par Mgr Choquette, professeur de physique à St-Hyacinthe, comme à Québec, par Mgr Laflamme, les conférences, très nombreuses sur le sujet, avaient la cote d'amour. Un public de plus ou moins grande culture s'y pressait, avide d'apprendre, et de s'amuser à observer au fluoroscope la structure intraabdominale d'un participant bénévole ou le squelette d'un ami.

Le 20 mai, dit le chroniqueur du Séminaire, grande séance

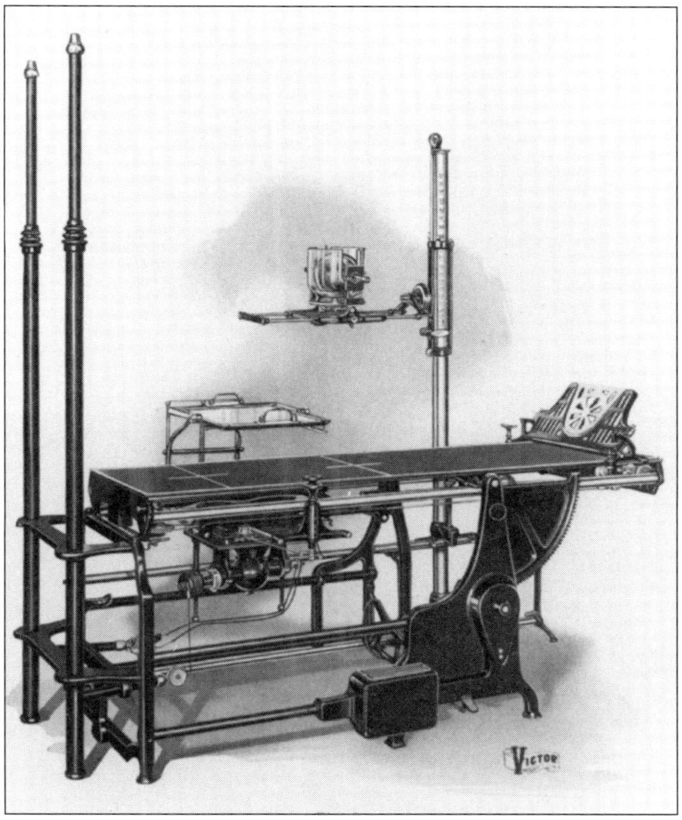

devant une assemblée d'archevêques, d'évêques et de prêtres. L'auditoire a été vivement intéressé. On a vu et regardé à travers un chanoine au grand amusement de tous.[18]

A votre prochain voyage, écrivait Mgr Laflamme à l'abbé Huard je vous photographierai l'intérieur.[19]

Il était alors de mise, lors de passage d'un visiteur distingué de lui radiographier la main *honoris causa*. C'est ainsi que lors de sa visite à l'Université Laval en avril 1897, la main de Mgr Merry del Val fut radiographiée par Mgr Laflamme et le document envoyé en hommage à SS Pie X.

En novembre 1896, nouveaux pas en avant marqués par le deuxième Congrès panaméricain de médecine à Mexico. Presque toutes les communications portent sur la radiologie: applications chirurgicales, recherches de corps étrangers, traumatologie, tumeurs, pathologie osseuse, anévrismes thoraciques, grossesses, etc...Pour la première fois, on constate que les rayons X ne détruisent pas les microbes.

Du domaine de la physique pure, la radiologie devient rapidement partie intégrante de la science médicale. Les physiciens s'en désintéressent quelque peu. M Gay écrit à Mgr Laflamme: "Vous recevez, je pense, régulièrement les communications de la Société de physique. Vous voyez que les rayons occupent toujours beaucoup de séances:... toujours, hélas" les rayons X..."[20]

Et un peu plus tard: "Ce sont les médecins qui en ce moment s'occupent partout des rayons X. Les physiciens paraissent avoir renoncé, pour le moment, à déterminer leur nature. Les médecins y trouvent un moyen pratique de voir dans l'intérieur du corps et d'éclairer ainsi leur diagnostic dans un grand nombre de cas."[21]

En juin 1897, M Marcy présente à l'Académie de médecine de Paris un appareil radiologique imaginé par Contremoulins pour le repérage des projectiles et corps étrangers. Le professeur Le Dentu qui l'a utilisé l'a trouvé merveilleux.

Mais tout progrès scientifique porte en lui-même sa rançon: dès le début de 1897, nous "avons" nos premiers "brûlés". "Sans que l'on sache exactement pourquoi, dit *L'Union médicale* [22] ces rayons provoquent de l'inflammation de la peau et même de la dépilation."

Le premier brûlé, note le docteur Edmour Perron,[23] un certain abbé O'Gara, fils du juge O'Gara, d'Ottawa, et professeur d'anglais au Séminaire de St-Hyacinthe, fut atteint d'une radiodermite grave de la paroi abdominale. On ignore s'il était un "patient" de Mgr Choquette et s'il fut "brûlé" à Saint-Hyacinthe. A la recherche d'un calcul rénal, on a sans doute tenté des radiographies abdominales avec des temps de pose fantastiques!

Si nous n'avons pas encore vu de médecins canadiens-français à l'oeuvre, c'est qu'en Europe même les applications proprement médicales de la Radiologie ne font que commencer; le "Traité de Radioscopie et Radiographie cliniques de Précision" de Guilleminot paraîtra en 1900, alors qu'arrivent à Québec les premiers appareils radiologiques de la maison Radiguet et Massiot.

D'autre part, il était normal, dans notre province que les premiers à s'intéresser à la nouvelle découverte fussent des professeurs de physique, puisqu'ils avaient à leur disposition, tel Mgr Laflamme, des cabinets de physique assez bien outillés avec tubes de Crookes, bobines de Ruhmkorff et interrupteurs. Il faut saluer avec reconnaissance ces prêtres qui ont été chez-nous, dans leur laboratoire de collège les vrais précurseurs de nos aînés médecins: Mgr Choquette à St-Hyacinthe, l'abbé Désilets à Nicolet, l'abbé Des Troismaisons—ô ironie—à Trois-Rivières; mais Mgr J-C-K Laflamme fut de tous le plus doué, celui qui par ses talents extraordinaires fut le levain dans la pâte et le véritable précurseur de notre Société.

De Blois, Charles Verge, fils et Lasnier (1902–1928)

C'est avec ces quatre noms que débute l'ère proprement médicale de la Radiologie canadienne-française.

Le docteur Charles de Blois était né à Québec en novembre 1867. Reçu médecin en 1892, il était parti pour l'Europe en 1895. Il était avec son ami Lasnier, au moment de la découverte des rayons X, interne bénévole à l'hôpital d'Auteuil. Désireux de se perfectionner en maladies nerveuses et en agents physiques, il passe l'année 1896 à Munich avec Baumgarten. Puis il revient au Canada et se fixe à Trois-Rivières où il organise la clinique d'électricité médicale et d'hydrothérapie la plus élaborée du pays pour l'époque. En 1900, en même temps que la ville de Québec, il procède à l'installation d'appareillage radiographique. Cette même année, il retourne en Europe où il suivra les cours d'Apostoli et d'Antoine Béclère. Il y retournera d'ailleurs plusieurs fois par la suite soit en 1908, 1917, 1927 et 1930, toujours désireux de joindre au plaisir de ses voyages celui de suivre quelques cours de perfectionnement en hydrothérapie, électrothérapie ou radiologie.

De Blois pratiqua toujours à Trois-Rivières où il acquit une réputation considérable comme électrothérapeute et hydrothérapeute. Bien qu'il fut moins préoccupé de radiologie proprement dite, il y consacrait quand même une part de ses activités.

Il fonda dans cette ville, avec le docteur Normand, la première école de garde-malade de la région. Dès 1902, l'année même où Antoine Béclère publie "La Radioscopie et la Radiographie des Organes splanchniques", à l'occasion du 2e Congrès International d'électrologie et de radiologie médicales à Berne, le docteur Charles De Blois publiait ce qui fut, sans doute, le premier travail du genre au Canada francais: "L'Hydrothérapie, I'Electricité et les rayons X". De nombreuses communications devaient s'échelonner durant cinquante ans, jusqu'à sa mort, sur ces diverses disciplines qui faisaient l'objet de ses préoccupations. Fervent chrétien, honoré de plusieurs décorations papales, ce pionnier de l'électrothérapie et de la radiologie médicales a laissé chez ceux qui l'on connu le souvenir d'un compagnon charmant et qui fut, de surplus avec le docteur Brochu, l'un des fondateurs de l'Association des Médecins de langue française de l'Amérique du Nord.

Je ne mentionne que pour mémoire, le nom du docteur Charles Verge, fils. Famille de Loyalistes anglais de la Nouvelle-Angleterre, les Verge étaient venus se fixer en Nouvelle-Écosse après le traité qui consacrait l'indépendance américaine. Son père, qui portait également le nom de Charles, avait eu le rare privilège d'assister au baptême du grand-père Nelson Verge, converti au catholicisme. Depuis lors, les Verge adoptèrent non seulement la religion, mais la langue du pays et le jeune Charles Verge, fils, après des études à Nicolet, avait terminé son cours de médecine à l'Université Laval. Il fit, de 1893 à 1903 plusieurs voyages en Europe pour des cours de perfectionnement et fit alors connaissance avec la radiologie. On le retrouve en 1902, à titre de trésorier membre du conseil des Médecins de langue française de l'Amérique du Nord.

Il entre à l'Hôtel-Dieu en 1904, pour y exercer, à temps partiel, la radiologie. Il était un grand voyageur qui sous son flegme demeuré britannique possédait, paraît-il, un goût prononcé pour les beaux-arts, la musique, la peinture... Il fut, lui aussi parmi les premiers de nos praticiens qui s'intéressèrent à la radiologie.

Le docteur Henri Lasnier. Reçu médecin en 1895, le docteur Lasnier part pour Paris où nous le retrouvons en compagnie de De B1ois et des autres s'apprêtant à fêter Noël 1895 en sablant le champagne, à l'Hôtel des Balcons de la rue Casimir-de-La-Vigne. Intéressé surtout à la médecine et à la chirurgie, le docteur Lasnier étudie à l'institut Pasteur avec Roux, Borel et Metchnikoff; mais il contracte lui aussi le microbe scientifique de l'époque: la radiologie. Après un stage dans cette spécialité à la Salpêtrière et un séjour de 2 ans comme House-Surgeon au London Hospital, il ne revient à Montréal qu'en 1900. Lasnier est probablement à titre officiel, notre premier radiologiste montréalais. Très au courant des dernières instrumentations européennes, il est équipé d'un tube portatif Gaiffe qui lui a coûté trente dollars; il fait paraît-il, avec succès beaucoup de diagnostic et de radiothérapie; ce qui ne l'empêcha pas de publier et de façon très consciencieuse nombre de communications à la Société de Montréal et que nous retrouvons dans l'Union médicale de l'époque. Il se rendit surtout célèbre en radiographiant en 1907 l'honorable Pérodeau pour une fracture de la rotule et le géant Beaupré. D'une stature d'environ 7 pieds 2 pouces, celui-ci voulait sans doute être rassuré de façon définitive sur l'activité de ses os "longs"!

En 1910, nous le retrouvons dans l'ouest canadien où il pratique pendant cinq ans. Il part, en 1915, à titre de médecin militaire pour Malte. Il y exerce ses remarquables talents de radiologiste, de même qu'à Londres en 1916 où il a charge d'un service radiologique considérable. Il séjourne encore quelque peu dans l'ouest, après son retour en 1917. Puis il pratique ensuite à Québec de nombreuses années. Jadis ami de Sir Wilfrid Laurier sur les bancs du collège de l'Assomption, Lasnier avait, paraît-il, un goût naturel pour la polémique de caractère politique. Il est impossible, à distance, de démêler l'écheveau de ces prises de becs, qui nous apparaissent avec le recul du temps, plutôt comiques dans leur indignation furibonde. Il écrit un jour au docteur Edmour Perron: "Je subis en ce moment l'étreinte de la féroce politique libérale. Je me débats et râle entre les mains du régime de la dynastie qui ne m'aime pas parce que je me suis rangé du côté de Baptiste". Le docteur Edmour Perron est souvent son confident, dans des lettres d'une indignation élégiaque. Les deux cibles les plus familières et les plus honnies dans ses poèmes (il rimaille même des couplets vengeurs qu'il déclame aux amis) semblent avoir été le ministre de la Marine et Robert Taschereau. Même dans les dernières lettres que j'aie pu trouver de lui, il continuera de les vouer aux gémonies dans des quatrains emportés:

Ils mènent le pays à leur guise.
Se prennent tous pour des ducs de Guise,
Mais ils trouveront leur Cyrano
Lavergne leur passera l'anneau.

Malgré l'impétueuse originalité de son talent, Lasnier demeure pour nous inoubliable à un titre spécial: celui d'avoir publié en 1910 une revue de spécialité intitulée " Les rayons X, revue mensuelle illustrée", alors qu'il était radiologiste à l'hôpital Ste-Justine de Montréal. Malheureusement, elle ne fit pas long feu et mourut après parution de sept numéros qui sont pratiquement introuvables aujourd'hui.[24]

Léo Pariseau, Edmour Perron et Léglius Gagnier, père

Frère de Lasnier par la truculence, Léo Pariseau a beaucoup plus de droits que lui à notre reconnaissance. Docteur en médecine de Laval de Montréal en 1904, il fut de 1906 à 1909 le radiologiste de l'hôpital Notre-Dame. Après quelques années comme professeur à l'École Polytechnique, il devient hygiéniste à la ville de Sherbrooke où il exerce en même temps comme radiologiste à l'hôpital St-Vincent. Radiologiste durant la guerre à l'hôpital militaire Laval de St-Cloud, il devient en 1919 directeur du service d'électroradiologie de l'Hôtel-Dieu, poste qu'il occupa jusqu'à sa mort en I938.

"Léo Pariseau," écrit Paul Dumas,[25] "arborait une barbe carrée, tigrée, batailleuse, un nez bourbon couperosé par les rayons X et par les grands crus et derrière ses lunettes, des petits yeux pétillants de vivacité et d'esprit auxquels rien n'échappait du spectacle du monde...Toute sa vie, (il) demeura l'exemple vivant du non-conformisme."

Un coeur d'or dans une peau de lion. Il demeura toujours un humaniste impénitent passionnément intéressé à toutes les manifestations de l'esprit et de la culture où qu'elles fussent dans le monde; il a péniblement amassé, à travers toutes les heures laborieuses de sa vie une bibliothèque scientifique et littéraire qui est sûrement avec celle du regretté docteur Edmour Perron la somme culturelle la plus considérable qui se soit jamais vue au Canada."

Son impétueux tempérament n'avait d'égal que sa droiture. Toutes les causes justes pouvaient faire appel à son dévouement sans limite. Pouvait-on lui démontrer l'existence d'une manoeuvre sournoise, qu'aussitôt, visière baissée, il partait en guerre contre l'oppresseur, qu'il clouait au pilori par son verbe châtié, incisif, dans des

POUR FAIRE DES OISEAUX SANS TÊTE[27]

Procurez-vous du veau qui ne soit point mort-né.
A ce choix, cependant personne n'est borné;
Mieux que du méchant veau du bon boeuf fait l'affaire,
Et l'important en somme, est de savoir quoi faire.
Coupez donc la "bidoche " en lanières très minces,
Grandeur quatre par deux. Et puis, augustes princes,
Sachez que vos morceaux, tailladés à merci,
Doivent, pour leur bien même, être battus aussi,
Pour les battre employez le rebord d'une assiette.
Dites, tout en battant: "A devenir paupiettes
Vous êtes condamnés, mais en plus d'être arcis,
Pour notre bon plaisir vous serez tous farcis.

Avant de prononcer la sentence terrible,
S'assurer qu'une farce est vraiment disponible.
On en fait de très bonne avec du porc haché
Des pommes ou du pain, le tout bien rabâché.
Au succulent mélange, en guise d'aromate,
S'ajoutent céleri, poivre, persil, tomate.
Il n'est pas de rigueur que tout cela soit cuit
Mais on sait qu'en cuisine "abondance ne nuit".
Ainsi donc laisser frire au moins un bon quart d'heure,
Dans une poêle où l'on a fait frire du beurre.

Lors donc que vous avez sous la main votre farce,
Soumise, prête à tout comme une simple garce
Et vos morceaux de veau encore tout pantelants
D'avoir été battus...avec les gestes lents
D'un bourreau coréen vous roulez vos paupiettes
Comme après un repas on roule les serviettes.

Le veau se débattra, cherchant à se détendre;
La farce voudra fuir, mais craignez d'être tendre.
Pour mieux les contenir, bardez-les de gros lard
Ou de bacon fumé. Transfixez-les d'un dard
Que vous improvisez avec un cure-bouche,
Ou bien ficelez-les. Qu'aucun cri ne vous touche!

Après quoi, frémissant d'un sadique plaisir
Laissant là vos paquets, vous les faites saisir
Par le chef-rôtisseur, sa femme ou sa..cocotte,
Et les faites jeter dans un pot dit "cocotte",
En voilà bien assez. Vous vous imaginez
A combien de tourments ces malheureux damnés,
Peuvent être soumis. C'est ainsi, par exemple,
Qu'on les fait..."revenir", et puis qu'on les contemple
En train de grésiller. Ceci fait, froidement
L'on doit lâcher ces mots: "Je veux qu'à ce tourment
Par le feu, l'on ajoute un bon ébouillantage
Avec du bouillon gras"—N'en dirai davantage.

Ma recette provient d'un livre canadien
Publié par Lauzon. Las! la femme de bien
Qui l'écrivit n'est plus.—O bonne Jeanne Anctil
Dieu vous garde avec lui. Amen, ainsi soit-il.

— *Dr Léopard*[28]

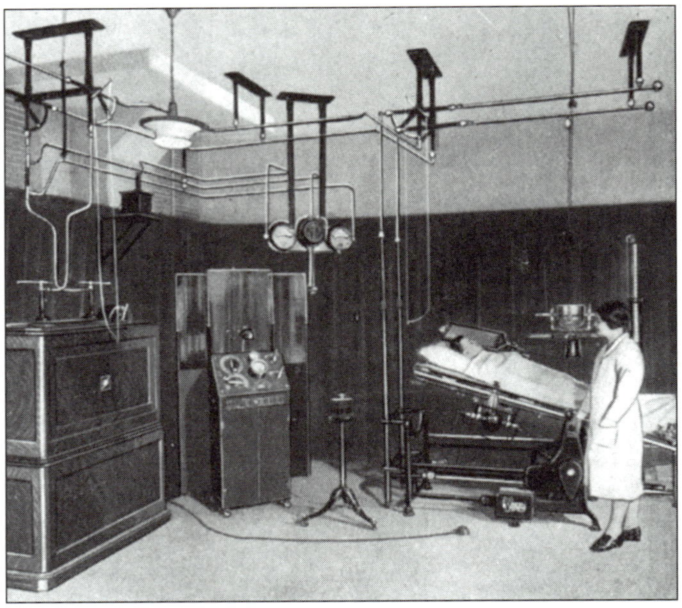

conférences fiévreuses, dans des lettres de polémiste de grande grande classe, ou dans d'impétueuses conférences de presse...Telles ces mises au point catégoriques qui ont caractérisé son intervention au cours de l'incident Dioclès dont plusieurs d'entre-vous, sans doute, se souviennent encore.[26] Mais ce polémiste vigoureux ne reniait jamais chez-lui le bon vivant. Dans le "Journal de l'Hôtel-Dieu" qu'il avait fondé et qui devait, malheureusement, disparaître à sa mort, on retrouve toute la gamme de son oeuvre littéraire remarquable, depuis les allusions vengeresses contre certains confrères charlatans jusqu'aux délicieuses miettes gastronomiques où nous retrouvons à la fois un fin lettré et un érudit souriant.

Je ne puis résister ici au plaisir de reproduire à l'intention des gourmets cette recette **[reproduced at left]**.

Fondateur de l'ACFAS dont il fut le premier président en 1924, Léo Pariseau a joué un rôle de premier plan dans la fondation de notre Société canadienne-française d'Electrologie et de Radiologie. "Les quelques médecins canadiens-français qui s'occupaient de ces spécialités, écrit le docteur Origène Dufresne, sentaient le besoin de se tenir pour étudier les nombreuses possibilités de leur spécialité. Mais d'autre part, il fallait rassurer les médecins et les chirurgiens de la province de Québec sur la valeur des agents physiques, que certains investigateurs trop zélés avaient discréditée."

Le pourfendeur de charlatans qu'était Léo Pariseau ne pouvait qu'acquiesser à ces arguments dont il s'entretenait souvent, depuis quelques années, avec le docteur Gagnier, père; et c'est au retour de celui-ci d'un voyage en Europe en 1927 que les pourparlers reprirent de plus belle et que fut décidé, en pratique, la fondation de la Société. Il restait à obtenir l'assentiment des collègues de Québec. Pariseau

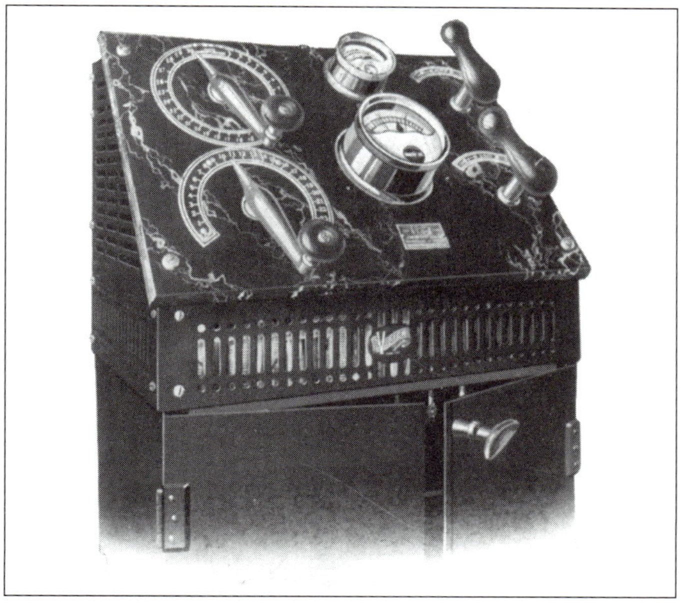

Extrême gauche
Equipement radiographique typique des années 1920

Gauche
Détail d'un tableau de contrôle qui démontre le cadran du transformateur automatique et la manette en position

Sous
Unité portative avec tube de Coolidge (circa 1920)

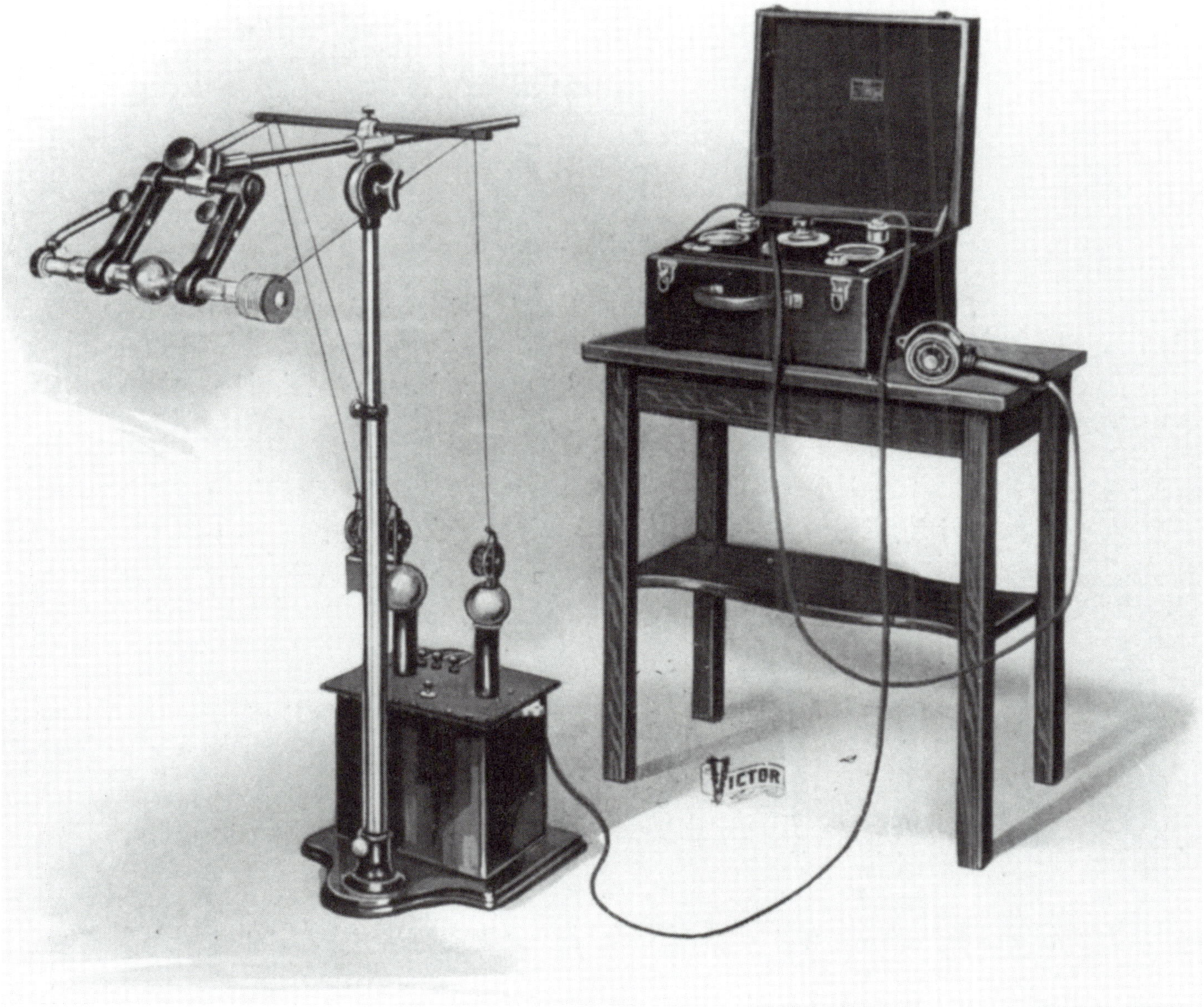

rédigea à leur intention une lettre adressée au docteur AR Potvin et qui constitue la charte fondamentale sur laquelle s'appuiera la rédaction de 1928: "La requête rédigée par le docteur Gagnier et signée par sept d'entre-nous parle par elle-même. Le but de la nouvelle société y est clairement défini. D'autres parts, vous connaissez la situation ici. Il s'agit d'empêcher notre profession de tomber aux mains d'une bande de farceurs qui lui fera plus de mal encore que les chiropraticiens et autres de la même farine," etc.

Pariseau, dès lors, n'abandonne plus la Société; ce rêve cher, qu'il partage avec son ami Gagnier prend lentement forme au cours des séances fiévreuses qui les réunissent tous les deux pour la rédaction des règlements, de la requête d'affiliation aux Sociétés françaises, etc. Familier des choses de l'héraldique, il dessine même l'insigne de la future Société. Enfin tout est à point; mais voilà que Comtois, lui aussi l'un des signataires de la requête, en route pour Québec où il doit les montrer à Perron, perd dans le train tous les documents, fruit de longues soirées d'étude. Pariseau est furieux; mais qu'à cela ne tienne, l'on recommence...

Et c'est le 22 mai 1928 que devait se tenir dans l'enthousiasme général la première séance de notre Société canadienne-française d'Electrologie et de Radiologie médicales. Pariseau, qui fut un fervent dès le début, devait peu à peu, la maladie aidant, s'isoler et ne plus marquer sa présence. Mais nous avons envers lui, comme envers Gagné et Perron une lourde dette de reconnaissance.

Autant Léo Pariseau était impétueux et impulsif, autant Edmour Perron était calme, mesuré, méticuleux... Sous le signe de l'amitié, le Cap Diamant souriait au Mont-Royal en bataille. Fils d'un médecin de campagne qui avait pratiqué jusqu'à 90 ans, dans les rangs les plus reculés de St-Charles de Bellechasse, le jeune Perron étudie la médecine à Laval et reçoit son diplôme en 1915. Neuf ans, il pratique son art dans le populeux quartier de Limoilou. Cette expérience humaine, ce contact avec la misère ne font qu'enrichir ses dons de naissance, qu'aiguiser le flair clinique aigu dont il fera preuve plus tard, autant que d'une maîtrise remarquable des sèches données mathématiques inhérentes à la physique des radiations. Parti pour Paris en 1924, il y coudoie les docteurs A-R Potvin, Albert Comtois et Hervé Lacharité. Il en revient en 1929 non seulement avec un appréciable bagage de radiologiste averti, mais féru de tout ce que l'humanisme de la vieille Europe avait de séduisant pour sa "teste bien faicte."

Il dirige durant 25 ans le service de Radiologie de l'hôpital du Saint-Sacrement. On lui confie la chaire d'Electrologie et de Radiologie médicales de l'Université Laval. Il suit de près tous les mouvements scientifiques, devient président de l'ACFAS dont il était l'un des membres fondateurs. Il y présente: "La merveilleuse découverte de Röntgen et son écho au Canada français", travail très au point où j'ai puisé nombre de renseignements qui figurent ici. A l'instar de Pariseau, il a amassé avec le goût sûr du fin lettré une bibliothèque remarquable. Il avait de l'érudit curieux de tout, les manies absurdes et délicieuses. S'il était parfois en retard au cours de Physiothérapie ou dans la correction des concours, c'est qu'il avait oublié l'heure à la lecture du "Quart livre" de Rabelais ou à la contemplation des planches de Clarence Gagnon dans l'édition Mornay de "Maria Chapdelaine".

Avec le docteur Perron, écrivait le docteur AR Potvin[29] *au lendemain de sa mort, disparaît un des pionniers de la Radiologie canadienne-française et québécoise. Il fut à la fois témoin et artisan de ses progrès depuis 25 ans. Ses collègues de la Faculté, de l'hôpital et de la spécialité, conserveront le souvenir du médecin instruit, de l'humaniste un peu dilettante, du radiologiste compétent et aimablement bohème que fut notre ami.*

J'ai gardé pour la fin, de vous parler d'un gentilhomme aux cheveux blancs, que vous avez tous connu et aimé, autre pionnier de la radiologie au Canada français. Histoire de vous amuser, devinez, si vous le voulez bien:

En dépit de ses vieux ans
Il fut jeune très longtemps
Pour lui
L'appareil radiologique
Était la cure magique
Qui luit
Pour tous, il était tout comme
Le plus parfait gentilhomme
D'antan.
Combien de nos tristes sires
Gonflés, ne peuvent en dire
Autant
La vie fut une aventure
Pour lui toute de droiture.
Il brille
Toujours deux mots dans sa vie
Ensemble: Radiologie—
Famille

Vous l'avez sans doute deviné: c'est le docteur Léglius Gagnier, père. Charade trop facile, pour les amis du fils qui reproduit dans sa vie avec tant de fidélité les belles qualités paternelles. Je ne le chicanerai pas, lui, débordant de jeunesse, pour ses cheveux blancs; c'est la rançon bien minime qu'il paie pour avoir voulu mouler trop parfaitement son image à l'effigie de son regretté père.

Membre d'une famille de 27 enfants, le docteur

Gagnier était né à Sainte-Martine de Châteauguay en 1871. Son grand-père, en 1812 avait servi de messager aux recrues des troupes de Salaberry. Après des études classiques à Ste-Thérèse et St-Hyacinthe, il reçoit son diplôme de médecine à Laval de Montréal. Parti en 1909 pour étudier la radiologie, il travaille sous A Béclère et Jaugeas à St-Antoine, sous Huet à la Salpêtrière, et à la clinique Apostoli avec Laquerrière qui deviendra par la suite l'un de ses fervents amis. De retour au pays, il fonde rue Saint-Denis une clinique électro-radiologique où Léglius fils devait plus tard lui apporter l'appoint de sa collaboration.

Le docteur Gagnier, père, n'était pas très grand de taille; mais il portait bien haut une tête altière déjà blanche où se lisait dans de fins yeux bleus, une déférence souriante pour l'interlocuteur. Travailleur, rangé jusque dans sa mine extérieure, il était la droiture même; d'allure avenante pour tous, il avait pour ses amis une dévotion véritable. Car l'amitié était pour lui "ce trésor qu'on cache au plus grand nombre et qu'on distribue sans réserve aux privilégiés."

Voilà donc tous les rôles distribués: Pariseau l'impétueux érudit à Montréal; Perron le souriant érudit de Québec; entre les deux, Gagnier, père, le gentilhomme amène, le médecin très digne auquel ses cheveux blancs confèrent un particulier prestige. C'est dans l'axe de ces trois Grands que s'inscrit la gestation et la naissance de notre Société.

Mais Gagnier en est véritablement la cheville ouvrière. Car il faut avant de les grouper, pressentir les confrères; leur arracher, pour la mise en nomination la promesse d'un travail scientifique. Et Québec est bien loin pour les consultations répétées qu'il faudrait avoir avec les collègues de la Capitale. Pariseau est peu fait pour convaincre en douceur et sa verve épistolaire est aussi capricieuse qu'incisive, se tarissant parfois comme le flot d'un geyser, sans qu'on puisse en prévoir le rejaillissement.

C'est ainsi qu'il écrira parfois au docteur AR Potvin. Mais c'est dans les innombrables lettres de Gagnier à Perron que nous retrouvons non seulement l'esquisse du rêve cher d'une Société caressée par les trois, mais aussi le reflet de cette grande amitié qui les unissait, et par dessus tout, les traits de ce noble coeur, de ce gentilhomme exquis qu'était le docteur Gagnier. "Quel beau rêve, écrivait-il à Perron, nous pourrions réaliser de fraternisation dans une même Société et d'émulation dans notre travail scientifique!" [30]

Lors de l'incident Dioclès, sa grande délicatesse d'âme éclate. Il ne veut blesser personne tout en recevant convenablement l'illustre visiteur. Quant à sa grande amitié pour Perron, lui qui couvait de sa tendresse son fils Léglius, il ne trouve pour lui nul bien plus désirable que de lui souhaiter un fils: "N'y a-t-il pas un petit Perron à l'horizon?...Je devrais être le parrain de ce futur radiologiste!" [31]

Premier président de notre Société, le docteur Gagnier en avait été vraiment le principal artisan...Je dépose au pieds de son fils, mon cher ami Léglius le témoignage d'estime et d'admiration que je viens de rendre à la mémoire de son père. Sans lui et tous les pionniers que j'ai fait revivre devant vous, notre Société qui a trente ans aujourd'hui n'aurait pas trente ans et ne serait pas ce qu'elle est.

APRÈS LA FONDATION—DUC IN ALTUM—PROLOGUE

Enfin la Société était née...Mais pour qu'elle vive, que d'écueils à surmonter, dans cette immense province de Québec où les distances sont un sérieux obstacle pour les pionniers clairsemés qui voudraient se tendre la main.

Nous entrions alors dans une ère de développement hospitalier sans précédent: dès 1922 le doyen Rousseau avait approuvé un gigantesque projet de modernisation du service de radiologie de l'Hôtel-Dieu de Québec, à la demande du docteur Potvin.

A Montréal naissait en 1923 l'Institut du Radium, alors que Notre-Dame déménageait dans ses nouveaux locaux de la rue Sherbrooke.

Il faut faire vite et le temps presse pour les fondateurs et les membres de la Société dont l'idéal est de fournir à tous ces nouveaux services radiologiques qui réclament leur aide, un personnel qualifié; d'organiser dans les deux grandes villes l'enseignement universitaire de la spécialité; de préserver, en contrepoids de la technologie américaine, nos contacts culturels avec la France, etc...

1922 nous avait ramené de France un contingent de recrues sérieuses: Potvin, Perron, Lacharité qui ont étudié à St-Antoine et à l'Institut du Radium. L'année suivante, de chez Delherm et Maingot: Dufresne, Gagnier, fils, Gosselin, Grondin, Léonard.

Dans les années 30, c'est Pailleurs, Jutras, Brodeur et Samson, qui sont en stage à Paris.

Enrichie de tous ces nouveaux membres, la Société progresse, tient des séances régulières où des communications d'une belle tenue témoignent de la vitalité et de l'enthousiasme des jeunes spécialistes, maintenant responsables de services hospitaliers bien organisés. (Je m'en voudrais d'oublier ici le "moins jeune" le docteur Grenier, notre premier radium-thérapeute qui, à 82 ans révolus, se rend régulièrement tous les jours depuis 1923 à sa clinique de l'Institut du Radium!) Ils assistent et participent parfois de façon active aux Congrès Américains de Radiologie et même en Europe, tel le docteur Gendreau, directeur de l'Institut du Radium, jusqu'à sa mort en 1949, que nous verrons à Londres, au premier Congrès International de la spécialité et que nous retrouverons à Zurich en 1928, à Paris en 1931 (président de la délégation canadienne) et à tous les autres...Fière des services rendus à la médecine canadienne-française, la Société sait qu'elle peut à bon droit compter sur son respect et sa reconnaissance. Soucieuse de contacts scientifiques stimulants, elle s'honore d'avoir accueilli depuis sa fondation un grand nombre de visiteurs et de conférenciers distingués: Del Regato–Lenz–Caffey–Pendergrass...Mais la France, on le comprend, avait et conserve la cote d'amour: les professeurs Dioclès, Belot, Cottenot, Maingot, Lacassagne, Lamarque, Baclesse, Claude Béclère, Gauducheau et plus récemment le Dr Lachapèle, de Bordeaux reçurent ici non seulement l'honneur de la tribune, mais l'accolade fraternelle, juste écho de la tendresse dont la radiologie française avait entouré nos aînés.

Dans cette évocation rapide de l'ère des débuts, je n'ai pu rappeler en détail le souvenir de tous. Que ces chers disparus: Mayrand, Comtois, Jules Gosselin, Panneton, Gendreau me pardonnent mon silence. Ils sont au même titre que les autres les artisans d'une oeuvre dont ils ont de leur vie d'homme façonné la charpente. D'autres, encore à la tâche, ont pris une part insigne à l'élaboration de l'oeuvre commune, mais j'ai préféré ne parler que des disparus: ils ne peuvent relever mes erreurs. Je crois avoir agi sagement en préférant piller "historiquement " le tombeau des morts que de m'exposer par mes inexactitudes à l'ire des vivants.

Remerciements:
Reproduction gracieuseté de l'Union médicale du Canada 1959; 88: 40.

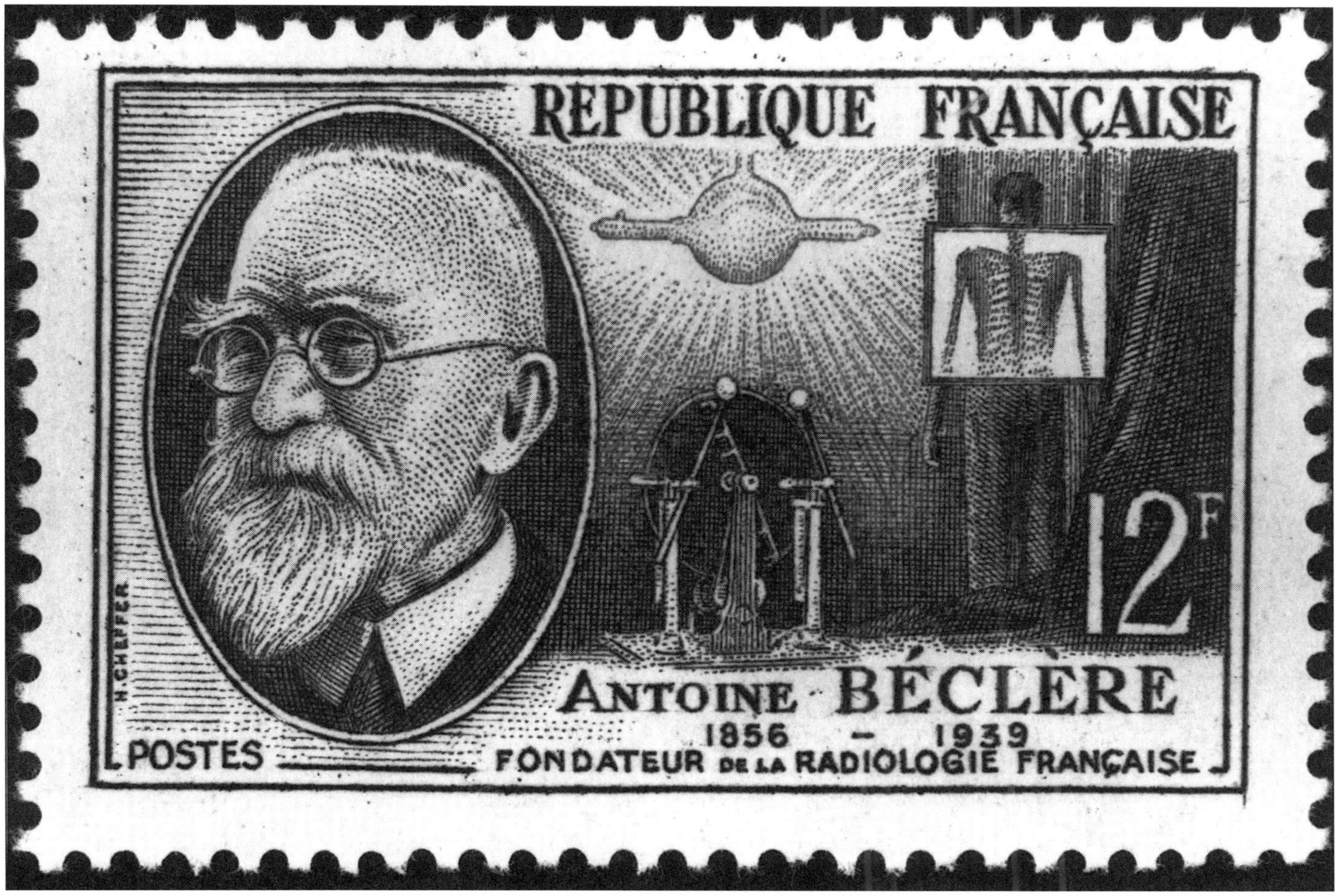
REPUBLIQUE FRANÇAISE
12F
ANTOINE BÉCLÈRE
1856 - 1939
FONDATEUR DE LA RADIOLOGIE FRANÇAISE
POSTES

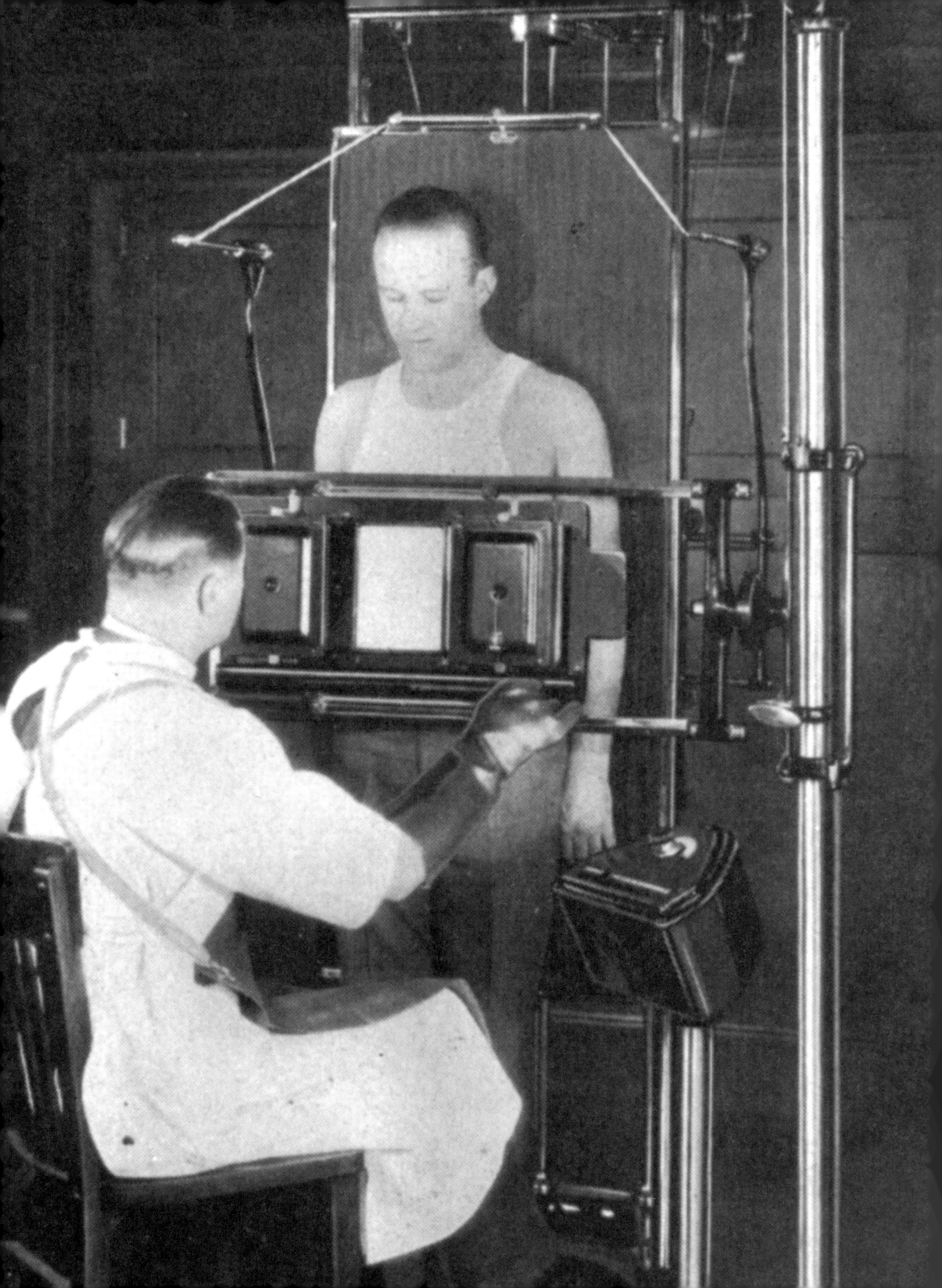

Chapter VI • La Réception des

Rayons X au Québec:

Radiographie des Pratiques Scientifiques

Yves Gingras

Il est bien connu que du milieu du 19e siècle jusqu'à la Première Guerre mondiale, et même au-delà pour certaines disciplines, les Canadiens français étaient, à toutes fins utiles, absents des carrières scientifiques. Pour ne donner qu'un exemple, en 1901, moins de un et demi pour cent des effectifs étudiants inscrits à l'Université Laval ou à sa succursale de Montréal sont en sciences alors qu'à McGill la proportion est de près de 19%.[1] Ces chiffres reflètent évidemment la structure des collèges classiques de l'époque qui privilégie les carrières religieuses et les professions libérales au détriment des carrières de scientifiques ou d'ingénieurs.[2]

Sans doute est-il possible de rendre compte de la différence d'attitude à l'égard des sciences entre les Canadiens français et les Canadiens anglais en invoquant la position économique dominante de la bourgeoisie canadienne anglaise qui lui donne un accès privilégié aux quelques emplois existant dans les industries ou les institutions fédérales telles que le *Geological Survey,* le *Biological Board ou* les *Dominion Experimental Farms.*[3] L'existence de débouchés sur le marché du travail est sans doute un facteur important dans le choix de carrière des étudiants. Le fait, par exemple, que les postes d'enseignant étaient occupés par les membres des communautés religieuses limitait énormément les possibilités d'emplois des diplômés de la Faculté des sciences de l'Université de Montréal dont la formation préparait à l'enseignement.

Un bon nombre des premiers diplômés de la Faculté étaient d'ailleurs membres de communautés enseignantes. Cela étant dit, il ne faut pas oublier que les polémiques des années 1920 sur la position

gauche
Radiologiste portant tablier et gants de plomb utilisant un appareil de fluoroscopie vertical (circa 1920)

marginale des sciences dans l'ensemble du programme d'enseignement des collèges classiques montrent clairement que les structures sociales ont une inertie que les seules forces économiques ne peuvent vaincre facilement.[4]

Il faut donc délaisser la simple mécanique de l'offre et de la demande économique, qui court-circuite la spécificité de tout système d'éducation, et porter notre regard sur les aspects culturels de la pratique scientifique. On verra ainsi que le choix d'une carrière scientifique et la manière d'envisager les objets de la science sont fortement conditionnés par la structure du système d'enseignement qui favorise certaines dispositions au détriment de certaines autres. Comme l'écrit Pierre Bourdieu, "ceux qui ont pour 'culture' (au sens des ethnologues) la culture savante, véhiculée par l'école, disposent d'un système de catégories de perception, de langage, de pensée et d'appréciation qui les distingue de ceux qui n'ont pas connu d'autre apprentissage", ou, pourrions-nous ajouter, qui ont été formés dans un système scolaire différent.[5]

Partant de cette observation, nous nous proposons ici de jeter un regard quasi "ethnologique" sur les pratiques des scientifiques de façon à voir comment l'attitude face à un objet scientifique donné diffère selon la trajectoire scolaire des agents. Dans cette optique, l'étude de la réception des rayons X constitue un choix privilégié, car il est peu fréquent que les scientifiques des deux principales universités québécoises du début du siècle, Laval et McGill, s'intéressent au même objet, quoique pour en faire un usage différent.

Notre approche du cas des rayons X au Québec part donc d'un certain nombre de faits déjà connus de façon à illustrer un problème plus large, à savoir les déterminants institutionnels et disciplinaires des différentes pratiques scientifiques.[6] Nous croyons que cette problématique permet d'éviter l'éternel (faux) problème du "retard du Québec", qu'il soit de nature économique ou scientifique. En effet, la problématique du "retard" est fondamentalement évolutionniste en ce qu'elle suppose toujours que ce qui est arrivé était nécessaire et que, conséquemment, ceux qui sont arrivés "deuxièmes" étaient "en retard".

Avant de décrire les différents usages auxquels ont donné lieu les rayons X et de chercher ensuite à les relier à l'itinéraire scolaire des acteurs ainsi qu'au niveau de développement des institutions universitaires de l'époque, rappelons brièvement les événements qui entourent la découverte de ces rayons.

LES RAYONS X: DÉCOUVERTE ET DIFFUSION

Le 8 novembre 1895, un physicien allemand, Wilhem Conrad Röntgen, étudiant les propriétés des rayons cathodiques, découvre par hasard un nouveau type de rayonnement possédant des propriétés inconnues jusqu'alors. Le 28 décembre, après avoir étudié certaines propriétés de ces rayons, il communique ses résultats à la Société de physique et de médecine de Würzburg. C'est alors qu'on apprend que les rayons X, ainsi nommés parce que Röntgen en ignorait la nature, traversent le bois et plusieurs métaux comme le cuivre, l'argent et l'or, mais sont arrêtés par le plomb. Chose plus intéressante encore, les rayons X traversent la chair et non les os et agissent sur une pellicule photographique. De cette façon, Röntgen a pu photographier—on dira plus tard radiographier—la main de sa femme et voir clairement sa structure osseuse. Pour le savant, la photographie était un moyen pour étudier les propriétés des nouveaux rayons et non une fin mais, écrit-il, "les journaux en ont fait la chose la plus importante."[7]

C'est l'aspect spectaculaire des radiographies, et non les rayons X en eux-mêmes, qui est à l'origine du battage publicitaire qui a rapidement suivi la découverte. Dès le 5 janvier 1896, *La Presse* de Vienne publie à la une un article sur la nouvelle découverte et prédit l'influence qu'elle aura sur l'étude des maladies. Le lendemain, la nouvelle se propage à travers le monde comme une traînée de poudre et des articles paraissent dans le *Daily Chronicle* de Londres et *Le Matin* de Paris. Dès le 7 janvier, par exemple, le *Frankfurter Zeitung* discute de l'intérêt pratique des nouveaux rayons et écrit:

> *Les biologistes et les médecins, spécialement les chirurgiens, seront très intéressés par l'utilité pratique de ces rayons... [Le chirurgien] pourrait trouver la position d'un corps étranger, comme une balle ou une pièce d'obus, beaucoup plus facilement qu'il n'était possible jusqu'à maintenant.*[8]

Ce genre d'application ne tardera pas à venir et un mois plus tard les rayons X seront utilisés, à l'Université McGill, pour localiser une balle dans la jambe d'un patient.

LES RAYONS À L'UNIVERSITÉ MCGILL: LA PRODUCTION DU SAVOIR

Depuis 1893, les professeurs de physique de McGill possèdent leur propre édifice, le *Macdonald Physics Building,* fruit des largesses du roi du tabac William C Macdonald. A l'époque, c'est un des laboratoires les mieux équipés au monde[9] et dont l'une des fonctions, quoique la moins importante aux yeux des dirigeants de McGill[10], est la production de nouvelles connaissances. John Cox, un savant britannique formé à l'Université de Cambridge, avait été engagé en 1890 pour superviser la construction du nouvel édifice et agir à titre de directeur. Au moment de l'ouverture du laboratoire en 1893, Cox engage un nouveau professeur en la personne de Hugh L Callendar. A l'instar du directeur, Callendar est formé à Cambridge mais, comme nous le verrons plus loin, il fait partie d'une nouvelle cohorte d'étudiants, ce qui le distingue de Cox sur plusieurs points.

Quoique le *New York Times* ait annoncé la découverte de Röntgen dès le 9 janvier, ce n'est que le 5 février que le *Montreal Daily Star* nous informe que des expériences utilisant les nouveaux rayons ont lieu à l'Université McGill. On y mentionne que, la veille, le professeur Cox a fait un exposé des découvertes du savant allemand et qu'il a répété ses expériences, en prenant une "photographie" de sa main gauche, laissant clairement apparaître les os du savant montréalais. Le journaliste décrit l'expérience avec minutie. On apprend que la main a été exposée vingt minutes aux rayons et on donne même le type de plaque photographique employée, ainsi que leurs dimensions. A la fin de la séance, Cox ajoute qu'il veut maintenant utiliser le procédé en chirurgie, car les hôpitaux environnants lui ont plusieurs fois demandé d'utiliser la photographie aux rayons X pour des fractures des os difficilement localisables à l'aide des outils dont disposent alors les médecins.

Le lendemain de cette séance publique, Cox tente déjà de radiographier une lésion à la hanche d'un patient qui avait donné beaucoup de mal aux médecins. Comme le rapporte le *Star:*

> *The best surgical skill in the city has so far been unable to completely reduce the fracture, although the injured one is able to get around with the assistance of a cane and a crutch.*
>
> *One of the leading surgeons of this city, who has become deeply interested in the case, and who has been closely following the experiments in Dr Röntgen's discovery thought that the latter, if applied to the present case, might be able to reveal what the surgeons had been unable to discover, namely, the causes which hindered the fracture from being properly reduced.*[11]

Malheureusement, après une exposition d'une heure aux rayons, la plaque ne laisse rien apparaître. Cox pense que cet échec s'explique par une durée d'exposition trop courte, ou par la présence de plomb dans la peinture noire recouvrant la plaque photographique, ce qui serait suffisant pour bloquer les rayons X. Il compte donc utiliser la prochaine fois une plaque différente composée d'aluminium qui, selon lui, laissera passer les rayons. Même si elle fut un échec, cette expérience marque le début d'une nouvelle collaboration entre physiciens et chirurgiens.

En collaboration avec le docteur Robert C Kirkpatrick, chirurgien à l'Hôpital Général de Montréal, Cox multiplie les expériences et, le matin du 7 février, il réussit à localiser une balle dans la jambe d'un patient. La jambe était placée entre un tube de Crookes—appareil de verre scellé contenant un gaz à basse pression dans lequel on fait passer un courant électrique alimenté par une bobine à induction de Ruhmkorff—et une boite de carton contenant la plaque photographique. Après un temps d'exposition de 45 minutes, le négatif montre clairement la présence d'une balle, ce qui permet une localisation précise. Une légère incision est alors pratiquée par le docteur Kirkpatrick et la balle est extraite sans difficulté.

Cette application précoce des rayons X est présentée le soir du 7 février à la séance de la *Montreal Medico-Chirurgical Society.*[12] Pour saisir toute l'importance de cette expérience, il faut noter qu'à l'époque il était souvent difficile de localiser une balle et on devait alors se contenter d'appliquer des antiseptiques. L'importance de l'événement est aussi marqué par l'éditorial du *Montreal Medical Journal,* de mars 1896, où il est dit:

> *Ce n'est pas sans plaisir que nous attirons l'attention sur l'article du professeur Cox décrivant et illustrant la première application, à des fins de diagnostic, sur ce continent, de la remarquable découverte de Röntgen.*[13]

Le journal adopte une attitude favorable à ces nouveaux développements et termine en mentionnant que, même si le nombre d'applications est peut-être restreint, il faut saluer cordialement la venue de chaque découverte permettant un diagnostic plus précis. Par la suite, on retrouvera souvent des comptes rendus d'applications médicales des rayons X dans des journaux comme *l' Union médicale du Canada.*[14]

A la suite de ces expériences d'une grande utilité mais techniquement élémentaires, Cox s'associe avec Callendar pour approfondir les connaissances des propriétés physiques des rayons X. Quelques mois plus tard, ils présentent les résultats de leurs recherches à la Société royale du Canada lors de la séance du 31 mai 1896. Publiée dans les *Mémoires de la Société,* leur communication passe en revue plusieurs propriétés des nouveaux rayons.[15] Les auteurs y discutent des effets physiologiques qui commencent à être rapportés de tous les coins du monde et qui décrivent l'assèchement de la peau, semblable à un coup de soleil, qui résulterait d'une exposition prolongée aux rayons X. Cox et Callendar mentionnent cependant que ces descriptions sont le fait d'observateurs peu réputés et que leurs propres expériences n'ont montré aucun effet physiologique, même après une exposition très prolongée. Ils présentent aussi les résultats de leurs expériences sur les propriétés germicides des rayons et concluent que les rayons X n'ont aucun effet sur la croissance de cultures de bacilles. Ce n'est que quelques mois plus tard que des expériences plus précises confirmeront l'existence d'effets physiologiques nocifs liés à l'exposition aux rayons X.[16]

Les deux physiciens s'attaquent aussi au problème de la nature des rayons X et tentent de mesurer leur vitesse. Reprenant la méthode qui avait permis au savant français Hippolyte Fizeau de mesurer la vitesse de la lumière[17], ils concluent que les rayons X ne peuvent être des atomes électrifiés en mouvement, car la vitesse mesurée, plus de 200 kilomètres par seconde, est beaucoup trop grande. Il s'agit alors probablement d'un genre de mouvement dans l'éther et des méthodes plus raffinées montreront peut-être que la vitesse des rayons est la même que celle de la lumière. Cette conclusion est intéressante, car elle suggère que les rayons X sont des ondes transversales comme la lumière, contrairement à l'opinion de Röntgen qui, à la fin de sa première communication, émettait plutôt l'hypothèse qu'il s'agissait de vibrations longitudinales de l'éther, milieu qui devait servir de soutien à la propagation de la lumière, comme l'air est le soutien à la propagation du son.

Au moment même où les physiciens de McGill effectuent leurs recherches, John Cunningham McLennan, alors assistant démonstrateur de physique à l'Université de Toronto, s'affaire lui aussi à reproduire les expériences de Röntgen et à améliorer l'état des connaissances sur ce nouveau rayonnement. Dès le 8 février 1896, le *Daily Mail and Empire* de Toronto fait état de ses travaux et mentionne que dans l'après-midi du sept, il a réussi avec quelques étudiants à photographier l'ossature d'une main après une période d'exposition aux rayons de dix minutes.

Au mois de mars, le *Century Magazine* publie un article de McLennan intitulé "Photographing the Unseen," réimprimé par la suite sous le titre "Röntgen Radiation."[18] La lecture de ce document montre que McLennan met en application un plan de travail similaire à celui de ses collègues de McGill. Assisté de deux étudiants, il prend une série de photographies à l'aide des rayons X et s'efforce systématiquement de diminuer le temps d'exposition qu'il réussit bientôt à rendre "presque instantané." Rappelons que Cox et Callendar durent exposer la plaque quarante-cinq minutes aux rayons avant d'obtenir un négatif permettant de localiser la balle dans la jambe du patient. McLennan étudie aussi les propriétés de ces rayons. Discutant ensuite de l'intérêt chirurgical de la découverte, il décrit comment il a réussi à localiser une aiguille dans le pied d'une patiente, ce qui permit au chirurgien de l'enlever dès la première incision.

En somme, on voit que le jeune physicien de Toronto, qui deux ans plus tard se rendra au laboratoire Cavendish pour parfaire sa formation de chercheur,[19] approche les rayons X d'un point de vue semblable à celui de ses collègues de McGill: ils travaillent tous en fonction d'un programme de recherche précis dont la logique est dictée par la structure du champ scientifique de l'époque. En effet, la découverte des rayons X pose le problème de leur nature corpusculaire ou ondulatoire et les scientifiques sont aussitôt amenés à concevoir des expériences par analogie avec celles effectuées auparavant pour connaître les propriétés de la lumière. D'où les multiples tentatives à travers le monde de mesurer la vitesse de propagation des rayons, leur réflexion et réfraction sur des surfaces diverses ou encore leur polarisation. D'où aussi les nombreuses "découvertes simultanées". Ainsi, uniquement au cours du mois de février 1896, on compte une quarantaine d'articles de journaux en Amérique du Nord rapportant à peu près le même type de résultat.[20]

Le fait que les appareils de base nécessaires pour produire des rayons X étaient disponibles dans la plupart des cabinets de physique, facilitait de beaucoup la reproduction des expériences de Röntgen tant par des physiciens professionnels que par des amateurs. De ce point de vue, les rayons X constituent peut-être l'une des dernières grandes découvertes de la physique directement accessible à un large public et aussitôt utilisée à des fins culturelles. Produits par des appareils de plus en plus complexes et coûteux, les phénomènes physiques découverts après 1900 pourront difficilement être intégrés à des pratiques culturelles et, en un sens, n'existeront que pour les spécialistes.

Avant de préciser les conditions institutionnelles qui rendent possible le regard savant posé par Callendar et McLennan sur les rayons X, voyons tout d'abord comment la découverte de Röntgen fut reçue à l'Université Laval.

LES RAYONS X À L'UNIVERSITÉ LAVAL: LA REPRODUCTION DU SAVOIR

Au moment de la découverte des rayons X, l'enseignement de la physique à l'Université Laval est dispensé par l'abbé Joseph-Clovis-Kemner Laflamme. Il avait succédé à son maître l'abbé Thomas-Etienne Hamel qui avait enseigné cette discipline de 1858 a 1874. Formé au Séminaire de Québec, Hamel avait dû parfaire sa formation scientifique à la Sorbonne où il avait préparé une licence ès sciences mathématiques. A son retour, il est chargé de l'enseignement de la physique, de la minéralogie et de la géologie.[21] En 1870, ces deux dernières disciplines sont confiées à Laflamme qui s'occupe aussi de la physique à compter de 1875.[22]

Sur le plan strictement scientifique, Hamel contribua peu à l'avancement des connaissances. Membre fondateur de la Société royale du Canada, les quelques communications qu'il présenta aux réunions de cette société relevaient davantage de l'exercice de rhétorique typique d'une formation classique que de la communication scientifique proprement dite.[23]

Bien qu'il ait reçu une formation plutôt axée sur la géologie, Laflamme suit de près les développements de la physique et profite de ses conférences publiques pour entretenir la bonne société de Québec sur "L'électricité à Québec" ou sur les propriétés des accumulateurs électriques.[24]

Alors qu'à McGill les cours de physique s'adressent en premier lieu aux futurs ingénieurs, ceux dispensés à Laval par Laflamme (et avant lui par Hamel) s'adressent plutôt à une clientèle qui se dirige vers les professions libérales et le sacerdoce de sorte que le niveau d'enseignement de la physique, et des sciences en général, demeure élémentaire. Malgré cela le cabinet de physique est toujours bien équipé et l'annuaire de l'Université ne manque pas de le signaler:

> *Le cabinet de physique à l'usage de la Faculté des Arts est très complet. Il renferme sur toutes les branches de la physique plus de 1000 instruments, comprenant la plupart des appareils qui servent à démontrer les découvertes les plus récentes.*[25]

Les cours ne comportant pas de séances de laboratoire, une telle collection est évidemment sous-utilisée et fonctionne surtout comme marque de prestige et de distinction. Elle semble d'ailleurs perçue davantage sur le mode de "l'oeuvre d'art" que de "l'outillage" scientifique comme le suggère les adjectifs employés dans la description de la collection: "une très belle machine électrique de Ramsden", "de splendides modèles de roues hydrauliques", "une jolie machine de Wimhurst", "de magnifiques échantillons de soudure électrique", etc. Ce discours "mondain" et émerveillé face aux objets de la science se retrouve aussi dans le *Journal du Séminaire:*

> *Le spinthariscope, commandé aux États-Unis par Mgr Laflamme, est arrivé cet après-midi. C'est une merveille. Tout lilliputien qu'il est, il nous donne le spectacle d'une ébullition d'étoiles et d'étincelles. Les confrères qui l'ont examiné en sont émerveillés.*[26]

À la même époque, McGill possède elle aussi une riche collection d'instruments scientifiques qui est rapidement utilisée par Callendar pour faire avancer des projets de recherche qu'il avait amorcés lors de son séjour au laboratoire Cavendish. Anticipant déjà les contributions de Callendar à la recherche scientifique, Cox note dans son rapport annuel de 1893 que la collection exceptionnelle d'instruments électriques, de thermométrie et de pyrométrie permettra au laboratoire de faire des travaux

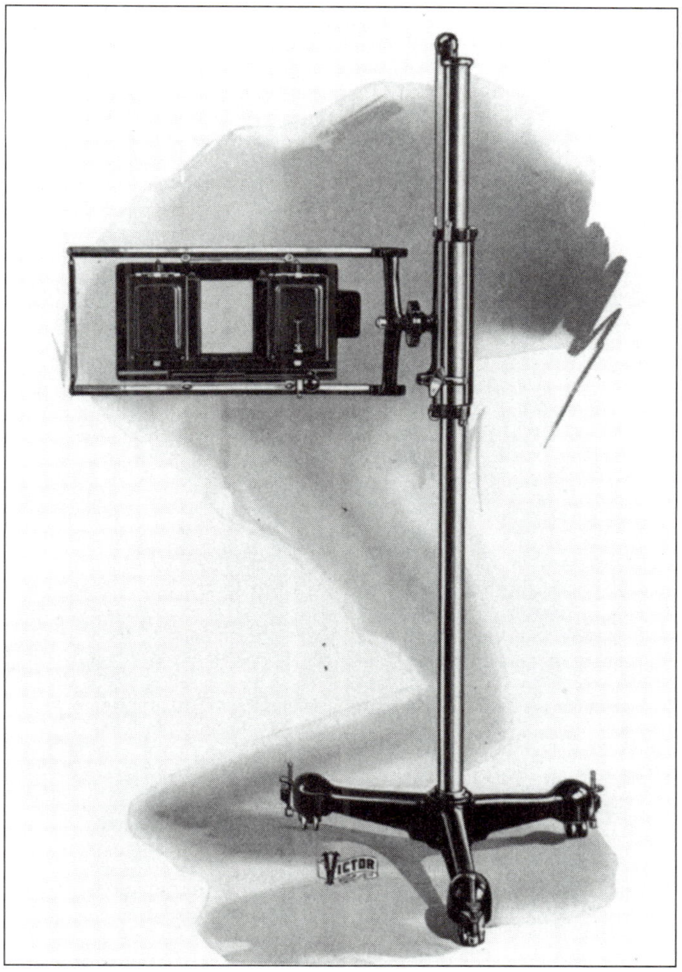

Écran mobile de fluoroscopie Victor, circa 1920.

utiles dans ces branches de la physique dans un avenir rapproché.[27]

C'est dans un contexte de culture générale que Mgr Laflamme effectue quelques expériences avec les rayons X et discute de leurs propriétés devant divers auditoires. Il commence ses expériences avec les rayons X vers le 12 février, soit une semaine après les premiers essais de Cox. Ses premières photos ne sont pas réussies mais son ami Jules Guay, trésorier de la Société française de physique, lui écrit le 17 février suivant pour lui donner quelques précisions, ce qui lui permet par la suite d'obtenir d'excellents clichés.[28] C'est ce qu'indique le journal du séminaire en date du 2 avril où il est noté que les clichés reçus de la pharmacie Livernois, située sur la rue de la Fabrique à Québec, "sont admirablement réussis."[29] Trois semaines plus tard, le journal *La Vérité* nous apprend que Mgr Laflamme a obtenu de nouvelles photographies "qui sont exposées chez Livernois."[30]

Le 29 avril 1896, Mgr Laflamme fait une démonstration des propriétés des rayons devant les élèves et professeurs de la Faculté de Médecine, et le 20 mai, il présente une "grande séance d'expériences avec les rayons X...devant un tout petit comité formé presque exclusivement d'archevêques et d'évêques [qui ont] regardé à travers un chanoine au grand amusement de tous."[31] Notons que la notion "d'expérience" dont il est question ici est assez différente de celle de Cox, Callendar et McLennan. Elle s'apparente davantage aux "expériences de Gala" du 18e siècle, qui visent un public de curieux, qu'aux expériences scientifiques proprement dites, faites dans le privé du laboratoire et dont les résultats sont ensuite rendus publics dans les revues scientifiques.[32]

Un an plus tard, Laflamme s'adresse aux médecins devant la Société Médicale de Québec. Discutant cette fois devant un auditoire plus savant, il aborde le problème de la nature des rayons X et note que "malgré la valeur très grande qu'il convient de donner à l'opinion du professeur de Würzburg, l'opinion la plus commune est que les rayons X sont absolument analogues aux rayons lumineux ordinaires...mais que leurs longueurs d'onde sont comparables aux dimensions moléculaires."[33] Mgr Laflamme exprimait ainsi de façon très claire l'interprétation qui sera finalement retenue. Cependant, son rôle est ici encore celui du vulgarisateur qui *diffuse* des connaissances et non celui du chercheur qui *produit* des connaissances.

L'HONNÊTE HOMME ET LE SPÉCIALISTE

Les sections précédentes ont montré dans quel contexte les rayons X ont été utilisés par les professeurs de physique à l'Université Laval et à McGill. Comparant ces deux attitudes face à la découverte des nouveaux rayons, on ne peut manquer de constater qu'à Québec, on se limite à diffuser les connaissances produites par d'autres. Par exemple, Laflamme fait essentiellement de la vulgarisation scientifique et ses opinions sur la nature des rayons X circulent parmi les étudiants, les médecins et la haute société de Québec, et non dans les milieux scientifiques concernés comme la Société royale du Canada. Ses conférences renseignent les médecins sur les possibilités d'application des rayons X à la médecine sans toutefois contribuer à concrétiser une collaboration efficace entre médecins et physiciens. À McGill, au contraire, l'étude des rayons X fait partie d'un programme pour "étudier les conditions de production des rayons de Röntgen et les meilleures méthodes pour obtenir des photographies claires et rapides", comme l'indique Cox dans son rapport annuel de 1896 soumis au président de l'Université McGill.[34] Cox et Callendar publient d'ailleurs les résultats de leurs travaux dans des revues savantes comme *Nature* ou les *Mémoires de la Société royale du Canada,* s'adressant ainsi spécifiquement à la communauté scientifique.

Les raisons de cette différence d'attitude face aux nouvelles découvertes scientifiques doivent être cherchées tout d'abord au niveau de l'organisation de la recherche scientifique dans les universités à cette époque et ensuite dans l'itinéraire des agents formés par ces institutions.

Pour comprendre les conditions d'émergence de la recherche scientifique à l'Université McGill, il faut tout d'abord rappeler brièvement certaines transformations survenues au sein des principales universités britanniques au début des années 1870.

L'enseignement de la physique à l'Université de Cambridge, dispensé sur une base régulière depuis 1851, année de la création du *Natural Science Tripos,* demeurait trop théorique (ou livresque) et devint la cible, vers la fin des années 1860, de critiques de la part d'un groupe de réformateurs réunis principalement autour d'anciens élèves tels Georges Gabriel Stokes, Georges Biddell Airy et James Clerk Maxwell. Les discussions avec les autorités conduisirent à la création, en 1871, d'une chaire de physique expérimentale confiée à Maxwell. Entre 1866 et 1874, une dizaine de laboratoires de physique furent créés à Glasgow, Édimbourg et Londres, ouvrant ainsi la voie à une nouvelle forme d'enseignement davantage centrée sur le laboratoire par opposition à la salle de classe.[35]

Grâce à ces nouvelles institutions, il devint possible d'inculquer systématiquement à un certain nombre d'étudiants des dispositions favorables à l'égard de la recherche expérimentale. Ainsi, le nombre de chercheurs formés à Cambridge seulement passa de quatre ou cinq en 1875 à plus d'une quinzaine par année au cours des années quatre-vingt.[36]

Hugh L Callendar fait partie de la génération de physiciens formés à la recherche par JJ Thomson, qui succéda à Maxwell à la direction du laboratoire Cavendish en 1879. Lorsqu'il arrive à McGill en 1893, Callendar ne conçoit plus son rôle comme étant limité à l'enseignement et compte bien poursuivre ses travaux de recherche. Débutées en 1885, ses expériences sur la thermométrie sont déjà connues par la communauté scientifique et en 1894, il est élu membre de la *Royal Society* de Londres, ce qui indique la position importante de Callendar dans le champ scientifique de l'époque. Entre 1893 et 1898, année de son départ de McGill, il publie régulièrement, seul ou avec des collaborateurs, dans plusieurs journaux scientifiques dont les *Mémoires* de la Société royale du Canada.

La trajectoire scolaire de Callendar est intéressante car elle constitue un bel exemple de transition d'une formation classique à une formation scientifique. En effet, ses études

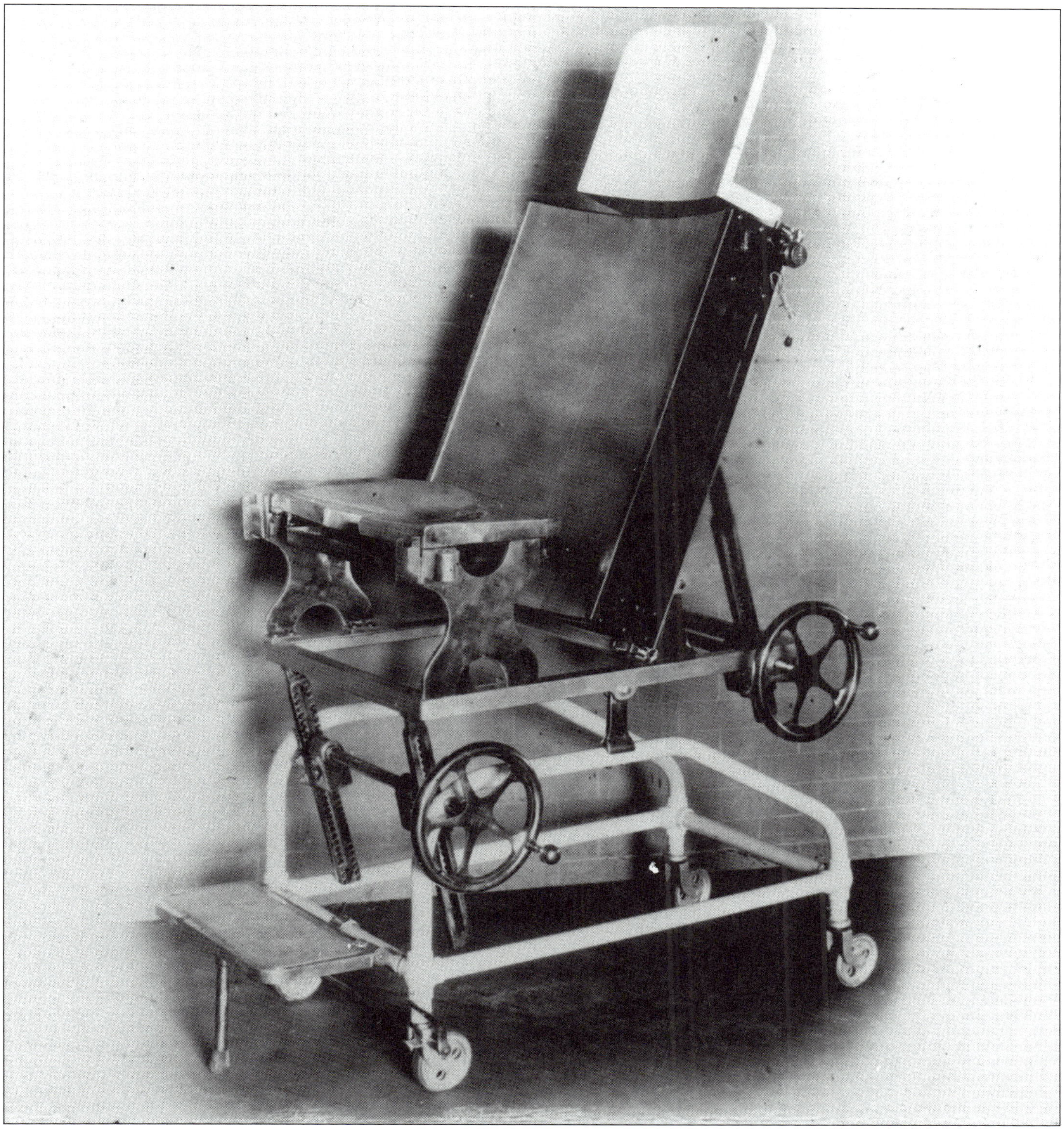

Table Braasch-Bumpus pour examens urologiques, cystoscopiques, et radiographiques, équipée d'un diaphragme Potter-Bucky (ici en position verticale) (circa 1920)

ne le préparaient nullement à la recherche en physique et c'est sous l'habile direction de Thomson qu'il a pu minimiser les désavantages de sa formation initiale. Comme le note ce dernier dans son autobiographie:

> *HL Callendar's career at the Laboratory was in some respects the most interesting in all my experience. He was on the classical side when at school and did not any physics. [...] He had never done any practical work in physics, nor read any of the theory except in a very casual way. [...] The problem was to find a subject for his research which would give full play to his strong points and minimise as much as possible his lack of experience. [...] It seemed to me that the most suitable research would be one which centered on the accurate measurement of electrical resistance.*[37]

Le départ de Callendar de McGill en 1898 n'est d'ailleurs pas sans liens avec sa carrière de chercheur.[38] Comme ce sera le cas dix ans plus tard pour son successeur Ernest Rutherford, il est certain que Callendar était affecté par son éloignement de l'Europe, véritable "centre de gravité" du champ de la physique, et qu'il ne pouvait que saisir toute occasion de rejoindre la métropole.[39]

À la différence de Callendar, John Cox, diplômé en 1874, ne reçoit aucune formation de chercheur et se destine plutôt à l'enseignement. Ses écrits se conforment d'ailleurs à ce rôle d'enseignant: il publie deux volumes dont un manuel de physique, *Mechanics,* et un petit ouvrage de vulgarisation, *Beyond the Atom,* présentant les travaux de JJ Thomson et de Ernest Rutherford (ce dernier ayant été son collègue à McGill entre 1898 et 1907).[40] Son seul article scientifique est celui sur les rayons X publié avec Callendar dont nous avons discuté plus haut. Bien adapté à son rôle, Cox n'hésite pas à donner plus de cours de façon à laisser du temps à Callendar pour faire de la recherche. Il agira de même avec Rutherford qui prend la relève de ce dernier en 1898.[41] La carrière de Cox est donc celle d'un professeur dont le temps est essentiellement consacré à l'enseignement et à la préparation des cours, ce que remarque d'ailleurs la revue *Nature* au moment de sa mort en 1923:

> *While keenly interested in all developments of physics, Cox had not the practical training requisite for research in experimental physics, but devoted himself to the teaching and administrative side.* [42]

Dans une certaine mesure, les commentaires de la revue *Nature* s'appliquent aussi à Mgr Laflamme ainsi qu'à ceux qui, avant lui, ont suivi une trajectoire similaire. Avant de s'initier à la recherche scientifique au laboratoire Cavendish, Callendar était d'ailleurs dans une position similaire à celle de Laflamme et des finissants du Séminaire de Québec. L'absence d'institutions de recherche permettant une "retraduction" des intérêts est donc un facteur à ne pas négliger pour expliquer l'absence de Canadiens français dans des disciplines scientifiques. Au début du XXe siècle.

DISCIPLINE ET EXCLUSION

La possibilité d'accès à une discipline scientifique dépend du degré de spécialisation de cette discipline. Par exemple, depuis le milieu du XIXe siècle, la physique s'est institutionnalisée et spécialisée de telle sorte qu'il faut un apprentissage précis et assez long pour *devenir* physicien. Hamel par exemple n'a jamais reçu une formation de physicien. Sa présence au sein de la section III (physique, chimie, astronomie et mathématique) de la Société royale du Canada à titre de membre fondateur, par exemple, s'explique davantage par des considérations politiques—présence de francophones au sein de la Société—que par des motifs strictement scientifiques. Au tournant du siècle cependant, la section III sera surtout composée de chercheurs qui n'éliront que leurs semblables.[43] Cette professionnalisation fera en sorte qu'après la disparition de Hamel et de Laflamme—qui, avec l'ingénieur Charles Baillargé, sont les seuls Canadiens français au sein de la Société—les sections scientifiques de la Société royale ne compteront plus aucun Canadien français jusqu'au milieu des années 1920. Ainsi, l'abbé Henri Simard, qui succède à Laflamme au poste de professeur de physique en 1893, ne sera jamais élu au sein de la section III et devra se contenter de faire partie de la section I (littérature, histoire et sciences humaines) qui regroupe les francophones.[44]

D'autres disciplines comme la botanique et l'entomologie ont, au milieu des années 1870, une structure qui laisse encore place à des recherches basées sur l'observation directe ou la cueillette de données, travail accessible à des "amateurs". À compter du milieu du siècle cependant, l'étude de la physiologie végétale prend de plus en plus d'importance, contribuant ainsi à marginaliser les amateurs ou les simples collectionneurs. Il n'est donc pas surprenant que les quelques individus, qui ont fait de la science au Québec au cours du XIXe siècle se sont retrouvés dans des disciplines ou il était encore possible de faire des contributions sans avoir à passer par un long apprentissage spécialisé alors inexistant au Québec. Ainsi, l'abbé Louis-Ovide Brunet se consacre à la botanique alors que son confrère l'abbé Léon Provancher choisit plutôt l'entomologie, sans ignorer la botanique.[45]

Dans cette perspective d'accès à une discipline scientifique, Laflamme constitue un cas limite. Au moment où débute sérieusement ses travaux en géologie, en 1882—soit l'année même où il est choisi membre fondateur de la

Société royale du Canada—cette discipline est en pleine transformation et la possibilité de n'être qu'un fin observateur sur le terrain perd de la légitimité. Le développement des connaissances est tel que la formation devient de plus en plus spécialisée et nécessite l'utilisation accrue de techniques et d'instruments de précision.[46]

Laflamme fait partie de ces observateurs de terrain, et ses travaux portent la marque de sa formation théorique incomplète qui l'empêche d'être au centre des problèmes de sa discipline.[47] Son intérêt pour les problèmes théoriques ne se manifeste que par la préparation de textes de vulgarisation comme celui qu'il publie dans le *Canada français* en 1891 sur un débat qui, dans le champ scientifique, se fait plutôt dans des revues savantes comme *Science, American Journal of Science,* etc.[48]

En somme, si la présence de scientifiques francophones se fait plus rare à partir du tournant du siècle, ce n'est pas parce que les trajectoires possibles se sont modifiées mais bien parce que les rares portes sur lesquelles elles débouchaient se sont fermées: la géologie s'est professionnalisée et la description "à l'oeil nu" des plantes ou des insectes a cessé, au XXe siècle, d'être une pratique scientifique légitime: l'ère des amateurs doués, tels que les Laflamme, Brunet et Provancher, était terminée. Les difficultés qu'éprouvera le Frère Marie-Victorin, un autodidacte, à se faire élire au sein de la section de biologie de la Société royale du Canada pourraient aussi être interprétées comme un effet de la marginalisation de la taxonomie dans le champ de la biologie. De ce point de vue, cet épisode de l'histoire des sciences au Québec ne se résume plus à un simple cas de conflit ethnique.[49]

BRISER LE CERCLE DE LA REPRODUCTION

À l'Université Laval, le fait que les professeurs de sciences étaient toujours choisis parmi les membres du clergé, anciens étudiants du Séminaire de Québec, rendait difficile sinon impossible la production d'un nouveau rapport aux sciences permettant la formation de chercheurs et non plus seulement d'enseignants. Hamel, par exemple, avait formé son successeur, Laflamme; ce dernier a enseigné à l'abbé Henri Simard qui lui succéda en 1893 et qui enseigna la physique à Laval jusqu'au milieu des années 1920. Tous ont ainsi reçu la même formation générale, suffisante pour un membre du clergé, un futur avocat ou un notaire, mais n'ouvrant aucunement la voie à une carrière scientifique. Lorsque la Première Guerre mondiale rendra évidente l'urgence de former de véritables scientifiques, il faudra importer de Suisse les premiers professeurs laïques de l'École supérieure de chimie, seule possibilité de briser le cercle de la reproduction.[50]

À McGill, le passage de l'enseignement à la recherche fut plus simple et s'est même fait, en partie, à l'insu des dirigeants: les professeurs étant recrutés en Angleterre, la deuxième génération de ceux qui ont quitté la métropole pour enseigner au Canada, en Australie ou au Japon,[51] n'avait déjà plus la même vocation que la première et sut imposer sa nouvelle vision des choses et prendre le temps de faire de la recherche. Ce faisant, elle fut à l'origine de la première génération des chercheurs canadiens-anglais formés à McGill qui, au tournant du siècle, prirent la relève de leurs maîtres lorsque ceux-ci regagnèrent la métropole.

Pour comprendre la différence d'attitude face aux rayons X—ou à la recherche scientifique en général—que l'on observe au tournant du siècle en sciences physiques, entre les savants de McGill et les professeurs de Laval, il est donc nécessaire de tenir compte du rôle de l'institution scolaire comme agent formateur *d'habitus,* c'est-à-dire de schèmes générateurs de pratiques et de critères d'évaluation des pratiques.[52] Cette approche des pratiques scientifiques permet de distinguer différents usages sociaux des sciences dont les pratiques de "recherche" et de "vulgarisation" ne sont que deux exemples. En reliant ces différents usages aux contextes social, institutionnel et disciplinaire qui les rendent possibles, on peut ainsi comprendre leur émergence et leur transformation sans préjuger de leur valeur respective comme le fait toujours implicitement la problématique du "retard".

Remerciements:
Je tiens à remercier Raymond Duchesne pour ses commentaires sur une version préliminaire de ce texte et pour avoir mis à ma disposition ses notes prises dans les archives du Séminaire de Québec.

Remerciements des rédacteurs:
Reproduction gracieuseté de l'auteur et de l'Institut national de la recherche scientifique (dans M Fournier, Y Gingras, O Keel [eds]. Sciences et médecine au Québec: perspectives sociohistoriques. Institut québécois de recherche sur la culture, 1987, pp 69–86).

DR SAMUEL CUMMINGS

The story of Dr Samuel Cummings is one of the enigmas of Canadian radiology. Being fluent in German as well as his native tongue he studied in that country with Professor Röntgen. Indeed he returned to Germany every year for a period at the turn of the Century. This eventually resulted in an ornately carved chair being given to him by the German government for his assistance to the Professor. The nature of that assistance remains to be discovered.

Born in Hamilton, of which city his father was twice mayor, Dr Cummings was a surgeon who graduated from the University of Toronto and who practised in Hamilton and Toronto. His experience in Germany led to him being a pioneer in introducing the clinical use of x-rays into Canada. He published some of his early experience on the radiological diagnosis of bone tuberculosis (see Appendix 1) and there is anecdotal evidence that his technique was so excellent that his rivals suspected him of retouching his radiographs.

Dr Cummings was involved in organized radiology and was a vice-president of the American X-ray Association. He declined the presidency having an aversion to anything which might make him a public person.

As a surgeon Cummings was an innovator and his services were simultaneously in demand in both Hamilton and Toronto. He studied under Dr William Mayo who remarked the Canada would never fully appreciate what in had in Dr Cummings as a surgeon. A colleague, Dr Douglas Storms, noted that Cummings was a quarter of a century ahead of his time.

A man of some complexity and many dimensions Dr Samuel Cummings was also a noted music critic and a connoisseur of good food. His home was a refuge for musicians visiting Toronto and Hamilton. Dr Cummings died in Havana in late 1933.

It would complete the circle to be able to recover this definitive "chair of radiology."

Beautiful Chair Recalls Doctor's Aid To Roentgen

A magnificently carved chair was the centre of interest yesterday as the estate of the late Dr. Samuel Cummings, internationally-famous surgeon, and his sister, Miss Alice Cummings, was closed with an auction at the old home, a chair that recalls the doctor's brilliant work in the discovery of the X-ray. The chair is a beautiful example of the furniture-maker's skill, with two German eagles poised regally on either side of the ornate back, but it is as a tribute to a Hamilton man by the German government that the chair has its greatest value.

It was presented to Dr. Cummings for his brilliant work and assistance to Professor Roentgen after whom the roentgen-ray was named, better known as the X-ray.

Tension mounted in the evening as swarms of people crowded through the spacious old downstairs rooms, cautiously bidding on crystal chandeliers, Napoleonic chairs, beautifully-carved bookcases and gold-framed paintings.

Sole surviving member of the family is a younger sister, Dr. Louise D. Cummings, brilliant mathematician who is teaching at Vassar College. Since her departure from Hamilton a year and a half ago, the house, which has been purchased by the McGregor Clinic, has been uninhabited. Many of Dr. Cummings' more beautiful objets d'art were taken with him when he moved to Queen's Park, Toronto. He was an ardent collector of Persian rugs, oil paintings and bric-a-brac.

The German chair was knocked down to George Sharples, local florist, for $36.

Extract from "Hamilton Spectator", 1930's

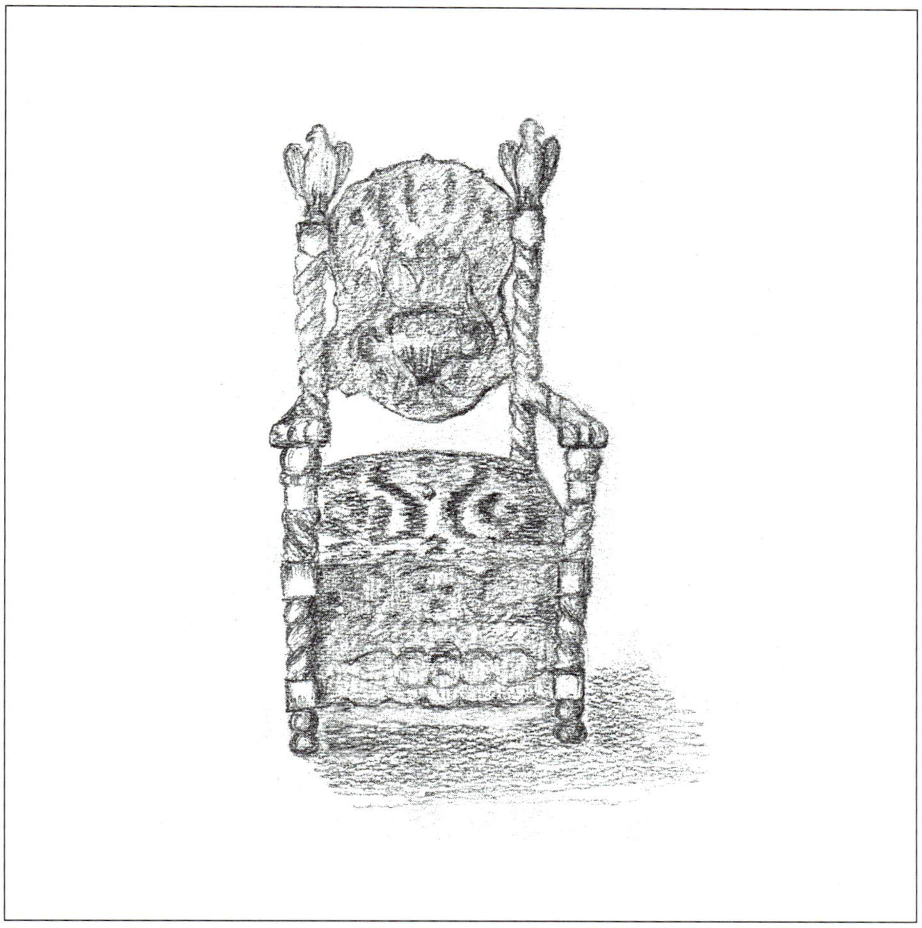

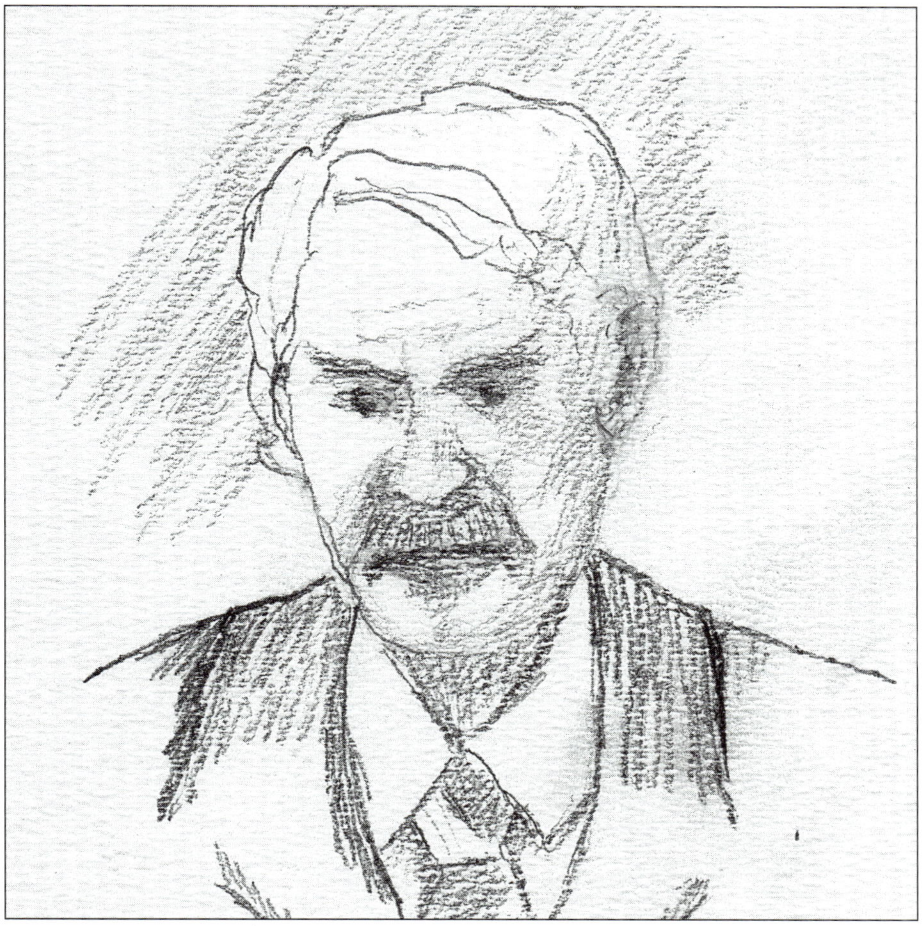

Left
The chair presented
to Dr Samuel Cummings

Below
Dr Samuel Cummings

EVENING TELEGRAM

February 25, 1896.

PRICE ONE CENT

THE DEFICIT IS HID IN THE SAFE

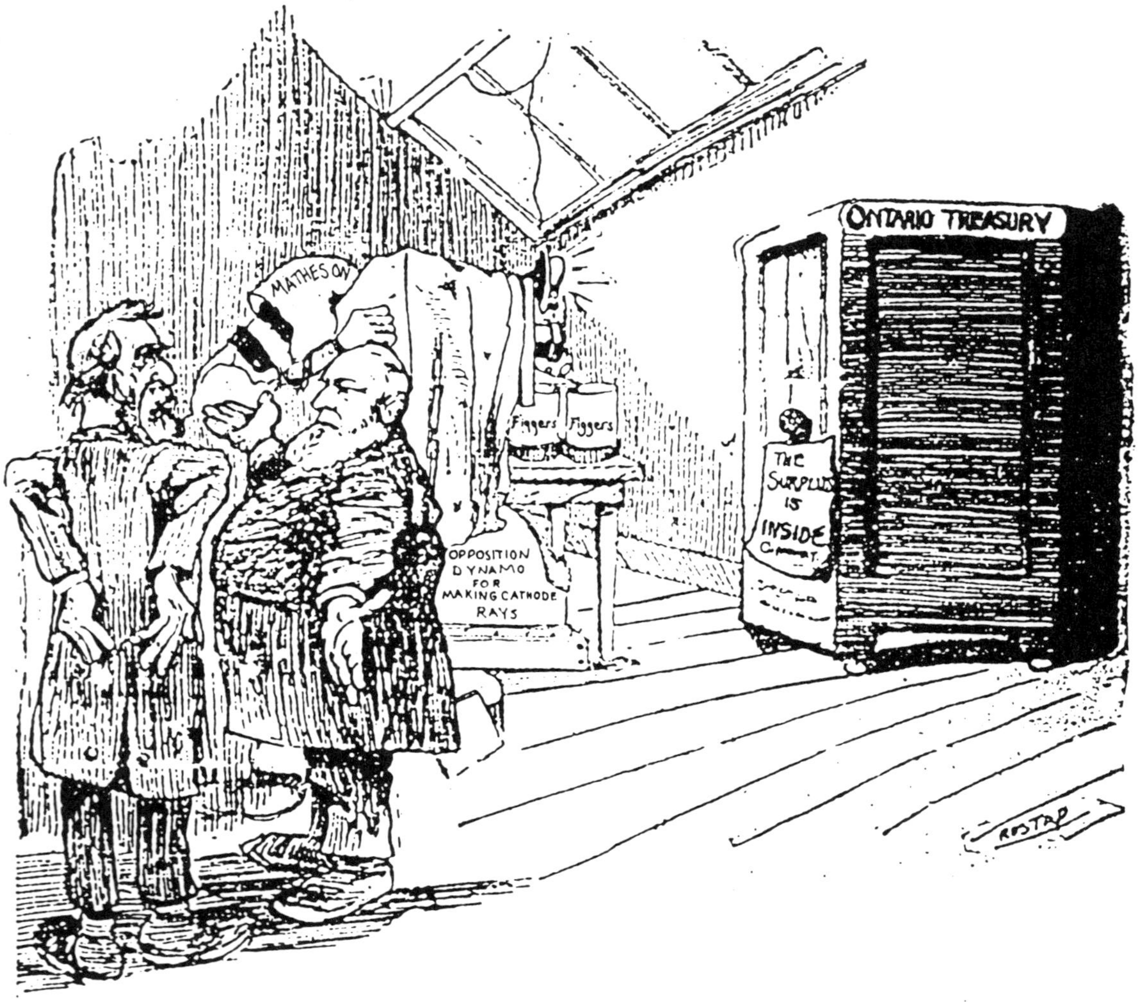

JOE L. HAYCOCK, M. P. P.— "I'm amazin' anxious to see that Deficit get its pickter took."

G. F. MARTER, M. P. P.—"Just keep yer eye on Prof. Matheson.

NOTE.—Col. Matheson, M. P. P., of South Lanark, in answer to the budget speech, insisted that there was no surplus inside the Ontario treasury.

Chapter VII • The Adoption and Effects of

X-rays in Ontario

JTH Connor

During the latter half of the 19th century, medical innovations—such as anaesthesia, antiseptic and aseptic surgery based on the germ theory of disease, and x-rays—transformed medicine in Ontario, as elsewhere, into a recognizably modern form.[1] Although there are detailed studies of the first two of these innovations in Ontario,[2] no analysis of the adoption of x-rays in the province has yet been undertaken. Medical histories of the province, as well as national surveys, pay scant attention to this subject; likewise, no systematic account of x-rays is contained in hospital histories, which make only scattered reference to the development of radiology in Ontario. Finally, general histories of radiology, while they provide much technical information, concentrate primarily on events in Europe and America.[3] Accordingly, this study presents an overview of Ontario's experience, particularly around the turn of the century, with the "new photography," as x-rays were first called. Through an examination of both the popular and professional responses to x-rays in Ontario, I will show that x-rays captured the public imagination as no other medical innovation had before and altered the nature and structure of the province's medical profession and its general hospitals.

In November 1895 the German scientist Wilhelm Conrad Röntgen discovered x-rays; by January of the following year all major European newspapers and professional journals had published articles about the "Röntgen Rays."[4] From an analysis of newspapers throughout the province, one can conclude that most Ontarians would have been familiar with the discovery of x-rays by February

1896. Readers of local papers in London, Stratford, Ottawa and Fort William-Port Arthur, for example, could all avail themselves of information on x-ray developments in Europe, the United States and Canada.[5] Arresting titles such as "The Mysterious New Ray," "Wonderful! Wonderful!", "Wonders of X-rays," and "Through Live Flesh" likely ensured that Ontarians read the news articles. However, the single richest source of material is the Toronto newspapers. The first information published in Toronto (and indeed in Canada) about Röntgen's discovery appeared in the January 30, 1896 issue of the *Mail and Empire*.[6] A brief piece, entitled "Prof Röntgen's New Photography," informed readers of the "probable great value of the discovery to medicine and surgery." Commencing February 5, the story of x-rays truly broke when the *Evening Star* published a front-page story under the title "Cathode Rays—The Discovery Tried In Toronto." This article quoted Dr Charles Sheard, the city's Medical Officer of Health, as saying that several local doctors were about to be "engaged in experimenting on their own account in as complete a way as the incomplete details of the discovery will permit them."

But while this group prepared for their experiments, another was already "photographing the invisible." A University of Toronto team consisting of members from the School of Practical Science (Charles Wright and J Keele) and from the Department of Physics (JC McLennan and WW Nichol) produced Ontario's first x-ray photographs, which demonstrated the skeleton of a hand as well as a variety of other objects such as spectacles in a case;[7] this work received a warm reception. The *Globe* editor commented:

> *Researches in bacteriology or in applied electrical science may be more important, or, to the scientific mind more wonderful. But the possibility of photographing the bones in a living body, the bullet imbedded in a tree or the coins in a purse will awaken a popular interest such as has greeted no invention of recent years.* [8]

The editor of the *Mail and Empire* placed the Toronto team's efforts in the context of civic and national pride:

> *As the scientific world is thus moving with the speed of this age of express trains and rapid transit generally, it is satisfactory to find that Canada, and especially that Toronto are not behind the times.... The university has a regiment of explorers...[which] is enough to show that the university is up-to-date with what is passing in the world of science. An institution that thus places itself abreast of the times does honour to the earnest labours of those who have striven in the past to bring it to its present grade of effectiveness, and to those who are now responsible for its holding of the position it has attained.* [9]

Similarly, a subsequent article in this paper further congratulated these Ontario scientists on their research, which "brought fame to themselves and honour to their university."[10]

Two other features characterized the way that the Toronto (and to a lesser extent, the Ontario) press presented x-rays to the public.[11] The first was the profuse use of illustrations. Initially, such illustrations were merely sketches of objects that had been photographed "by the new process" and were impressionistic and lacking in detail. However, by mid-February actual photographs were reproduced that illustrated more detail of their subjects. Clearly the inclusion of such illustrations was popular, for during the last week of February both the *Globe* and the *Mail and Empire* published weekend illustrated supplements that included many x-ray photographs produced by McLennan, Wright and Keele as well as scenes of the Toronto researchers at work with their electrical apparatus.[12] The significance of photographs in newspapers is likely to be lost on the modern reader as their appearance is now standard, but for the late Victorian reader photographic illustrations were a novelty. It was not until the 1890s that a wholly satisfactory technique for reproducing photographs on newsprint was devised; indeed, the general use of photographs in newspapers was a practice not widely adopted until after 1900.[13] Hence, the x-ray story allowed publishers to employ these new modes of journalistic expression to their fullest; and, in turn, such means conveyed information about Röntgen's work in a most compelling and informative fashion to Ontario readers. Humour constituted another feature of the popular response to the "new photography." One indirect example was a series of display advertisements for "The Textile Wonder 'Textile Buckskin'-The Perfect Dress Interlining," which was certified to be "impervious to the Röntgen rays." Reinforcing the advertising copy, which informed readers that this material afforded "an impenetrable shield against the mortifying possibility of the surreptitious use of this new photographic wonder," was the revealing illustration of the skeleton of a woman clad in an unprotected dress; by her side was an uncompromised woman wearing "Textile Buckskin."[14]

More overt examples of x-ray humour pertain to political matters. For example, an editorial note in the Conservative *Mail and Empire* stated laconically that a "Röntgen photograph of Premier Greenway would show that he has a Liberal quantity of backbone." (Thomas Greenway was the first Liberal Premier of Manitoba from 1888 to 1899.) Another noted that if a Röntgen ray were applied to the head of the Liberal politician Richard

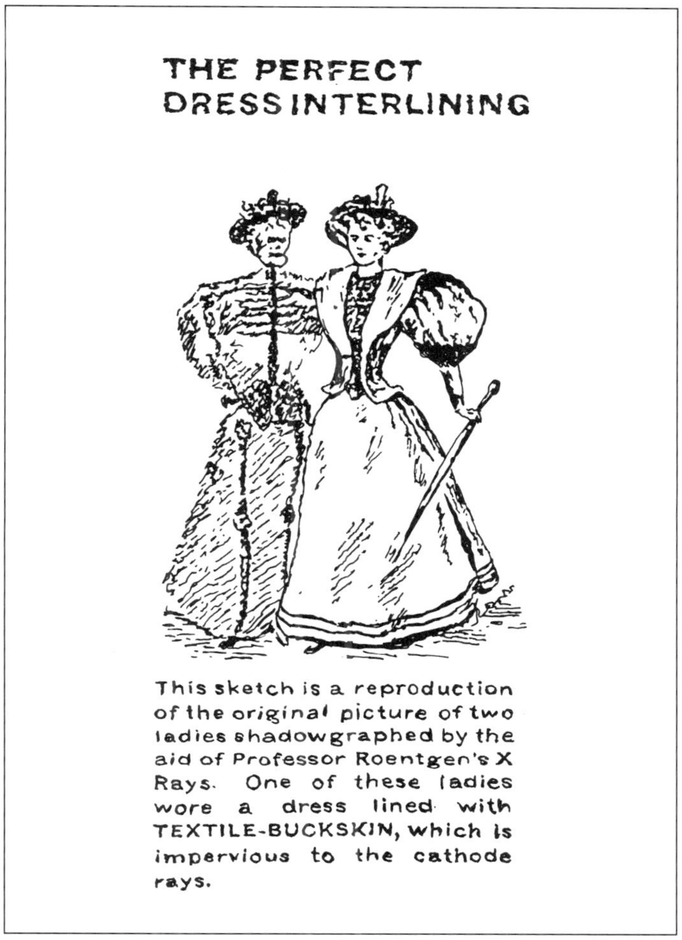

Cartwright, it would "reveal the real trade policy of the Liberal party, viz, out-and-out free trade and destruction to Canadian agricultural and industrial interests."[15] And the *Evening Telegram* published a front-page political cartoon that depicted an Ontario opposition MPP (identified as Matheson) operating a "Dynamo for making Cathode Rays," which was directed at a large safe identified as the Ontario treasury. On the door of the safe was a note reading "The Surplus is inside." The cartoon also showed two other Ontario politicians—Joe L Haycock and GF Marter—with the former remarking, "I'm amazin' anxious to see that Deficit get its pickter took," to which the latter politician replies, "Just keep yer eye on Prof Matheson." Certainly, the opposition was sceptical of the provincial government's claim that it had generated a surplus in its finances.[16] Indeed, in the Ontario legislature itself another opposition member quipped across the floor that it "would be an interesting experiment to apply cathodic photography to the Treasury Department to find the surplus."[17] Perhaps the most satirical lampoon told of a professor who took several "Röntgen photographs" of some Ottawa "notables." But upon developing the plates, he found the results baffled him, for while they contained many fine details of the subject, the area defined by the skull was completely empty.[18] It is not surprising that Ontario commentators seized upon the metaphoric use of x-rays for purposes of political satire. At last, here was a discovery that could penetrate matter to reveal the underlying reality of a situation—what better technique to apply to politics, where illusion and rhetoric invariably seemed to mask true intentions. Moreover, like the use of photographs, the front-page political editorial cartoon was a relatively new way for newspapers to attract readers' attention; thus, the joining together of a topical discovery, political comment, and illustrative material was an effective combination.[19] In sum, then, the marriage of humour and the "new photography" allowed newspaper publishers to inform their readers further of the existence of x-rays, attack their political opponents and, no doubt, increase newspaper sales.

The final manifestation of the popular interest in x-rays was the many public demonstrations, discussions and lectures concerning them. Various societies and groups, particularly in Toronto, sponsored evening meetings where the wonders of Röntgen's discovery were revealed to audiences. For example, the Canadian Institute (an association concerned with literary as well as scientific matters), the Toronto Camera Club, the Toronto Engineering Society and the Toronto Astronomical and Physical Society all held such events.[20] To be sure this account of the popular response to x-rays centres on events that occurred in Toronto, but as has been noted, other Ontario newspapers also reported pertinent information. A question that needs to be answered, however, is why so much excitement was generated over the introduction of x-rays.[21] To some extent, the answer may be that the x-ray story was, simply stated, a good one, for while it was mysterious in some aspects, the results of the rays were tangible and readily appreciated by all. Moreover, here was an international event with a local angle, which meant that the reader's interest would be high and that material for print was readily available. In addition, one suspects that a more general historical force was also at play. A clue to identifying such a force is afforded in a study of the late Victorian press in Canada by Paul Rutherford, who notes that the "daily press popularized...a particular dogma of modernity" based in part upon the notion of progress—a concept that he considered the "most hallowed maxim of the age."[22] Indeed, if we recall the editorials quoted above in the *Globe* and *Mail and Empire* that referred generally to the work of the new photography, and specifically to the notion that the "scientific world [was]...moving with the speed of this age of express trains and rapid transit", it is clear how the reception of x-rays was consistent with

Rutherford's evaluation of the age. Finally, it should be borne in mind that x-rays were a special case of the then-current electrical revolution, and if anything exemplified modernity, electricity did. Even the president of the staid Royal Society of Canada declared in his 1896 address, "Electricity . . . bids fair to revolutionize" almost all aspects of life from domestic affairs to warfare. And the "newest and most remarkable" application of electricity, the Society official noted, was the "production of cathode rays, by which photographing through opaque substances has been made possible."[23] There can be little doubt, then, that for many Ontarians x-rays were a symbol of a new, modern conception of society and, as Ontario was not merely a spectator to, but a participant in, the Röntgen revolution, by implication the province too was modern and progressive. Not surprisingly, the popular reception of x-rays did not go unnoticed by members of the medical profession. The editor of the journal the *Canada Lancet,* published in Toronto, commented that the daily press had "gone daft over the possibilities" of x-rays.[24] However, other representatives of Ontario's doctors were almost as enthusiastic about x-rays as the lay segment of society. One writer assured his medical colleagues that they should "expect revelations of very great interest which will, when practically applied, be of incalculable benefit."[25] Another editor prophesied that "the rapid strides already made from this most wonderful discovery will continue to go on until the art of surgery . . . will become almost a play toy in the hands of the most ordinary physician."[26]

Such optimism, however, had to be tempered by accurate technical knowledge in the use of the rays—a subject not covered in popular reports. At this early stage, of course, there were no textbooks or experienced teachers; thus, articles in professional journals and meetings of medical societies were the primary means for communicating information about x-rays. Central to this process was the activity of the prominent Toronto physician Edmund E King, who based his knowledge on his own pioneering experience and disseminated it to his colleagues at annual meetings of the Ontario Medical Association as well as meetings of the Toronto Clinical Society. At these gatherings King introduced and demonstrated to his audience the latest equipment and discussed how to interpret the resultant skiagraphs (the term then usually used to describe x-ray photographs—from the Greek *skia,* meaning shadow). Usually these discussions centred on the diagnosis and detection of foreign bodies and un-united fractures.[27] At the same time retailers began to sell complete x-ray outfits of varying sizes: large units were capable of any work, while smaller

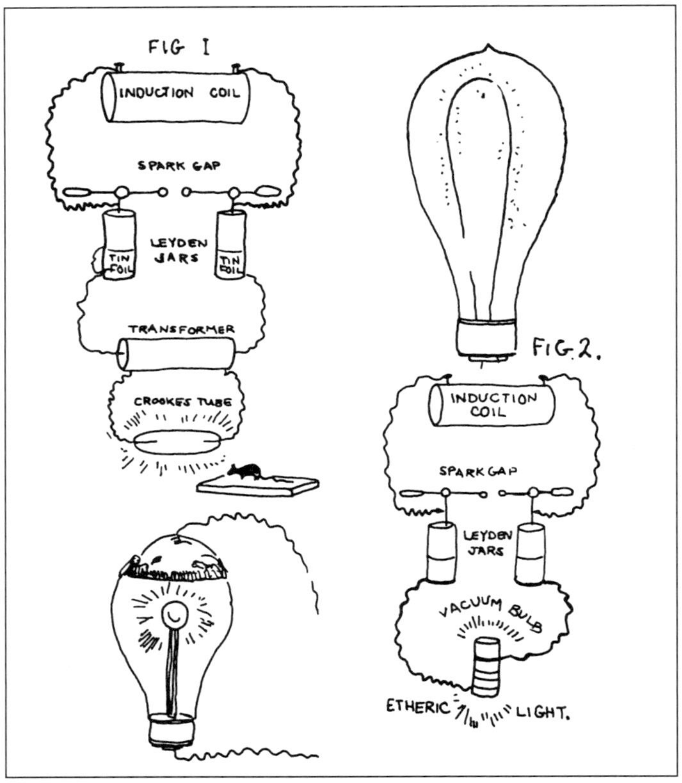

ones were limited to hands, feet, joints and so on. Depending on the unit chosen, a doctor could spend up to $100 for a full x-ray kit.[28]

In mid-February 1896, the first documented clinical use of x-rays took place at Toronto's homeopathic Grace Hospital, when a needle embedded in a woman's foot was removed, once the foreign body had been located with the aid of x-rays. Whereas the operation took only a few minutes, a fifteen-minute exposure to the rays was necessary in order to produce a clear negative.[29] The application of x-rays in similar cases soon became commonplace; contained in the contemporary medical literature are details of the removal of objects such as bullets, coins, and buttons, which were located with x-rays.[30] X-rays were not without their dangers, however. For example, Dr Edmund King reported the case of one of his patients—identified as Mr "R"—who had capitalized on the public excitement about x-rays and had engaged in public demonstrations of them. From May until July 1896, "R" had been exposed to the rays for periods of up to ten hours daily. An examination of "R" by King, presumably in September, revealed that the entire left side of the patient's face around the temple and ear was devoid of hair, and that his left eyebrow and left half of his moustache were missing; so too the "whisker on left cheek, chin and neck [was] almost gone," King further noted. In assessing this case King was "perfectly satisfied that no extraneous agents were at work," and thus he concluded that "R"'s lesions were solely the result of the x-rays.[31] Of course, "R"'s experience was an extreme case, for very few people would amass five hundred hours exposure to the rays in a few months, but such conditions brought to the fore the possible harmful effects of prolonged exposure to this new force. Notwithstanding the problem of x-ray burns, radiological methods quickly became standard medical and surgical practice, owing to their utility. James Third, a leading Kingston physician writing in 1901, summed up the situation:

> *The Röntgen ray, as a diagnostic agent, is no longer an experiment. Its growth has been phenomenal. It came up through the stage of criticism with unprecedented rapidity, receiving few scars and for these it is therapeutically the richer.... Some physicians would limit its use to the detection of foreign bodies and the recognition of certain fractures and dislocations but these are the limitations of its natal day; as well we might limit the use of the microscope to the recognition of the grosser tissue elements.*[32]

Indeed by the early 1900s, owing to better equipment, refined technique and more experienced operators, physicians were using x-rays to diagnose conditions as diverse as heart disease, stones in the kidney and bladder and diseases of internal organs. Similarly during this period x-rays were used as a therapeutic agent in the treatment of skin, bone, lip and breast cancer. For physicians of the time it mattered little *how* malignant cells were destroyed; rather, the issue was to be assured that this new force did indeed destroy tumour cells. Moreover, x-ray therapeusis was painless; scarring was minimal; only diseased tissue was destroyed; pain was relieved; the offensive odour of rotting tissue was eliminated; and, finally, patients no longer feared a major operation (extirpation of a tumour was the most likely treatment before the development of x-ray therapy).[33] During the following two decades both the therapeutic and diagnostic efficacy of x-rays increased with the development of more powerful equipment. In particular

Left
Dr WJ Morton's arrangement for cathode rays

Below
Making an early radiograph (early 1900s) in the Hospital for Sick Children, Toronto

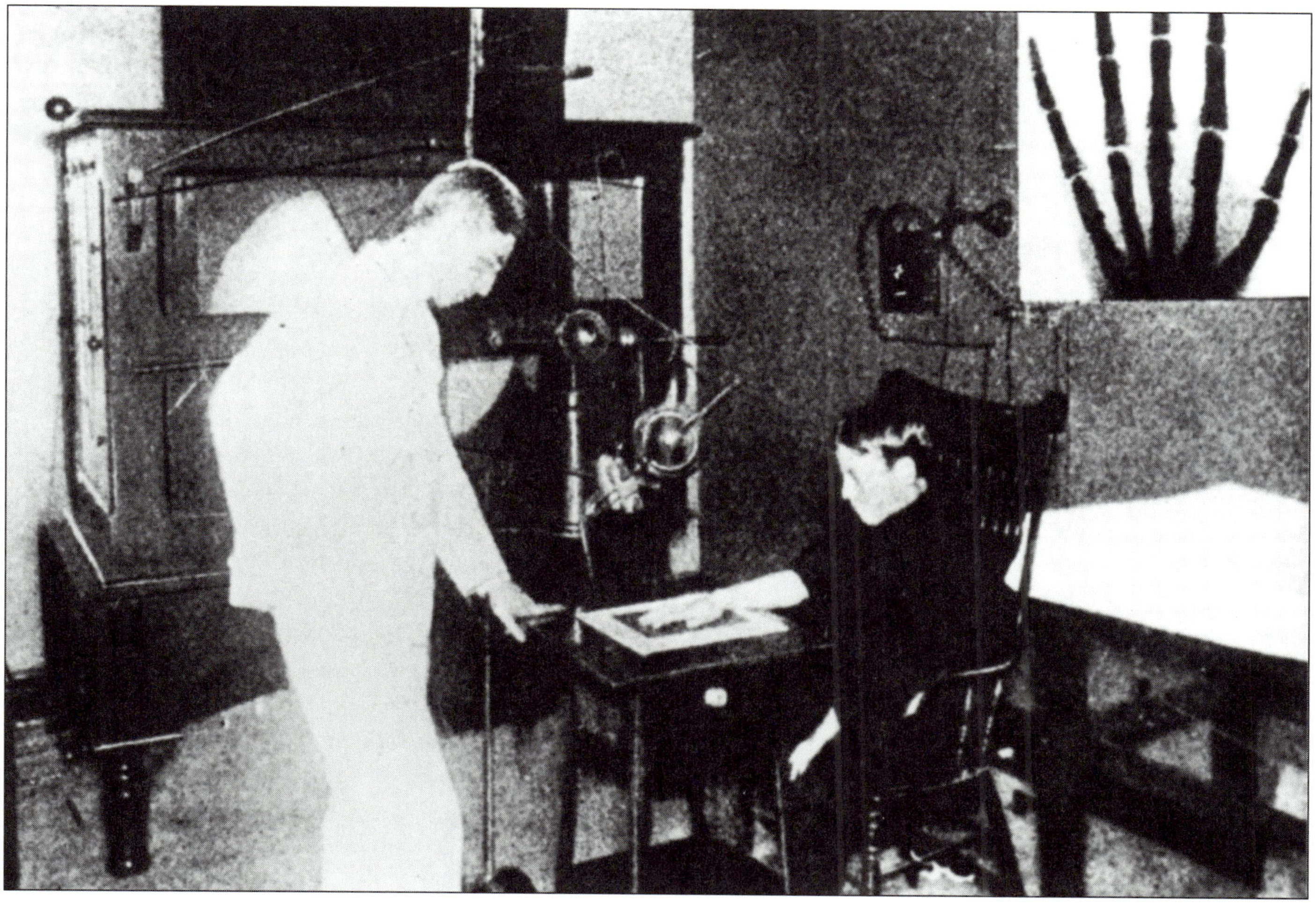

the use of cellulose acetate film (around 1916) rather than the old-fashioned glass plate greatly aided in producing sharper negatives. By the 1940s, however, x-ray therapy was being replaced by new radiotherapeutic techniques based upon the use of radium and, later, cobalt-60.[34]

Because new x-ray methods put increasing demands on physicians who routinely used them, changes occurred in the structure of the Ontario medical profession: a new specialty was created as some practitioners began to limit their practice to x-ray activity. Later these specialists formed their own professional societies, such as the Ontario Society of Radiographers, founded in 1935, and the Canadian Association of Radiologists, founded two years later by Gordon E Richards of the Toronto General Hospital. By 1946 this trend towards specialization was formally recognized by the Medical Council of Canada when examinations in radiology were required for certification.[35] A corollary of this process was that what was once a fairly homogeneous profession during the 19th century became increasingly heterogeneous or compartmentalized in the 20th. And, while such "branching" was taking place, a "layering" process also was underway during the 1920s and 1930s, with physician specialists becoming the elite within the profession at the expense of what was perceived to be the lowlier general practitioner.[36]

While many private practitioners continued to perform their own radiological examinations and established their own clinics—a practice that continues today—hospitals also installed x-ray facilities. The process was not an even one, however; some institutions acquired equipment almost immediately, while others did not. For example, when the newly built Sarnia General Hospital opened in October 1896, it was described as "one of the best-equipped institutions of its kind in Canada" with full facilities for aseptic and antiseptic surgery, and yet there was no x-ray apparatus.[37] And, when a new general hospital in Wingham opened its doors in February 1907, it too was equipped with modern operating and surgical facilities but no x-ray equipment.[38] On the other hand, the Kingston General Hospital installed a machine in 1896 (albeit homemade); the Toronto General and the Hospital for Sick Children obtained their equipment in 1900, and the St Catherine's General in 1903; hospitals in London first offered x-ray services during 1915–16; and the Oshawa General did not begin x-ray work until 1920.[39] It was not until 1926 that St Joseph's Hospital of Parry Sound installed its x-ray equipment.[40] Generally speaking. one can assume that by the late 1920s most Ontario hospitals were equipped with x-ray facilities.[41]

Although many factors may account for the time it took Ontario hospitals to acquire x-ray equipment, certainly the most significant one was cost. As technological developments increased the sophistication of the apparatus, so too did prices escalate. Contrasting with the cost of the $100 outfit of 1896 was the $10 000 unit that the Toronto General Hospital purchased in 1910.[42] Hospitals coped with this problem in three distinct ways. First, through dramatic increases in provincial support: in 1902 hospitals in Ontario received aid in the amount of $110 000; by 1932 this sum had risen to just under $2 million.[43] Second, hospital patients increasingly had to pay for services received. For example, in 1895 at the St Catherine's General Hospital there were two free patients for every paying one; but by 1904 this ratio was just short of a full reversal.[44] Similarly, at the Kingston General Hospital in 1892, 20 per cent ($3100) of the hospital's income was derived from paying patients; by 1913 this figure had risen to 60 per cent ($24 649); and ten years later $95 013 was derived from this source—70 per cent of the total income for the hospital.[45] X-rays played a specific role in this process, for larger urban hospitals usually ran their radiological departments on a profit basis, as was the case in London's Victoria Hospital and in the Toronto and Kingston General hospitals. In this regard a particularly instructive case is the Kingston hospital, which in 1919 established the Radiological and Radiotherapy Department. The radiologist directly charged his patients for services rendered; 90 per cent of the revenues went to the physician and 10 per cent to the hospital; within six years the cost of the new department had been recovered.[46]

The final technique that hospitals employed to offset the cost of x-ray equipment was to rely on public and corporate benefaction. This approach was successful for several institutions, especially those in smaller towns. The community hospitals of Cobourg, Hanover and Kenora, for example, received sums in the thousands of dollars from prominent local citizens specifically to purchase x-ray equipment; in Sarnia the Imperial Oil Company donated eight thousand dollars for this purpose.[47] These donations stand out as novel events in the development of hospital–society relations, for although citizens had previously supported hospitals with small gifts such as food, linen and other minor supplies, none was comparable to the gift of x-ray equipment. One reason for these acts of benevolence was probably the wave of public excitement over x-rays: to purchase x-ray apparatus for a local hospital could well have been considered by all as a sign of the donor's personal progressiveness as well as his generosity. Similarly, to be so equipped meant that the community hospital, once a constant reminder that poor and needy people existed in the region, now stood as a symbol of that community's modernity.[48]

One last ramification of the relationship that was forged between the hospital and medical technology in general, and x-rays in particular, should be considered. Owing to the increased sophistication of apparatus, it was no longer possible to have radiological equipment or laboratories located where there happened to be free space in the hospital, for as these services became established they had to be fully integrated into the overall concept of the institution. That is to say, the layout of hospitals now had to conform to, or was greatly influenced by, the requirements of the services, and not the reverse. Similarly, as diagnostic and therapeutic services increased, such departments became the focal points of hospitals, thus again affecting hospital design, especially with respect to traffic patterns. Accordingly, hospitals became "monolithic" and centralized in design, unlike the rambling structures they had been earlier in the 19th century and before.[49] Finally,. the layout of individual departments had to be carefully planned in order to coordinate patient, operator and equipment in an effective manner. For example, in the early days of x-rays in the Oshawa General Hospital, the equipment "rested" in the office of the lady superintendent; but in later years as the equipment increased in size and sophistication, properly designed quarters were obtained for it.[50] The culmination of this process can be seen in a mid-20th century Ontario government guide for the construction of hospitals, which devoted no fewer than twelve pages to the considerations, location, components, and plan of radiology departments. For example, according to the guide, the radiology department of a two-hundred-bed hospital should occupy approximately four thousand square feet and consist of numerous personnel areas such as offices and dressing rooms, film processing and chemical storage areas, separate photofluorography and general and gastric radiography sections, a cystoscopy room and a fracture room. Moreover, the department's location within the hospital required "careful study," for it was to be accessible to the inpatient department and be as close as possible to the emergency and out-patient departments. Finally, to ensure that the extensive electrical equipment was not affected by dampness, the department was not to be located in the hospital's basement.[51] Thus, the institutional effects of x-rays were twofold: they allowed hospitals to offer a particular service that generated needed funds for the institution, and hospital design and construction had to be rethought because of the constraints imposed by technological devices such as x-ray apparatus.

It is evident from this brief account of the adoption and effects of x-rays in Ontario that, through direct and indirect means, their discovery influenced the lives of the majority of Ontarians; for layman and professional alike, Röntgen's name became a household word. To be sure, the impact of radiology was felt most in the clinical and scientific worlds, where it fast became a useful diagnostic tool for revealing pathological conditions that, in an earlier era, would have gone undetected. Similarly, x-ray therapeusis proved beneficial until it was superseded by more effective means. And as we have also seen, as radiology became firmly entrenched in medical practice, it stimulated institutional change in the profession and the general hospital. But x-rays, in addition to being a sophisticated scientific discovery with important clinical applications, were also representative of the spirit of modernity and progressivism that prevailed in Ontario during the late Victorian period. In sum, the "new photography" marked the beginning of the fusion of medicine with high technology—a combination that contemporary Ontarians eagerly embraced and soundly supported.

Acknowledgements:

This article has been reproduced the from the *Quarterly Journal of the Ontario Historical Society* 1987; LXXIX: #1 with the permission of both publisher and author and after due payment of royalties.

"Re" 2½ in nail in rt. bronchus

I think the child's surname was Robinson.

He was about a year old (circa 1904) when he was playing by a slough on his father's farm in Saskatchewan with some gravel + 2½ in nails, when his mother saw that he was choking + black in the face. So she turned him up + smacked his back when only mucus was coughed up. From that time onward he had spasmodic cough on lying down for a few minutes. Medical opinion in Saskatoon + elsewhere favoured T.B. A sinus developed betw. 5th + 6th ribs. A year later he was brought to me. My diagnosis was F.B. in bronchus – Gravel? 2½ in nail??? Dr. Lehmann and I took him to Dr. J.H.R. Bond for X-ray wh. revealed 2½ in nail. Dr. Lehmann opened the trachea (circa 1904-5) + extracted nail. Child recovered but died at the age of 23 yrs. from infection due to Bronchiectasis

H. M. Speechly

Chapter VIII • *Early History of*

Radiology in Manitoba

Robert A McPherson and GF Boult
(Written in 1962)

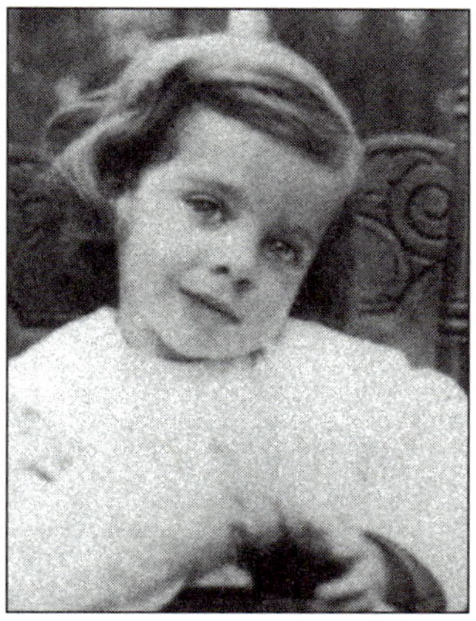

The patient described in the accompanying report (left)

The first recorded reference to radiology in Manitoba was in 1900. In that year John Gault donated a hand operated machine to the Winnipeg General Hospital. The cost of this machine was $296.00. In 1901 a rheostat was added and two fluorescent screens were also purchased.

In the minutes of the board meetings of the Winnipeg General Hospital at this time was the statement that this machine had been very satisfactory for therapy. This, however, seems to be somewhat at variance with the experience of one of the earliest patients treated. One of the older members of the Medical Profession in Manitoba recalls the case of the bank clerk who was treated for pruritus ani around 1905. The treatment was apparently much worse than the disease.

Dr MS Inglis was the first radiologist to be appointed to the Winnipeg General Hospital in 1905.[1] He was succeeded by Dr Walter Watt in 1912. In 1914 he left with the Third Field Ambulance for overseas and was succeeded by Dr Currie McMillan. Dr Watt reversed a later trend by remaining in Britain after the war where he opened a private practice in radiology on Harley St.

During this early period (from 1908 on) a Mr WA Martin was x-ray sales representative for Fisher & Chandler who represented the Victor X-ray Corporation in the West. He travelled extensively in the three Prairie Provinces at this time. At first he sold the portable x-ray (suitcase) unit to general practitioners. This, however, was soon replaced by floor-mounted machines (such as the Wantz Junior). One thing which stands out in his memory of the early days was the marked impression the fluoroscope had on patients. He mentioned that in Saskatchewan around Wadena, where there was a fairly large Ukrainian settlement they would ask for "glass" as they called the fluoroscope.

The patients believed that this was "a must" before anything else was done. Mr Martin also recalls the increased use of radiological examinations in the early 1920s for the diagnosis of fractures. This was done even then to avoid the possibility of a legal suit should a fracture be missed for want of a radiograph.

Dr G Bond and Dr W Hamilton were two of the first general practitioners in Winnipeg to have a "suitcase" x-ray outfit. A real individualist appeared on the scene in about 1908. He was Dr Cyril Burger, who was in private practice as a radiologist and "electric therapist". He had no hospital appointment.

Dr Currie McMillan succeeded Dr Watt at the Winnipeg General Hospital in or about 1914. He left shortly after his appointment for overseas service. He was invalided out of the Army in 1917. After some post-graduate study with Dr Louis Gregory Cole in New York and Drs George and Leonard in Boston he returned to the Winnipeg General Hospital and opened a private office in Winnipeg in 1919. Dr William Carr joined him as an assistant at the Winnipeg General Hospital in 1920 and later left to take a hospital appointment in Victoria, BC.

At about this time Dr Frank Smith was a radiologist at St Boniface Hospital as well as serving part time at the Children's Hospital. He also had a private office in the Somerset Building. Dr Herman Ferrier was radiologist at the MacLean-Gunn clinic for a short time in the 1920s and then left for Fort William and an appointment at the McKellar Hospital.

The successor to Dr Smith at St Boniface Hospital was Dr R Michaud who also had a private office in the Medical Arts Building. Later he worked at the Misericordia Hospital and from there moved to Moose Jaw and then to Ottawa. His successor at St Boniface Hospital was Dr Omar Hague who also had a private office in Winnipeg.

Dr Digby Wheeler joined Dr McMillan in 1926 and in the early thirties opened his own office in the Medical Arts Building. He later became chief at St Boniface and Deer Lodge Hospitals and was also consultant to several other hospitals in Winnipeg until the time of his death in 1955. Dr Edmison joined the Winnipeg General Hospital group in 1932 and later left to join Dr Digby Wheeler and was radiologist at the Children's Hospital for some time prior to World War II. Following the war he moved to Victoria. Dr RA MacPherson joined Dr McMillan in 1938 as did Dr Childe in 1946.

At the end of World War II there were two radiological groups in Winnipeg who did most of the work both in private offices and the hospitals. Dr Omar Hage was the only independant radiologist in Winnipeg at this time.

In about 1948 the Provincial Government set up a diagnostic service which included radiology. This at first only involved two rural centres and was serviced by Dr Tom Dingle. However, as the service expanded and more centres opened up, they brought in radiologists from overseas and at the present time [1962] this service has two radiologists one of whom does some private practice in Brandon.

After the war, clinic practice boomed in Winnipeg. As a result, a great number of private clinics established their own x-ray departments. The two groups mentioned above have serviced the majority of these clinics over the years since their establishment.

Dr McMillan who was one of the remaining pioneers of radiology in Western Canada after World War II, suffered a stroke in 1948 and never recovered sufficiently to return to work. He died in 1950. He was the first radiologist in Manitoba to have a University appointment. Dr Wheeler took over his University position as head of the department of radiology and held this post until his death in 1955. Dr RA. MacPherson then became the Professor of Radiology at the University of Manitoba. Drs McMillan & Wheeler were the last of the early radiologists to pass from the scene in Manitoba and their going meant the loss of a direct link with the early history of radiology in this province.

After the death of Dr Digby Wheeler, one major change which did take place several years later, was the hiring of a full time radiologist with two assistants at St Boniface Hospital. This took place in about 1958.

By 1962 there were two independent radiologists in Winnipeg besides the two large groups while in rural Manitoba Dr Sykes practices as a full time radiologist in Brandon.

Top right
Dr JC McMillan, director of radiology 1914-1944

Right
Drs WJ Elliot, GF Boult and MK Kiernan

Lower right
Dr DW MacEwan

Top far right
Dr Arthur R E Childe (international authority on pediatric radiology and neuroradiology)

Far right
Dr Robert MacPherson

Lower far right
Dr JB Sutherland

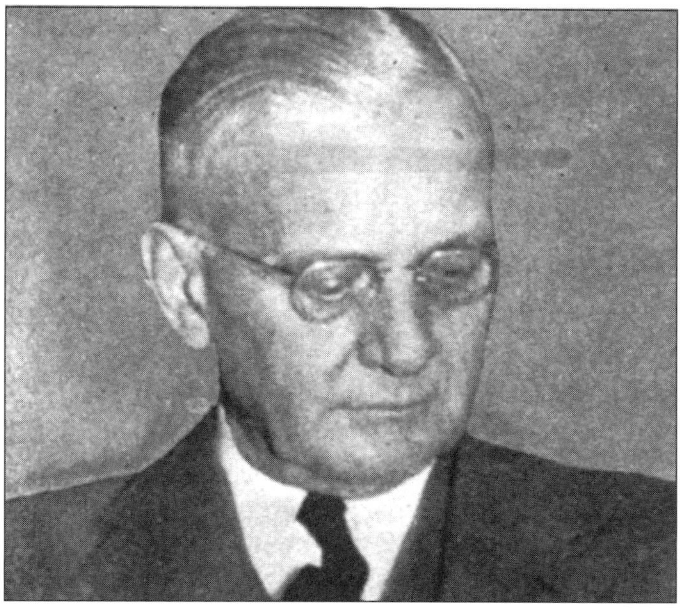

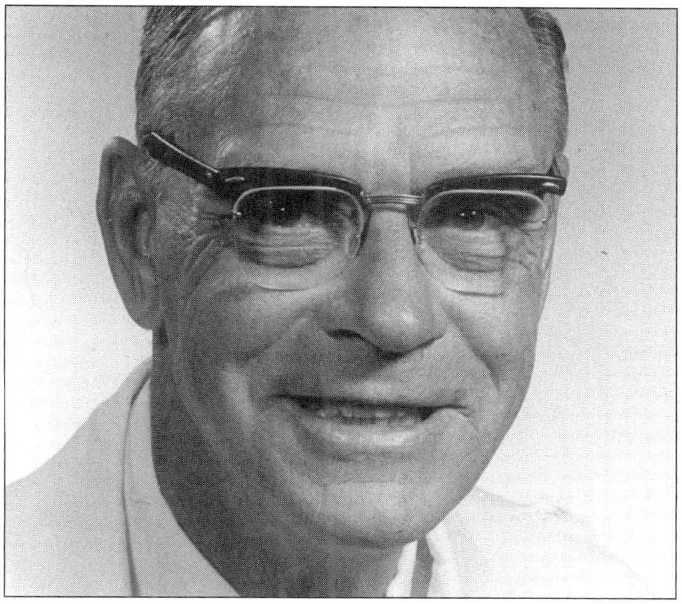

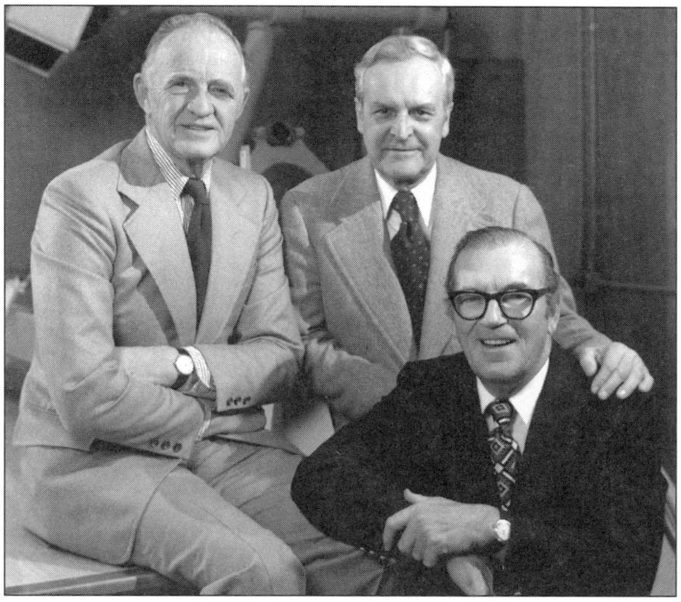

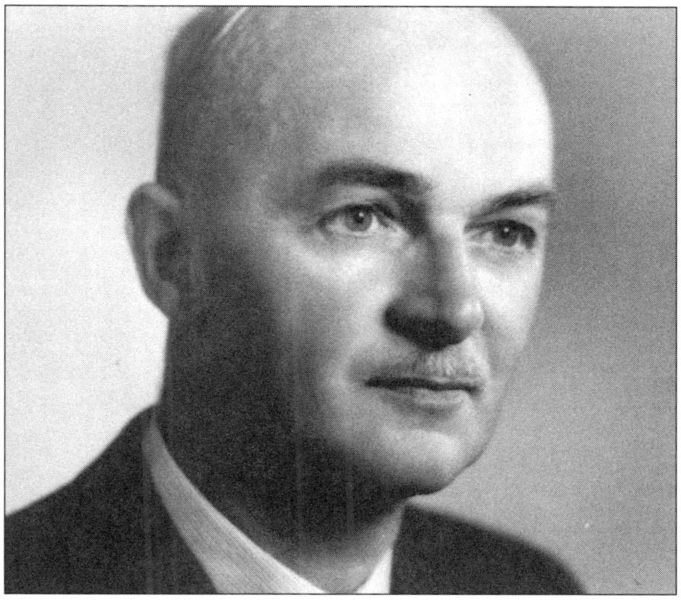

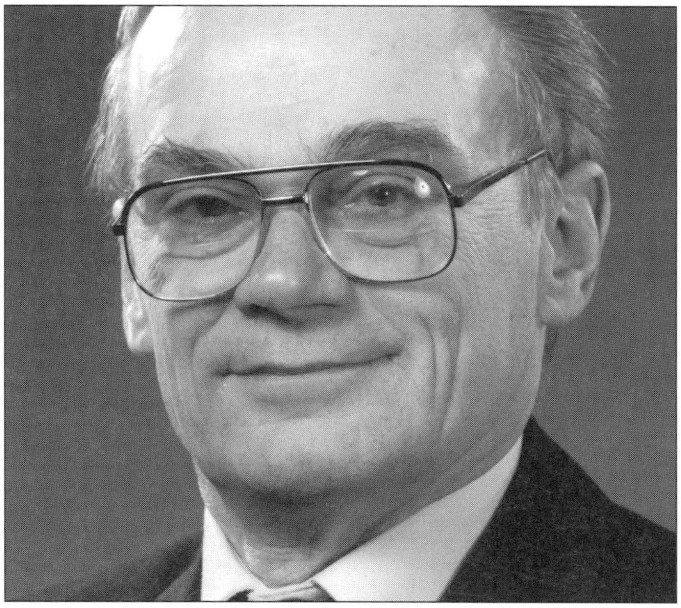

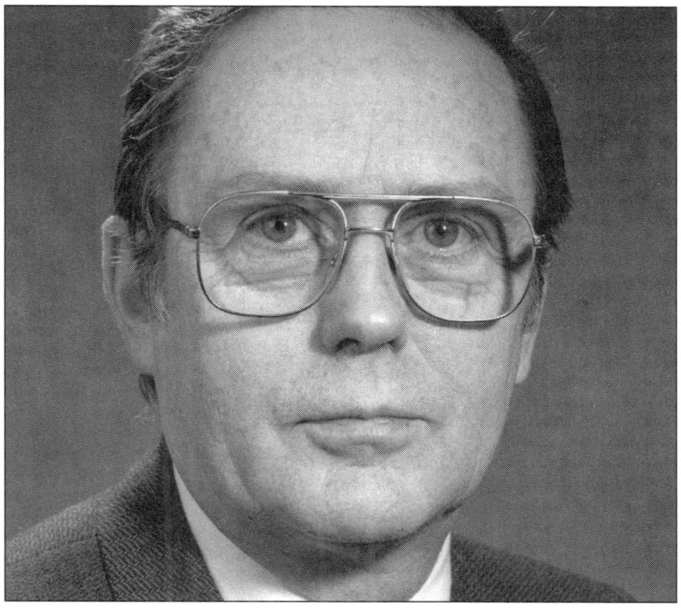

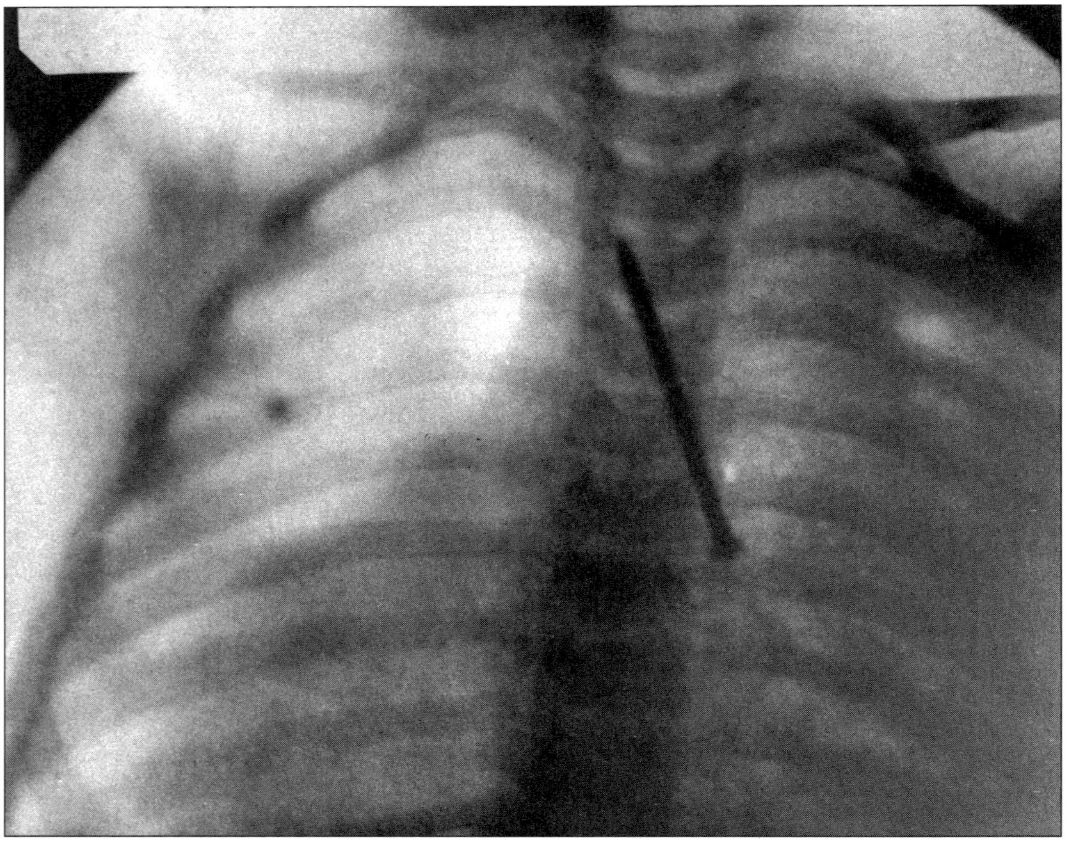

Chapter IX • History of

Imaging in Manitoba

Douglas W MacEwan

Individuals and groups of radiologists provided leadership as remarkable advances constantly expanded and altered imaging. This history only records the names of radiologists who received recognition outside Manitoba.

DR MAXWELL STEVENSON INGLIS: THE FIRST WESTERN CANADIAN RADIOLOGICAL SPECIALIST

Information about Dr Maxwell Stevenson Inglis suggests that he was the first radiology specialist in western Canada.[1] The sources are a recollection, the annual reports of the Winnipeg General Hospital from 1900–1910, newspaper items, and records from the University of Manitoba and the College of Physicians and Surgeons of Manitoba.

Just before World War II, Dr Robert Tait, a physician in Vancouver, met Dr Inglis and the following recollection was recorded in 1974:

Dr Inglis, apparently a very fine and intelligent gentleman, told me (RT) he had been a Canadian Pacific Railway surgeon since 1904 in Winnipeg—I imagine he had a private practice as well but I do not know.

I noted he had skin changes, not very noticeable, on both temples which looked as if they had been caused by excessive irradiation at some previous date but he was not a radiologist then nor apparently had been for some time. At our second meeting I asked about these changes. He courteously asked me to sit down and told me why they had occurred.

[His account was that] in 1895, he had started to practice in Winnipeg. He was married and had his home there but wished to study surgery as

Left
A chest radiograph described on page 126 and showing a nail in the airways

a postgraduate student. His wife was pregnant so they deemed it advisable that she should stay in Winnipeg instead of going to London where, early in December, he read Professor Röntgen's paper on x-rays. This, to him, seemed very important so he left immediately for Germany to see Professor Röntgen who treated him in a most courteous and kindly manner and told him he had the same idea, and Professor Roentgen taught this little class—apparently out of the goodness of his heart.

Dr Inglis left for home at about the end of April, 1896 and resolved to assemble an x-ray machine and dark room. This was not easy as the machines were not being manufactured and he picked up bits and pieces and tubes from various places—he mentioned, as I remember, Boston and Kansas City.

By the spring of 1897 he had a laboratory and had started to make prints on glass for a few patients. He suggested that the Winnipeg General Hospital should have an x-ray department but the Board, after due consideration and advice, decided it might be useless. I think that Dr Inglis was quite depressed over the reception that [the use of] x-rays was being given.

However, fate intervened. A patient had gone to a doctor with an injured wrist. [The doctor] told him that he had a sprained wrist and treated him accordingly. The patient became dissatisfied and went to another physician who told him that his wrist had been fractured. The patient sued the first physician and was finally referred to Dr Inglis for an x-ray [examination]. A fracture was quite plainly seen and the case went to court. After much argument concerning symptoms, findings, etc. Dr Inglis was called to the stand and he reported his findings. The judge asked to see the plate and had Dr Inglis demonstrate the fracture. The judge said that the evidence was good enough for him and awarded damages to the patient to be paid by the first physician. As the case had caused some interest reporters were present and it was written up in the papers. From then on arguments regarding the value of x-rays ceased and the Winnipeg General Hospital started to assemble an x-ray department.

At that time, [Inglis] was using a static machine and would estimate when a sufficient charge was built up by how his hand showed up under the fluoroscope as well as assessment of the thickness of the part to be [imaged]. Meanwhile he was becoming busier as the profession began to use x-ray [examinations] to a greater extent and he had noticed reddening of the skin on his hands with some itching.

Inglis said a "one man commission" arrived from Boston. He had been asked to visit all people using x-ray machine to see what physical changes they had noticed due to x-rays. Dr Inglis told him about the reddening of his skin and the loss of his Van Dyke [beard] which had taken him much time and care to develop, and of which he was quite proud. He had been sitting at his desk one morning and his face felt itchy so he gave it a vigorous rub with his hand. To his surprise and chagrin, half of his beard came away in his hand. It was quite a shock. He looked at his beard and thought he was rotting away.

The "one man commission" said, "Yes, yes, the changes you mentioned have all been reported by the eastern radiologists, but are you sterile?" [Inglis] was quite astounded, but said that as far as he knew he was not, and certainly he did not feel any different. Anyway, he was tested and live spermatozoa were absent. He said the "one man commission" sent by the doctors using x-rays in the East was apparently correct as he had never used contraceptives and they had one son—an infant born shortly before or just after his return from Europe.

The following items in the annual reports of the Winnipeg General Hospital give insight into the successful growth of the department under his leadership. In 1900, through the kindness of Mr J Galt, and a number of friends, a valuable static electrical machine with a complete outfit of electrodes and x-ray apparatus was added to the equipment of the Hospital.

During the latter part of 1902 x-rays were used in a few patients for their therapeutic effect and the results obtained warranted an extension of the radiology department shortly after. In November of the same year, Dr J Halpenny, Medical Superintendent, visited New York and other eastern cities to ascertain what work was being done in this line in the hospitals in those places. Though much of the therapeutic work was done by physicians in private practice, treatments had been done in some of the best hospitals. This made it essential that such work be carried out in our hospital and proved the value of x-rays when used in conjunction with surgery..

In 1903 the maintenance report indicated that expenditure for Roentgen ray supplies was in the vicinity of $100. The first x-ray burn was received in this year. It was located on the eyelid—the patient recovered.

Dr MA Inglis was formally recorded as x-ray specialist to the department in 1905. New equipment purchased in this year cost $80.

In 1906 an induction coil was installed. The number of skiagraphs taken was 129 and 443 electrical treatments were given including x-ray and high frequency treatments. The maintenance costs for this year were $39.

In 1907 the department proved much more effective

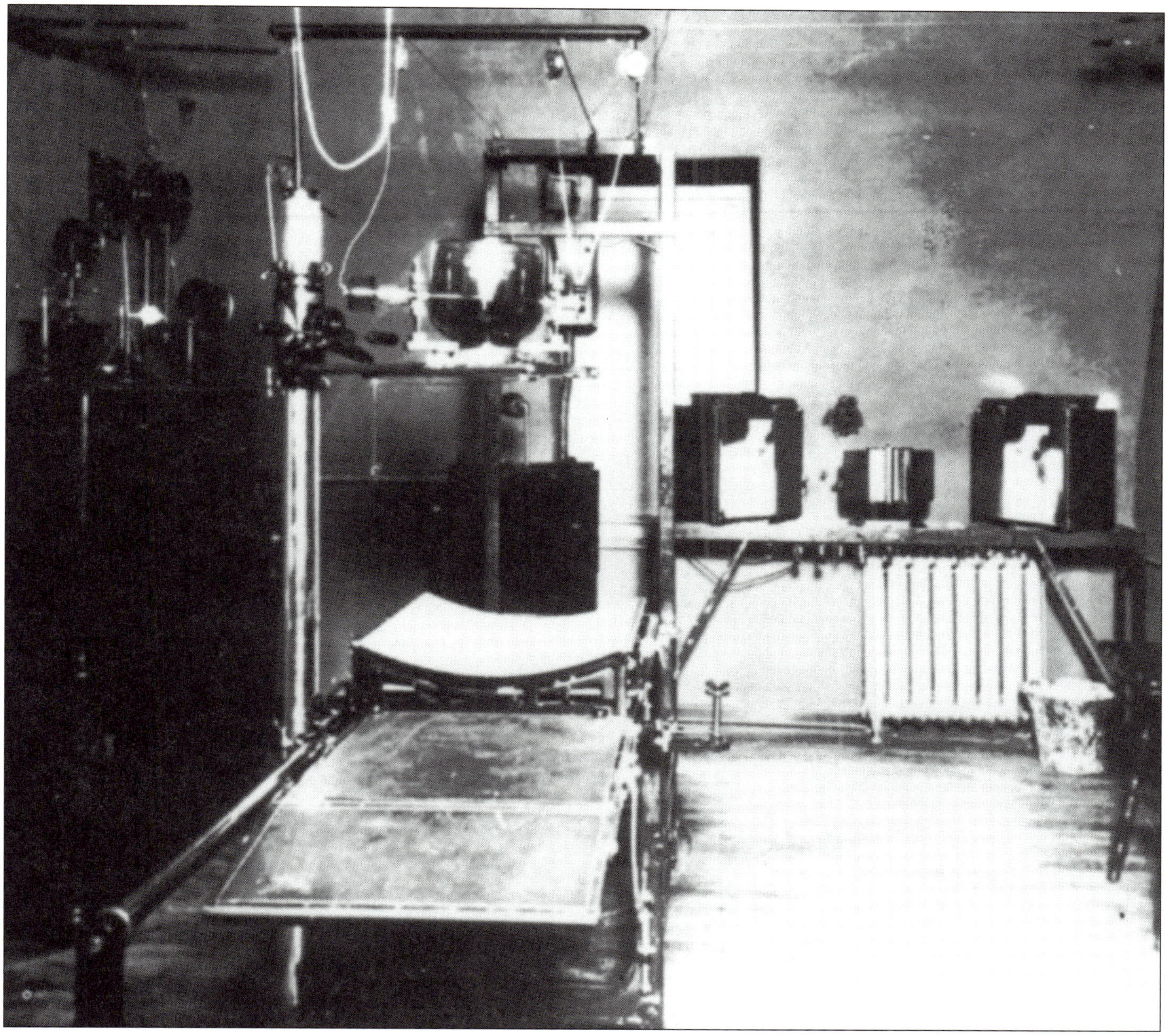

A photograph of an x-ray department as it was in 1927. On the left of the picture is a "Snook" mechanically rectified generator of the cross-arch type. The tube, mounted on a movable tube arm, is an air-cooled radiator type and is surrounded by a lead glass bowl, which offered some protection from scattered rays. This tube, known as a 5-30 radiator tube, carried a maximum load of 30 milliamps at 85 KVp. The control panel is located at the rear of the table and the overhead wiring, with bare leads from the main and filament transformers is shown above the tube. On the table is a curved "Bucky" diaphragm. A stereoscope is in the background.

(Photograph kindly supplied by CAMRT and the Archives of the Manitoba Association of Medical Radiation Technologists, and published with the permission of the Dept of Radiology of the Misercordia General Hospital, Winnepeg).

when a staff nurse was hired to assist Dr Inglis. The work of the department was handicapped by insufficient accommodation, so in 1908 two additional rooms and further equipment were added to the electrical department. In that year maintenance cost $438 and supplies $456. By 1910 the number of radiographs taken annually increased to 1290 whereas the number of treatments increased to only 1771. In that year revenue amounted to $1204 and expenses $1384.

Dr Inglis was also involved in other medical responsibilities, as recorded in the *Manitoba Free Press* in 1899, in a report on infectious disease in the city of Winnipeg.

The archives of the Medical Library of the University of Manitoba contain two interesting letters concerning the use of x-ray examinations in Winnipeg before the turn of the century.

Electrical Department
City of Winnipeg

March 2nd, 1926

Professor H E Bletcher,
Department of Pharmacy

Dear Sir:

In reference to your enquiry as to the first use of the x-ray in Winnipeg, I have been able to trace this up through the kindness of Dr A D Carscallen, whose letter I enclose.

Dr Carscallen is, however, not quite correct in attributing the taking of the x-ray photograph to the writer. A Mr Hilliard made this plate and all I had to do with it was the manipulation of the x-ray apparatus.

It might be of interest to you to know that the x-ray outfit the North West Electric Company had in 1897 was made up of a step-up transformer and a Tesla coil together with the usual spark gaps, tubes and other paraphernalia. It might also be of interest to you to know that about the time Dr Carcallen speaks of, a number of medical practitioners used to come down to the office to experiment with the rays and I well remember Dr H H Chown on several occasions bringing down a number of medical students for the same purpose.

Yours truly,

F A Cambridge
City Electrician

Sunnyside Hospital
530 Balmoral Street
Winnipeg

February 24th, 1926

Mr F A Cambridge
City Electrician

Dear Sir:

I think it was in the year 1897 that I took a patient to the North-West Electric offices to obtain radiographs of a lady's foot, who had previously had two operations in Toronto and then two in this city, to find a broken needle. Needless to say that all of these operations were unsuccessful.

We could see the two pieces of the needle plainly in the radio picture, consequently we hung the picture along the side of the patient's foot while we operated and succeeded in extracting the two pieces of the needle without much trouble.

I may say that I have had many x-rays taken of my patients and seen many others also but I never saw a more perfect picture than the one you took for me.

It is a great pleasure for me to give you this information and considered it a great favor when you did this for me.

A D Carscallen

The records of the College of Physicians and Surgeons of Manitoba reveal that Dr Inglis graduated MD CM in 1893 and was registered with the college on October 23, 1893. He was listed in the Manitoba Medical Registers of 1905, 1912 and 1916. He is understood to have moved to Victoria, British Columbia, and he died on January 19, 1938.

DAVID ALEXANDER STEWART: A TUBERCULOSIS PIONEER

The fight against pulmonary tuberculosis (TB) was greatly enhanced by chest radiography used for detection and in management of the disease. DA Stewart was the founder of the anti-tuberculosis movement in the prairie provinces.[2] Manitoba was the first to have compulsory TB training for all medical students. A prolific writer and a skilled administrator, Stewart lowered death rates when the only treatment was rest, sunlight and good food.

Stewart graduated from Manitoba Medical College in 1906 and soon after a senior internship in the Winnipeg

General Hospital he was appointed executive director of the Manitoba Tuberculosis Society. In his work he developed tuberculosis himself, but after treatment he became the medical supervisor of the 60 bed Ninette Sanatorium and he devoted his life to that institution. He was one of the leading Manitoba physicians and of great interest to radiology is membership in the Radiological Society of North America, during their seventh annual meeting in Chicago, 1921, upon recommendation of the Board of Governors and Censors, as he was considered to be qualified in the science of radiology. As chest disease changed, a specialized chest hospital was named in his honour, the D A Stewart Centre, now part of the Health Sciences Centre, where all radiology residents learn respiratory radiology.

W L WATT, J C (CURRIE) MCMILLAN: EARLY RADIOLOGISTS

The most complete early records are annual reports of the Winnipeg General Hospital. In 1912 the department reported 1840 radiographs and 2619 treatments, 1914 an illuminator was purchased to hold 30 glass plates, 1915 Coolidge tubes replaced old tubes, 1917 dressing rooms were added, 1921 a Potter-Bucky diaphragm was purchased, 1922 18,044 radiographs were made and intensifying screens were brought into use, 1927 the first portable unit was purchased, the work fell during the depression but began to increase 1935, the cost per examination was $0.92, and in 1939 Macpherson joined the staff.

DIGBY WHEELER, ROBERT (BOB) MACPHERSON, ARTHUR (ART) CHILDE: FOUNDERS

Radiology became more important with advances in gastrointestinal, respiratory, nervous, pediatric, obstetrical, and skeletal diseases. The services were provided in private facilities and hospitals. Those that could not pay were examined in the public hospital clinics. Wheeler and Macpherson were excellent organizers and very good clinical radiologists. Wheeler built an empire of Winnipeg Hospitals, several offices and clinics, and as well services to many rural hospitals. Prodigious work output, a Rolls Royce, spats, two bull dogs and a gold tipped cane were his trademarks. He left a large legacy to the St Boniface General Hospital radiology department which is very important in its role as a teaching hospital. Macpherson built a similar empire at the Winnipeg General Hospital, Winnipeg Childrens Hospital, a private office, and services to the Winnipeg and Manitoba Clinics, the largest two in Canada. Macpherson recruited Childe in 1945, who from 1934 was the first radiologist at the Montreal Neurological Institute and Montreal Childrens Hospital. He was a world giant in radiology, writing the neuroradiology section of Golden's Loose Leaf Textbook of Radiology and providing clinical services to children on a par with his contemporary John Caffey of the New York Bavies Hospital. Through the depression and after World War Two, radiology services were very good in spite of limited funds. All became presidents of the Canadian Association of Radiologists and Childe Vice-President of the American Roentgen Ray Society. In co-operation with the Picker X-ray company an unique stereoscopic biplane angiographic unit was developed in Winnipeg.

RURAL AND NORTHERN RADIOLOGY AND MEDICAL PHYSICS SERVICES

Rural diagnostic services had its origin in 1948, when the first Laboratory and X-ray Unit was established in Dauphin. The problem for Manitoba is the large number of small scattered communities and a central administration enabled the development of local radiology services. By 1973 offices in the Cadham Provincial Laboratory located in Winnipeg and the Westman Laboratory in Brandon co-ordinated facilities in 59 Manitoba hospitals for itinerant radiologists from Winnipeg and Brandon. In 1995 there are 5 rural radiologists and there are 72 rural and northern radiology departments with ultrasound services in the larger departments.

Dr Richard Walton, reorganized and opened the new Manitoba Cancer Treatment and Research Foundation building. The Foundation provided leadership under the direction of Dr Art Holloway in organizing provincial radiation protection programs and Dr Mervyn Billinghurst established the first licenced hospital-based radiopharmacy service in Canada. Gamma cameras for world sale were manufactured in Winnipeg by CoNuclear Enterprises following local research and development.

Acknowledgements:

Some of the material in this report was presented at the Canadian Association of Radiologists annual meeting in May 1975 at Toronto. It was published in the *University of Manitoba Medical Journal*[1] and is reprinted in a slightly edited form with permission.

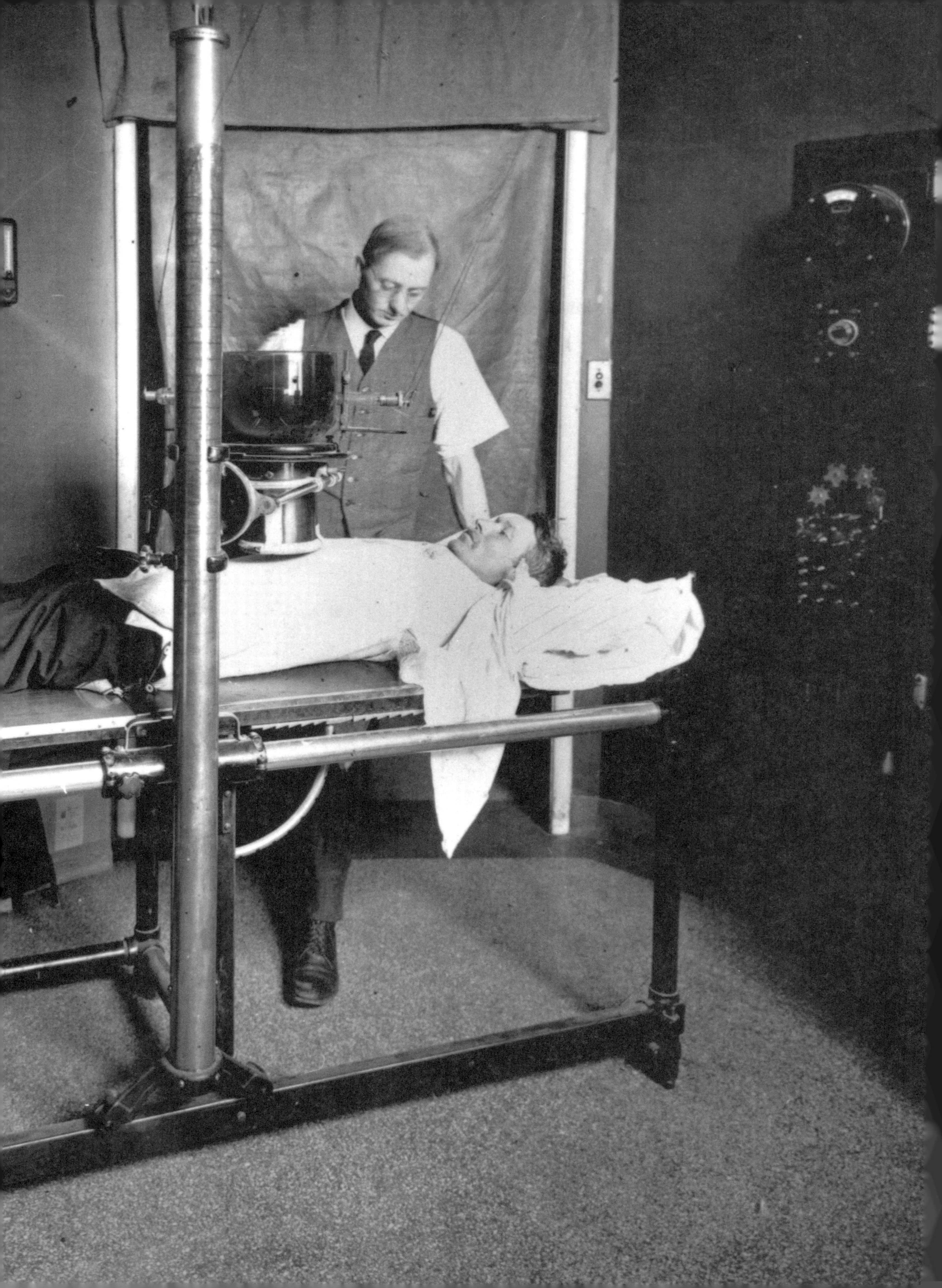

Chapter X •

Radiation Oncology in Manitoba

JAMES GILLIES

With the 1930 appointment of Pat MacDonald, a medical physicist, to head the newly formed Manitoba Cancer Treatment and Relief Institute, the province moved hesitantly towards establishing a cancer service. Assisted by Earle Campbell, the institute offered advice to the group of surgeons in private practice who had pooled their resources to purchase a small amount of expensive radium; it also lent its technical expertise to the operation of a deep therapy machine that had been installed in Winnipeg General Hospital (WGH) some 5 years previously. Those involved set about building their own 400-kV deep therapy machine, fondly known as the "pump," since the tube had to be evacuated continuously.

The institute greatly expanded its activities when in 1935 Mr John Forlong donated $30 000 in memory of his late wife, who had died of cancer, to build the Forlong Annex to house radiotherapy equipment. The Annex was operated by the WGH x-ray department, whose physicians had taken training in both diagnostic and therapeutic radiology, and the machines were run by nurses who had taken only brief, hands-on training.

In 1944 the institute became the sole provider of cancer radiotherapy, offering treatment to all Manitobans. A follow-up program was begun. A Westinghouse 250-kV machine was added to the Forlong Annex, and a radon seed plant was set up in one of the temporary wartime buildings on Broadway near the Legislature.

Left
Radiographic room patient and radiologist, 1914, Winnipeg General Hospital

The treatment of skin conditions—mostly benign—remained in the hands of dermatologists for many years to come, but in 1950 a retiring dermatologist donated a Mattern superficial x-ray machine to the Forlong unit.

By this time cobalt-60 teletherapy was on the horizon. In Saskatoon Sandy Watson had started using the home-built unit that Dr Harold Johns had designed. Atomic Energy of Canada Limited (AECL) then started producing its Eldorado model and installed the first unit in London, Ontario for Dr Ivan Smith. Manitoba placed an order for their production model #2, to be installed in 1953 in an extension to the Forlong Annex. Since the institute would operate the expanded service, two radiotherapists were recruited from Glasgow, Scotland (Jim Bennett and Jim Gillies).

Cobalt teletherapy was state of the art treatment. With sparing of the skin from excessive radiation doses, a large dose deliverable to deep organs and high dose rates, who worried about penumbral effects? We were at last able to treat the true pelvis uniformly by using four oblique fields, and this procedure became our standard, prior to the use of radium insertions.

The Eldorado came with a Lucite pyramid used to define the 80-cm long beam direction by means of a protractor scale on the gantry, a C-arm backpointer and a pin-and-arc. Body casts were made of plaster of Paris bandage with "windows" cut at entry points to preserve skin sparing, and localization films to verify the treatment volume were taken in the x-ray department.

A set of cobalt-60 needles was obtained for interstitial use, and the use of radon was discontinued; radium was, however, available for intracavitary use.

In 1954 Dick Walton of New Zealand was appointed Medical Director of the Cancer Institute, and that same year St Boniface General Hospital (SBGH) ordered a Picker cobalt-60 machine which the institute was expected to operate.

Simon Kramer came at that time from London to head that department, but a year later he departed for Philadelphia (Jefferson), leaving Jim Bennett to take over at SBGH, where he was joined by Alex Meikle. The Manitoba Cancer Treatment & Research Foundation replaced the old Institute in 1957, with a broad mandate covering research, professional education and comprehensive cancer care. Art Holloway joined as head of an expanding physics section. A technologist-training program was started locally as part of a Canada-wide movement.

When in 1959 medicare was introduced in Manitoba, the funds in the hands of the dissolved Blue Cross Medical Insurance plan ($2 000 000), were turned over to the clinic to build a cancer center. It took two years to build the new four-storey building, which opened in 1963. The radiotherapy floor at basement level housed a 38-MeV Brown-Boveri betatron, an AECL Theratron F, the original AECL Eldorado cobalt-60 unit, a Siemens deep x-ray therapy machine and a Chaoul contact unit. There was a mould room, a treatment planning department and an operating room for radio-cesium insertions and biopsies.

The betatron room was described as "huge and awe-inspiring." The 12-ton betatron was suspended from the ceiling on a massive yolk which allowed vertical movement and rotation through a 180-degree arc. It could be coupled to the treatment stretcher platform which moved laterally on a floor track. A fluoroscopy unit built into the head provided "simulation" for planning treatments. In addition to closed-circuit TV (an innovation at the time) and two-way intercom, the patient could be observed by the technicians through a water-filled window. The photon beam was of limited field size and had a distressingly low output. Electrons produced ranged in energy from 10 to 35 MeV.

The sub-basement housed a total body irradiation (TBI) room. This unique shielded room, about 35 feet square, was designed to hold six cobalt-60 sources, one in each corner of the room, one in a pit about 10 feet below the wooden floor and the sixth directly overhead. The 10-foot-square "treatment room" in the center was defined by curtains; the patients were to have been seated comfortably reading or watching television while they received uniform irradiation of their entire body at low dose rates. The six cobalt source housings were designed and built in our own workshops, and we had planned to use inexpensive "pre-owned" cobalt sources from AECL. With this facility we had hoped to determine the role (if any) of TBI as an adjuvant therapy and its place in the management of lymphomas and leukemias. Unfortunately, for whatever reason, the sources were never installed, and the room still exists serving only as a storage space.

The use of hyperbaric oxygen (HO) to increase tumor oxygenation in the hope of reducing local recurrences was the first research program to get underway. Because of the oxygen effect whereby cells are more sensitive to radiation when oxygenated compared with being cultured in a nitrogen atmosphere it was believed that treatment failures might be due to anoxic cells present in a tumour during their irradiation. Richard Johnson whose special interest was in such a use of HO joined us. We had obtained two pressure chambers capable of operating at 30 psi above ambient atmospheric pressure and had run high-pressure oxygen lines to all treatment rooms. We chose to study locally advanced cancer of the cervix, using a box technique on the Eldorado cobalt-60 machine. Since each treatment —compression, irradiation and decompression—took about an hour, hypofractionation was inevitable. Looking back, we would say that patient compliance was unbelievable. These ladies were confined in a narrow Lucite-walled chamber and were scantily clad, since we constantly feared combustion of oxygen-soaked bedding and body hair from static sparks when the chamber was opened. Happily, this never occurred. Stan Dische continued this study on his return to England.

Investigators at the clinic joined in the Stage C prostate cancer study designed by Juan del Regato, the first of a flood of cooperative studies that were to follow. We attended the inaugural meeting of the Radiation Therapy and Oncology Group in Chicago, but were prevented from participating since the National Institute of Health had ruled that only United States centres would be funded. We scrapped the Eldorado cobalt-60 unit in 1969 and replaced it with an SHM linac 4. Drs Marshall Tulloh and Bill McLellan joined us from Edmonton in tht year.

In 1970 we cooperated with Picker design engineers in developing a prototype simulator which they installed in Winnipeg in 1972 at a cost of $80 000. Dr Dick Walton left to join the Health Sciences Center as Vice President–Medical. Dr Jim Gillies took over as head of radiation oncology while Dr Kamal Malaker was recruited from the Hammersmith Hospital in London to run both educational and research programs.

In 1973 additional treatment rooms were added to house a Therac 40/Sagittaire linac. Installation took over 12 months since the gantry had to be reinforced to carry the additional shielding called for by AECB, while still retaining isocentric accuracy. The Sagittaire more than lived up to expectations.

In 1980 the Cancer Centre building expansion opened; the floor area was essentially doubled to accommodate the medical oncology unit and additional clinic space was provided for gynecological and surgical oncologists. The cell and biology laboratories were greatly enlarged. A second simulator was installed in 1981 and an AECL treatment planning computer added. SBGH started planning a new cancer wing and requested a linac to replace the aging Picker cobalt-60 machine. This suggestion was resisted, since the main purpose of radiotherapy at this location was to serve the excellent palliative care unit. An AECL Therac 25 was installed when the new centre opened 2 years later. The WW Cross Clinic in Edmonton later donated to us their retired Picker simulator, which we overhauled and continue to use in SBGH. We had kept our pledge to the Hospital Commission never to duplicate services.

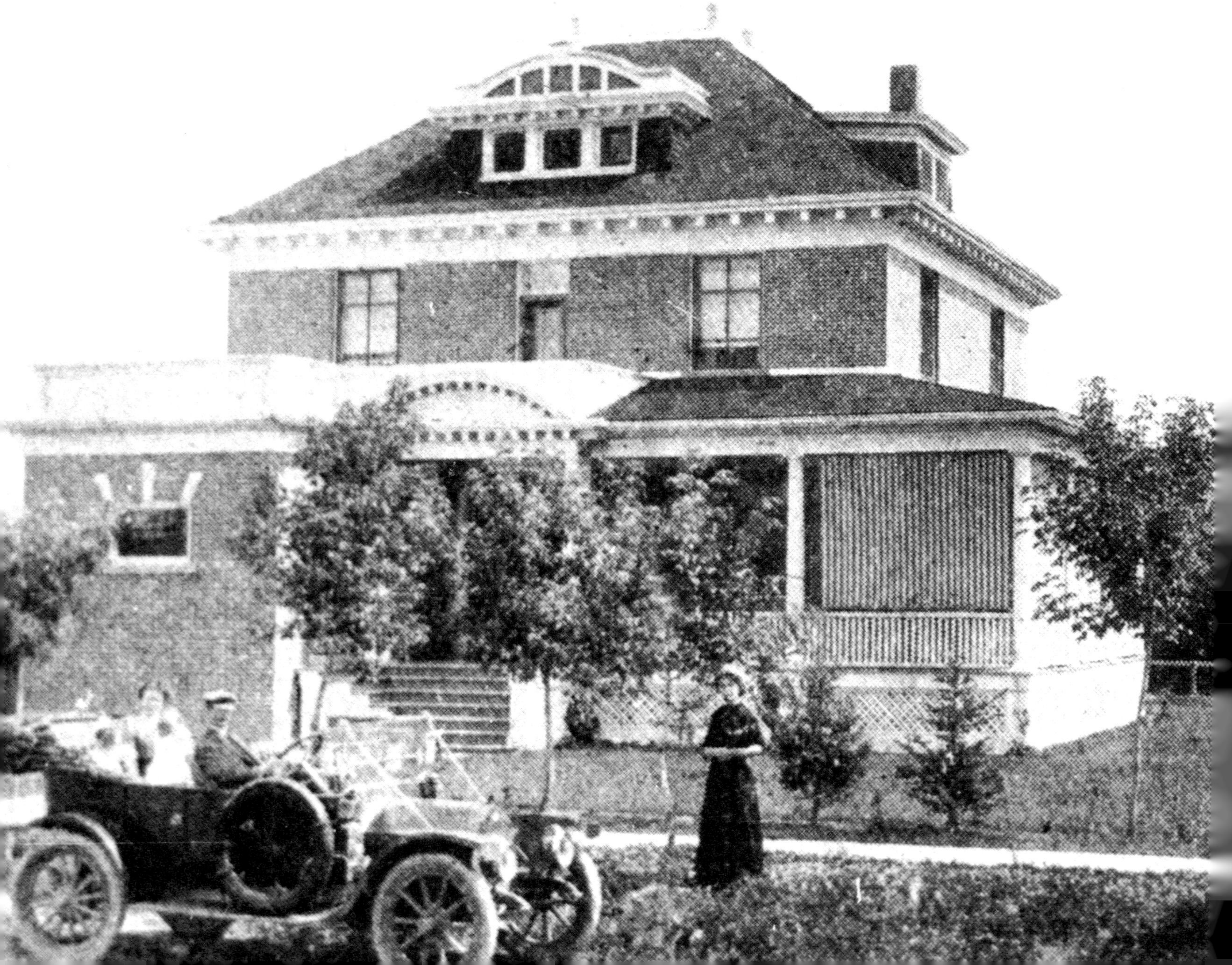

Chapter XI • The History of

Radiation Therapy in Saskatchewan

C Stuart Houston and Sylvia O Fedoruk

Saskatchewan has led all other jurisdictions in North America in many aspects of health care service. Saskatchewan's list of firsts includes:

— the first municipal doctor (in the rural municipality of Sarnia, 1914);[1]
— the first union hospital district legislation (1916);[1]
— the first municipal doctor legislation (1919);[1]
— the first universal, free tuberculosis treatment (1929);[2]
— the first legislation in the British Commonwealth concerning cancer diagnosis and treatment (1930);[3]
— the first statistically controlled Bacillus Calmette Guerin prophylaxis in Indian infants (1933) and student nurses (1934);[2]
— the first province-wide chest radiographic survey for tuberculosis (1941–1946);[2]
— the first province-wide medical care plan for indigents, old age pensioners and mother's allowance recipients (1945);[1]
— the first regional medicare medical plan in Canada (Swift Current region, 1946);[4]
— the first province-wide hospital plan (1947);[1]
— the first province-wide medicare plan (1962);

Such developments arose from the highly developed cooperative spirit and mutual help necessary among pioneer settlers, who were sparsely distributed in a relatively hostile environment. House-raising, barn-raising and the building of community amenities such as schools and rinks made it logical for more sophisticated cooperative developments to occur. Although money was scarce, an unusually high

Left
The home of Dr CM Henry in Yorkton, now the Henry Block. Courtesy Provincial Archives of Saskatchewan, photograph S-A147

priority was given to health matters by the public and especially by farm women. "It was this pervading spirit of cooperation and acceptance of public responsibility which led to the emergence of a whole range of tax-supported health services."[5]

Tuberculosis was the first disease targeted for attention. On January 1, 1929 under the leadership of Dr RG Ferguson, Saskatchewan became the first jurisdiction in North America to offer free treatment for tuberculosis, eight years in advance of the second province, Alberta.[2] Disproportionately large amounts of money were expended on three large sanatoria. Saskatchewan led in BCG research funded by the National Research Council and in community-wide radiology surveys, funded mainly by community amateur hours on radio stations. Some rural municipalities, reflecting the priority given to health by their farmer constituents, spent more money on one disease—tuberculosis—than they did on roads.[2]

The cooperative impetus, which had been so successful in the fight against tuberculosis, carried on in Saskatchewan for several decades, with cancer as the next priority. Eventually, this working together led to the development of the first universal programs for hospitalization and medicare in North America. Governments of all three political persuasions, Conservative, Liberal and Cooperative Commonwealth Federation (CCF), played their parts in this leadership role.

The University of Saskatchewan's interest in the radium treatment of cancer was first expressed on October 6,1922 when University President Dr Walter Murray wrote to Premier Charles A Dunning to offer the services of the physicists at the university if the province planned to offer cancer treatment to its citizens.[6] Dr WS Lindsay, professor of pathology, had visited the Radium Institute in New York; Dr Ellice McDonald from the Memorial Hospital in New York (a brother of DH McDonald, the member of the Saskatchewan Legislative Assembly for Qu'Appelle) had visited Dr Murray at the University. McDonald informed Murray that the province of Québec had just purchased a gram of radium for $75 000.

Dunning responded to Murray's offer promptly on October 11,1922, pointing out that tuberculosis "affects a very much larger proportion of the people and affects more directly and seriously the life of the community; on the principle, therefore, of putting 'first things first' we feel we must give first importance in public health work to tuberculosis...The view of the Government at the present time is that the possibility of successful use of radium in any large way in the treatment of disease has not been fully demonstrated, and in any case, the population of this

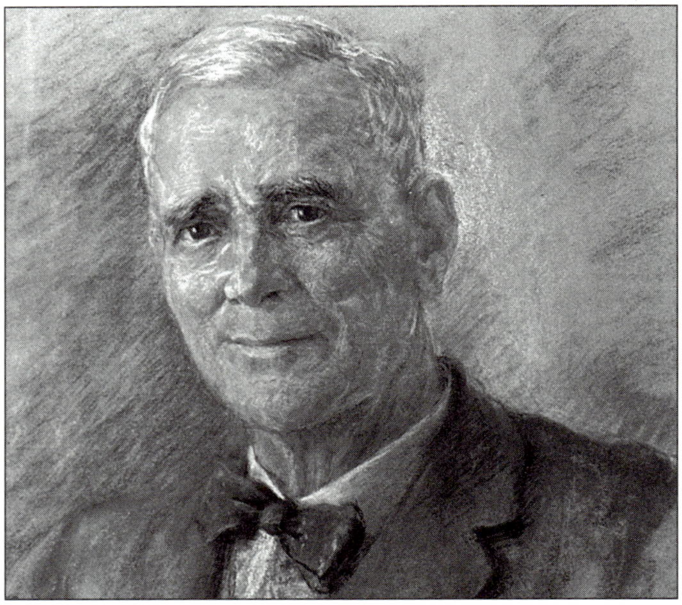

province has not yet reached a point either in numbers or wealth which would justify the erection of an Institution..."[7]

Eventually, President Murray's dream came true, through Dr Ertle Leslie Harrington (1887–1956), professor of physics at the University of Saskatchewan. Harrington, a native of Missouri, had obtained his BSc from the University of Missouri in 1910, an MA from Harvard in 1915 and a PhD from the University of Chicago in 1916. He was subsequently a post-doctoral fellow at the University of Chicago under RA Millikan. Harrington, famed as the ultimate example of an absent-minded professor, joined the Department of Physics at the University of Saskatchewan in 1920 and was appointed head in 1924.[8] In 1929 he was the only non-medical member of the Cancer Committee appointed by the Saskatchewan Medical Association. The medical association was concerned about a few private doctors who had purchased small amounts of radium, giving little more than homeopathic doses in treating cancer, yet attracted additional patients to their practices. The medical profession, according to Dr CC Burkell, felt it would be better to have the government purchase larger amounts of radium for use in Regina and Saskatoon. Harrington's advice led to the drafting of the Saskatchewan Cancer Commission Act, passed by the Conservative government of JTM Anderson in 1930.[9] This act established the Saskatchewan Cancer Commission, the first cancer control agency in Canada and probably the first in North America.

SASKATCHEWAN CANCER COMMISSION

North America's first government-sponsored, part-time

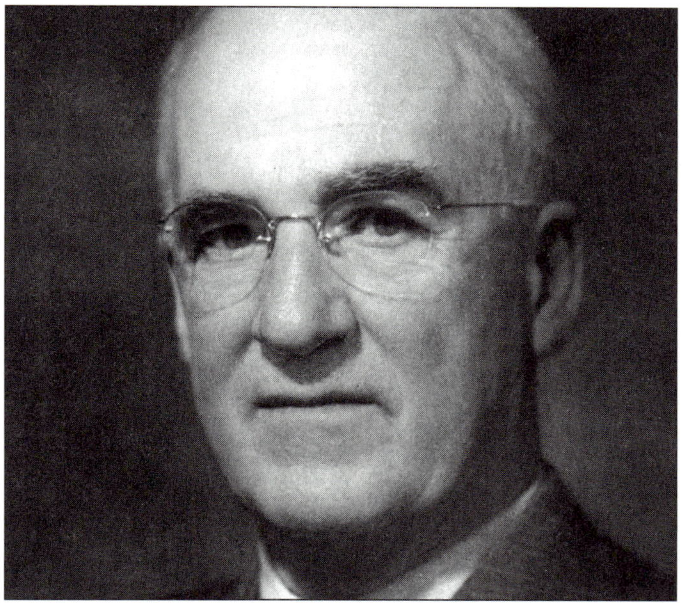

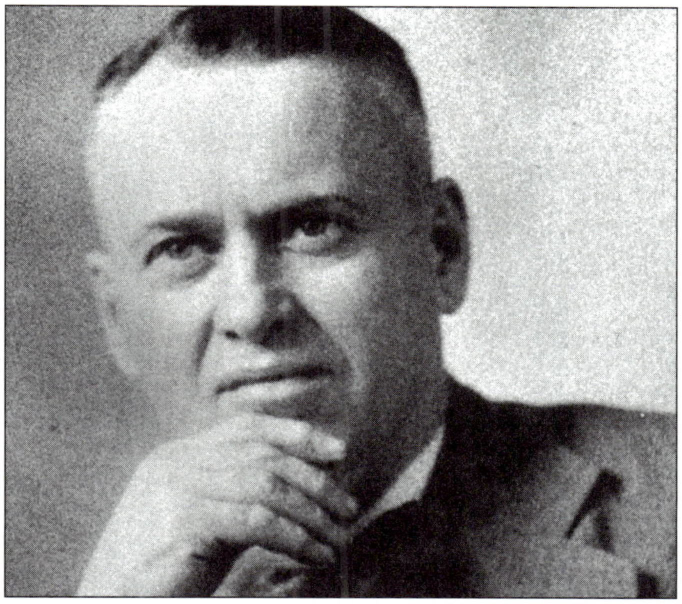

(2 mornings a week) consultative, diagnostic and treatment clinics were held at the Saskatoon City Hospital under Dr Earle E Shepley in 1931, and at the Regina General Hospital under Dr CM Henry in 1932.[10–12] Treatment and hospitalization were the financial responsibility of the patient. Nevertheless, the average number of patients referred per year increased from 575 to 735 to 1065 to 1470 in each of the first four three-year periods, until the end of 1943.[3] The radiotherapist was also the hospital radiologist and only a part-time Cancer Clinic employee, in Regina until 1939 and in Saskatoon until 1945.

Therapy with radon seeds began in 1931, particularly for cancers of the cervix, uterus and tongue, and was possible because of the collaboration of Dr Harrington, who supervised and distributed radon in small gold tubes or "seeds" which had a 3.8 day half-life. The radium source was purchased by the government and delivered in two parts in February and July 1931. Harrington was a proficient and enthusiastic glass blower who constructed the apparatus with the help of Dr JWT Spinks of the Chemistry Department (Spinks later became president of the university). This radon plant was in operation until 1962.[13] Patients were also offered treatment with what were then called high voltage radiotherapy machines. A General Electric 400-kVp x-ray radiotherapy unit was installed in the Saskatoon City Hospital in 1935.[14] Because of pressure from Liberal MLA Dr George Dragan, on the very last day of the Liberal government of WJ Patterson, before the legislature prorogued on April 1, 1944, a bare-bones cancer act was proclaimed: *Chapter 78, An Act Respecting the Control and Treatment of Cancer.* It remained for the new CCF government, led by TC Douglas, to flesh out the details and promulgate a more complete program.

Far left
Portrait of Dr RG Ferguson by Nicholas de Grandmaison, 1962
Courtesy of the Ferguson Family

Left
Dr Ertle Harrington
Courtesy of the University of Saskatchewan Archives

Above
Dr Earle E Shepley
Courtesy the late Dr AW Becker

CANCER CONTROL ACT, 1944

In 1944, the Cancer Control Act replaced the Saskatchewan Cancer Commission Act, and patients were no longer charged for services. As Acker and Watson reported in 1960,

> *The underlying philosophy of the [Cancer Control] Act and its regulations is unmistakable. In effect it says: Cancer is a serious disease, and it is costly for the individual to obtain all the care he requires. The diagnosis and therapy of this disease are often very difficult and complex and require special skills and modern, expensive equipment. The specialized services can best be provided in central clinics associated with major hospitals where the family physician can readily and confidently refer his patients...[T]he people must...seek care early.*[5]

With the amendments and regulations passed in October 1944 by the new CCF government, any person who had resided in Saskatchewan for three months was eligible for all services necessary for the diagnosis and treatment of cancer, without charge, including all specialized diagnostic and radiotherapeutic services and all surgical operations for the treatment of cancer. Patients were free to choose their attending surgeon, in most cases with the advice of their family physician. Each clinic, one in Regina and one in Saskatoon, had a medical staff of seven physicians. Between 1944 and 1946, with free treatment, there was a twofold jump in the volume of patients seen to 2626 per year. Because there was a rising proportion —reaching 62.2 per cent in 1947–49—of non-malignant disease referred to the Cancer Clinics, the Commission in 1950 reimposed a $10.00 fee on any patient who proved not to have cancer.[5] The proportion of non-cancer patients then declined to between 55 and 60 per cent of patients seen. The program was entirely paid for from public revenues and soon emerged evidence that earlier diagnosis was being achieved. Family physicians had full confidence in the service.[5]

At the Regina Cancer Clinic, Dr Henry was succeeded in 1938 by Dr Herbert C George and the next year by Dr Allan Walker Blair, who became Director of Cancer Services for Saskatchewan. Dr Blair had taken his radiotherapy training under Dr Gordon Richards at Toronto General Hospital. Blair was promoted to Director of Cancer Services for the entire province in 1944 and served in this capacity until his death in 1948.[15] Before oncology was recognized as a specialty in the rest of Canada, Dr Blair desired a full-time staff of specialist oncologists. Blair also realized that Saskatchewan doctors must be sent away for appropriate training and sent Dr Charles C Burkell to Manchester, England, one of the world's foremost radiotherapy centres, on half pay, his funds given in part by the United Farm Women of Saskatchewan. Dr Arthur JS Bryant took training in pathology and then qualified as a radiotherapist in 1948. Dr HF McKenzie went to Manchester with financial support augmented by the Women's Auxiliary of the United Commercial Travellers. Burkell returned to the Saskatoon Cancer Clinic and McKenzie to the Regina Cancer Clinic. Later, Dr Esther Brown and Dr Helen Bean were sent for training, Brown returning to Saskatoon and Bean to Regina. Following the death of Dr Blair on November 9, 1948, Dr Arthur JS Bryant became director of the Regina Cancer Clinic, and Dr Helen Bean later, Dr HF MacKenzie and Dr John Gibson was in charge of radiotherapy.

In Saskatoon Dr Earle E Shepley was the therapeutic radiologist from 1932 until the end of 1938 when he was succeeded by Dr EW Spencer. When Spencer enlisted in July 1940, Dr AB MacDonell continued this work until Spencer returned from war service in 1945 and became director of the Saskatoon Cancer Clinic and director of therapeutic radiology. In November 1946 Spencer was succeeded in both positions by Dr Thomas Alastair Watson, who had obtained his MD from the University of Otago in New Zealand in 1937.[15,16] With the appointment of TA Watson as Director of Cancer Services in November 1946, Saskatchewan developed "a more comprehensive cancer program than any other province or state on the North American Continent."[17] Cancer records for Saskatchewan were more complete than for any other jurisdiction, in part because of a relatively stable population, but even more because doctors were paid for care of cancer patients only if the patient was registered with the Cancer Clinic. Dr Watson assembled a talented staff.[18–20]

In Saskatoon Dr Charles C Burkell, a radiotherapist and clinical oncologist, succeeded Watson as head of the Saskatoon Cancer Clinic when Watson moved to the University of Western Ontario in April 1963. Other radiotherapists included Esther M Brown, who later succeeded Burkell as head of the Saskatoon Clinic, George Cowan and Donald A Fee. Sylvia O Fedoruk became Chief of Physics Services for both the Saskatoon and Regina clinics.

The following account deals with the improbable achievement whereby Saskatchewan led the world in the development of high-technology cancer treatment.

THE BETATRON

The Saskatchewan radiotherapy story accelerated because of the foresight of Dr Blair. Blair's first letter to Harrington, on December 12, 1944, suggested that a full-time physicist should be hired jointly by the Saskatchewan Cancer

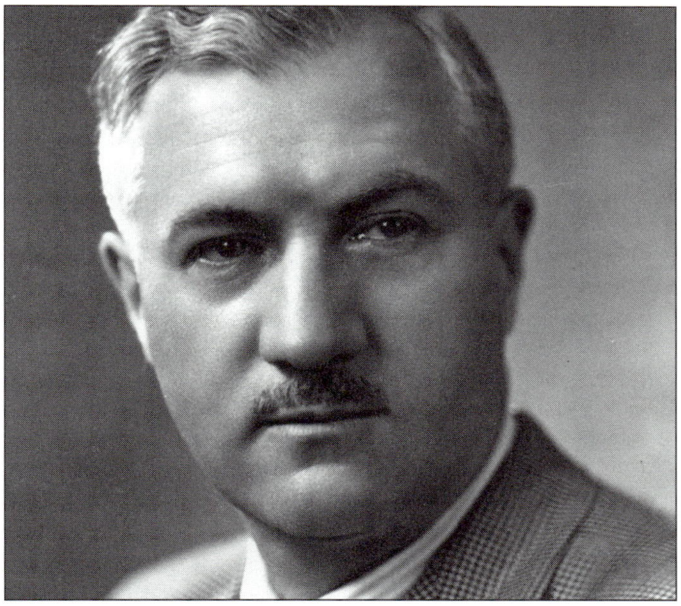

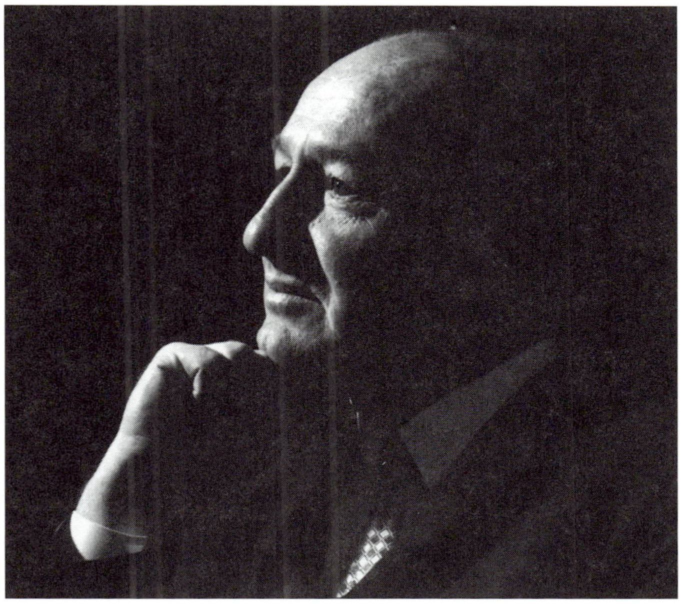

Above
Dr Allan W Blair
Courtesy Provincial Archives
of Saskatchewan, R-B 11015

Top right
Dr TA Watson.
Photograph by Karsh
Courtesy Saskatchewan
Cancer Foundation

Right
Dr Harold E Johns

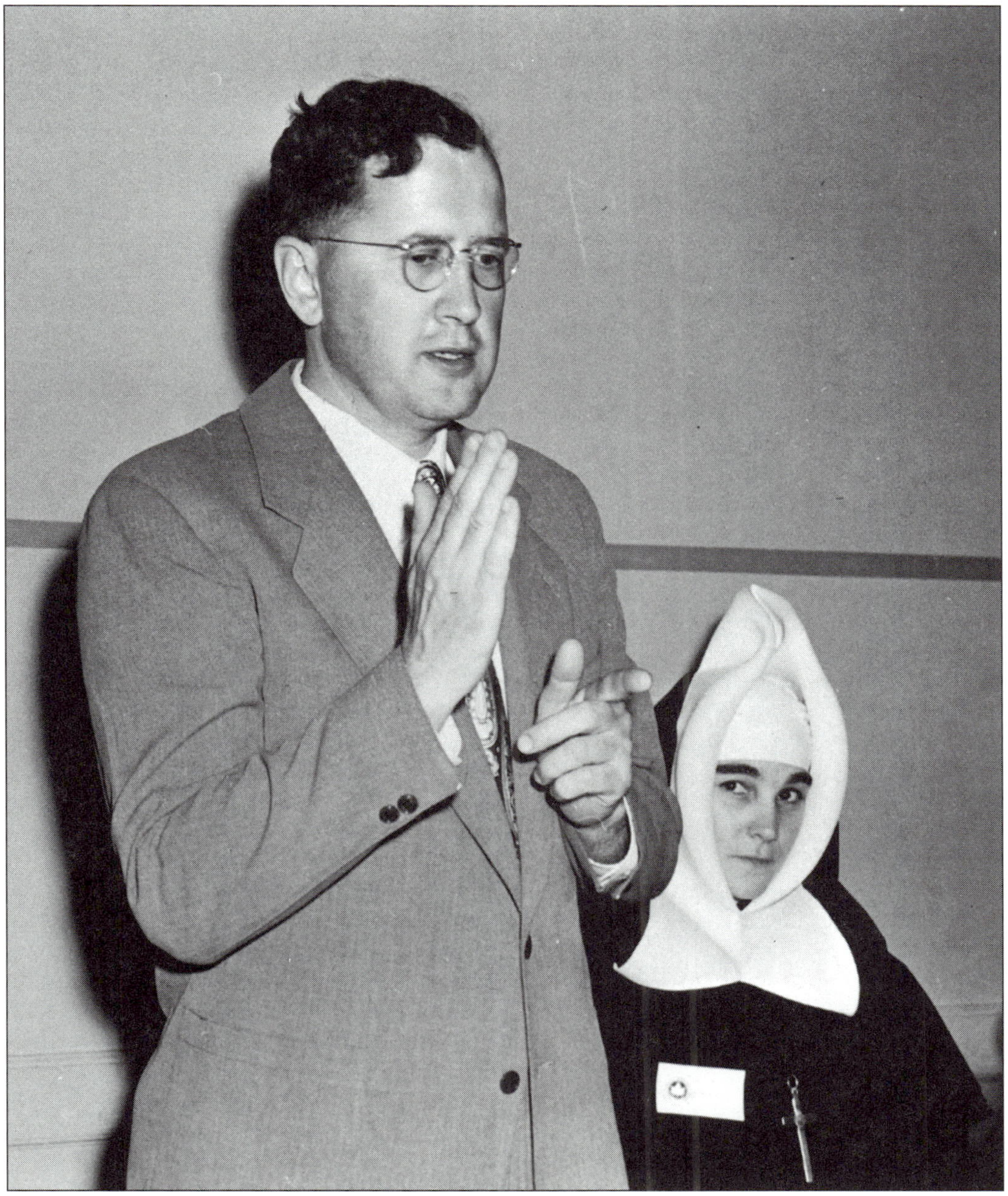

Right
The Betatron installation, Department of Physics University of Saskatchewan

Far right
Bob Mauchel, installing Betatron donut, with Harold Johns. From *Saturday Night* 18 October, 1949

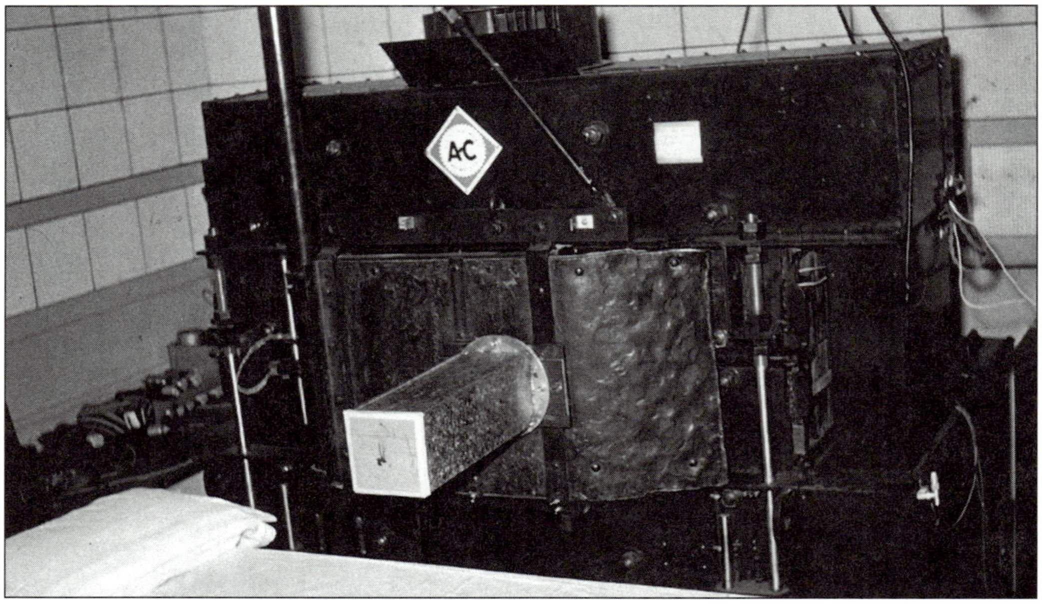

Commission and the university. Six days later, Harrington offered his full cooperation. Harrington displayed great wisdom when he hired Dr Harold E Johns on March 26, 1945 for the joint position at $3600 per annum. Johns was a thirty-year-old instructor at the Radar School at the University of Alberta, where he used a radium needle on the ceiling to obtain industrial photographs of steel propeller shafts. Johns had received his bachelor's degree in Physics from McMaster University in 1936, his master's degree from the University of Toronto in 1937 and his PhD from Toronto in 1939.[21] Johns was made an assistant professor of physics at the university and was to "give half time to supervision of the radium and x-ray therapy equipment of the two cancer clinics." Johns later told Lauriston Taylor that he thus became Canada's first full-time cancer physicist.[22]

In May 1946 Johns was awarded a travelling scholarship of $800, allowing him to visit the leading centres of radiation physics in the United States and Canada. Johns also attended a series of lectures in Toronto given by Professor MV Mayneord, a senior medical physicist in England who mentioned the possibility of using cobalt-60 as a radiation source. Shortly thereafter, Johns gained permission from the University and from Saskatchewan Premier and Health Minister TC (Tommy) Douglas to purchase a betatron.

The betatron project required further support from national agencies. University of Saskatchewan President James S Thomson wrote to Blair on November 18, 1946: "I called last week upon Dr CJ Mackenzie, President of the National Research Council, to discuss with him the use of a betatron in connection with the cancer treatment in this province. Dr MacKenzie . . . expressed some doubts as to whether research was fully advanced to make such a project practicable...Matters affecting the use of atomic energy are really under the control of the Atomic Energy Commission of which General AGL McNaughton is the chairman." Blair then wrote to Mackenzie on December 11, 1946 concerning the possible betatron installation: "It is not planned to use it for any actual treatment until the physical measurements have been completed to everyone's satisfaction." (This principle of exact calibration before patient treatment became the cornerstone of all future development of radiation treatment facilities in Saskatchewan and demonstrated the benefit of full collaboration between medical physicists and therapeutic radiologists. Depth-dose data produced in Saskatoon were used widely throughout the world for many years.) When the university requested $80 000 from the Atomic Energy Control Board but received only $30 000, Johns was disturbed, but Blair was jubilant. "Spend that money, Johns," he said, "when it is gone more will be found."[23]

Meanwhile, other centres viewed this development in Saskatchewan with suspicion, as indicated in a letter from Harrington to President Thomson on February 10, 1947: "In the earlier part of the discussion regarding the betatron, it appeared that a certain member of the Atomic Energy Commission, to which this matter must be referred for decision, had expressed the belief that if the reason for the betatron was mainly medical it would be in the interest of the country as a whole to locate it in a large medical centre, say, in Toronto. In the mind of Dean Mackenzie, the chance of obtaining a favourable action on our request for this equipment would be better if any possible uses in medicine of the betatron were given but little emphasis."

At the end of April 1948 Johns, accompanied by Drs

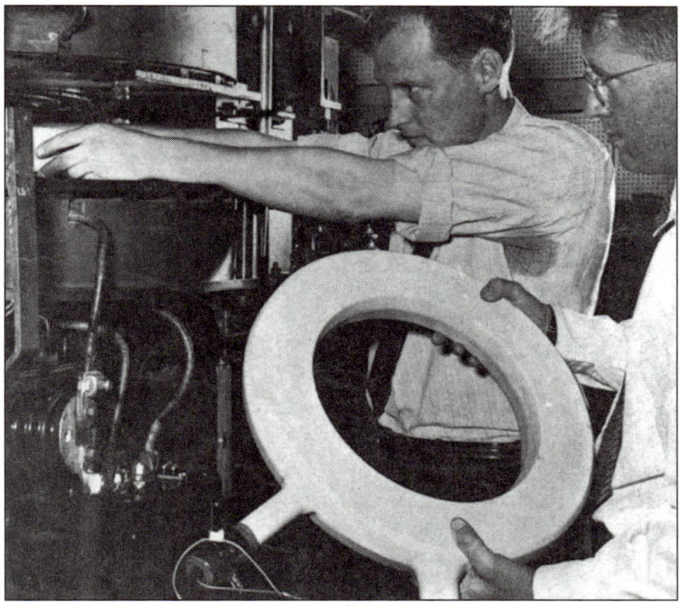

RNH Haslam and L Katz of the physics department, left Saskatoon to visit the Allis-Chalmers Plant in Milwaukee, Wisconsin, where they examined "their" betatron. Where else could an agricultural province have found a manufacturer of heavy duty machines more suitable than an agricultural equipment company? Johns wrote back to Blair on May 12, 1948: "The betatron is finished but has not been tested. The machine which we are getting is the one ordered by the University of Pennsylvania, but they have no building finished to house it and have allowed us to have it...We reached the University of Illinois on Monday, May 3 [1948] where we have been since... Professor Kerst has been more than cooperative. First he introduced us to all his men and gave us full access to *all* blueprints, *all* reprints, keys to the building...Kerst then presented us with two donuts for nothing and one electron donut for a nominal sum . . . Dr Kerst is amazed at the rapidity with which we have pursued our program and in the fact we are getting the first betatron to be installed in any university or hospital...The University of Illinois medical school gets the third betatron (second to the University of Pennsylvania) and I heard yesterday that the University of California medical school is getting one, at Berkeley."[24]

Dr DW Kerst of the physics department of the University of Illinois at Urbana had developed a small 2.3-million-volt betatron by 1940 and 2 years later had developed a device which accelerated electrons to 20 million volts, the prototype of the Allis-Chalmers machine.[25] Kerst had, with Dr Henry Quastler, treated his first patient just four days before the Saskatchewan physicists arrived.

An addition to the University of Saskatchewan physics building was built quickly. The 24-million-volt betatron was installed in the summer of 1948 and the first Saskatchewan patient was treated on March 29, 1949.[26–32] As MD Schulz said in a historical review in 1975, "...thus started the really first concerted clinical investigation of the usefulness of multimegavoltage as a radiotherapeutic tool."[33]

The Saskatchewan betatron installation was used as much for physics research as for patient treatment. Until the new University Hospital was completed in 1955, patients were brought across the South Saskatchewan River from Saskatoon City Hospital. Even after it was built the shorter distance of several hundred metres, outdoors, across the campus from the hospital to the betatron in the physics building still presented difficulties. The operating costs of the betatron were considered exorbitant in the 1940s. TA Watson reported on November 10, 1949 to Dr OH Warwick of the National Cancer Institute that each donut cost $3800 and, although guaranteed to last for 150 hours, "No doughnut (sic) which has so far been used has lasted nearly as long as this...[T]he cost of the doughnut alone is $25.70 an hour...[E]leven patients were treated at an average cost of $224 per patient." In 17 years, only 301 patients were treated with the betatron.

Nevertheless, Johns reported to the president of the Saskatchewan division of the Canadian Cancer Society that the betatron offered "a method of delivering easily a high dose to tumours at a depth, without appreciably affecting the overlying skin...Radiation sickness and blood changes are much less likely."

COBALT-60 THERAPY

Johns and his co-workers were not content with developing the betatron for clinical use. Their greatest achievement was the development of the so-called cobalt bomb. Dr Harrington in his 1947 Presidential Address to the Royal Society of Canada, Chemical Mathematical and Physical Sciences Division, followed Professor Mayneord in predicting that cobalt-60 "may become a more suitable source than radium itself in the treatment of cancer."[34] In June 1949 Johns visited the Chalk River reactor in Ontario, the only installation in the world capable of producing large quantities of radioactive cobalt, where he had discussions with Drs AJ Cipriani and WB Lewis of the Atomic Energy Project. Johns agreed with Harrington that cobalt would offer even better and more economical opportunities for cancer therapy.

Johns wrote to University of Saskatchewan President Walter P Thompson on July 15, 1949, presenting his proposal. He wanted an effective source of 1000 curies of cobalt-60, about 100 times the activity of any radium unit,

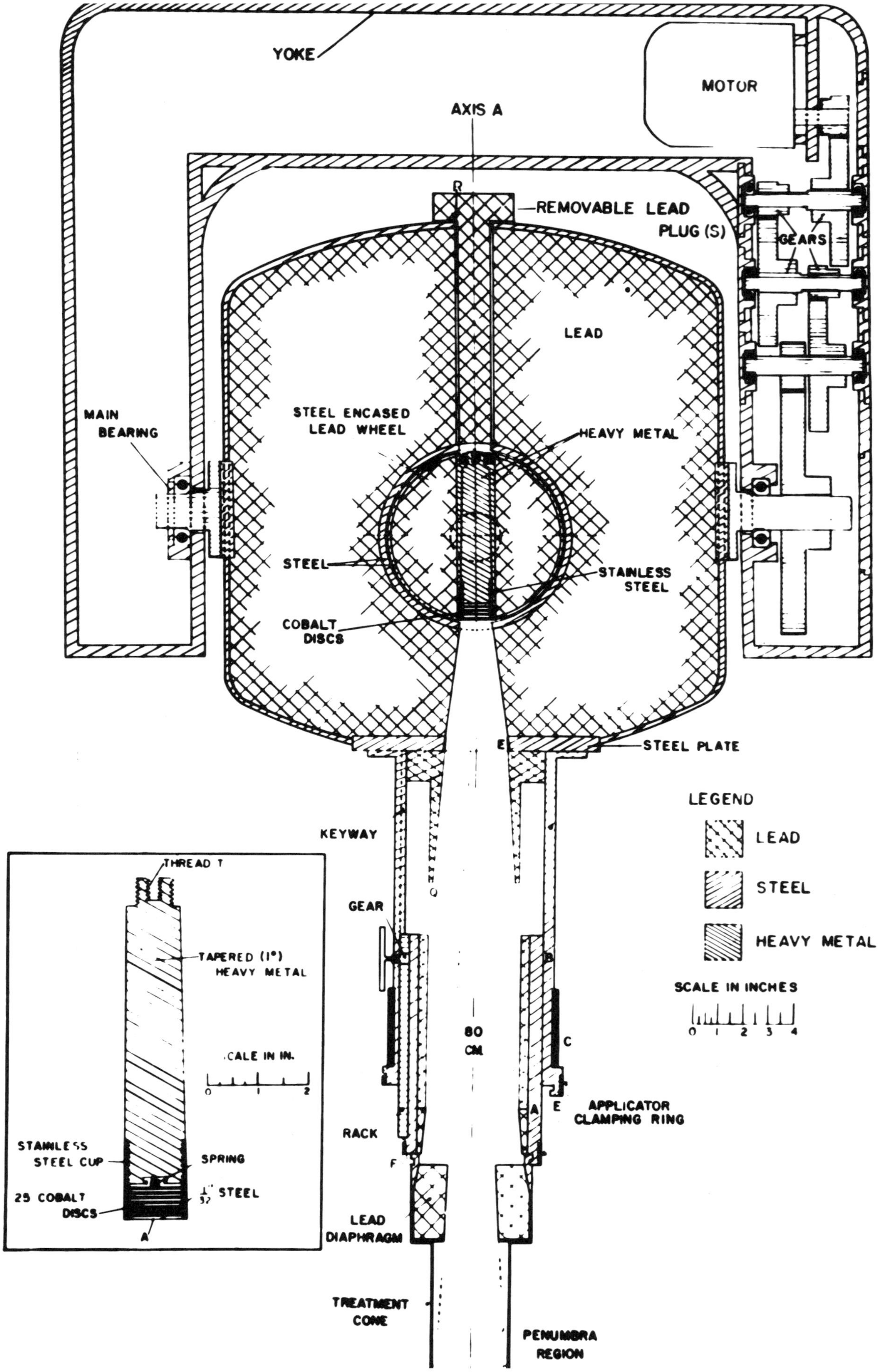

YOKE
MOTOR
AXIS A
R
REMOVABLE LEAD
PLUG (S)
GEARS
LEAD
MAIN
BEARING
STEEL ENCASED
LEAD WHEEL
HEAVY METAL
STEEL
STAINLESS
STEEL
COBALT
DISCS
E
STEEL PLATE
LEGEND
LEAD
STEEL
HEAVY METAL
SCALE IN INCHES
0 1 2 3 4
KEYWAY
THREAD T
TAPERED (1°)
HEAVY METAL
SCALE IN IN.
0 1 2
STAINLESS
STEEL CUP
SPRING
25 COBALT
DISCS
1/32" STEEL
A
GEAR
B
80
CM.
C
A
E
APPLICATOR
CLAMPING RING
RACK
F
LEAD
DIAPHRAGM
TREATMENT
CONE
PENUMBRA
REGION

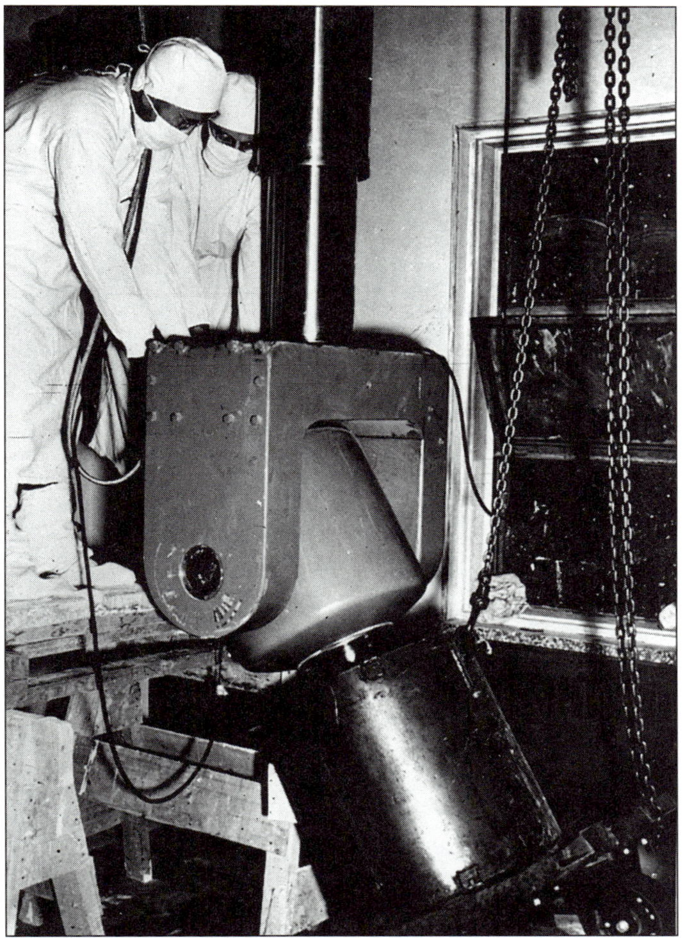

Left
Diagram of Cobalt-60 unit with 180° rotation[38]

Above
Installation of cobalt unit by HE Johns and JA MacKay, August 17, 1951

which would allow treatment of a patient at a large focal-skin distance. Johns asked for "between $2500 and $7000 to cover the total cost of construction." Johns, Cipriani and Lewis agreed that this project would receive greater priority if it were considered as a research project. A quick visit to Premier Douglas in Regina obtained assent for this expenditure. The cabinet, the treasury and the University Board of Governors were bypassed; there were no visits from outside reviewers. Saskatchewan's simple two-page, three-copy application for the isotope was sent to the National Research Council at Chalk River on August 13, 1949.

Lewis, the father of the Canadian nuclear energy program, praised the strong case made in the application but in his letter to Johns dated August 23 he expressed scepticism: "Doubts have been expressed in some quarters about the wisdom of applying Cobalt in this way for therapeutic work."

Three radioactive cobalt sources had been put in the Chalk River pile to "cook" in the fall of 1949. The first of these sources was delivered to the University of Saskatchewan on July 30, 1951 and the second to the University of Western Ontario (UWO) on October 16, 1951. The third source, destined for the United States, was not released until 1952.

Each cobalt source was 2.5 cm in diameter and 1.25 cm thick, described by Sybil Johns, Harold's wife, as "a little half-inch stack of these cobalt discs about the size of a quarter,"[35] and, as Johns had forecast, had an approximate strength of 1000 curies (37 GBq). The Saskatoon unit was designed by Johns and Lloyd Bates, a graduate student, and was built by Johnny MacKay, the proprietor of Acme Machine and Electric in Saskatoon. It was installed in Room 167 in the newly constructed cancer wing, adjacent to the medical college, on August 17, 1951. The room was hardly ready for use; the walls were still being plastered and the concrete floor had not yet been poured. Rigorous depth-dose measurements, using phantoms, soon began.

The unit, weighing approximately 0.9 tonnes, consisted of a steel-encased cylinder suspended from an overhead carriage; a rotating, circular platform, flush with the floor, permitted rotation therapy. A variety of treatment fields could be obtained by using interchangeable lead plugs which were manufactured by MacKay. How to turn the machine on and off caused problems, but the MacKay-Johns solution rediscovered the wheel. The radioactive cobalt source was mounted on the circumference of a wheel near the centre of the head. By rotating the wheel, the source could be moved 180° from its shielded resting position until it was opposite an opening through which

(*Reprinted from Nature, Vol.* 168, *p.* 1035, *December* 15, 1951)

1,000-Curie Cobalt-60 Units for Radiation Therapy

TELETHERAPY units using radium are limited in usefulness by the low radiation intensities produced by the small amounts of radium which can be used. To secure an adequate dosage-rate, the distance between the source and the tumour cannot be more than a few centimetres, and therefore the dose delivered to the skin lying between the source and the tumour is much higher than that delivered to the tumour. The dose-rate below the surface, expressed as a percentage of the dose-rate at the skin, decreases very rapidly with increasing depth. Thus the percentage depth-dose is influenced primarily by the inverse square law, and one of the chief advantages of high-energy radiation, namely, its small attenuation by the tissue between the source and the tumour, is not realized.

Any attempt to obtain an improvement in the depth-dose by increasing the amount of radium, and correspondingly improving the ratio between the source-to-tumour distance and the source-to-skin distance, is limited by the high cost of radium, and by the required increase in the volume of the source. If the diameter of the source is increased, it is harder to get a well-defined beam; if the thickness is increased, much of the radiation is lost by absorption within the source.

With the high density of neutron flux of the Canadian nuclear reactor at Chalk River, sources of cobalt-60 having specific activities of 20–60 curies per gm. can be prepared. One gram of this isotope will give about the same radiation output as 32–96 gm. of radium. The gamma-rays from cobalt-60 have energies of 1·17 and 1·33 MeV.; thus the average energy is about the same as that of the gamma-rays from a sealed radium source.

Two identical sources of cobalt-60 were made available by the Atomic Energy Project of the National Research Council of Canada in the summer of 1951 for experimental and clinical use. Each source is 1 in. in diameter and half an inch thick, and has an effective strength of 1,000 curies. Two quite different units have been designed to use these sources for radiation therapy.

One of the units, designed by two of us (H. E. J., L. M. B.) for the Saskatchewan Cancer Commission, was installed in the University Hospital, Saskatoon, in August 1951. This unit consists of a steel-encased lead cylinder, with rounded ends, 20 in. in diameter and 22 in. in length, and weighs about 2,000 lb. The source is mounted on the circumference of a wheel near the centre of a head, so that by rotating the wheel it can be brought opposite an opening in one end of the head through which the radiation can emerge. The head is suspended from an overhead carriage. It can be moved in a horizontal direction, raised and lowered, and rotated through 120° in a vertical plane. A rotating circular platform, flush with the floor, is provided for rotational therapy. A variety of treatment fields can be obtained by the use of interchangeable lead diaphragms. Light stainless-steel cones, attached to each of these, indicate the size of the field and fix the treatment distance. Circular fields and rectangular fields up to 20 cm. × 20 cm., at 80 cm. source-to-skin distance, can be obtained.

With the source rotated to the 'off' position, the dosage level 1 ft. from the head is less than 7 mr./hr. With the machine turned on, dosage-levels outside the treatment room, for the severest scattering conditions, are less than 5 mr./hr. Other measurements on this unit were carried out by members of the Saskatchewan group, and details of these will be found elsewhere[1].

The second unit, designed by R. F. Errington and D. T. Green, of the Development Division of Eldorado Mining and Refining (1944), Ltd., is installed in the clinic of the Ontario Cancer Foundation in the Victoria Hospital in London, Ontario. This unit consists of a head pivoted between the arms of a horizontal 'Y', so that it can be rotated downward in one plane through about 105°, that is, from a few degrees above the horizontal to a few degrees beyond the vertical. The horizontal arm can be moved up and down a vertical column by a motor-driven screw mechanism. The vertical column is supported from the floor by a base extending forward under the head.

The radiation beam emerges through a conical opening in the head. When the beam is 'off', this opening is filled with mercury. When the beam is turned on, an air compressor built into the horizontal arm is started, and air pressure forces the mercury up into a reservoir. If the beam is turned off, or if there is a power failure, the reservoir valve opens and the mercury returns, under gravity, to cut off the beam.

Field-sizes are varied by means of diaphragms in front of the opening in the head. Four lead blocks at right angles to each other can be adjusted by levers on the outside of the head to yield square or

N.R.C. No. 2589

the radiation emerged.

The *Saskatoon Star Phoenix* on August 18, 1951, printed a photograph of the installation with the caption: "Wearing specially treated smocks and masks as protection against deadly gamma rays, Dr HE Johns, physicist to the Saskatchewan Cancer Commission (left), and Mr J A MacKay of the Acme Machine Shop, are shown here carefully transferring a small piece of radio-active cobalt from a lead container to a treatment head..." The Saskatoon unit was officially commissioned on October 23, but even more rigorous measurements continued until November 8 when the first patient was treated by Watson. Watson played down attempts to publicize the importance of Saskatoon's achievement, saying this was merely a device that might provide more efficient and economical cancer treatment.

Depth (cm.)	Field, 100 cm.². Distance, 100 cm.		Field, 100 cm.². Distance, 70 cm.	
	Cobalt-60	2 MeV. (ref. 2)	Cobalt-60	3 MeV. (ref. 3)
0·5	100	100	100	100
1·0	99	98	98	98
5·0	80	79	77	76
10·0	58	54	54	53
15·0	41	37	37	36
20·0	29	25	26	25

rectangular fields between 4 cm. × 4 cm. and 20 cm. × 20 cm., at 100 cm. from the source. The diaphragm system can be moved along the axis of the beam so that any source-to-skin distance between 70 cm. and 100 cm. can be utilized. In any position, the end of the diaphragm system is 13 cm. or more from the patient. A beam of light from a source at the same distance from the patient as the radiation source, and limited by the diaphragm in the same way as the radiation beam, is used as a field localizer. A detailed discussion of the unit, and of the depth-dose measurements made on it at the Radiology Laboratory of the National Research Council by some of us (National Research Council group), will be found elsewhere[1].

Depth-dose measurements were carried out in Saskatoon and in Ottawa, using D.C. amplifiers with small ionization chambers and water phantoms. The results were in excellent agreement. A summary of the percentage depth-dose data is given in the accompanying table. The maximum dose occurs 5–6 mm. below the surface of the phantom. The surface dose and the dose at any given depth depend on the size of the field. A distance of at least 15 cm. should be used between the limiting diaphragm and the surface of the phantom to reduce the electron content of the gamma-ray beam.

In the first two columns of the table, depth-dose data for the cobalt-60 units, using a 100 cm.² field at 100 cm. source-to-skin distance, is compared with data obtained by Miller[2] for a 2-MeV. Van de Graaff type X-ray unit. In the last two columns a comparison is presented between the cobalt data and measurements obtained by Trump[3] for a 3-MeV. Van de Graaff type X-ray machine, for 100 cm.² fields and for a source-to-skin distance of 70 cm. It is apparent that the percentage depth-doses for the cobalt are considerably higher than for 2-MeV. X-rays, and slightly higher than for 3-MeV. radiation. This indicates that the average energy of the photons from a 2-MeV., or even a 3-MeV., X-ray generator is lower than the average photon energy of a cobalt-60 source.

The cobalt units are flexible, simple to operate, and should require little servicing. They may prove to be very convenient sources of high-energy radiation for therapy.

H. E. Johns
L. M. Bates
E. R. Epp
D. V. Cormack
S. O. Fedoruk

Saskatchewan Cancer Commission, and
Physics Department,
University of Saskatchewan,
Saskatoon.

A. Morrison
W. R. Dixon
C. Garrett

Radiology Laboratory,
Physics Division,
National Research Council,
Ottawa.
Oct. 26.

[1] Brit. J. Rad. (in the press).
[2] Miller, H., Brit. J. Rad., 23, 731 (1950).
[3] Trump, J. G., and Cloud, R. W. Amer. J. Roent. and Rad. Ther., 49, 531 (1943).

Printed in Great Britain by Fisher, Knight & Co., Ltd., St. Albans.

Eldorado Mining and Smelting had completed the second unit for installation at Victoria Hospital in London, Ontario on October 23. Their unit, using a somewhat different design, consisted of a head pivoted between the arms of the horizontal "Y" which could be raised and lowered. The beam was turned on and off by an air compressor that forced mercury in and out of the reservoir. The radiation beam was turned off when a pool of mercury was introduced between the source and a conical opening in the head. The field size was varied by means of four lead blocks at right angles to each other. This was the prototype of the Atomic Energy of Canada Limited (AECL) cobalt unit. Dr Ivan H Smith quickly treated the first patient in London, Ontario on October 27, four days after installation.

This first cobalt treatment at London was widely publicized in the Canadian press. The *Saskatoon Star Phoenix* commented on the "cobalt race" in an editorial on November 7, 1951:

> *We hope Messrs Truman, Stalin, Peron et al won't think someone is trying to steal their thunder, but we think they ought to know theirs is not the only atomic race going on in the world. Another has been declared by* The London Free Press *which claims, editorially, 'the world's first cobalt bomb' for…the Ontario city. With all due respect to the preservation of national peace and goodwill, that is a boast which this newspaper cannot allow to go unchallenged—especially since the* Free Press *is brazen enough to remark that a cobalt bomb 'is also being installed at Saskatoon, Sask.' One is indeed. Or, to be more accurate, one has been installed.*

Historians can assess the relative merits of the two claims (Table 1). Suffice it to say that the first patient at

London was treated with a machine which had not been fully calibrated, and soon afterwards the patient died of advancing disease. The first patient treated at Saskatoon had advanced carcinoma of the cervix at age 40, unlikely to be cured by any then known-treatment regimen. She received a precise dose, carefully calibrated. Not only was she cured of her cancer, but she was alive and well in Victoria, British Columbia in 1992.

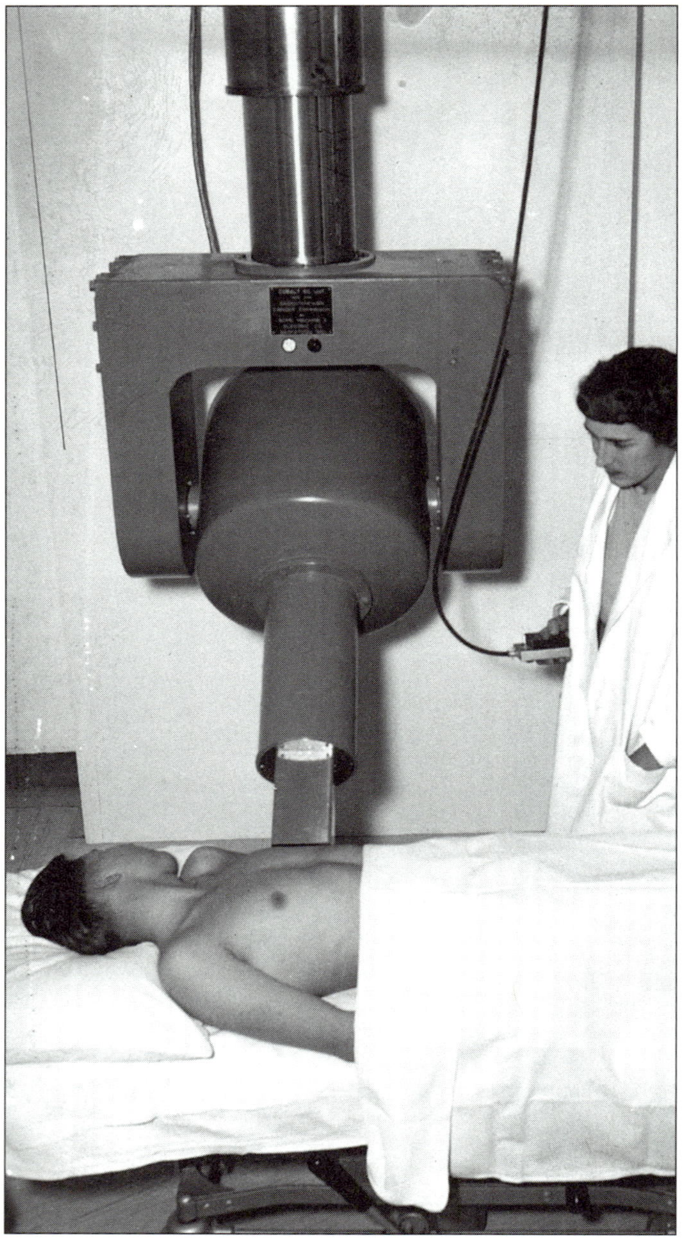

Sylvia O Fedoruk arranging a field for radiotherapy with cobalt-60 machine, early model

Table 1

The First Cobalt-60 Treatments in the World, 1951

	Saskatchewan	W. Ontario
Cobalt-60 source delivered	30 July	16 October
Unit installed	17 August	23 October
Calibration	11 weeks	—
First patient treated	8 November	27 October

The first formal publication giving details of cobalt therapy was brief and to the point. It appeared in the December 15, 1951 issue of *Nature*. The authors, sometimes referred to as the "Saskatchewan mafia," were HE Johns, LM Bates, ER Epp, DV Cormack and SO Fedoruk, all from Saskatchewan, and three University of Saskatchewan physics graduates (A Morrison, WR Dixon and C Garrett) from the radiology laboratory in the physics division of the National Research Council in Ottawa. This paper describes both Canadian cobalt units and concludes, "The cobalt units are flexible, simple to operate, and should require little servicing. They may prove to be very convenient sources of high-energy radiation."[36] A second paper by the same authors appeared in *Science* in March 1952.[37] More detailed papers on the calibration and use of the two units and the Saskatchewan betatron filled an entire issue of the *Journal of the Canadian Association of Radiologists* in March 1952.[38,39] Isodose curves were made available and the Saskatchewan cobalt-60 depth-dose data were included in the *British Journal of Radiology* in July 1951[40] and a special supplement to the *British Journal of Radiology* in June 1952.[41–43] Additional papers on dosimetry appeared in *Radiology*,[44–46] *The Journal of the Faculty of Radiologists*,[47] *American Journal of Roentgenology*,[48] *Acta Radiologica*,[49] *The British Journal of Radiology*[50] and the *Journal of the Canadian Association of Radiologists*.[51] Watson told a meeting of the International College of Surgeons of the benefits of cobalt-60 therapy.[52]

MacKay turned his attention to designing a new collimator system, using a large number of interleaved diaphragms rather than a single diaphragm in one plane to achieve a smaller penumbra and eliminate the interchangeable lead plugs that were 5 cm to 8 cm thick

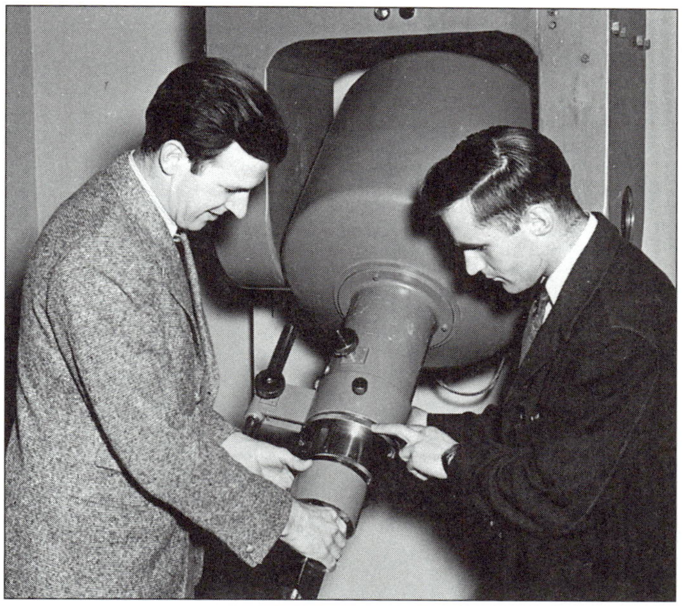

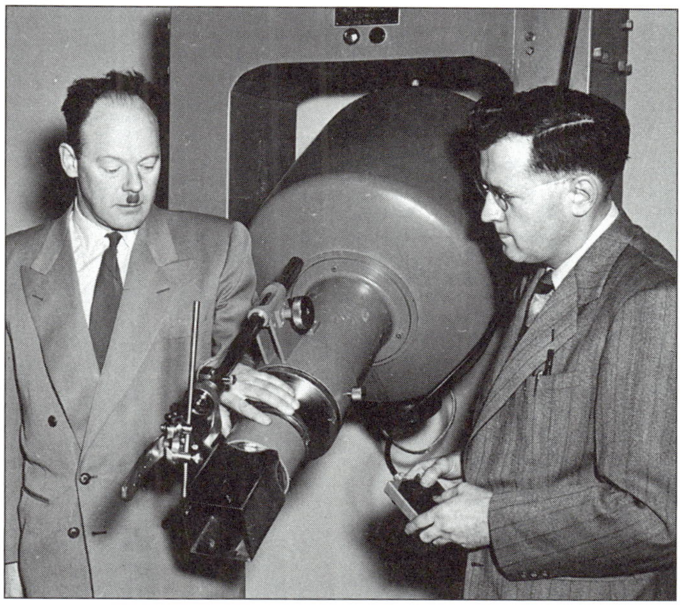

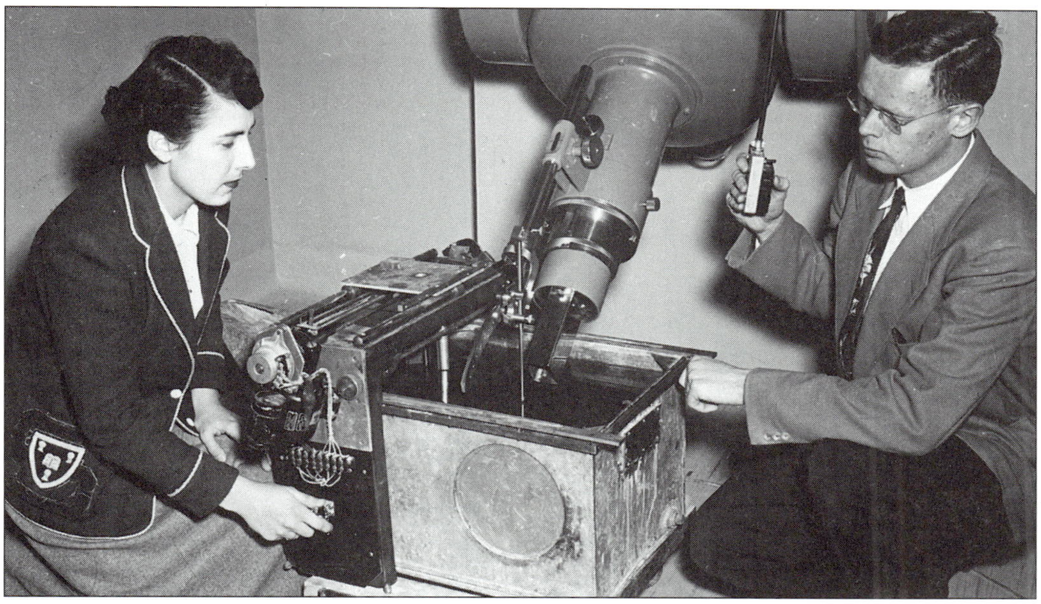

Top left
Dr L Bates and Dr DV Cormack, Physicist, Saskatchewan Cancer Commission with Cobalt-60 machine

Above
TA Watson, JA MacKay and HE Johns with Cobalt-60 machine and collimation

Left
Sylvia O Fedoruk and E Epp testing collimator of Cobalt-60

and very heavy. The final version of the MacKay-Johns collimator was a system of fixed and moving steel-encased lead bars that provided rectangular and square fields from 4 cm x 4 cm to 20 cm x 20 cm by simply twisting two dials. MacKay's small engineering firm in Saskatchewan produced these collimators for over 100 Picker Cobalt units that were distributed worldwide.

Another special issue of the *Journal of the Canadian Association of Radiologists*, in June 1957, presented the medical world with the first five-year report on the clinical application of cobalt-60 therapy units.[53] Harold Johns summarized his work when he presented the Gordon Richards Memorial Lecture, "Impact of Physics on Therapeutic and Diagnostic Radiology," to the 1979 annual meeting of the Canadian Association of Radiologists.[54] The original Saskatoon cobalt-60 unit was in service until 1972, treating 6728 patients over 21 years. Finally, it was replaced by a commercial AECL cobalt radiotherapy machine.

Although one highly respected commercial consultant predicted in 1952 that in 10 years there would only be 30 cobalt machines in use worldwide, these machines proved to be not only compact but economical to purchase and maintain. By 1984 there were about 2500 units in routine use in the free world, 1500 of which had been built in Canada by AECL.[55]

One of us (CSH) had many times heard the story of how Allan Blair and Harold Johns had visited Premier and Health Minister Tommy Douglas in his office, without any prior appointment. Was this apocryphal folklore? The opportunity to satisfy my curiosity presented itself in February 1983. Douglas was scheduled to visit Saskatoon for what proved to be his last major speech here. I phoned

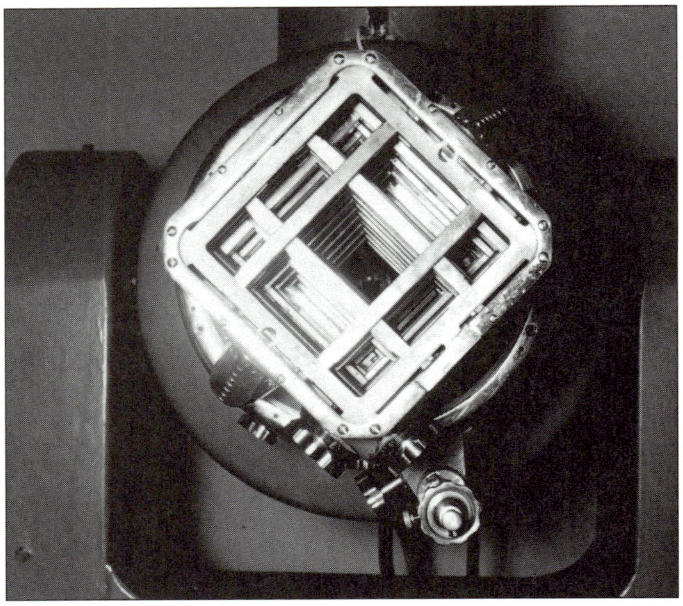

Final collimation system developed by McKay and Johns: a system of fixed and moving steel-encased lead bars that provided rectangular and square fields by simply twisting two dials

Peter Prebble, the New Democratic Party MLA for my constituency, and asked whether it would be possible to have ten minutes with Douglas during his visit. Although his schedule was extremely tight, Peter arranged for me to drive Douglas back to the Bessborough Hotel after his banquet speech at the Elks Hall, on condition that my wife, Mary and I purchase tickets to the banquet.

The story was true. But how, I asked Douglas, did he have the courage to give carte blanche approval "off the cuff," with no consultation with his cabinet, the provincial treasurer or an outside review agency? Douglas explained to me that when he attended Brandon College as a student his favourite professor was his mathematics teacher, Dr Alfred Edward Johns, the father of Harold Johns. AE Johns had been a missionary in Chengtu, West China until 1924. Indeed, the Johns family had taken pity on the little student with chronic osteomyelitis in his femur and sometimes had him over for Sunday supper. On such occasions Douglas observed that Harold already showed promise as a scholar. Later, as premier, Douglas knew that Allan Blair's Cancer Clinic was a leader in North America.

At their impromptu visit in his office, Blair and Johns persuaded Douglas that high voltage radiotherapy offered great promise for the people of Saskatchewan. Their estimate of the possible cost Douglas felt was within reach. It was because of his close personal knowledge of both Johns and Blair and his *faith in their integrity* that Douglas gave such ready assent. There were no site visits, no consultations with experts, no forms to fill out in quintuplicate or more.

Ed and Pemrose Whelan, in their compilation of Douglas anecdotes, *Touched by Tommy*, have cited a number of instances of how the first CCF Premier's informal grassroots operation created a constant headache for his personal secretary, Eleanor McKinnon. In her words:

> *There were hundreds of farmers coming who wanted to talk to Tommy and he had an open door policy. Our office was full of people all of the time. And he sat back just as cheerful and relaxed as if there was just one man in the world, the man he was talking to, and he had lots of time. We did have to screen people a bit, but if he were free, he was always willing to see people, especially if they had a problem...The phone rang just about every five minutes. We never let anybody with a problem go.*[56]

This policy of availability contributed greatly to Douglas' popular appeal. In the case of betatron and cobalt research, the rapid approval and unfettered support from the Douglas government helped to put Saskatchewan in the forefront.

Though born of war-time nuclear research, the cobalt bomb was in practice a ploughshare rather than a sword and a largely Canadian contribution to medical care. With its flair for trend-setting performance in medicine, Saskatchewan had led the way.

Acknowledgements:

This chapter has benefited from constructive criticism offered by Dr AJS Bryant of Regina, Dr Charles C Burkell of Saskatoon, and Dr Harold E Johns of Toronto. We thank them for their suggestions.

Note:

Photographs in this chapter are courtesy of the Saskatchewan Cancer Foundation.

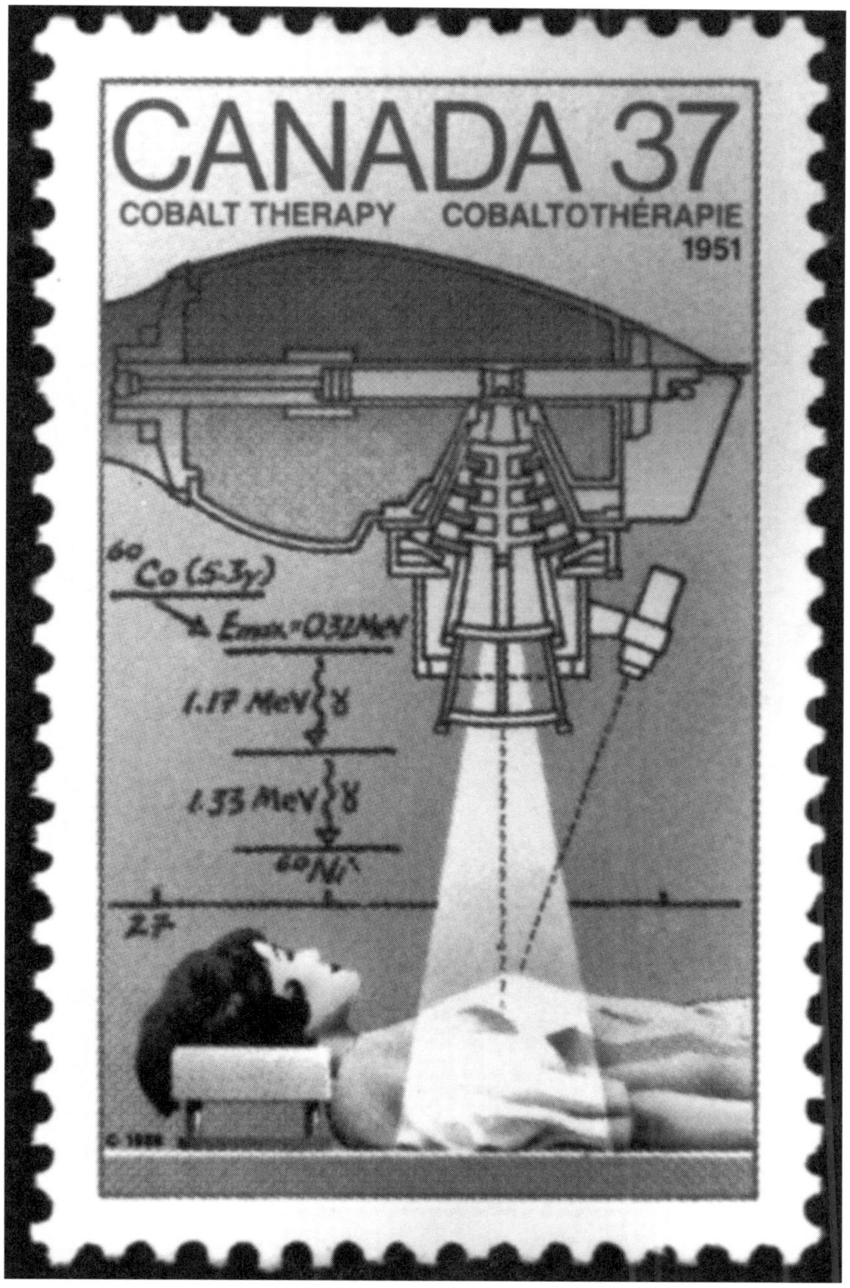
CANADA 37
COBALT THERAPY
COBALTOTHÉRAPIE
1951
60Co (5.3y)
Emax=0.32MeV
1.17 MeV γ
1.33 MeV γ
60Ni
27

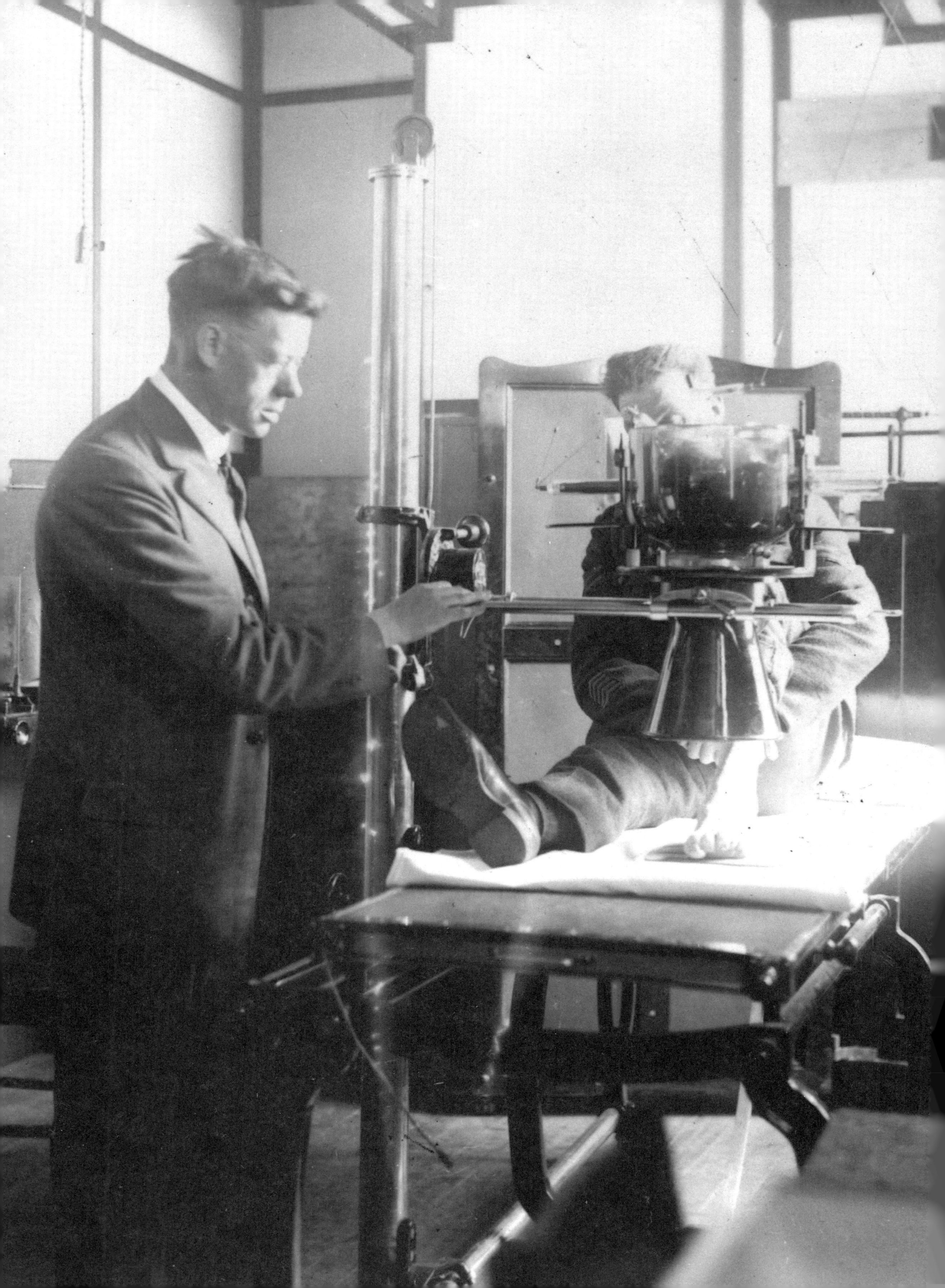

Chapter XII • *Information on the Early Days of*

Radiology in Alberta

WB (Bill) Parsons

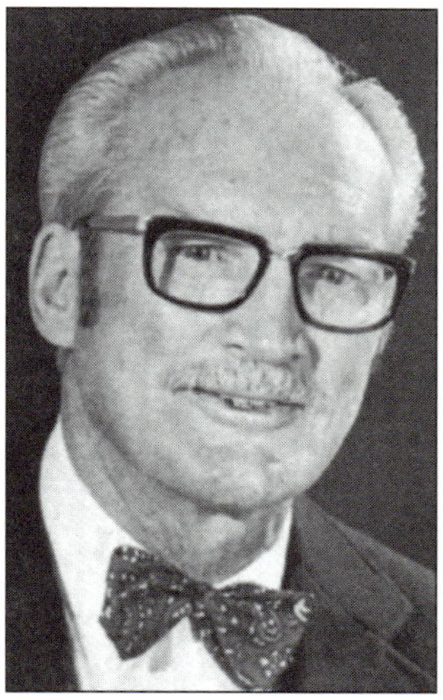

Dr WB (Bill) Parsons

Left
X Ray Dept at the Belcher Hospital Calgary, circa 1928 (Photography courtesy of the Glenbow Museum and Archives)

Some of the background and much of the detail of the early days of radiology in Alberta lie with those who made this history. Although it is only 51 years since the arrival of the first x-ray unit in Alberta, none of those who were first to introduce this technology into their own communities in this province is still alive as I write in 1974.

The first radiographs were not made in Alberta's larger cities. The province was but three years old and cattle were of more interest than science when news of Röntgen's discovery (thirteen years previous) came to the prairie town of Medicine Hat. This was not Medicine Hat's medical "first." In 1884 the first hospital between Winnipeg and Victoria was opened in Medicine Hat to care for those building the railroad. Through the years, the Canadian Pacific Railroad (CPR) and its officials were generous to this pioneer hospital; the local railways superintendent was usually president of its board, and it was the CPR employees who demanded x-rays. Back in Winnipeg they had become used to examinations in a darkened room where sparks flew and sizzled. It fell to Dr J H Woodland to buy the x-ray unit and set it up in space donated by the hospital. This unit was a Sleidal Western consisting of an induction coil with a mechanical converter which for a time used gas tubes. Like the majority of early users of x-rays, Dr Woodland was his own technician. He did not restrict the use of the unit to his own patients but would examine those of other doctors for a small fee, though the only abnormalities examined for the first few years were fractures. As word spread, the unit saw very active use. As far as is known, Dr Woodland got his radiological knowledge from books. He may have seen x-rays in use before he graduated from Dalhousie University and came west to register, first in the Northwest Territories in 1905 and then in Alberta in 1906.

However, Dr Woodland did not stay on in Medicine Hat, and some use of the unit was made by Dr F W Gershaw, who, after graduating from Manitoba in 1908 and interning at the Winnipeg General Hospital, came to Medicine Hat in 1910. Dr Gershaw also purchased and used to a limited extent a small suitcase set which could be plugged into a standard wall socket, the tube being set up on a platform contained in the carrying case. However, Dr Gershaw was often busy and persuaded Dr J S McLeod to carry out most of the radiology.

Apparently Dr McLeod's interest in x-rays was rather casual; although Medicine Hat had the first x-ray unit in Alberta, it was quite a number of years before the city had a full-time radiologist. Dr SF McEwen graduated from the University of Toronto and practiced in rural Alberta communities from 1909 to 1918, then moved to Medicine Hat as Dr Gershaw's assistant. After one year in this capacity, Dr Gershaw convinced him to go into x-ray practice, which Dr McEwen did, after first taking a short course in Toronto. Dr McEwen served the Medicine Hat Clinic and hospital in the capacity of radiologist until his retirement in 1954. Dr Gershaw remained in part-time practice and was a member of the Canadian Senate.

The second x-ray unit was not established in Edmonton, the capital, nor in thriving Calgary. Back at McGill Dr JE Lovering had become acquainted with x-rays, and on a trip to Toronto, where several instruments were on display, his interest became enthusiastic. His first subject was his fiancée, whom he impressed by looking into her purse. Dr Lovering moved to Alberta, where he registered in 1908 and practiced at Cardston until 1909. He then moved to Lethbridge where he immediately ordered an x-ray machine. Whether the hazards were not publicized or they were ignored is not known, but Dr Lovering was said to have frequently tested the intensity of the x-ray with his hand in the fluoroscope, so that by 1920 he was showing advanced skin changes from radiation exposure.

Dr FH Mewburn, who later achieved fame as the first professor of surgery at the University of Alberta, also purchased an x-ray unit not long after Dr Lovering. The year he acquired it is not known, but Dr Mewburn left Lethbridge in 1913 to go to Calgary, from where he went overseas in 1914. Later on, between 1919 and 1921, a unit was installed in the offices of the Campbell Clinic with Dr W Bryans acting as technician.

Lethbridge's first radiologist was Dr SM Rose, who went to the city in 1933 to operate the unit which the Galt Hospital had installed in 1930. Dr Rose later leased space at this hospital and worked there, as well as serving some of the clinics in Lethbridge, until ill health forced his retirement in 1955. This marked the year of the opening of the Lethbridge Municipal Hospital with Dr M Marshall as radiologist. St Michael's Hospital had been built many years earlier, with Dr Rose serving both hospitals until Dr BO Black came to the Sisters' Hospital as radiologist after World War II.

In Edmonton an electrician named Edwards was fascinated by the accounts he had read of x-rays. He went to see his friend, Dr EA Braithwaite, who had been a police surgeon in the west since 1892, and persuaded him to order a new unit. Each evening Edwards would visit the doctor and check the unit, and together they would examine any plates that had been made.

Dr Braithwaite's interest in x-rays was not sufficient to prompt him to pursue its study very vigorously. This work fell to Dr GH Malcolmson, who became Edmonton's first radiologist and its senior one until his death in 1944. Dr Malcolmson graduated from the University of Toronto in 1897 and registered in the Northwest Territories in 1898, practicing for some years at Pincher Creek, later moving to Frank in the Crowsnest Pass. He and his family survived the Frank slide, when half of a mountain fell and buried most of the town. Dr Malcolmson later moved to Edmonton where he was found to have a tuberculous kidney which was removed. Returning to practice, he found the pace very hard. He went overseas to attend an international conference in Sweden and became very interested in the radiographs he saw there. He stayed on to take a course in radiology and on his way back to Edmonton ordered a unit which he set up in his home. During World War I Dr Malcolmson moved into the McLeod Building and soon joined the Allin Clinic, though he did work for others in the building. Dr Malcolmson, Edmonton's first hospital radiologist, was appointed to Edmonton's city hospital, the Royal Alexandra, in about 1924. He was first given a room in the basement, and later, one in the attic. In 1928 great indignation arose when the new medical superintendent, Dr AF Anderson, gave Dr Malcolmson considerable space on the main floor. The other staff members felt this was a great waste of valuable space. However, here a high kilovoltage unit Dr Malcolmson had ordered was installed—the first such unit in Alberta—and its installation marked the beginning of the era of modern treatments in Alberta.

Meanwhile, across the river at the Strathcona Hospital (South Edmonton), Dr Richard Proctor arrived. He had joined the Soldiers' Civil Re-establishment (SCR) [what might be called a veterans' hospital—editor's note]. Dr

Proctor had graduated from the University of Manitoba, where his first experience with x-rays was hand cranking a generator as a student. He had first gone to Edmonton, then overseas in 1915 on military service. Back at Moore Barracks in England in 1918 he ran into Dr Howard Pirie, the first radiologist at McGill, who had written the first Canadian textbooks on diagnostic and therapeutic radiology. Dr Proctor then went to the Granville Special Centre in Buxton, where he studied radiology, and returned to Edmonton on September 1, 1919. From there he went to Edson, where he spent a year in general practice, and then returned to Edmonton to the SCR, a hospital of 85 beds. Here he gave anesthetics and ran the radiology department, replacing Dr Malcolmson, who had operated it during the war. Dr Proctor looked after radiology and physiotherapy, as well as giving anesthetics, for two years at the Strathcona Hospital. This hospital was later taken over by the University in 1923 and became the University Hospital. Dr Proctor remained on the staff at the hospital until ten years after his retirement age. Dr Proctor also developed troublesome dermatitis of the hands.

Dr Proctor reports that his first unit was made by Meyer. He he paid $5000 to $6000 for it and replaced it with a Victor in 1925. The units were much simpler than those in use today, and he said that he serviced them largely himself. If he couldn't, it was necessary to bring in an expert from Winnipeg. One or two extra tubes were always kept on hand in Edmonton. Dr Proctor's Meyer's unit was a spark gap set with open wires. Dr Proctor does not recall any x-ray burns; he thinks they came later with higher power. At the SCR he was alone at first and did his own technical work, but later a patient came who proved to be a technician who had worked with Pirie overseas. This man stayed on for many years as chief technician. Dr Proctor had to train his own technicians and, apart from the one mentioned, only employed nurses in this capacity.

The second radiologist who moved to Edmonton was Dr Dixon, who practiced in the Tegler Building after World War I. Dr Mooney, Dr AB Irving, Dr Marshall Mallett and his son have followed.

Dr Malcolmson was joined by his son, Dr PH (Pat) Malcolmson, in 1938, but Pat died in 1955, and the radiology office in the McLeod Building was closed. However, another office was opened by Dr RM Hall in the Northgate Building. Dr Hall is the son of Dr Morton Hall, who was the first pathologist at the Royal Alexandra Hospital. Dr Hall, after returning from overseas, had practiced in Regina and then joined Dr Mallett in Edmonton, but left to open his own office and was later joined by Dr SC Windle of Winnipeg.

At the university after Dr Proctor's retirement, Dr Hector E Duggan became director of the department. Some time after the war, Dr RM Clare became a full-time radiologist at the Misericordia Hospital. In 1957 he became administrator of this hospital, still working as director of radiology but with an assistant.

Soon after World War I Dr Walter Morrish, who practiced both diagnostic and therapeutic radiology and was trained in diseases of women and dermatology, came from England. Dr Morrish also served for some time as Liberal member of the provincial legislature.

The first x-ray unit in Calgary was purchased by the nuns at the Holy Cross Hospital in 1912. The sisters asked Dr CF McGuffin, who had been practicing general surgery in Calgary since 1907, to run the machine. Dr McGuffin did not wish to, so the task fell to his brother, Dr W H (Herbert) McGuffin. Dr Herbert McGuffin graduated from the University of Western Ontario in 1909 and spent a year in the Victoria Hospital in London before joining his brother. Dr Herb ran the service from 1912 until he left general practice in 1918 to devote his full time to radiology. Like many other early radiologists, for a long time he was both radiologist and his own technician and, again like many of the early radiologists, he acquired his knowledge little by little. He attended many radiological conventions in Canada and the United States and took several short courses at hospitals, including Cook County Hospital in Chicago, and a three-week course in New York on diagnosis and therapy.

During the war Dr CF was away on military service, while Dr Herb a major in the army stayed in Calgary. He had both an army and a civilian practice and provided radiographs for soldiers. He did not work in the Colonel Belcher Hospital: during the war Dr Walter Quint had become the radiologist for the SCR. Subsequently, Dr Quint entered practice in the Greyhound Building, until his practice was taken over after World War II by Dr KD Symington. After World War I, Dr Quint was appointed radiologist at the General Hospital, which post he held along with his practice until he left. Dr WH McGuffin was radiologist for the Holy Cross Hospital through the years. He started his private practice in 1918 when he bought a unit similar to the one at the Holy Cross. The type is not known, but it had a mechanical rectifier. In 1929 he expanded his practice and built a radium and x-ray institute, which he sold in 1947 to Drs J Porter and D Florendine, though he practiced with them until his death in 1949. The institution was operated by Drs Porter and Florendine, but not as a private hospital as in Dr McGuffin's day.

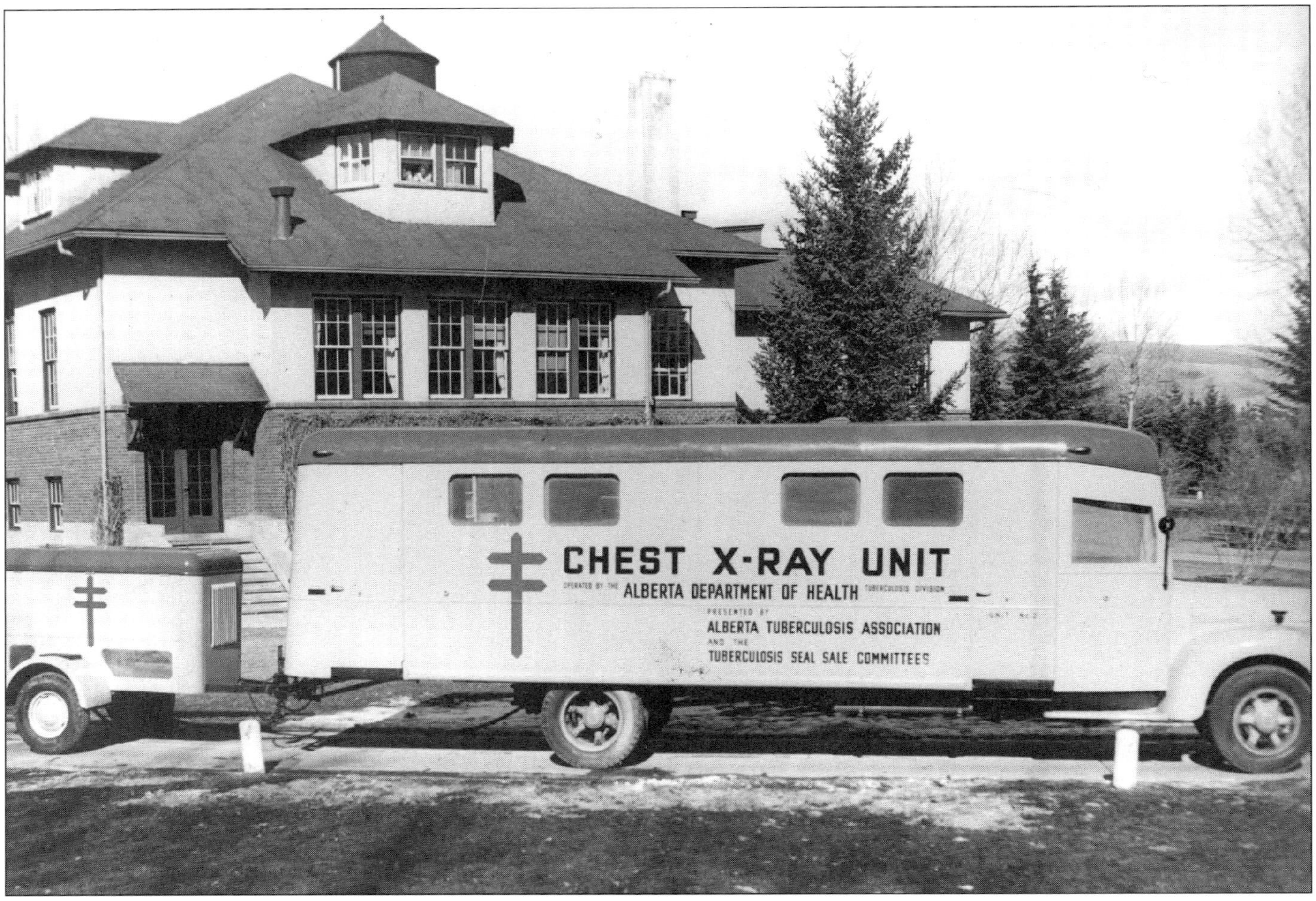

Not much is known about the advent of radiology in other small communities in Alberta, though Red Deer, which then had a population of 2900, had an x-ray unit installed in 1911 in the office of Dr Richard Parsons. Dr Parsons graduated from Trinity Medical College in Toronto in 1901 and came to Red Deer in 1903. He was in general practice, but his chief interest was surgery, and he made frequent visits to the larger centres, including the Mayo Clinic, which was then becoming prominent; Johns Hopkins University; and the Polyclinic Hospital in New York. These visits convinced him that an x-ray unit would be a valuable additon to his practice, and in 1911 he purchased a Victor machine. The machine was not shock-proof, and the wires were strung about the room. The spark gap was a source of wonderment to those examined. After the glass plates were exposed, they were taken two blocks to the local photographer to be processed. Apart from the four larger Alberta cities, Red Deer was the only community with a resident radiologist, Dr Richard Parsons' son, Dr WB Parsons (the writer), who had been with his father and brother in general practice since 1935 but had taken up radiology in the army.

Not long after the World War I a great number of x-ray units were placed throughout Alberta in various hospitals and doctors' offices. Many were placed in chiropractors' offices as well. Dr Graham of Ponoka reports that during the early twenties he used to take his patients with suspected fractures to the dentist's office. He recalled that the dentist would take a film and then say, "You'll just have to move it a little more, doctor." Some doctors would bundle patients with severe fractures into a car and drive them as much as sixty or eighty miles, set the fracture with x-ray guidance and drive home.

Much of the early setting of fractures was done fluoroscopically. Dr McEwen reports his first unit was a Victor with a rotary convertor, which could be adapted to lying or standing fluoroscopy. The tube under the table did not have shock-proof cables, and Dr McEwen recalls that once while attempting to set a difficult fracture, the surgeons and he were working in the dark pulling on the fractured limb when one of them backed into one of the cables. All of them got a shock and were scattered about the room. The anesthetized patient knew nothing of the accident.

Public opinion of x-rays had changed, moving beyond the Victorian reaction of horror at the possibility of

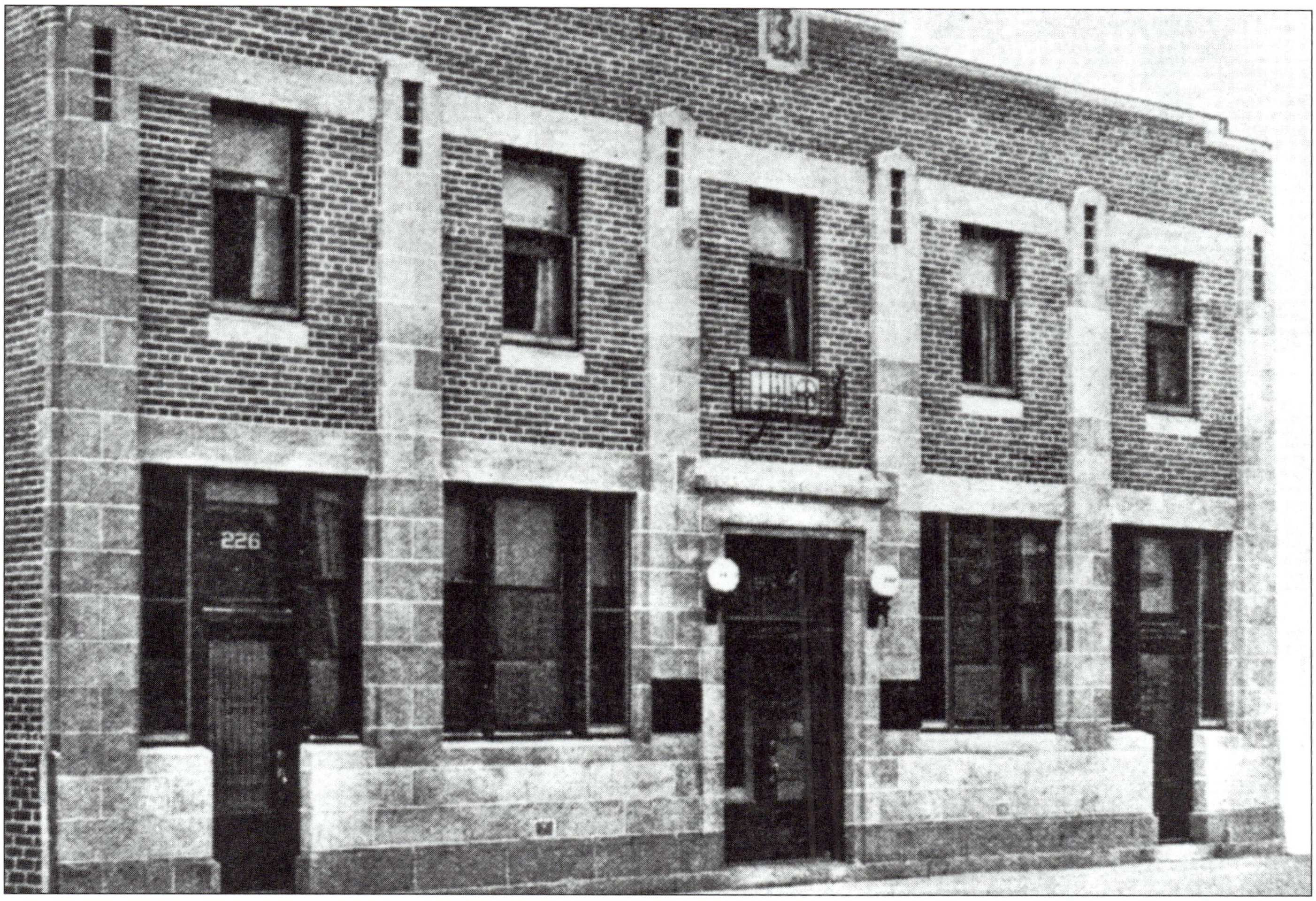

Left
Mobile chest photofluorographic unit (date uncertain—possibly the late 1950s or early 1960s)

Above
The X-ray and Radium Institute, Calgary, Alta, founded by Dr McGuffin. (Photographs courtesy of the Glenbow Museum and Archives, Calgary)

looking through people's clothes, so the technology was welcome in Canada. That is, until the appearance of radio. I can remember people calling up my home to see if the x-ray unit was turned on, because there was such a terrible noise due to interference with reception. Unquestionably, the early x-ray units did cause a great deal of static, though they were probably unfairly blamed for a great deal of noise they did not cause. Mrs AL Chute, who is a doctor and married to Dr Chute of Toronto Sick Children's Hospital, was born Helen Reid, daughter of Dr Reid of Vegreville, Alberta. She recalls that her father acquired his first x-ray unit between 1918 and 1920. It was an awesome piece, made of solid oak and varnished, except for a big white panel in the front, a "man-sized tube—about 5 1/2 feet tall and 3 feet square." Much of her letter is worth quoting:

> *I think it cost him $750.00 which in those days was not inconsiderable. He always vowed it paid for itself on just one case. A visitor to our town fell and sustained a Colles' fracture. Father was accustomed to set this sort of thing without x-ray, but the new machine and his love for all things mechanical proved irresistible. He took "before and afters" as he called them, and she went her way. He was most distressed some months later when a lawyer from the States threatened suit for damages. He blessed the old machine because he had the pictures to prove that when she left his office her fracture had been reduced.*
>
> *Only his love of gadgets, I am sure, kept him using the thing—for all that time an x-ray was a major production. The machine stood in the corner of a back room at the local drugstore. He had a table made to accommodate patients. We still have this long, narrow table in the family. I think he didn't take many pictures but used it more as a fluoroscope. The tube hung all unguarded and silvery from a crane arrangement at the top. The two brass rods with the brass ball on each were adjustable and were moved back and forth until the spark crackled and ran between*

them. While I am sure my father was in danger of being electrocuted or developing radiation sickness, I think his greatest danger was from the local citizenry. Radio was just coming in at this time and those fortunate enough to own the then massive knobs and sets of ear phones were convinced that he deliberately waited until the programme began and then rushed to operate the infernal machine. A local promoter had arranged a demonstration in the Elks Hall in which a radio with loudspeakers was on the stage and a broadcast from Edmonton was picked up and heard by those assembled. They had paid admission; me too. I shall never forget the chaos. The programme was nicely underway when it was suddenly halted by the screeches and howls of first-class static. People demanded their money back. I can see the promoter now, rushing down the aisle and blasting at the top of his voice "Dr Reid and his —, —, x, —, — x-ray." My father was Scottish and the practice of medicine was the practice of medicine, a great art. I don't think he ever really felt the fuss and language were justified. Radio would be with us always, it was only beginning, but Bill Miller wouldn't be and his foot had been crushed by a binder.

Mrs Chute continues, "This unit required the agility of an acrobat, the patience of Job, and the ability of an engineer to understand her foibles—that's right, he always referred to the x-ray as 'she.'"

Dr Morley Young reports that when he arrived at Lamont in 1922 Dr Archer already had an old Victor machine with some name such as Snook. It operated with a gas x-ray tube and used glass plates. A chest plate required a 25-second exposure. In 1923 this was traded for a Wappler machine, and by then film was being used. The current at Lamont was direct, so they made use of a rotary convertor losing about 25 per cent of their energy in the process. The first Wappler machine had a mechanical rectifier with a spark gap.

Acknowledgement:

This material was obtained by discussion or letter so is only as reliable as the memory of those who supplied it. There was no documentary material that I could find.

Editorial Acknowledgements:

This article is published posthumously with only minor editorial changes, although in an abbreviated form; it had been published in *Illuminator* when that newsletter was not included with the *Journal*. It was given in manuscript form to one of us (BCL) in 1974 by Dr Parsons and is used here with the permission of the estate of Dr Parsons. He had himself contributed immensely to the development of radiology in Alberta, in general, and in central Alberta, where he practiced in Red Deer, in particular. The photograph of Dr Parsons, obtained with some difficulty, has been contributed to the archives by Dr John Radomsky.

SIR WILLIAM OSLER AND EXPERIMENTAL RADIOLOGY

A physician treats the disease but a good physician treats the patient.

— Osler

At the eleventh Annual Meeting of the Association of American Physicians held in Washington, DC on April 30th, May 1st and 2nd 1896 it is recorded [1] that Dr Osler took some gallstones both in his hand and rolled up in a beefsteak and made radiographs. The stones were not visible on the image.

[Sir William was unfortunate in his choice of stones because we now know that a minority containing calcium are indeed radio-opaque.]

1. Williams FH. The 'x'-ray in medicine. Med Rec NY 1896;49:665. [Osler's comments are included in the discussion which also includes reference to experiments by Dr George Sternberg in which he reported that bacilli grew in culture while exposed to "the 'x' ray" as freely as those not so exposed: all this within months of Röntgen's original report.]

Sir William Osler graduated from McGill University in 1872. He has been described as "the most influential physician since Hippocrates". He was one of the first ten inductees into the Canadian Medical Hall of Fame in 1994. At that time the selection committee noted that he had achieved eminence as a clinician, researcher and teacher, and that he "drew many traditions together to alter traditional approaches to medicine". Osler worked in Montreal and Baltimore (Johns Hopkins) and was then Regius Professor of Medicine at the University of Oxford, England before his death in 1919[1]

1. OReilly M. Canada's new Medical Hall of Fame pays homage to medicine's giants. Canad Med Ass J 1994;150:2022-2023.

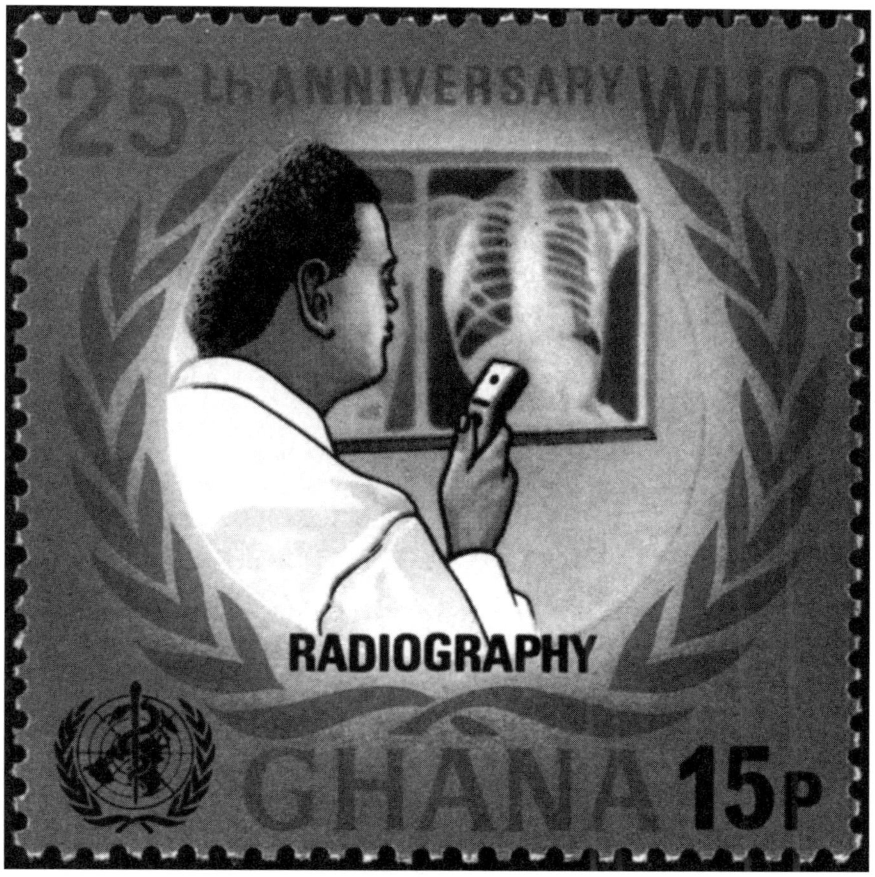
25th ANNIVERSARY W.H.O
RADIOGRAPHY
GHANA 15p

Chapter XIII •

The New Tesla Machine

Makes the Patient Transparent at the City Hospital

The Vancouver Province, December 29th, 1900.

A blinding flash of violet coloured flames leaped from one to another of the little brass knobs on the top of a box about 16 inches square by two feet long. The shrill scream of the interrupter reminded one of the cry of a savage animal.

Deadly? A thousand deaths leaped and sported in the arc spanned by the rays of light. It takes 250,000 volts of electricity to develop the spark in the new x-ray machine which was yesterday installed in the City Hospital by Mr R Hutchison, the Victoria expert. It is a Tesla "high-frequency" apparatus built by the LE Knott Company of Boston.

By the aid of the fluoroscope and this machine the interior anatomy of the patient can be examined in a leisurely manner by the physician and should anything be found wrong a photograph will render the details more definite. Foreign substances in the body need no longer be probed for or sought more or less hap-hazard [sic] with the knife. Obscure fractures can be studied in the most complete manner, and treated in a far more intelligent manner than would be possible under any other method.

Mr Hutchison toyed with his little pet, which spluttered and hissed like a thing of life.

"We take the ordinary house current," said the expert, "with a voltage of 110 and after passing it through a rheostat it goes to the step-up transformer, which raises it to 10,000 volts, thence it passes through what is known as the Nicola Tesla oil coil. This gives a perfect insulation, and by the time the current reaches the sparking point an intensity of 250,000 or more volts has been developed."

When one looked at the four or five inch steady stream of blue fire

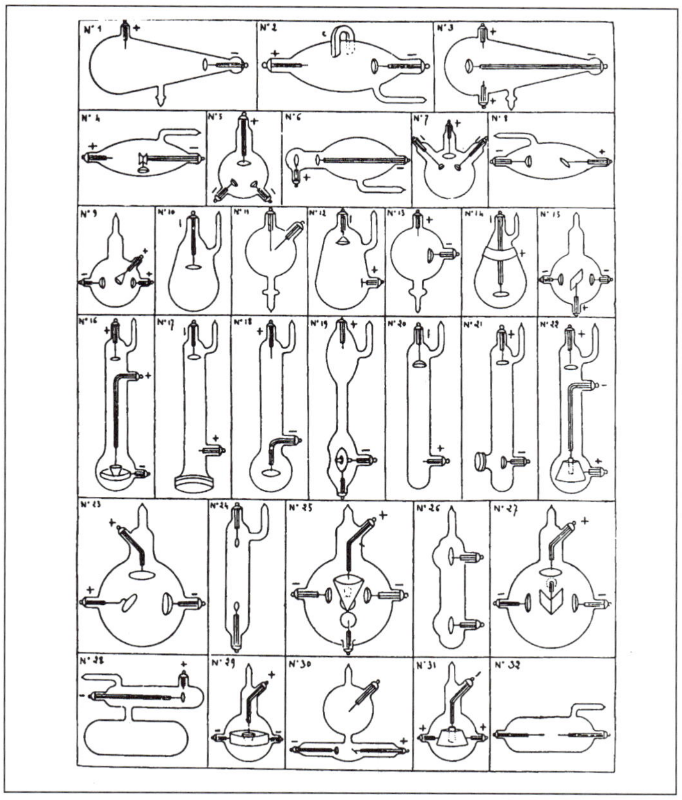

Left
Gas tubes

Acknowledgement:
This extract from *The Vancouver Province* is published with permission.

which zigzagged from one of the points to the other, there was no difficulty in believing the statements of Mr Hutchison about the voltage.

"You may not know it," he continued, "but in fact you are stealing my electricity at the present time."

The Province man felt in all his pockets and finding nothing was about to make an indignant denial when the man of sparks placed a pair of pincers in the "patient's" hand.

"Now point that at the brass rod on the top of the Machine."

A spark nearly two inches long was the result.

"Do you know that there is now passing through your body some 75,000 volts?"

The writer remembered that it only required from 1,500 to 2,000 volts to effect the electrocution of murderers at Sing-Sing, and even allowing for the extra toughness of reporters, the 75,000 volts seemed a little high.

"It is the high frequency developed by the interrupter which renders such a voltage safe," said Mr Hutchison. The explanation was so clear that it removed at once all feelings of uneasiness.

A Crookes' x-ray tube was then attached to the machine, and the expert handed the reporter a pyramid shaped box, about ten inches square on the base, and with a curved opening at the small end. This opening was found to shut off all light except that received through the screen at the other end. This is called the fluoroscope, by the aid of which it is possible to look through the body or limbs.

When the hand is placed between the screen and the tube the flesh appears like a faint grey shadow and the bones stand out in startling distinctness. Every joint can be clearly seen, a fracture instantly located, and any foreign substance detected without the slightest difficulty.

A coin tightly grasped in the hand can be clearly seen and the denomination made out. When the fluoroscope is turned on the face and head of a patient, the effect is ghastly in the extreme. Only a dim outline of the face appears, and in dark relief the grinning skull stares through the screen.

The immense advantage of such an instrument in the hand of the surgeon can scarcely be over-estimated.

The usual x-ray photographs are produced by exposing the sensitive plates to the rays from the Crookes' tube, after they have passed through the portion of the anatomy under treatment. These plates are then developed in the ordinary manner.

The complete plant as installed by Mr Hutchison will cost the city $375, and will form a most valuable addition to the equipment of the hospital.

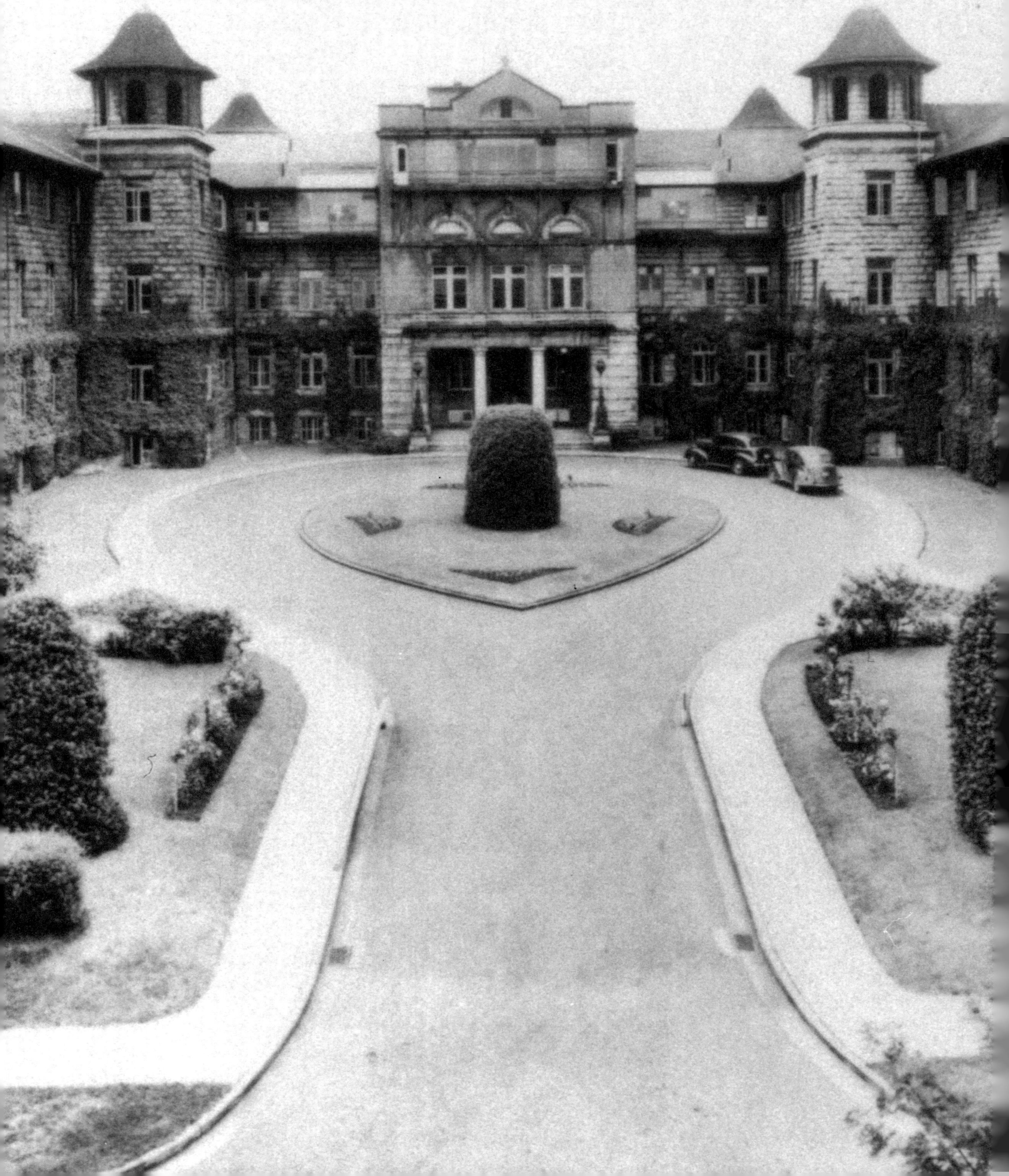

Chapter XIV • Radiology at

Vancouver Hospital

and Health Sciences Centre

Elwood Wylie and Brian Lentle

BEGINNINGS

On June 6, 1900 the medical staff at the Vancouver City Hospital passed a resolution reminding the city's Board of Health of the "urgent necessity of procuring an x-ray apparatus for the use of the Hospital." Its cost was estimated to be $300.00, and the secretary was instructed to write to manufacturers for information. The Vancouver Hospital had begun life as the City Hospital, becoming the General Hospital before receiving its present name in 1994.

On July 23, 1900 a *Tesla* high-frequency machine was purchased from a Mr R Hutchison of Victoria. In December of that year the machine was installed, and the first radiograph made was of the hand of the matron, Ms Clendenning. The actual cost of the machine was $375.00.

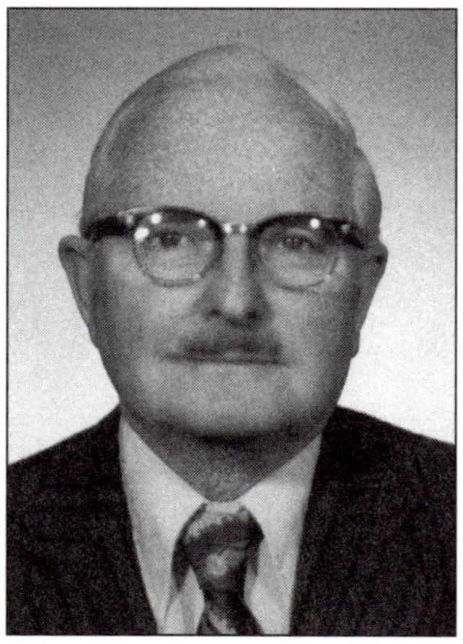

Dr RW Boyd

Left
Heather Pavilion, Vancouver General Hospital

In April 1902 the Vancouver *Daily World* reported the radiation treatment of a sarcoma of the jaw by Dr Alfred Poole of the City Hospital. The minutes of the Board of Trustees subsequently record that a new x-ray machine was donated to the hospital in September 1906 by Mr AC Flumerfelt. Later that month the medical staff discussed the appointment of one of its members to be in charge of the x-ray service. It then recommended to the board that the hospital pharmacist be given full charge of the machine and its maintenance. His services were to be available whenever the use of x-rays was required. The board was asked to send a letter to physicians in the city indicating the need for an x-ray and electrical specialist.

Subsequently, a search committee of Drs Brydon-Jack and Weld was formed to look for a family physician to take charge of the service. Some interest was shown by Dr Alison Cumming, but Dr HH McIntosh was appointed. He expressed a willingness to travel for study and presented his ideas about a scale of fees. Dr McIntosh had been appointed superintendant of the hospital in 1907, and the board minutes indicate that he resigned in May 1909, presumably to pursue x-ray studies. By August of that year Dr McIntosh was back and was appointed skiagrapher to the hospital, a position he held until he left for military service in France in 1914 or 1915. In the previous year he had been given "membership of the hospital's medical staff" which must have meant something different from being given admitting privileges.

Dr WA Whitelaw had served as superintendent from 1909 to 1913. He took charge of the x-ray service during Dr McIntosh's absence and submitted a list of revised charges, which prompted a survey of fees in other hospitals in Canada. The medical staff sent a petition to the board recommending adoption of the suggested fee revisions and advocating larger and better quarters than those they had then in the basement. The 1916 annual report indicates that the department was removed to the southwest wing, although it remained in the basement. The issue of larger and better quarters was to remain fundamentally unresolved for 80 years.

In 1919 Dr McIntosh returned from war service to resume his former position, which he held until his resignation on December 31, 1930.

The first full-time chief of radiology at the Vancouver General Hospital (VGH) was Dr Bede Harrison, whose grandson, Dr Philip Harrison, is a radiologist at St Paul's Hospital in Vancouver. Dr Bede Harrison whose life is briefly described elsewhere in this volume,[1] served as President of the British Columbia Association of Radiologist and authored one of the the first textbooks of radiology by a Canadian, in 1936.

THE BOYD ERA

Dr RW Boyd was appointed director of the department in 1946 and also served as Director of Residency Education. The program of that era graduated such radiologists as Drs Don Longley, Jim Knickerbocker and Nigel Clark. Dr Knickerbocker would later become the head of the Department at University Hospital and a president of the Canadian Association of Radiologists. Dr Nestor Müller, when he had become an internationally recognized chest radiologist, was to tell one of us, as Dr Clark's retirement approached, that he occasionally still asked Dr Clark for an opinion about a chest film.

By 1965 there were sections of pediatric radiology (chief, Dr Betty Wood) and neuroradiology (chief, Dr Gordon Trueman), but specialization was not then the norm. Apart from Drs Wood and Trueman all the radiologists rotated through the department. Radiological services were also spread over many of the hospital pavilions—a situation which persisted until the building of the "tower" in the eighties and its occupancy in the late nineties.

One of us (EW) was appointed to the Department in January 1965 and writes, "I was shocked at the status of the equipment...it was not as up to date as [that] I had left in Saskatoon." All of the equipment had been manufactured by General Electric, and manual bucky cocking devices were still in use.

Dr David Garrow was the first angiographer, and he designed a chair for pneumoencephalography. He left the hospital in 1991 and has since written a very personal account of his life and the evolution of radiology at the hospital.[2]

By the mid-sixties there were only two automatic film processors. At that time, with no government-sponsored medical care, the hospital was divided into beds for those who paid privately and beds for"staff patients," who were uninsured or on welfare, and who were the subjects of much of the teaching activity.

In 1968 the Division of Nuclear Medicine was created under the directorship of Dr RT Morrison. It occupied space in Heather Pavilion vacated by radiation oncology, which had separated from the department with the creation of the BC Cancer Agency.

TECHNOLOGY EDUCATION

The British Columbia Association of Medical Radiation Technologists (BCAMRT) was created, largely at the initiative of Mr William Stirling, in 1942. It was then known as the BC Society for X-ray Technicians.

The School of Radiography at Vancouver Hospital was started in 1936 and the 50th anniversary was duly celebrated in 1986. By 1964 the model for technology education had come to require collaboration with a community college and in June of that year the last class of technologists to be fully trained in hospital was enrolled. In August of the same year the first class to be jointly trained at the British Columbia Institute of Technology (BCIT) and the hospital was enrolled.

At first the program leading to certification was 27 months long comprising five months of academic instruction at BCIT and 22 months at the hospital. In 1967 this was changed to a three year course of instruction, two years of which were spent at BCIT. From 1989 to the present, formal technology education has extended over 27 months with the BCIT component reduced to 15 months. Ms Phyllis Wasylyshyn has served as the Clinical Instructor for the past six years at the Vancouver Hospital.

In 1968 a technology education program in nuclear medicine was initiated at the British Columbia Institute of Technology (BCIT) with Ms Brenda Clarke as program head. The first students graduated in 1970. At that time the students spent their first year at BCIT and in the second year alternated between a week at the Institute and a week at a hospital with the summer off. Now the students work right through that year.

In 1973 Ms Joan Miki joined Brenda Clarke as laboratory supervisor and in 1979 Mr Randy Singer became clinical supervisor, later replacing Ms Clarke.

THE DUNBAR ERA

After 25 years of service as director of radiology, Dr Boyd retired in 1971, and in that year Dr Scott Dunbar was appointed to the first joint headship of a hospital department (in this case at the VGH) and the Department of Radiology at the University of British Columbia. In 1972 the first equipment for special procedures (angiography etc.) was installed. Dr Dunbar came, having had a distinguished career in radiology in Montréal, and after having served as editor of the *Canadian Association of Radiologists' Journal.*

At the instigation of Dr Dunbar, the first computed tomography scanner, manufactured by EMI (Electrical and Musical Industries of the UK), was purchased in 1974 and finally installed in 1976. Also in 1974, the Division of Nuclear Medicine separated from the Department of Radiology, becoming a Division of the Department of Pathology. This was prompted by irreconcilable differences between Drs Dunbar and Morrison. In the same year a seminar room and teaching facility was created to be named after Dr Dunbar when he left in the fall of the same year. Dr Gordon Trueman became acting-director and subsequently kept an active interest in the department, attending some of its social functions and endowing a prize for resident research.

Dr Dunbar had brought a distinctive leadership style and was greatly respected. He started the Department down a more intensive academic path which was to come to even greater fruition under Dr Joachim Burhenne.

In 1975 Dr Peter Cooperberg became section head of Ultrasonography and was to raise his section to international prominence before becoming Head of the Department of Radiology at St Paul's Hospital in 1987.

THE BURHENNE ERA

In 1978 Dr Joachim Burhenne was appointed as head of the department as well as head of radiology at the University of British Columbia. He was to fashion the department much as it exists towards the end of the 20th century, short of its final coming together as a cohesive unit in the once-and-never tower. This tower was built to house a redevelopment of much of the hospital including the Department of Radiology. The shell of this structure had been built in the early eighties, only to stand empty through no fault of Dr Burhenne, because of political change, lack of money and administrative uncertainties, until the late 1990s. A planning committee was established in 1980 to design the Department to be built in the tower. None of its members were in active practice at the hospital as the tower approached completion some twenty years later. It is, however, a Vancouver landmark.

In 1978 a General Electric computed tomographic (CT) scanner with a body sized aperture had been installed. By 1979 plans were underway to establish a Division of Neuroradiology, of which Dr Bill Robertson was to be the first head. In 1980 an arsonist, perhaps driven to desperation by the ageing facilities, set fire to the film library. Those film files not burned were destroyed by water used in extinguishing the conflagration. Not satisfied, the arsonist attempted an encore two weeks later and was sufficiently unsophisticated to leave the fuel can behind. He or she has never been caught.

In 1982, with the opening of the BC Children's Hospital, the pediatric section moved. Dr Newman was to become the head of this department and associate head of the university department, both of which he was to serve with exemplary loyalty and devotion for more than the next decade.

A second CT scanner was installed in 1982, replacing the now-obsolescent EMI unit. A management information system then installed proved to be a failure and was replaced by the ADAC Mars system and its software.

With high academic standards and an international perspective, Dr Burhenne shaped the department much as it was to remain for two decades. Dr Burhenne had a great interest in the newly developing interventional radiology. A renowned radiologist in his own right he brought fame and prestige to the hospital and university when asked to fly to New York and extract a retained common-duct gallstone from the deposed Shah of Persia (Iran) using a device he had designed.[3] This was done by a radiological method that avoided open surgery. In keeping with this thrust a lithotripter was installed in late 1985 to treat kidney stones non-invasively (i.e., without requiring surgery) using a focused beam of ultrasound waves.

After the precipitous departure of Dr Morrison the nuclear medicine service was repatriated into the department in 1986 by virtue of the foresight of Dr David Hardwick, then Head of Pathology, and Dr Burhenne. In 1986 one of us (BL) was recruited to head this division and to create a residency education program in nuclear medicine. The department then had two university-affiliated residency educational programs, in radiology (Program Director, Dr Douglas Graeb) and nuclear medicine. A program in bone densitometry was developed jointly by the nuclear medicine physicians and radiologists.

A building was begun in 1988 to house a newly purchased magnetic resonance imaging (MRI) machine. The first magnet was faulty, and a second one was installed by the end of January 1989. Meanwhile the government again announced that funding was to be made available to finish the tower. A new committee was struck to plan the department, and five of its eight members were still members of the department six years later, although occupancy of the podium level in the tower was still several years in the future. The MRI system did not come into clinical use until November 1989 because of a province-wide dispute over the payment of professional fees.

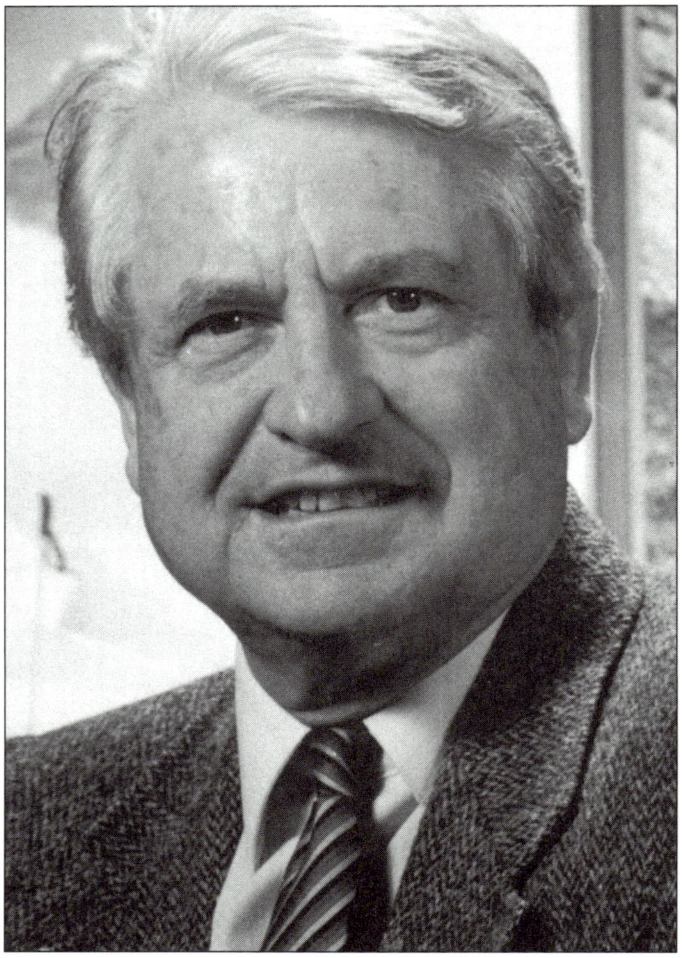

Dr H Joachim Burhenne

RECENT TIMES

Dr Burhenne stepped down from the headship at the end of 1990, providing an opportunity for family, residents, former colleagues such as Dr Alex Margulis, members of the department, the faculty and hospital administration to celebrate his many contributions to radiology, to the university and the hospital. One of us (BL) was appointed to succeed him on February 1, 1991. Dr Nestor Muller, who had been acting-head, became associate head; he gave the Radiological Society of North America Annual Oration later in that year.

In 1991 another committee was struck to plan the tower. Meanwhile Mr Ron Wood was recruited from Winnipeg to serve as Administrative Director succeeding one of us (EW).

In 1993 the University Hospital on campus, after flirting with the Shaughnessy Hospital, consummated a union with the Vancouver General Hospital. To save money Shaughnessy Hospital had been precipitously closed. The new corporate entity became the Vancouver Hospital and Health Sciences Centre. Work on the tower continued...slowly.

Editorial acknowledgement:

After 25 years of immense service to the hospital, Mr Elwood Wylie retired in 1992. He had lectured at the 25-Year-Long Service Dinner in 1991 on the history of the department.

Chapter XV • St Paul's Hospital

ANON

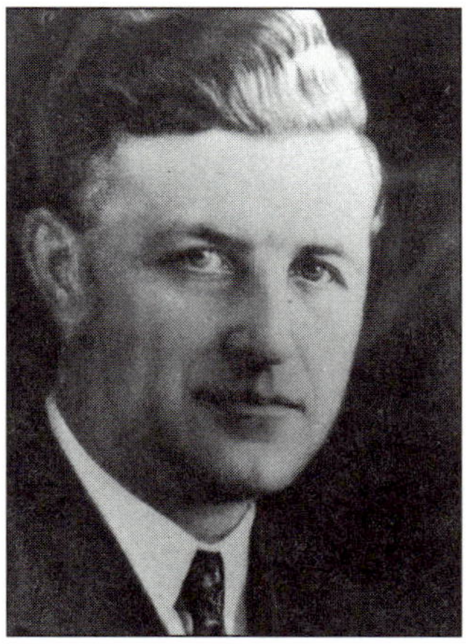

Dr CW Prowd

In 1906 when St Paul's Hospital radiology department opened, it included in its equipment a small, coil-type machine. Although very up to date at the time, this machine could record extremities only on primitive glass negatives, and that with great difficulty as exposures took from 15 to 35 minutes, and there was the ever-present danger of burning the patient or giving the operator a shock because of uninsulated wiring. Dr DeVerteuil of Edinburgh, one of the first clinicians in British Columbia to become interested in x-ray therapy, had charge of the operation of this machine. He was succeeded by Dr George V Lockett, a graduate who brought his own machine from England, and who was very much interested in the physics of the new rays. On his retirement the department was closed until 1912 when it moved to the new building erected in that year. Dr GE Richards, later professor of radiology at the University of Toronto and radiologist-in-chief of Toronto General Hospital, and Dr CW Prowd, later the head of the department, supervised.

In 1920 St Paul's was the first hospital in Vancouver to have a supply of radium. The department was, after 1933, under the management of Sister Charles Spinola. In 1937 Dr Fred Bonnell of Kingston was added to the staff as assistant radiologist. Dr CG Campbell of Dalhousie replaced him when Dr Bonnell enlisted for overseas service in World War II. Dr Campbell came to Vancouver after postgraduate studies in Boston and Kingston.

With the increasing demands on the radiology department a move to a new location in the north wing, erected in 1931, was very necessary. Built exclusively for the use of x-rays and radium, the department came to offer full protection for both patient and operator and was equipped with the most modern machines. These included a serialograph fluoroscopic machine, the first of its type in the Pacific Northwest.

Subsequent chiefs of the Department included Dr Richard Pitman and Dr Peter Cooperberg.

Acknowledgement:
This account was found in the archives of CAR along with the terms of the contract between Dr Prowd and the hospital. The account is of uncertain provenance.

"The major figure in nonsurgical stone extraction was H Joachim Burhenne of Canada, who developed a remote-controlled catheter through which extraction baskets of several sizes could be introduced (1). Using this technique, Burhenne has succeeded in removing 95% of retained calculi under fluoroscopic control."

---

1. Burhenne HJ. Nonoperative retained biliary stone extraction: a new roentgenologic technique. *Am J Roentgenol* 1973;117:388.

Eisenberg RL. *Radiology. An illustrated history.* St Louis: Mosby Year Book, , 1992:301

Heretofore, radiology was a record of still-life and usually illustrated various pathological states. Physiologic abnormalities could only be inferred. With the newer techniques, altered physiology can be recorded and studied at leisure.

R Brian Holmes *Canad Med Ass J* 1968; 99: 1159.

Right
Radiation oncology in BC former buildings of cancer clinics

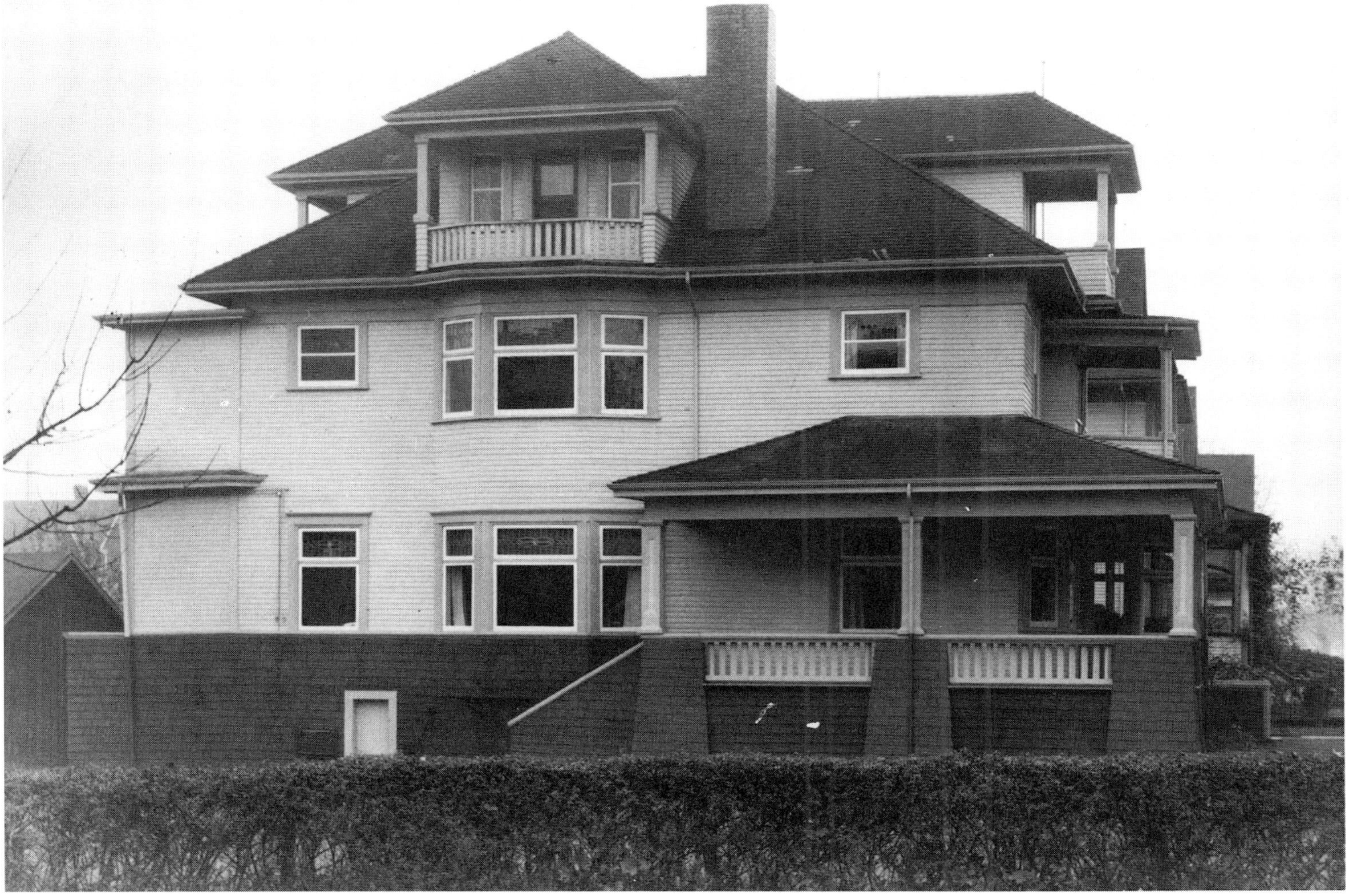

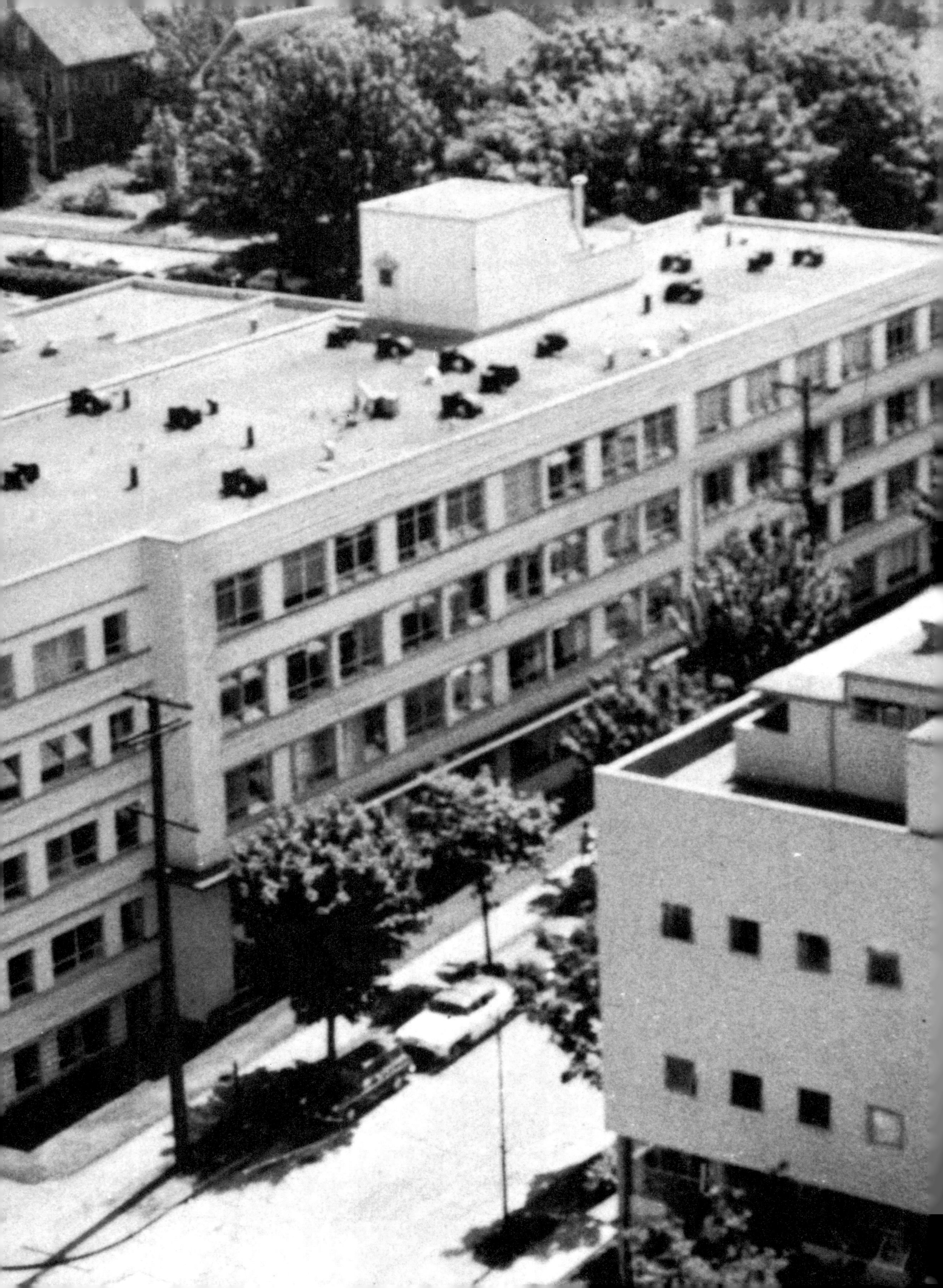

Chapter XVI • *The Evolution and Development of*

Radiation Oncology in BC

George Goodman

INTRODUCTION

The first radiation therapy in BC was practiced by general radiologists, a few of whom continued dual practice into the 1950s. However, this gradually ceased with the growth of organized cancer centres and the splitting of radiology into subsections of diagnosis and therapy for specialist certification. The name of the specialty was changed to radiation oncology with the approval of the Royal College of Physicians and Surgeons of Canada in 1976. The new name emphasized that the specialty was cancer focused and, while de-emphasizing its technological orientation, linked it to its traditional roots in radiology.

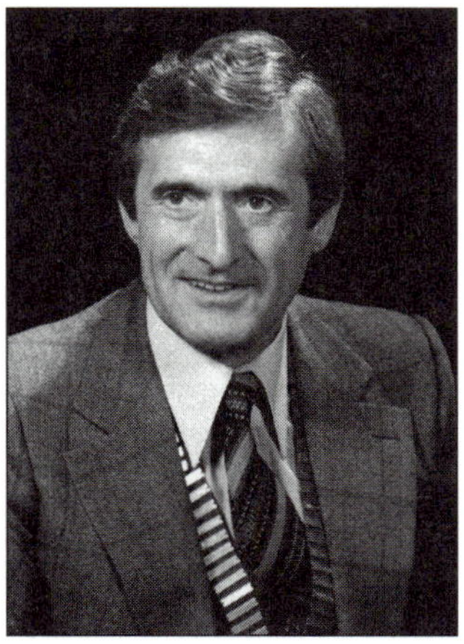

Dr George Goodman, author and former president of the Canadian Association of Radiologists

Left
Former buildings of cancer clinics in BC

EARLY RADIATION THERAPY IN BC

The first report in BC of the use of radiation in cancer treatment was by Dr CW Prowd, Head of Radiology at St Paul's Hospital, Vancouver. He published an "Analysis of Radium Treatments in 600 cases in the period 1921–1926." Of the patients he reported 84 per cent had malignant disease, and a wide spectrum of tumour sites was treated. A majority of patients had epitheliomata of skin (147), lip (72), mouth (84) and the uterine cervix (93). Survival benefits were immediately obvious. In the same era, Drs HH McIntosh and WA Whitelaw, radiologists at Vancouver General Hospital, (VGH) used 140-KV x-ray therapy to treat enlargement of the thymus gland in infants, as well as other types of benign disease. It was Dr Bede J Harrison, a radiologist from Melbourne, Australia who introduced "deep x-ray therapy (200–400 KV x-rays)" to the city. He was appointed Head of Radiology at VGH in 1931. Rumour had it that appreciable radiation doses could be measured outside VGH on Heather Street next to the unit.

Dr Ethelyn Trapp was BC's first radiation oncologist. After graduation from McGill in 1927, she travelled extensively in Europe and the United States studying radiation therapy. Later, she worked with Dr Prowd at St Paul's Hospital. She spent a large part of her considerable personal fortune developing a private radiation treatment centre in Vancouver, which opened in 1937. During the war years she functioned as Acting Director, BC Cancer Institute until the return of Dr Evans in 1945.

It is also noteworthy that Dr HH Murphy, Head of Radiology, Royal Jubilee Hospital, Victoria from 1931, was appointed as the first Director of the Victoria Cancer Clinic under the BC Cancer Foundation. The renowned Dr Gordon E Richards of Toronto started his medical career in BC. After graduating in medicine (MB) from the University of Toronto in 1908, he was entered in the BC medical register as resident in 1909 at Port Simpson, later at Stewart and finally in Vancouver. He relocated to Toronto about 1920.

THE DEVELOPMENT OF ORGANIZED CANCER TREATMENT SERVICES (CANCER CENTRES) IN BC

In 1931 the British Columbia Medical Association formed a cancer committee to address the diagnostic and therapeutic needs of cancer patients in the province. The BC Cancer Foundation was formed in 1935 and raised monies to purchase radium and x-ray equipment. In 1938 it established the BC Cancer Institute (BCCI) to provide a central radiation treatment centre for cancer patients in the province.

Dr AM Evans was appointed director, a staff of full-time radiation therapy specialists was recruited, Dr HF Batho was appointed as head physicist. Services were available to all citizens upon referral by private physicians, and patients were expected to pay if able to do so. The BC Division of the Canadian Cancer Society (also founded in 1938) in addition to its primary commitments to research and education, assisted needy patients with transportation costs to Vancouver and accommodation in the city.

In the early 1940s a 14-bed boarding home was built adjacent to the BCCI to house some out-of-town patients during their treatment. Simultaneously, an extensive Consultative Clinic (Outreach) Program was inaugurated, including the Okanagan and Kamloops clinics, Prince George, Prince Rupert, Dawson Creek, Nanaimo, Chilliwack and the Kootenay clinics including Cranbrook. These clinics were held in public health facilities or in local hospitals, and new and already treated patients were seen. In addition, the foundation opened a diagnostic clinic in Victoria at the Royal Jubilee Hospital in 1948. This clinic was expanded to a radition treatment unit about 1950, with the appointment of Dr Lockyer (radiation oncologist) as director.

External consultants Ralston Paterson, Simon Cantril and OH Warwick proffered advice about future expansion of cancer services. Federal health grants were introduced in 1948 and the BC Government requested an expanded program for the diagnosis and treatment of cancer in the province. As a result, it was recommended that the BC Cancer Foundation be made the agent of the BC Provincial Health Branch for the care of cancer patients in the province. Other recommendations included professional and lay education; free diagnostic biopsy services; co-ordination of records and follow-up of all centres interested in the diagnosis and treatment of cancer, under the direction of the Division of Vital Statistics. This plan was approved by the federal Department of Health and Welfare.

The University of British Columbia medical school was established in 1950. The Vancouver General Hospital (VGH) served as the parent teaching hospital. BCCI was physically linked to VGH by a tunnel under Heather Street, and 30 beds within VGH were allocated for patients attending BCCI. This close association fostered the development of excellent multi-disciplinary clinics for patient management, the development of conjoint treatment policies and the inauguration and support of the cytology services, initially for cervix cancer screening and later for cancer cytology at other sites.

From 1952 onward there was a continuing redesign and expansion of physical and treatment resources at the BCCI. A cobalt-60 teletherapy unit (the third to be installed in Canada) was acquired in 1952. Assisting with its installation was a young physicist, Raymond Bush, who would later study medicine and become Director of Princess Margaret Hospital in Toronto. Boarding home beds were increased to 36 in 1955 by constructing a second floor, and a third floor was added in 1965, making a total of 54 beds. At this time BCCI was designated a hospital facility by the Hospital Insurance Service, providing hospital insurance coverage to inpatients. In 1966 hospital benefits were extended to cover outpatient radiotherapy and chemotherapy at BCCI as well as at the Victoria Clinic.

In 1970 the BC Cancer Treatment and Research Foundation operated the BCCI and its adjoining hospital, the Victoria Cancer Clinic, and 15 consultative clinics throughout the province. In 1969 the Department of Health Services and Hospital Insurance appointed a review committee, chaired by Dr D Williams, to study cancer care and control. It recommended establishing a comprehensive, coordinated, province-wide cancer control program with the services to prevent, detect and treat all forms of cancer. In 1972 the New Democratic Party came to power with "a new vision of social justice and large increases for consumption programs." Shortly thereafter, in October 1974, the BCCI was transferred back to the provincial government by the BC Cancer Treatment and Research Foundation, and the institute property was leased for a nominal sum to the Cancer Control Agency of BC (CCABC). The agency was a non-profit society created to carry out the expanded province-wide program of cancer care and control. The agency board managed the BCCI (Vancouver) and its Victoria Clinic and appointed Dr T Hall (medical oncologist) as director in 1976. He was later replaced by Dr D Boyes.

With vastly increased financial resources promised in late 1974, planning for a new Vancouver Clinic proceeded. Initially intended to be constructed at Shaughnessy Hospital, changed circumstances eventually located it at the old BCCI site. Subsequently, the Vancouver hospital was named the A Maxwell Evans Building. A cancer clinic for the BC interior was started at Royal Inland Hospital, Kamloops to provide regional chemotherapy services and to ensure close cooperation between medical oncologists in the Okanagan region and the central Vancouver facility. This plan has been abandoned for a future cancer centre in Kelowna. The CCABC opened a new treatment facility in Victoria in 1986. The BC Cancer Agency (formerly CCABC) will soon provide a new cancer treatment facility in Surrey in 1995. Apart from these new physical resource developments, the agency has expanded chemotherapy and drug services, initiated a bone marrow transplant program and developed active applied research programs in biophysics, pharmacokinetics, endocrinology and immunology.

As a result of these changes, the BC Cancer Foundation has assumed responsibility for support of applied research programs and basic science workers and created the BC Cancer Research Centre, juxtaposed to the Vancouver treatment facility. At the same time, the Canadian Cancer Society (BC Division) constructed high-quality, low-cost hostel accommodation in Vancouver and Victoria for patients undergoing treatment at these centres.

RADIATION TREATMENT SERVICES

As stated, Evans centralized radiation treatment services in facilities in Vancouver (BCCI) and Victoria and provided extensive outreach programs.

An ex-army colleague, Ms Dorothy Findlay, became Head of Nursing at BCCI. With a coterie of registered nurses (formerly of the Canadian Army Nursing Corps), she assumed responsibility for nursing care of patients in the boarding home and the outpatient department, and she operated the treatment machines. Together, Dr Evans and Ms Findlay established a strong training school for radiation therapy nurse technicians. Financial support for nurses in training was provided by the Canadian Cancer Society (BC Division).

Dr HF Batho, who was later joined by Margaret Young, developed an excellent department of clinical physics. Both enjoyed international reputations and provided valuable advice concerning the development of facilities, choices of treatment equipment and treatment planning systems. Today, the pi-meson treatment facility at TRIUMF is named in honour of HF Batho for his role in the development of the particle therapy program in Vancouver. Batho, an extremely modest, retiring man, was a superb teacher, and his physics notes were widely sought after throughout Canada by technicians and residents in training. Upon his retirement he was succeeded by Dr RO Kornelsen, a worthy successor, who continued to make significant contributions to the TRIUMF program and the practice of medical physics in Vancouver and Victoria and across Canada.

The initial medical staff at BCCI (R Moffat, R Nash and M Hardie) had moved elsewhere or retired by about 1960. Trained specialists in radiation oncology from the United Kingdom and a few Canadians sent there for training replaced them and modern treatment equipment was provided. Evans developed a record system which permitted him to analyse treatment results. His publication "British Columbia Cancer Institute Treatment Results 1946–1954 and Policy 1961" received wide international acclaim. Late in the 1960s, when better drugs became available, he expanded the scope of the cancer chemotherapy service under Dr DM Whitelaw. He also accommodated Dr HK Fidler, his cytology screening staff and the screening program in the BCCI. Evans unquestionably laid the foundations for today's cancer services in BC. He was succeeded by Dr JM Gibson in 1971.

Over the years steady improvements have continued to be made in radiotherapy. The Vancouver centre, under Dr S Jackson, head since 1976, is an extremely strong department with excellent staff and a large resident training program. Present therapy equipment includes seven linear accelerators with x-ray energies in the range of 4–25 MeV, with some also providing electron beams; two kilocurie cobalt units; the first low-dose Selectron and MicroSelectron afterloading units in Canada; two simulators; and one orthovoltage and one superficial x-ray unit. In addition, 3-D treatment planning is also available. In 1958, by contrast, equipment consisted of one Eldorado cobalt unit, two orthovoltage units, one superficial unit and one gram of radium.

Today, there are 22 staff radiation oncologists in Vancouver and five in Victoria. For comparison, in 1958 there were (including the director) five radiation oncologists in Vancouver and one in Victoria. There is no doubt that improved radiation treatment exists today in BC, and all the radiation oncology staff have played a part.

MAJOR CONTRIBUTIONS TO RADIATION ONCOLOGY IN VANCOUVER

Charged Particle Radiotherapy[1]

We were fortunate in Vancouver that the world's largest cyclotron was installed at the University of British Columbia at the Tri-Universities Meson Facility (TRIUMF) in 1969, for nuclear physics research. This instrument was used to produce negatively charged pi-meson particles (pions) considered to be of possible value in radiotherapy. Because of their unique properties, such particles could be stopped in tumour tissue where they caused "millions of mini-atomic explosions." The dose could be selectively concentrated in the tumour and its effect was enhanced because the radiation was densely ionizing and more locally destructive than conventional radiation. It seemed possible that this new radiation might increase the local cure rate for tumours, whereas failure to cure still occurred in about one-third of patients treated with conventional radiotherapy. A major research program was started, and it was high profile because only two other such facilities in the world existed or were being developed (at Los Alamos, USA and Villigen, Switzerland).

Dr L Skarsgard, biophysics, was recruited to develop the preclinical program—including beam line construction—and the conduct of dosimetry measurements, both physical and biological (*in vitro* and *in vivo*). Dr BG Douglas, a young radiation oncologist, was much involved in the *in vivo* work. The first human patient, with cancer nodules which had spread to skin was treated in 1979. All of Skarsgard's preliminary work indicated that pi-meson therapy was more effective than conventional radiation in achieving a given biological effect (and this eventually led to innovative approaches to multi-fraction treatment with conventional radiation therapy).

Clinical studies of deep-seated tumours of the brain and pelvis began in 1982 under the direction of Dr GB Goodman. Because of the fixed, horizontal pion-beam-line, it was necessary to develop a beam-scanning system consisting of a treatment couch for lateral scanning of the patient relative to the beam and a range shifter. The treatment couch was designed and built at TRIUMF at a cost of $140 000. Techniques for patient immobilization were developed together with a 3-D treatment planning system. A series of studies was undertaken to determine optimum dose and to select tumour sites for prospective comparative trials of pions and photons. Randomized trials were begun in 1989 for high grade (grade 3 and 4) astrocytomas and for prostate cancer stages C and D in 1990. These are the only trials of their kind in the world and should be concluded in 1995.

Efforts to expand the Charged Particle Radiotherapy Program to include proton beams began in 1984. In 1994 the first proton facility in Canada became available for eye tumour treatments at TRIUMF.

Cancer Screening Programs

The approaches available in BC for screening are cervical cytology for cervix cancer and mammography, physical examination and breast self-examination for breast cancer.

The cervix cytology screening service in BC has achieved a model for excellence and is internationally renowned. Dr D Boyes, a radiation oncologist and gynecologist, ably continued to develop and expand this program. Today, this method has been widely credited with making a major contribution to the reduction in mortality from uterine cancer.

Another radiation oncologist, Dr V Basco, has been largely responsible for the development of a mammography screening program in BC for the early detection of breast cancer. Nowhere in Canada is screening mammography as well developed as it is in BC.

CANADIAN SOCIETY OF RADIOLOGICAL TECHNICIANS

In 1895 William Roentgen discovered the mysterious form of radiant energy which he called the X-ray. Over the next twenty-five years tremendous accomplishments were made in adapting this energy for medical purposes. The hot-cathode vacuum tube and the nitrate-base X-ray film were two key developments which facilitated the widespread use of X-ray equipment in hospitals by 1920.

The first technicians were trained to handle films and care for equipment in military hospitals during the first world war. In the early 1920s the Radiological Society of North America and the American Roentgen Ray Society set up a registry for X-ray technicians. Many Canadian were registered by this American Registry of Radiological Technicians. There was no Canadian Association before 1929, when the Western Society of Radiographers9 was organized in Winnipeg. The Ontario Society of Radiographers, formed in 1935, took steps in the late 1930s to bring about the formation of associations for X-ray technicians in the other provinces (except for Manitoba where one already existed) as a preliminary step to a national federation. In 1942 the provincial societies in co-operation with the Canadian Association of Radiologists formed the Canadian Society of Radiological Technicians. At the end of 1943 active membership was 386. Claude J.Bodle of Winnipeg was the first president.

The prime function of the society has been to improve the qualifications of technicians by holding registration examinations for graduates of approved two-year courses in radiologic technique. Curriculum standards were set up and after extensive negotiation with the Canadian Medical Association and the Canadian Association of Radiology, a joint committee on technical training was established in 1959.

The society's excellent journal *Focal Spot*, originally founded as the *Ontario Radiographer* in 1939, became the national publication four years later."[1]

---

1. Agnew GH. *Canadian hospitals, 1920 - 1970: A dramatic half-century*. Toronto:University of Toronto Press, 1974.

SHOE FITTING

"Three viewings should be adequate to select a pair of shoes, and four pairs of shoes is a generous yearly average. On this basis it is possible to recommend that the number of viewings be limited to three in one day, or twelve a year.

"Only authorized sales persons should operate the machines. To make it difficult for others to do so, the starting mechanism should be fairly complex.

"Shoes must be worn on both feet during a fitting."[1]

---

1. Sowby FD. The regulation of shoe fitting fluoroscopes. *J Canad Assoc Radiol* 1956;7:18.

"Every year nearly one million nuclear medicine procedures are carried out in Canada alone, while around the world, over a half a million cancer patients are treated annually with cobalt therapy units designed and developed by AECL [Atomic Energy of Canada Ltd]."

— Sylvia Fedoruk

Presentation to the Annual Conference of the Canadian Nuclear Association and the Canadian Nuclear Society, Ottawa, June 6, 1989.

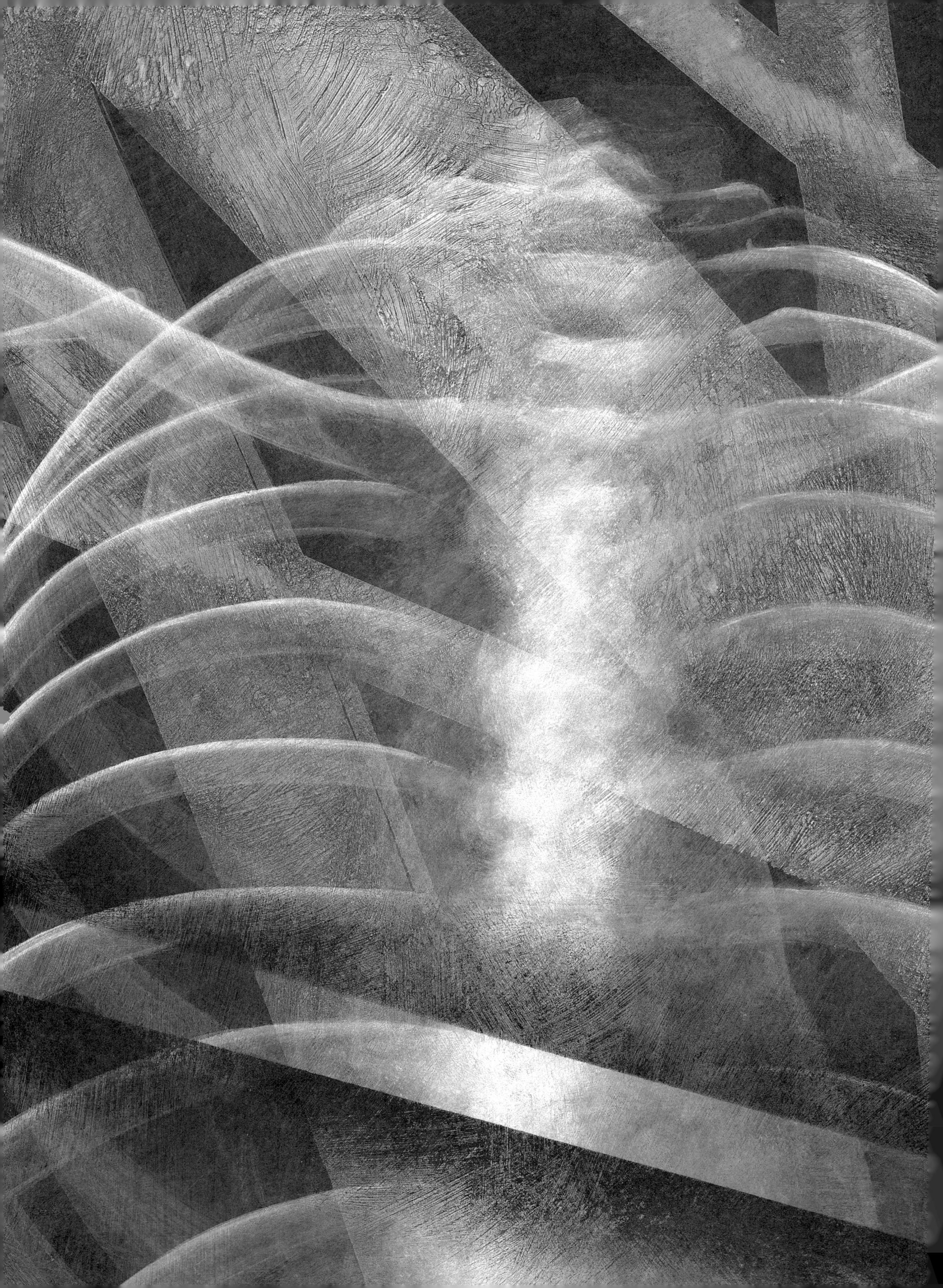

Part Four
Regions and the Canadian Academic Departments of Radiology

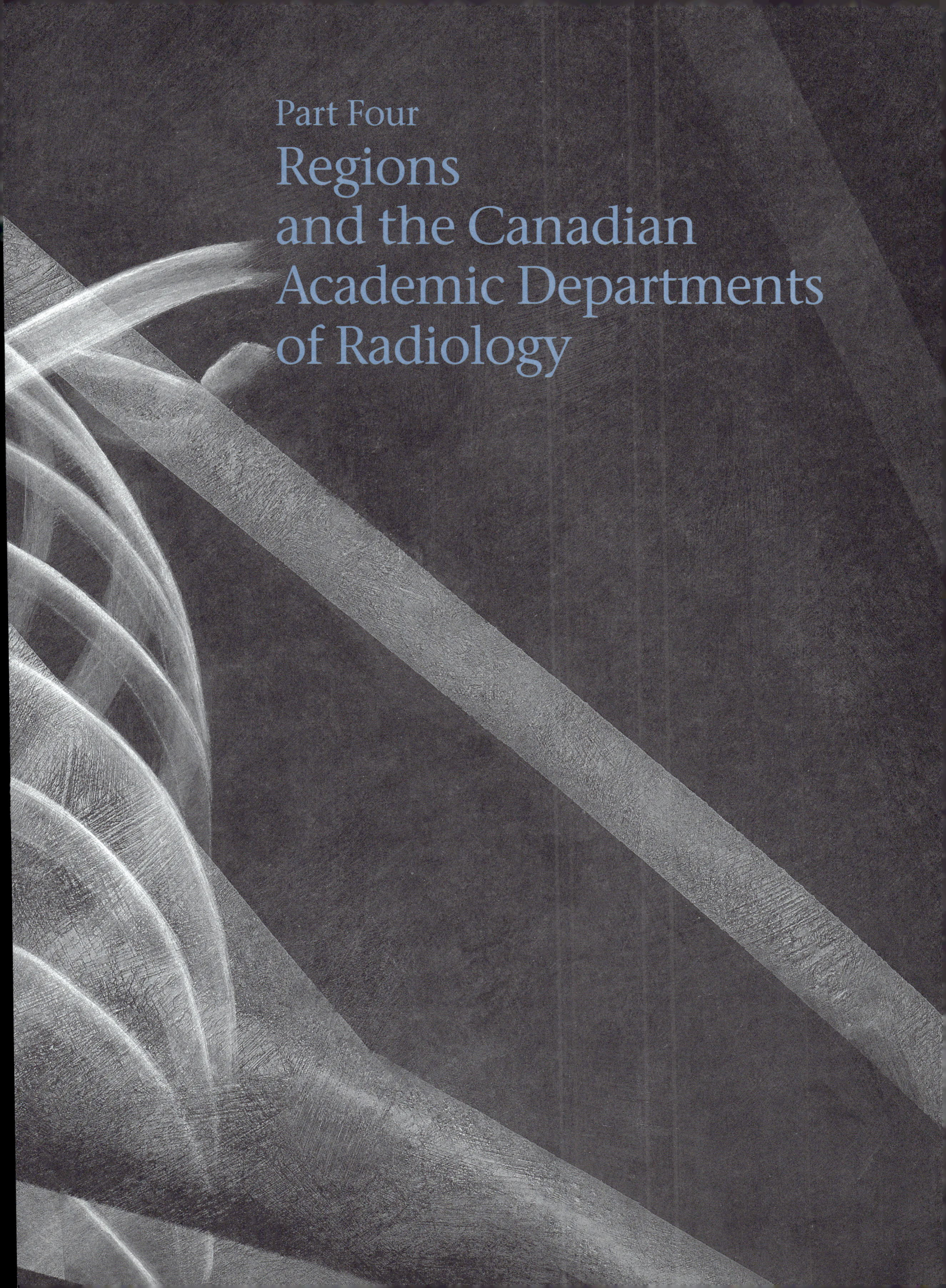

"Why is it," asked my charming hostess, "that medical schools are the only institutions of higher learning that give diplomas in omniscience."
— Morris Gibson

The radiological sciences are new on the scale of the history of medicine.[1] Moreover for much of its early development radiology has been seen, from the perspective of a dean of a medical faculty, as a rather technical and uninteresting specialty. Medical schools, most of which have never been at their best in leading change, have been particularly slow to recognise that radiology has altered out of all recognition in the past quarter of a century. As a result radiology departments are only modestly funded in many academic centres across Canada when compared with the longer established departments such as medicine and surgery.

Using modern methods of investigation such as echo-planar magnetic resonance imaging, *in vivo* magnetic resonance spectroscopy, positron emission tomography and tracer methods, it is now possible to do much more than applied clinical research in radiology. And yet Shorter describes below how the Dean at the University of Toronto, admittedly in the mid-1960s, remarked that he had never thought of research in connection with radiology. Methods like those now available to radiologists permit the investigation of fundamental mechanisms of disease. They also permit, for example, visualization of brain activation which precisely localizes cerebral function in life—information only available otherwise in a limited form from brain surgery. Just as strikingly they permit the teaching of detailed anatomy, physiology and pathology in life. Recourse to the anatomy laboratory for dissections or the morgue for post-mortems will not be made obsolete, but can be complemented and enhanced by radiological methods. As academic radiology departments adapt to the new reality of the radiological sciences in the 21st Century so must medical schools and curricula also change to recognise this reality.

Centres and programs of genuine excellence in the radiological sciences have emerged: the basic science group in the Robart's Institute at the University of Western Ontario; the imaging groups at the Montréal Neurological Institute and Montréal Heart Institute; the McMaster University positron emission tomography program; and the radiobiology division at the Cross Cancer Institute in Edmonton come to mind. At their best they combine multidisciplinary research with a clinical focus.

The challenge for an academic radiology department in the second century of the specialty goes beyond maintenance of physical plant, although that is likely to be difficult enough. The challenge will also be to consolidate its academic rôle in teaching to undergraduates and graduates, and to fulfil the research potential implicit in modern radiological methods. This will need medical schools and their affiliated clinical sites which are sensitive to an academic mandate. It will also need an acceptable level of capital re-investmment by governments. Such progress, if it occurs, will increasingly move radiology into the mainstream of academic medicine.

— Brian Lentle

Chapter I •

University of Alberta:

The Department of Diagnostic Imaging

Alexander JB McEwan

INTRODUCTION

The University of Alberta was established by a bill introduced in the first session of the legislative assembly of the province.[1] In 1908, Henry Marshall Tory was appointed president of the university and the first faculty established; the Faculty of Arts and Sciences began teaching in the autumn of 1908 with four professors and a class of 45 students. This first class graduated in 1912. In 1913 the Faculty of Medicine was established as the fourth university faculty, preceded by those of Arts and Sciences, Law, and Applied Science.

The medical school was the first to be established west of Winnipeg and the eighth school in Canada. The population of the province of Alberta was approximately 400,000, and approximately 400 medical practitioners were in active practice.

The first dean of the faculty was appointed in 1920.

In the first years of the school, about 150 students completed the three year program and were subsequently admitted with advanced standing to the Universities of McGill, Toronto or Manitoba.

The practice of radiology was established in the associated hospitals in 1923 by Dr Richard Proctor, who provided almost single-handed practice from 1923 until his retirement in 1957. During this period, he was responsible for clinical work as well as for teaching. At that time, radiology was a division of the Department of Medicine.

THE DEPARTMENT OF RADIOLOGY AND DIAGNOSTIC IMAGING

The Department of Radiology was formed by the University in 1957 and was headed by the first appointed Professor and Chairman, Dr Hector E Duggan. In 1953, Drs Duggan and RE Bell from Laboratory Medicine, formed the first radioisotope laboratory in the province.

This laboratory was the forerunner of the division of nuclear medicine.

Dr Duggan was succeeded by Dr Fleming McConnell as Professor and Chairman in 1965, a position he held until 1970. Dr JDR Miller was appointed Professor and Chairman in 1970, stepping down in 1983. Dr Miller remains on staff at the University Hospitals as a neuroradiologist. He was largely responsible for the design and construction of the department in the Walter C MacKenzie Health Sciences Centre and for major improvements in imaging equipment during the period of his tenure including the introduction of many of the newer imaging modalities, such as computed tomography, ultrasound and in-house nuclear medicine capabilities.

Dr DB Russell was appointed Acting Chairman in 1983 and Professor and Chairman in 1986, a position he held until 1991. Dr. Russell remains on staff at the University of Alberta Hospitals as a neuroradiologist and as director of the undergraduate teaching program.

Dr AJB McEwan succeeded Dr Russell in 1992.

Until 1992, the Department of Radiology at the University of Alberta had three divisions, encompassing the following specialty areas:

1. The Division of Diagnostic Radiology
2. The Division of Radiation Oncology, and
3. The Division of Nuclear Medicine.

The Division of Diagnostic Radiology and the Division of Nuclear Medicine are sited at the University Hospital, the Royal Alexandra Hospital, the Cross Cancer Institute, the Grey Nuns Hospital and the Misericordia Hospital. The hospitals primarily involved in teaching at the undergraduate and postgraduate levels are the University Hospital, the Royal Alexandra Hospital and the Cross Cancer Institute. The Division of Radiation Oncology is sited entirely at the Cross Cancer Institute; in 1922 the university established a Department of Oncology.

Over the years, the number of radiologists and nuclear physicians at the University of Alberta Hospitals has increased from one to the current 16. There are presently two geographic full-time positions within the department with the balance of the academic responsibilities of the department being carried by part-time faculty.

Radiology at the Royal Alexandra Hospital was developed by Dr George Malcolmson, who was the sole radiologist at that hospital until 1939 when his son, Dr Pat Malcolmson, became head of the department. The chiefs of radiology at the Royal Alexandra Hospital since that time have been Drs C Hyndman, S Windle, R Keogh, L Dunbar, H Phillips, R Arnold and currently, Dr G Andrew, a neuroradiologist.

Radiology at the Edmonton General Hospital was performed primarily by Dr Marshall Mallett from the Misericordia Hospital until June of 1951, when Dr Rupert Clare became chairman, a position he held until 1975 when he was succeeded by Dr A McPherson. Dr Myron Babiuk (a University of Alberta graduate) was appointed chairman in 1979. The Edmonton General Hospital has largely been replaced by the Grey Nuns Hospital with relocation of the Department of Radiology into that facility; only a satellite operation remains at the original Edmonton General Hospital.

The Misericordia Hospital radiology services began under the direction of Dr Marshall Mallett. Dr Mallett was very involved in setting up and teaching in the technology training programs at the Northern Alberta Institute of Technology (NAIT). Dr Mallett was succeeded by his son, Dr Lawrence Mallett, who was then succeeded by Dr John Mason. The current chief of the Department of Radiology and Medical Imaging is Dr Eric Preville. The Misericordia Hospital is unique in that it has the only lithotripter in the northern part of the province sited in that hospital.

The first diagnostic radiologist for the Cancer Treatment Centre was Dr W Morrish in 1954, who was head of the department for one year; he was succeeded by Dr Zbignew Gutter who was also a radiologist and radiotherapist. The third head of the department at the Cross Cancer Institute was Dr William Castor, an Alberta graduate with qualification in therapy and diagnostic radiology. He was succeeded in 1994 by Dr Ian Birchall, as head of a newly formed Department of Oncologic Imaging, which includes radiology and nuclear medicine.

The Division of Radiation Oncology

The "Radiotherapy Department" of the Edmonton Cancer Clinic began in 1953 with Dr Marcus Marlborough as head. The heads of the department of radiation oncology since that time have been:

- Dr AL Dick, 1954–60
- Dr ME Tulloh, 1960–68
- Dr J Pearson, 1968–84
- Dr AAE Starreveld, 1984–91
- Dr R Pearcey, 1991–present

In July 1968 the WW Cross Cancer Institute (CCI) was opened. Academically, the department was a division of the University of Alberta Department of Radiology and remains so today. The division has grown to a large, well-staffed service and academic department which includes radiation oncologists, radiobiologists and physicists. This division is very productive in research and teaching as well as carrying a large clinical load.

The Division of Nuclear Medicine

Nuclear Medicine became a division of the Department of Radiology and Diagnostic Imaging in 1972, and the first director of that division was Dr Brian Lentle who was head of Nuclear Medicine at the Cross Cancer Institute. Dr Lentle was largely responsible for early development of this specialty in Edmonton and establishing research and teaching programs in this discipline.

Nuclear medicine has grown to become an integral part of clinical investigation and is extensively involved in research activities, largely through the CCI Department of Nuclear Medicine. Nuclear medicine services are part of the hospital Radiology Departments in all the affiliated hospitals except the Cross Cancer Institute where it is a free standing department (though it is still part of the Division of the University Department of Radiology and Diagnostic Imaging).

There are seven physicians in Edmonton with Canadian fellowships in Nuclear Medicine (three at the Royal Alexandra Hospital, three at the University Hospital and one at the Grey Nuns Hospital). The divisional director of nuclear medicine at the University of Alberta is currently Dr Conor Maguire.

RESIDENCY TRAINING

The residency training program at the University of Alberta was established in 1956 by Dr Duggan, and the first resident trained in the program was graduated in 1959. Between 1959 and 1969, a total of ten radiology residents graduated. Between 1959 and 1994 a total of 103 radiology residents have graduated from the program. These graduates have subsequently practiced in Alberta, British Columbia, Ontario, Québec, the United States, Brazil and Australia.

The nuclear medicine residency program was established in 1979 and since then, nine residents have graduated with nuclear medicine fellowships.

GRADUATE STUDENT PROGRAM

The MSc and PhD programs were established in 1983; since then nine graduate students have been granted degrees. In 1994, there were six students enrolled in the graduate programs. A medical physics residency was established in 1993 under the leadership of Dr L Filipow, head of the Division of Medical Physics.

SUMMARY

The history of the development of the Department of Radiology and Diagnostic Imaging at the University of Alberta is one of collaboration between the university and part-time faculty; one of collaboration between the many clinical institutions within the city; and a tribute to the foresight and hard work of a small number of dedicated individuals who had the vision to establish the department and to lead it into the 1990s. The department is currently poised to consolidate and build upon the successes of the early years, and to learn from the difficulties which have strengthened its structure.

Right
An X-ray requisition from 1933

X-RAY REQUISITION

V. G. H.

WARD A　　　　C 75855 HOSP. No.

NAME ____ SURNAME IN BLOCK CAPITALS　　　　W Wilson DOCTOR

AGE 54　　　　X-RAY No.

PROVISIONAL DIAGNOSIS Ca. liver

INFORMATION (OR TREATMENT) REQUESTED After administration of thorotrast 75 c.c

PREVIOUS X-RAY REPORT NUMBERS

PATIENT MAY GO TO DEPARTMENT ON FOOT__ WHEEL CHAIR__ STRETCHER✓ BED__　　　　AND MAY STAND__ SIT__ LIE__

DATE May 26/32　　　　SIGNED [illegible]

This Form to Be Sent in "Triplicate" to the X-Ray Department by the Ward or Department Requesting the Examination or Treatment.

DO NOT WRITE IN THIS SPACE

REPORT

FILMS USED 200K.V.P.　　　　DATE

DETAILS OF TECHNIQUE .5cu+2al 700 r.

FINDINGS

May 26 - 700 r to ant Abdomen.
" 29 800 r " post Rt. "
1400 r to R & L. anter
1400 r to R post.
12" 700 at 200 .5+2 200 700 at 200. 2cu+2al.
June 2 700 r ant liver
" 5 700 r " Left abd
" 6 much worse.
" 7 700 r post Rt Abd.
Deceased June 11 -

Chapter II • Department of Radiology:

University of British Columbia

Brian Lentle

ORIGINS

In 1872, within a year of the province entering the Canadian Confederation, it was suggested that a university might be needed in British Columbia (BC). Mr John Jessop, the newly appointed superintendent of education, wrote in his annual report of that year: "The fact, too, that British Columbia will soon require a Provincial University, capable of conferring degrees in Arts, Law and Medicine, should not be lost sight of..."[1]

It is perhaps unnecessary to point out that that idea was a long time in coming to fruition. Indeed, BC politicians of whatever conviction, with their passionate commitment to pragmatism, have always been persuaded that it is possible to attract sufficient physicians to the province irrespective of the contributions of the Faculty of Medicine.

Thus, Logan writes some 80 years after the founding of the University:

> *In spite of the inspired leadership of Dean Weaver, the Faculty of Medicine continued to lead a most difficult existence during the 1950s. Because the necessary funds could not be found to establish the Faculty in independence at Point Grey, the division of medical facilities between the University campus and the Vancouver General Hospital was assuming a disheartening aura of permanency.*[2]

The Faculty of Medicine had been created in 1950, although as Turnbull notes it is difficult to explain why a BC medical school took so long to come into existence.[3] A sustained effort to create the medical school had begun in 1944.

In 1920 the university was adjacent to Vancouver General

Hospital. With the transfer of the university to its present site on Point Grey the issue of a hospital to serve as the site for clinical instruction arose. As late as 1947 Dr CE Dolman, who had come to Vancouver to be in charge of bacteriology at UBC, wrote in the *News-Herald*: "The University and the province would do well to defer opening of a medical school until a more suitable teaching hospital than the Vancouver General is provided."[3] Turnbull comments: "It was unfortunate that in 1946 the hospital was weakly administered and its physical plant was in disrepair."[3]

Logan notes:

The Board found it necessary therefore [because of fiscal constraints] to give up, for the present, and for the foreseeable future, the ideal, set forth in the Dolman report and the Senate resolution, of a university teaching hospital on the campus. Its attention was then focussed on the existing and contemplated clinical teaching facilities of the Vancouver General Hospital, which had already offered its co-operation. The development of these facilities, however, to a point where they would be adequate for student needs had to wait on the advancement of the Hospital's own building programme...In the course of the summer, the Provincial Government...[declared that it] was willing to improve the ward facilities of the Vancouver General Hospital for the use of the University.[4]

When the medical school at the University of British Columbia opened in 1950 the Dean was Dr Myron Weaver. The Vancouver General served as the major teaching hospital but, in a compromise, a small "university hospital" was to be built on campus. After an independent life as University Hospital this institute merged with Shaughnessy Hospital as University Hospital on two sites in 1989. With the closure of the Shaughnessy site by government edict in 1993 it is ironic that the campus site then merged with the Vancouver General to form the Vancouver Hospital and Health Sciences Centre. In the meantime the BC Children's Hospital and Vancouver Clinic of the BC Cancer Agency had been created. With St Paul's Hospital these institutions provide the major part of the Faculty of Medicine clinical programs in general, and radiological teaching in particular.

The departments within the faculty at its creation were Anatomy, Biochemistry, Physiology, Medicine, Obstetrics and Gynecology, Pediatrics, Pathology and Surgery.

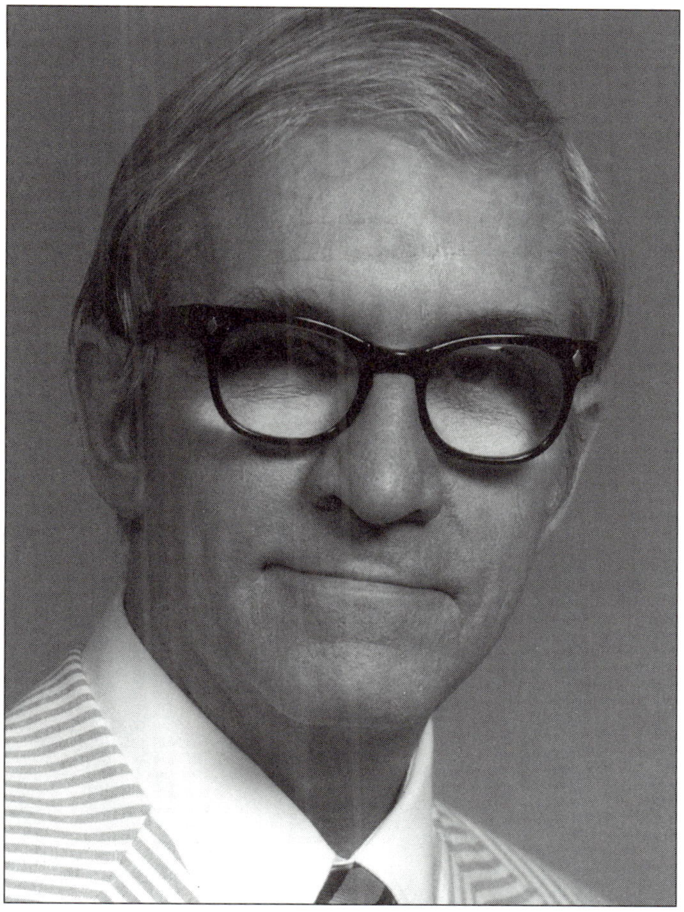

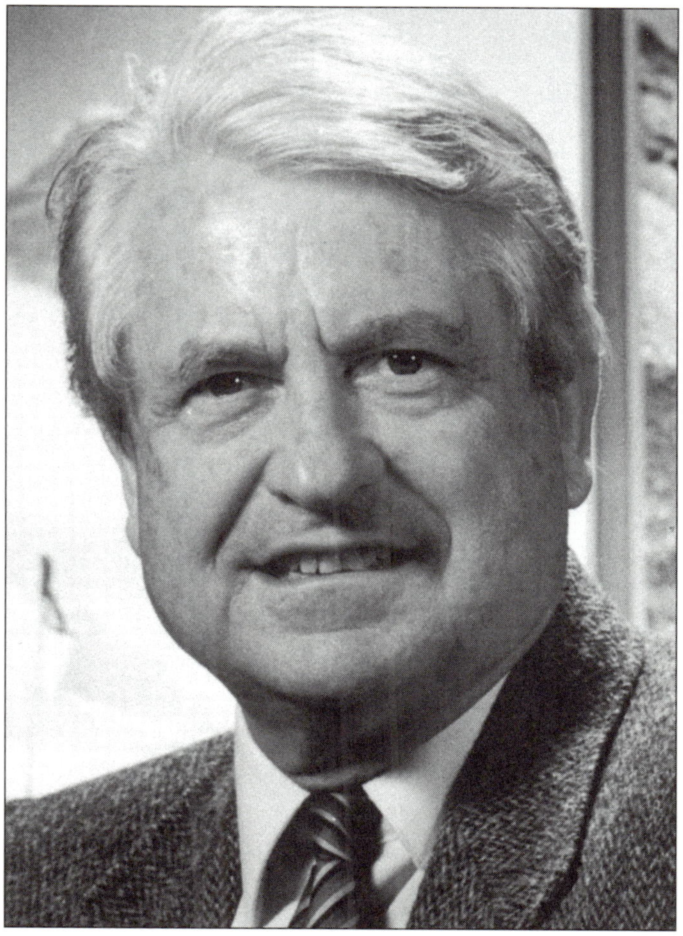

Top
Dr Scott Dunbar

Right
Dr H Joachim Burhenne

THE FIRST CHAIR OF RADIOLOGY

The creation of a chair of radiology had to await the arrival of Dr Scott Dunbar in 1971, although a hospital-based program of residency education had been started by Dr Boyd.[5] Dr Dunbar and his successor, Dr H Joachim Burhenne, created a department with a strong academic bent. Dr Dunbar had already been editor of the *Canadian Association of Radiologists Journal* while Dr Burhenne would be a gold medallist of the American Roentgen Ray Society, among the many honours he received. The residency education program in radiology was to be a strong one with Drs Peter Cooperberg, Weldon Hooge, Douglas Graeb, Nestor Müller and Bruce Forster among those serving as directors.

LATER DEVELOPMENTS

In 1986 a Division of Nuclear Medicine was created and in 1993 a Division of Basic Science with Dr John Aldrich as its first head. The Division of Nuclear Medicine under my headship developed a residency education program in that specialty, the second departmental program. The Division of Basic Science is forging enhanced links with the Tri-Universities Meson Facility (TRIUMF) and the Department of Physics in the Faculty of Science.

RECOGNITION

Dr Burhenne's distinguished career has brought him many awards including the gold medal of the American Roentgen Ray Society. He has been a visiting lecturer in both radiological and surgical departments in virtually every corner of the globe.

Dr Nestor Müller has been one of the pioneering radiologists in the development of thin-section computed tomography and its use in diagnosing lung disease. Dr Peter Cooperberg is likewise an international figure in having developed clinical applications of the use of diagnostic ultrasound in medicine. Both have taught and lectured, and continue to do so, world-wide. Dr David Li is a pioneering investigator in the use of magnetic resonance imaging (MRI) in evaluating multiple sclerosis. Dr John Mayo, working with his basic science colleagues Drs Alex McKay and Ken Whittall, has had his innovative research in the use of MRI in diagnosing lung disease recognized by the award of the Fleischner Society Medal. With Dr Mayo joining Dr Müller as members of the Fleischner Society the Vancouver Hospital and the University of British Columbia become one of the few such institutions to have two radiologists as members of that prestigious group. Dr Don Lyster, the second divisional head of nuclear medicine, has had his contributions to radiopharmaceutical science recognized by an award for scientific contributions from the Western Region of the Society of Nuclear Medicine.

Not least Dr Don Newman and his colleagues, Drs Gordon Culham, Helen Nadel, Kenneth Poskitt and David Stringer, have made internationally recognized contributions to developments in imaging disease in children.

SUMMARY

The foundations laid by the wisdom and foresight of Drs Dunbar and Burhenne continue to serve the department well. Under Dr Peter Cooperberg's guidance St Paul's Hospital, in a redeveloped department, is playing an enhanced and invaluable part in the educational programs. Dr Cooperberg has also administered, annually, two very successful courses in radiology, one at Whistler (in the footsteps of Dr Burhenne) and one in central Vancouver. These serve not only to attract visitors but also to enhance the academic life of the department and to bring to it resources for academic enrichment.

Dr Don Newman has equally developed a strong pediatric teaching group with its own record of accomplishments at the BC Children's Hospital. A more recent recruit is Dr Peter Poon. As Head of the Department of Radiology at the Vancouver Clinic of the BC Cancer Agency Dr Poon is redeveloping that service as a substantial component of the teaching programs and introducing interventional radiology at his hospital with the help of a re-recruited radiologist, Dr Peter Munk, who originally obtained his radiology education at UBC.

By way of unfinished business, Dr Burhenne has also invested an endowment in the department with which it is hoped to offer substantial support for a Scholar in Abdominal Radiology.

Contract research in magnetic resonance imaging and spectroscopy under the able leadership of Dr David Li, and in osteoporosis within the Division of Nuclear Medicine, promise to provide some relief in the resource-constrained context of the late 1990s.

Given the earlier recruitment of a strong faculty and the ground-breaking contributions of Drs Burhenne and Dunbar, the department can look forward to a future as rich in promise as any spring. This promise will receive further impetus when the once-and-never tower provides a new and consolidated home for the Department of Radiology at Vancouver Hospital and Health Sciences Centre.

Chapter III • *History of the Department of Radiology at*

The University of Calgary

Chen Fong

In 1966 the Foothills Hospital building was complete, and the Department of Radiology started its operation. The founding members of the Department of Radiology were Drs Hector Duggan, Hugh Morrish and Barry Evans.

The Faculty of Medicine at the University of Calgary was established in 1967. In the following year Drs Abe Zacharias and Leo Desautels joined the group. In 1969 a Division of Radiology was started under the Department of Medicine. Dr Hector Duggan was appointed Professor and Head of the Division of Radiology as well as the Director of Radiology at the Foothills Hospital. At the same time approval was received from the Royal College of Physicians and Surgeons of Canada for the establishment of a Residency Training Program in Radiology. Dr Abe Zacharias was made program director for the residency training program.

In 1970, following an outside survey by the Royal College, the Department of Radiology received full approval for its program using the Foothills Hospital and the Calgary General Hospital as training sites. Four residents were admitted to the Residency Training Program in 1971 under the direction of Dr David Lewell. He was succeeded by Dr Hugh Morrish in the same capacity in 1976.

In 1978, following the retirement of Dr Hector Duggan, Dr Hugh Morrish was appointed Professor and Head of the Department of Radiology at the University of Calgary and Director of the Department of Radiology at the Foothills Hospital. At the same time Dr Leo Desautels succeeded Dr Morrish as the Program Director for Residency Training.

In 1980 Dr Sam Share was appointed the Program Director of the Residency Training Program. He held this post until 1986.

In 1980, following a further review by the Royal College of Physicians and Surgeons of Canada, the Division of Radiology at the University of Calgary ceased to be a Division of the Department of Medicine, and gained full departmental status. This structure—the Department of Radiology of the Faculty of Medicine, University of Calgary—remains to this day.

In 1985 approval was received from the Royal College of Physicians and Surgeons of Canada for a residency training program in nuclear medicine. Dr Reinhard Kloiber was appointed program director.

In 1986 Dr David Reid became program director for the radiology residency program. He stepped down in 1992 and Dr Benny So succeeded him.

In 1990 Dr Robert Johns was appointed Professor and Head, Department of Radiology at the University of Calgary and the Director of Radiology at the Foothills Hospital. Unfortunately, Dr Johns passed away in 1992 after a brief illness.

Dr T Chen Fong was appointed as Professor and Head of the University of Calgary and Director of the Department of Radiological Sciences and Diagnostic Imaging at the Foothills Hospital in 1994.

Currently, the Department consists of 20 radiologists involved in the Residency Training Programs of both Radiology and Nuclear Medicine. There are two fellows and 12 residents.

"Thanks to anesthesia and to the development of aseptic surgery by WS Halsted of Johns Hopkins and Berkeley George Moynihan of Leeds, surgery had progressed so far and so fast by 1900 that Moynihan opined that not much further progress was to be expected. Yet surgery still had one serious handicap: the surgeon had to embark on his operation without knowing what to expect inside. There was an imperative need for some method of making human flesh transparent. Imagine now that a system of research funding such as that which prevails today were in operation in 1900 and imagine also the incredulous derision with which a research proposal "to discover a means of making human flesh transparent" would be greeted by any grant giving body. Yet as we all know, just such a procedure was discovered by a man primarily interested in studying electric discharges in high vacua. The medical potentialities of Roentgen rays (x-rays) for what is now called diagnostic radiology were recognized almost immediately."[1]

— PB Medawar

1. Medawar PB. *The limits of science*. New York: Harper and Row, 1984.

"Well I made the wave didn't I?" (In answer to the jibe: "Lucky fellow, Rutherford, always on the crest of the wave.")[1]

— Lord Rutherford

1. Quoted in: Snow CP. *The two cultures and the scientific revolution.*

Chapter IV • *A New Era in*

Nova Scotia Radiology

David B Fraser

Dr WH Eager was Chief of Radiology at Victoria General Hospital in Halifax in 1920. Dr SR Johnson became the head in 1926, and remained head until 1953. During this period the department installed for x-ray treatment of malignant conditions a new high voltage apparatus previously available only in Upper Canada or the United States. At that time radiologists were trained in diagnostic imaging as well as radiotherapy, and in fact, radiotherapy was carried out in the x-ray department at VGH until the late 1940s. The annual report of the VGH for 1931 states that 70 per cent of the department's cases came from outside Halifax County, and 7963 examinations were given during the year. In 1946 there was a new VGH and a new Department of Radiology. For the brief period 1953–54 Dr WM Roy was head of department, and he still practices radiology in Ontario.

In 1955 Dr JS Manchester became head of department as well as chairman of the Dalhousie University Department of Radiology. Dr Manchester was responsible for the major development and growth of the specialty in Halifax. In 1955 the VGH department installed its first angiocardiographic suite. The residency training program was revised, and three new residents were appointed for 1957. The department received approval for complete training for certification and fellowship with the Royal College of Physicians and Surgeons of Canada. By 1965 there were 10 residents in training, 27 student technologists, and the department performed 62,258 exams.

In 1974 the hospital installed its first computerized axial tomography (CT) system—the original EMI Head Scanner—and made plans for the purchase of new ultrasound equipment. Two years later, the department installed its first computerized management and scheduling system. In 1977 nuclear medicine was transferred from the Radiotherapy Department and formed its own imaging division.

The first body CT scanner was installed in 1981, and one of the first digital vascular imaging systems was installed for evaluation. After many years of negotiation, magnetic resonance imaging became a reality in 1988.

Dr JS Manchester completed his term as department head in 1975 and was succeeded by Dr James Standen from Toronto. Dr Standen remained head until 1979 and chairman at Dalhousie until 1981 when he was replaced by Dr DB Fraser.

"La radiologie ne remplissait pas toute seule l'existence très active, comme on sait, du Docteur Léo-E Pariseau; il accordait une bonne part de son temps à d'autres sciences et à d'autres œuvres. Néanmoins, c'est son titre d'électroradiologiste que ce grand médecin et ce savant préférait et c'est celui-là qui lui servait d'identité."

— *Albert Jutras*
Le Journal de L'Hôtel Dieu de Montréal
1943 (No. 6): 354

l'Université Laval de Québec

Laurent Aubé

MGR JOSEPH-CLOVIS K LAFLAMME

Mgr Joseph-Clovis K-Laflamme fut le pionnier de la radiographie à l'Université Laval de Québec. John Cox de l'Université de Montréal, l'avait précédé de peu, soit le 5 février 1896. Voilà ce que rapporte *Le Journal du Séminaire de Québec* en 1896:

> *Laflamme. Mgr JCK*
> *A fait cet après-midi des expériences de photographie à l'aide des rayons-X de Röntgen. Deux poses de 25 et 20 minutes. Les résultats sont attendus avec anxiété. Le procédé est simple, mais la lumière est si faible qu'on se demande comment les choses peuvent se passer comme on le dit.*[1]
>
> **14 Février 1896** *A essayé hier de photographier avec les rayons-X de Roëntgen, sans succès. Les expériences ont été tentées de nouveau.*[2]
>
> **2 Avril 1896** *Mgr Laflamme avait fait hier des expériences photographiques à la Roëntgen. A reçu les clichés aujourd'hui de la main de Livernois*. Ils ont admirablement réussi.*
>
> **5 Avril 1896** *Radiographie de la main et du pied d'un enfant. Le petit bonhomme a dû poser au delà d'une demi-heure et a trouvé le temps très long.*
>
> **23 Avril 1896** La Verite *de ce soir contient un excellent article sur les expériences faites sur les rayons-X à l'Université. C'est le premier journal qui en parle.*
>
> **29 Avril 1896** *Mgr Laflamme a donné ce soir devant les élèves en médecine et les professeurs de la Faculté, une causerie sur les rayons-X et leur application en médecine.*
> *Cette soirée a paru intéresser beaucoup les auditeurs, surtout les expériences faites avec le skiloscope.*[3]

18 mai 1896 *John Cox remercié pour photo aux Rayons-X.*
Uni. 64 no:118
20 Mai 1896 *Grande séance d'expérience avec les rayons-X, donnée ce soir devant un tout petit comité foumi presqu'exclusivement d'Archevêques et d'Évêques. Auditoire vivement intéressé. On a regardé et vu à travers un chanoine, au grand amusement de tous."*[4]
17 Sept 86 *Mgr Laflamme a fait quelques expériences avec les rayons-X devant un certain nombre d'Anglais protestants, médecins et autres. Ils ont eu l'air fort intéressés.*[5]

ORGANISATION DU DÉPARTEMENT

1955–56 Organisation du département d'Électroradiologie, de Physiothérapie et de Réadaptation aux fins de l'enseignement.[1]

Les départements de médecine, de chirurgie, de neuro-psychiatrie et d'Electroradiologie, de Physiothérapie et de Réadaptation ont été organisés aux fins de l'enseignement. Le docteur Renaud Lemieux a été nommé chef du département de médecine, le docteur Lucien LaRue, chef du département de neuro-psychiatrie, et le docteur Mathieu Samson, chef du département d'Electroradiologie, de Physiothérapie et Réadaptation.

MGR LAFLAMME (1849–1910)

Né à Saint-Anselme, le 18 septembre 1849, fut un professeur de physique reconnu universellement et de plus s'intéressa vivement à l'électricité, à la géologie, à la botanique, à la météorologie de même qu'à l'astronomie. Son laboratoire de physique était équipé d'un grand nombre de tubes de Crookes dont les uns étaient montés pour l'étude des rayons cathodiques et avaient été achetés chez Radiguet et Massiot (France).

Supérieur du Petit Séminaire il fut également secrétaire de l'Université Laval.

Chapter VI • *Radiology at the*

University of Manitoba

Douglas MacEwan

DOUGLAS MACEWAN, EDWARD (TED) LANSDOWN: ACADEMIC LEADERS

There were eighteen provincial radiologists in 1966 when the partnership of Macpherson and Childe, soon to become Kiernan, Elliot and Boult, recruited MacEwan to the newly created full-time post of university Head of Radiology in 1966. A giddy era of growth and expansion occurred in the next twenty-five years. The dean of medicine and the director of the hospital kept asking if more money could be spent to bring all of the advances of nuclear medicine, ultrasound, angiography, and computed tomography to the teaching hospitals. Soon there were more residents, with credentials hardly dreamed of, than attending staff. The plan was that after three years they would spend a final year at a leading world centre. In turn, many became leaders—four departmental chairs (Ted Lansdown, Ian Sutherland, Carl Zylak and Ted Lyons), two vice-presidents of medicine of teaching hospitals (Sutherland, Brown), three were to write textbooks (Lyons, Billinghurst, Martin Reed), and one was to found the Pakistan Journal of Radiology (Atiqur Rahman). The community radiologists established a visiting professor program with the luminaries of radiology lecturing and teaching in Winnipeg. Imaging advisory committees were established to advise government about equipment purchases and the conduct of imaging programs. MacEwan retired as head in 1982 and finished the decade by attracting 20 per cent of the medical school class to electives and thus flooding the radiology residency programs of Canada with applicants. On the way, the now over fifty radiologists in Manitoba shared in his work as editor of the *Canadian Association of Radiologists Journal*, president of the Canadian Association of Radiologists, the

Radiological Society of North America, and the Society of Chairmen of Academic Radiology Departments, Examination and Accreditation Committee work of the Royal College of Physicians and Surgeons of Canada, and Canadian Chancellor of the American College of Radiology.

GWILYM EVANS, JOHN (IAN) SUTHERLAND: ACHIEVEMENT

Evans filled many roles in Manitoba radiology, kept the country informed as editor of *Illuminator* (the newsletter of the Canadian Association of Radiologists), and served a term as president of the Canadian Association of Radiologists. Ian trained in Manitoba, built a strong section of nuclear medicine, opened a private office, became a leader in the evolution of nuclear medicine in Canada, and was appointed university head of radiology bringing order and stability following rapid growth. His greatest contributions to the Canadian Association of Radiologists were as chair of a committee making recommendations on reorganization and in serving as president during the Röntgen Centennial Year. He revitalized the Manitoba Medical Association and was rewarded with its presidency. His talents led to his appointment as Vice-President Medicine at the Health Sciences Centre, one of the largest teaching hospitals in Canada. Concurrently Dr Ross Brown, who had founded the clinical use of ultrasound in Manitoba, became Vice-President Medicine at the companion teaching hospital, St Boniface General Hospital. He had previously served as President of the American Institute of Ultrasound in Medicine.

EDWARD (TED) LYONS, BLAKE MCCLARTY: NEW DIRECTIONS

As a medical student Ted took night calls as a technician in ultrasound, then trained in radiology in Manitoba, had a fellowship with Professor Ian Donald in Glasgow, and, on his return in 1972 became section head of ultrasound. Ultrasound evolved as a province wide program with an emphasis on high training standards for technologist and radiologist. Companies tested and developed equipment on site and educational programs attracted world wide interest. His text, *Color Atlas of Sectional Anatomy*, was an instant success as cross-sectional anatomy for ultrasound diagnosis arrived at the start of computed tomography. He served as President of the Society of Radiologists in Ultrasound. He became university head in 1990.

A generous gift established the first MRI scanner at St Boniface General Hospital and McClarty soon established an important clinical and research presence in the field. He was trained at the University of Toronto under Dr Lansdown. Blake has been recently appointed Program Director of Neurosciences in the Faculty of Medicine of the University of Manitoba. There are to be approximately 10 such integrated medical science programs in the Faculty.

Chapter VII •

McGill University:

The Beginnings of the Department of Radiology

PATRICE BRET

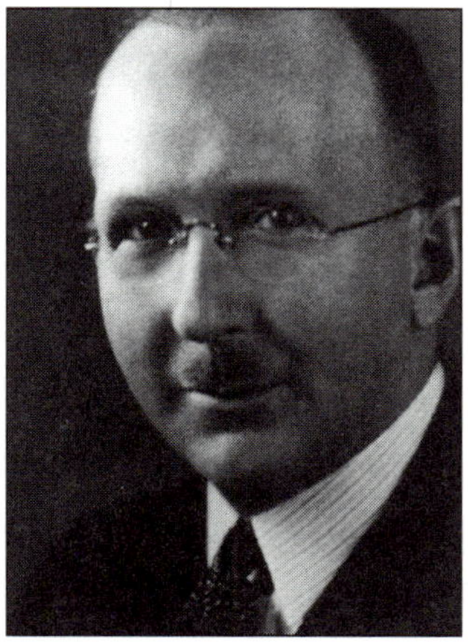

Dr William Lloyd Ritchie

In 1938 the Dean, Dr Grant Fleming, reported to Principal Lewis Douglas that the creation of a Department of Radiology was approved in the Faculty of Medicine and should allow for the better organization of teaching in this subject. However, it took two years for the department to come into being under the chairmanship of Dr Ritchie.

In the 1941–1942 annual report to Principal F Cyril James, the Dean, Dr JC Meakins, reports: "The department of radiology has at last come into being under the Chairmanship of Professor Ritchie. The final establishment of such a Department has greatly aided the teaching of this subject and will, I am sure, make the Faculty of Medicine one of the leading centres of radiology in Canada."

Right
A report signed by Dr WL Ritchie during his time in Ottawa

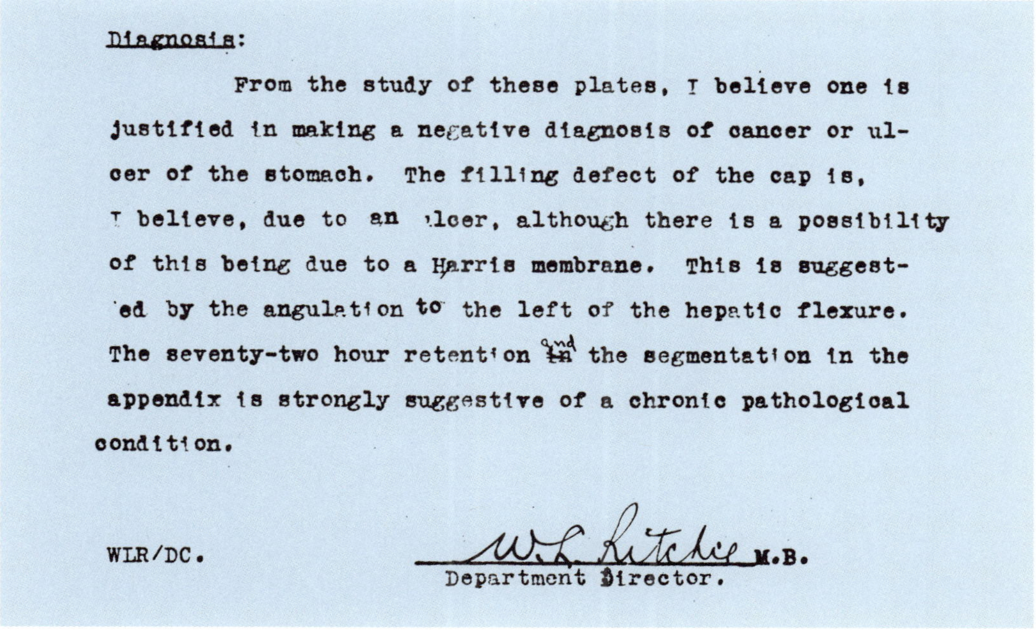

Diagnosis:

From the study of these plates, I believe one is justified in making a negative diagnosis of cancer or ulcer of the stomach. The filling defect of the cap is, I believe, due to an ulcer, although there is a possibility of this being due to a Harris membrane. This is suggested by the angulation to the left of the hepatic flexure. The seventy-two hour retention and the segmentation in the appendix is strongly suggestive of a chronic pathological condition.

WLR/DC.

W L Ritchie M.B.
Department Director.

DR WL RITCHIE

Dr William Lloyd Ritchie, FRCSC, was the first director of the department of radiology at Montréal General Hospital, and the first chairman of McGill University's radiology department. In his day he was doyen of the radiologists in Canada. Dr Ritchie was born in 1883 at Beamsville, Ontario, and attended school there before entering the University of Toronto from which he was graduated as a bachelor of medicine in 1910. He interned at the Toronto General Hospital.

During the years following his graduation, he was a general practitioner first in Saskatchewan and later in British Columbia. He then undertook training in radiology with Lewis G Cole in New York.

After completing his studies there he joined the Toronto General Hospital as assistant radiologist and, later, the Ottawa Civic Hospital as radiologist-in-chief.

He was appointed director of the department of radiology at the Montréal General Hospital in 1925 and served the hospital in this capacity until his retirement in 1948. He is credited with having built the department into one of the outstanding radiological departments in Canada. During this same period he was chairman of the Department of Radiology at McGill University with the rank of associate professor. On retirement from active duty in both these posts, he became radiological consultant to the Montréal General Hospital and served as radiologist at the Herbert Reddy Memorial Hospital—posts he held at the time of his death. He died at the Montréal General Hospital, after an illness of six weeks, in his 68th year.

Considered the senior radiologist in Canada, Dr Ritchie was a Fellow of the Royal College of Surgeons of Canada and contributed many scientific papers and articles to Canada's medical literature. He was at one time honorary secretary-treasurer of the Canadian Association of Radiologists.

Also as a member of the University club, he was an active badminton player in his younger years, being a charter member of the now defunct Cliffside Badminton and Squash Club.

Chapter VIII •

Nuclear Medicine at McGill

Douglas Wilansky

Nuclear Medicine at McGill began in 1952 at the Royal Victoria Hosital at the instigation of Dr Martin M Hoffman. Martin was without a doubt the outstanding clinical teacher of his era and he served as Professor of Medicine at McGill and Dalhousie universities as well as at the University of British Columbia.

In 1952, with the assistance of Dr Lloyd G Stephens-Newsham, a thyroid probe and rectilinear scanner were installed in the Department of Radiology at Royal Victoria Hospital for the investigation of thyroid disorders.

During the next two to three years, this equipment was used for routine clinical testing for thyroid disease. In addition, in 1953–54, Dr Maurice Dongier (later to become Professor of Psychiatry at McGill), served as a fellow under Dr Hoffman studying the effect of acute psychiatric syndromes on thyroid function. In addition, Dr Gilbert Rosenberg studied the effect of aging on thyroid gland activity in human beings and several papers were published by both of these fellows in collaboration with Drs Hoffman and Newsham. I also set up an *in vivo* Geiger counting system for studying thyroid function in senescent animals. This work, done in collaboration with Drs Bernard Grad and Martin Hoffman, resulted in an international award of the Ciba prize for the best research on aging in 1954.

By 1954, the isotope laboratory—the precursor of a nuclear medicine service—was well developed mainly for use by endocrinologists, hematologists and surgeons. In 1955 a second thyroid function diagnostic unit was established at the Jewish General Hospital when Dr Hoffman moved there to be chief of medicine.

Several clinical papers on the scanning of thyroid nodules and apathetic hyperthyroidism were published in the *Canadian Medical Association Journal*. In addition, thyroid function in nephrotic animals was studied and further papers on this subject published in significant journals.

Dr Norman Kalant, Dr Norman Nadler, Dr Joseph Wolfson and Dr D Wilansky were engaged in developing these programs at the Jewish General Hospital.

From these clinical and experimental beginnings, full scale departments of nuclear medicine soon developed at the Royal Victoria and Jewish General Hospitals. Dr Allan Gold started thyroid scanning at Montréal General Hospital in the late nineteen fifties. Subsequently, in the mid nineteen sixties, Dr L Rosenthall was instrumental in having the first gamma camera installed at the Montréal General Hospital in collaboration with, and upon the advice of Dr A Daniel Rotenberg who was then consulting physicist at the General. Subsequently he moved to the Jewish General where a gamma camera was also installed and, simultaneously, the Royal Victoria acquired its first gamma camera.

EE King records a case of exposure of the hands for three to four months for from two to six hours daily before x-ray effects developed * [1].

Cases of conjunctivitis from x-rays have been reported by King...* [1].

* King EE. Skin, hair and nail lesions produced by the action of x-rays. *The Canadian Practitioner* 1896; 21: 789.

1. Pusey WA, Caldwell WE. *Röntgen rays in therapeutics and diagnosis*. Philadelphia, WB Saunders and Co, 1903:241 and 244

Chapter IX • History of

McMaster University

Department of Radiology

GILES STEVENSON

McMaster University was founded by the industrialist of the same name in Toronto. The university moved in the 1920s to its present site in the village of Westdale, west of Hamilton. The city had four active treatment hospitals, each with a group of radiologists providing service and education for radiography students and clinical residents. The medical school opened in 1968, with a new building functioning as a fifth acute care hospital, as a campus base for the medical and nursing schools and as a university research centre for the new Faculty of Health Sciences.

The radiologists in the existing hospitals continued in their practice groups, accepted part-time appointments in the university and became integral to the success of the residency program. Geographic full-time salaried radiologists were appointed to the new hospital, which slowly expanded and now has the highest volume of clinical radiology of the city hospitals: 91 000 examinations a year.

Two geographic full-time nuclear medicine physicians were appointed in the new centre, within the radiology department administratively but on a separate floor and with a mandate to promote research. Within nuclear medicine a radiopharmacy was developed which soon supplied materials for use in nuclear medicine in the city and further afield. A cadre of scientists gradually accumulated. They had developed and built their own positron emission tomography scanner by 1979, have made some fundamental discoveries in neuro- and pulmonary physiology, and have made progress in image handling and transmission which will lead to the development of an internal picture-archiving and communication system.

Scientists at the Cancer Centre were recruited and provided with an academic base in the Department of Radiology. They have been very active in monoclonal antibody research and in exploring the fundamental aspects of interaction between light and tissue, which is now starting to lead into animal and human work in development of laser treatment.

A radiation biologist was recruited by the hospital in 1972; the position is funded jointly by the faculties of science and health sciences. The radiation biologist and the scientists in nuclear medicine have worked on the creation of a medical physics group within the Faculty of Physics. This group won its first appointment in 1991; a second is being recruited now. There is in 1995 a critical mass of physicists within the radiology department, with a large number of graduate and post-doctoral students. The medical physics group has regular monthly meetings.

The Department of Radiology has reached a strength of 55, with 10 physicists and two chemists, 10 geographic full-time radiologists, two geographic full-time nuclear medicine physicians and 31 part time radiology faculty.

Geographic full-time radiologists have been recruited predominantly according to organ system subspecialization, with four in abdominal radiology, two in chest, two in bone, one mainly in ultrasound diagnosis and one mainly in angiography. A neuroradiologist was in place from 1970 but left in 1986 for Saudi Arabia, and a replacement has had to wait for the advent of the magnetic resonance imager, just installed.

The city of Hamilton has regionalized its medical care as follows: the General Hospital has radiologists with particular interest in cardiac, neuroscience and trauma radiology; St Joseph's has expertise in renal imaging and respirolo gy; and the Henderson General Hospital with the adjacent Ontario Regional Cancer Centre, has radiologists with special interest in cancer imaging. Nuclear medicine in these hospitals is under the Department of Medicine.

The residency programe has 14 residents, and there has been a 100 per cent success rate in the Royal College of Physicians and Surgeons of Canada examinations for the last several years. There is an annual residents and graduate students research day competition, and the undertaking of a research project is a mandatory part of the programe. Starting in 1993, second year residents have been part of the faculty's team, teaching anatomy to medical, nursing, occupational therapy and physiotherapy students. Residents rotate between the city hospitals, with fixed rotations allocated in the first year. After the first year the rotations must be done as required, but residents can choose the hospital in which they wish to work, a market pressure that encourages faculty to keep the standards high.

Over the past fifteen years there have been numerous post-residency fellows, particulary from abroad, mainly at McMaster University Medical Centre, and mainly in abdominal radiology. They have been productive in writing scientific publications and have provided much stimulation and pleasure for the geographic full-time faculty. Many of them are from hospitals in Britain and Ireland where they practice general and abdominal radiology, in many cases with endoscopy.

Chapter X • *Le Département de Radiologie:*

Université de Montréal

Guy Hébert

Les rayons X ont été découverts en 1895 par Wilhem Conrad Röntgen. Dès le 7 février 1896, John Cox de McGill University réussissait la deuxième radiographie réalisée sur le continent américain. Entretemps à Québec, Monseigneur Joseph Laflamme, professeur de physique au Petit Séminaire, faisait ses premiers essais cinq jours plus tard, soit le 12 février de la même année. Au musée du séminaire de Québec, on peut d'ailleurs admirer plusieurs clichés réalisés par Monseigneur Laflamme. D'autres religieux également professeurs de physique ont précédé les médecins dans la réalisation de radiographies.

En 1900, à son retour d'Europe, Charles DeBlois ouvre une clinique d'électricité médicale et d'hydrothérapie à Trois-Rivières, où il installe un appareil de radiographie. La même année, Henri Lasnier, après des stages à Paris et à Londres, revient à Montréal avec un appareil radiologique. Il devient radiologiste à l'hôpital Sainte-Justine. Pour sa part, Léo Parizeau est de 1906 à 1909 le radiologiste de l'hôpital Notre-Dame. Après son service militaire, il accède à la direction du service d'électroradiologie de l'Hôtel-Dieu en 1909 et y reste en poste jusqu'à sa mort en 1938. Le Dr Albert Jutras lui succède alors et devient le premier titulaire de la chaire d'électroradiologie à l'Université de Montréal.

Cependant, le département de radiologie n'a été créé qu'en 1964 et la direction en a été confiée au Dr Jean-Louis Léger.

Celui-ci est resté en poste jusqu'en 1969, année où le Dr Roger Maltais a pris la relève qu'il a assumée jusqu'en 1977. Cette année-là, c'est le Dr Jacques Saltiel qui devenait le troisième directeur du département de radiologie de l'Université de Montréal.

Depuis la découverte de Röntgen, quel essor a connu la radiologie!

Des produits de contraste permettant d'évaluer les cavités naturelles et les structures vasculaires ont considérablement amélioré l'investigation des malades et des maladies. Puis, on a appliqué les principes des ultrasons à l'évaluation de plusieurs pathologies. Le perfectionnement des ordinateurs nous a également valu la tomodensitométrie et plus récemment encore la résonance magnétique. De plus en plus, par ailleurs, les radiologistes deviennent interventionnistes, que ce soit pour effectuer des biopsies transcutanées ou pour traiter ce qui autrefois nécessitait une intervention chirurgicale sous anesthésie générale: drainage d'abcès, extraction de calculs, embolisation vasculaire, etc.

Peu après la découverte des rayons X, on les a utilisés pour traiter un certain nombre de pathologies. Là encore, l'amélioration des appareils a permis une approche de plus en plus fine et efficace, permettant de traiter plusieurs formes de cancer et d'obtenir des résultats impensables quelques années auparavant.

La médecine nucléaire n'est pas en reste; en effet, depuis le développement des premières sondes à captation, on a vu apparaître les cartographies, puis les caméras gamma suivies par la tomographie numérisée par émission simple de photons. De plus en plus, par ailleurs, la tomographie par émission de positrons trouve des applications cliniques.

Chapter XI • *A Brief History of the Department of Radiology at the*

University of Ottawa

Conway Don

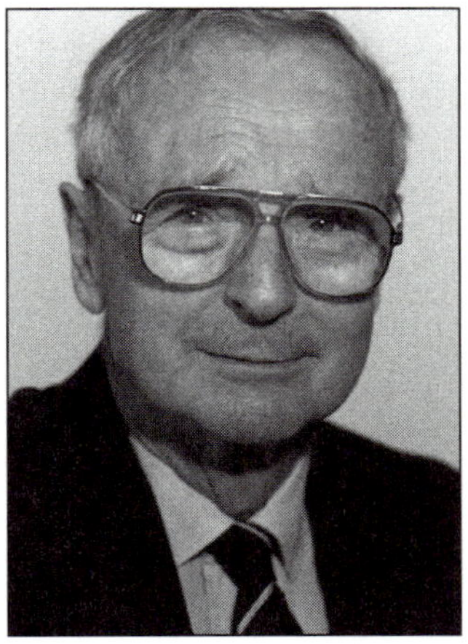

Dr Conway Don, first Professor and Chairman of Radiology, University of Ottawa

The University of Ottawa was founded by the Oblate Missionaries of Mary Immaculate in 1848 as a bilingual liberal arts college, the College of Bytown. Bytown was renamed Ottawa and became the capital of Canada in 1857. In 1861 the College was renamed the College of Ottawa, and it became the University of Ottawa in 1866. Although originally a liberal arts college, it nonetheless taught pure and applied sciences in both French and English well before the turn of the century. The 20th century marked a period of major expansion for the university, particularly in the science faculties. In 1965 it became a public, provincially funded institution, and expansion of the facilities continued. It is now the oldest and largest bilingual institution in North America.

During World War II, it became evident that Ontario needed to produce more physicians, and in 1945 the University of Ottawa founded its medical school.

The Ottawa General Hospital is the fifth oldest in Canada and was founded by the Grey Nuns of the Cross (now the Sisters of Charity of Ottawa) as a bilingual, community general hospital in 1845. Its first x-ray department was created in 1911 and then operated for three years by the Ladies Auxiliary at a total cost of $6000 (Fig. 1)! When the university decided to establish a medical school, the only clinical facilities available were at the Ottawa General Hospital, since the Ottawa Civic Hospital, a much larger institution, was then affiliated with Queen's University in Kingston. The Grey Nuns increased the bed quota by 200 to 449 in order to provide the required bed capacity for the educational programes of the new medical school.

In 1957 while I was doing a clinical fellowship at the Massachusetts General Hospital, I was approached to take over the x-ray department in Ottawa. I found that the new medical school considered its mission to be training general practitioners, and other than in pathology, which had been fully approved by the Royal College, there was virtually no postgraduate education. Medicine and surgery each had approval for one year of education. No such recognition had been granted other departments; radiology had none, and seemingly no prospect of it. One reason was the very poor relationship between the department's succession of radiologists and the administration, and the consequently poor relationship with the Canadian Association of Radiologists.

However, the mother superior, Sister Ste Philippe, convinced me that the hospital was very anxious to begin a new era in its relationship with its radiologists, and that if I came I would get every support. At the same time, the dean assured me that as soon as practicable a university department of radiology would be created. I therefore decided not to return to the University College Hospital London but to take up the challenge at Ottawa and its university, even though I was advised against this by the president of the Canadian Association of Radiologists. I may say that among my contemporaries in London my intention was regarded as evidence of profound mental instability! When I started in Ottawa, the staff in radiology at the university and the General Hospital consisted of Dermot Hurley (who left in 1967 to become chief of radiology at the newly built Riverside Hospital of Ottawa) and C. Hsu, and the total number of annual investigations was around 15 000. The assurances that the Grey Nuns had given me about supporting radiology proved very well founded, and they gave every support to the expansion of the x-ray department. Just before I left the Massachusetts General Hospital in 1957, that hospital had installed on a provisional basis the first automatic film processor, the Kodak M1; in 1958 one of the first in the world was installed at the Ottawa General Hospital, at the then inconceivable sum of $36 000 (a whole room could be equipped at that time for around $10 000). Similarly, when Dr Albert Jutras at the Hôtel Dieu Hospital in Montréal pioneered fluoroscopy by closed circuit television—now routine—the Grey Nuns provided the funds for one of the first installations in Canada; in 1975 they also funded one of the first computed tomographic scanners in Canada—the original EMI brain scanner—thus providing a service for the whole of eastern Ontario and western Québec.

The university also came through in turn, and the Department of Radiology was founded in 1958. The university, moreover, provided the department with a six-figure annual budget, unchanged for twenty-five years. Unfortunately, two of the figures were cents!

The Seldinger technique of arteriography was introduced at the Ottawa General in 1958—certainly the first in Canada and possibly the first in North America—and the workload increased dramatically from 15 000 examinations a year in 1957 to 45 000 a year in 1967 and 75 000 in 1971. In the current year (1994) the total will be about 145 000.

Recruitment of radiological staff in the early years was not easy since there was distrust of the General Hospital administration in radiological circles, but in 1964 we were able to recruit Allon Liver from the staff of the Montréal General Hospital, and in 1965 we recruited one of the only neuro-radiologists then practicing in Canada, Z Grahovac, from the University of Saskatchewan. In 1966, we added one of the first graduates from our own program, David Gray, who was on staff until 1976, when he moved to become Chief of Radiology at the newly opened Queensway Carleton Hospital; he has been Chief of Medical Staff there since 1984. Dr Gray has also been the distinguished Secretary Treasurer of the Canadian Association of Radiologists for the last seven years. In 1968 we were able to recruit Gerald Copestake, who had recently finished his term as Professor and Chairman of Radiology at the University of Western Ontario. By this time confidence in the General Hospital had been restored among the radiological community, and we had no further problems in recruiting.

In 1961 we obtained approval from the Royal College for the training of one resident per annum, and soon after that we became the second program in the university to receive full approval for training.

In 1958 Queen's University discontinued its affiliation with the Ottawa Civic Hospital (OCH), which, in 1959, became an affiliated teaching hospital of the University of Ottawa. Initially, this arrangement did not impact on the university department of radiology: In those days all training programs were approved by the Royal College on a hospital basis. The Civic Hospital had had for some years a fully approved resident training program in diagnostic radiology, and the program maintained its independent status under the direction of Glen Stoddart, Chief of Radiology at the Civic Hospital.

The Royal College, however, started to shift the basis of approval from hospital departments to university departments, and in 1971 they requested that the two hospital programs be merged in one university program. The new combined program was approved in 1972.

In the 1950s and 1960s it was difficult to find applicants of appropriate quality for an education in radiology, a problem across Canada but particularly acute in Ottawa. Nevertheless, steady progress was made, particularly after the integration of the hospital programs. Progress was greatly accelerated from 1981 when Ian Hammond became director of the Resident Training Program, a post which he held until 1989 when he was succeeded by Dr Hardy Tao of the Civic Hospital. The problem now, both in Ottawa and across Canada, is not how to find first class applicants for radiology, but how to select from so many.

In 1966, in what was perhaps an indication of the improving status of radiology in the hospital, I was elected Chief of Medical Staff, which post I held for five years, subsequently becoming the first Chief of Medical Staff at the new Ottawa General Hospital from 1977 to 1980. It has been said that busy people warrant no sympathy, as they seek their own level of stress. Practicing radiology and running university and hospital departments and the resident training program presumably did not provide me with enough stress.

In 1974 the Children's Hospital of Eastern Ontario was founded, and all pediatric facilities, including pediatric radiology, were transferred from the two general hospitals. The Chief of Radiology, recruited from the staff of the Sick Children's Hospital in Toronto, was Dr Peter McDonald, who was succeeded by Dr Mary Ann Matzinger in 1991.

In 1980 the Ottawa General Hospital was rebuilt in a new site on the Health Sciences Complex in the Alta Vista region, joining the medical school—which had been moved from the university campus—the Children's Hospital of Eastern Ontario, and the Rehabilitation Centre. At this time the order of Grey Nuns withdrew from governance of the hospital and transferred ownership to an independent corporation. Nevertheless, the change of administration did not result in any diminution of support for radiology, and the first cassetteless department in the world was installed at the opening, in collaboration with Siemens. This system is still functioning without a hitch in 1994, and the cassetteless general radiographic unit in the emergency room is still performing perfectly after functioning for twenty-four hours a day for fourteen years! In 1987 the board also provided one of the first MRI scanners in Canada; it was the only such scanner providing services for Eastern Ontario and Western Quebec for seven years.

In 1988, after thirty years of on-site training, I finished as Chairman of the Department of Radiology at the university and was succeeded by Peter McDonald, who was, in turn succeeded in 1992 by Ian Hammond. I also resigned in 1988 as Chief of the Department of Radiology at the General Hospital and was succeeded there by the present incumbent, Ian Hammond.

From its start in 1958 with a single hospital and a faculty of three radiologists giving 15 000 examinations a year, the university department now has three hospitals with a faculty of 44 diagnostic radiologists performing 350 000 examinations a year. The improved standing of radiology in the university is perhaps reflected in the fact that 12 per cent of University of Ottawa graduates applied this year to the residency matching service for radiology, as opposed to the national average of 3.8 per cent. Also, the Radiological Society of North America has awarded faculty members two international visiting professorships, the first to myself in 1993 to spend four months in the University Hospital, Kuala Lumpur, Malaysia, and the second in 1994 to Steve Millward of the Civic Hospital to spend a similar time at the Kenyatta Hospital, University of Nairobi, Kenya.

I believe the expansion in diagnostic radiology in Ottawa reflects two things. One is the staggering technological developments in radiology, with an unbelievable increase in the scope and accuracy of radiological investigations. The other is local change, namely the remarkable expansion of postgraduate training in the University of Ottawa Faculty of Medicine, from one fully approved program in 1956 to its present status as one of the larger postgraduate training institutes in Canada with 44 Royal College accredited programs in the medical specialties and subspecialties.

In Ottawa radiation oncology is the exclusive province of the Ontario Cancer Foundation. The Ottawa Clinic was founded in 1934 and was based at the Ottawa Civic Hospital, where Glen Stoddart was Chief of Radiology. He headed the Ottawa Clinic from 1952–1978. In 1958 a small branch of the cancer clinic was founded at the General Hospital under the direction of Alfred Crook, who became responsible for undergraduate teaching in radiotherapy. Radiotherapy (radiation oncology) was then and still is part of the Department of Radiology, despite several efforts I made to have it declared a separate department. The medical school faculty council has hitherto taken the view that the number of faculty involved in radiation oncology does not warrant a separate university department, but the number of faculty in the specialty has increased remarkably in the last few years, and some change seems inevitable as well as desirable.

When I arrived in Ottawa, the Civic Hospital had a fully approved program for training in radiation oncology, but recruiting in Ottawa, as elsewhere in Canada, was very limited.

In 1980, when the General Hospital was rebuilt, there was a considerable expansion in the General Hospital division of the Ottawa Cancer Clinic, in terms of facilities, equipment, staff, and patient treatments, and the two divisions now are approximately equal in size, each treating approximately 1400 patients a year.

As facilities and staff in the Ottawa Cancer Clinic grew, interest increased in radiotherapy training, under the aegis of successive directors of the clinic Dr Michael Tulloh, Dr Gordon Catton and, since 1988, Dr Bill Evans. The resident training program also made great progress, particularly when Dr André Girard became program director. He had been named the first head of the newly formed Division of Radiation Oncology in the Department of Radiology in 1991. The radiation oncology training program, now under the direction of Bernd Esche, is currently one of the largest in Canada, with 13 residents, and a faculty of 27 radiologists and physicists.

At both general hospitals nuclear medicine had been part of the departments of internal medicine; radiology residents rotated through these departments during training. In 1982 Dr Brian Lentle, when he arrived to succeed Dr Randy Patterson as Chief of Radiology at the Civic Hospital, developed nuclear medicine services in radiology. In 1984 he left Ottawa (presumably and, perhaps, rather surprisingly not finding running the Civic Hospital department sufficiently stressful) and proceeded by way of the Cross Cancer Hospital in Edmonton, to Vancouver to become Chief of Radiology at the Vancouver General Hospital and Chairman of the Department of Radiology at the University of British Columbia. Hopefully, he has managed to find sufficient stress by also becoming Chief of Medical Staff at the General Hospital. He continues to hold all three posts.

Dr Garry Belanger, one of our former residents, served five years as chief at the Civic Hospital following Dr Brian Lentle and did some valuable recruiting to the radiological staff. He was succeeded in 1989 by Dr Karen Gulenchyn, and she has further consolidated nuclear medicine within the Department of Radiology. Among other accomplishments, she has recruited Dr Michael Chamberlain from the nuclear medicine staff of the University of Western Ontario.

Queen's University

William A Jones

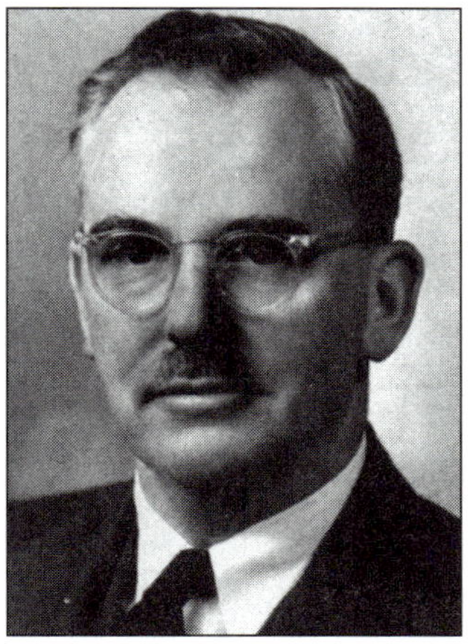

Dr Ronald G Burr

The early history of radiology at Queen's is bound up with the Kingston General Hospital and the name of Dr James Third. The memory of Third's contemporaries is short, and the records of the time are sketchy. However, a few facts stand out which reflect much credit on Third.

Professor Röntgen had announced in December 1895 the discovery of a new ray, the x-ray, invisible light, or "light that was never on land or sea."

When this discovery was announced, Third was a young medical graduate, and he became enthusiastically interested. At his instigation, in 1896 the first x-ray machine was placed in the hospital. Dr GW Mylks Sr recalled that in the late summer or fall of 1896 Third coated a piece of cardboard with a fluorescent medium which had been recommended and made his own fluoroscope. Mylks was a third year medical student at the time and an undergraduate intern. The day came when Third demonstrated his new fluoroscope, and that day Mylks saw a wonder: he observed the bones of his own living hand and watched their movements on the screen.

Third retired from his position as medical superintendent of the hospital and its first radiologist in 1897. Later, a succession of medical superintendents was responsible for operating the x-ray machine. Dr HA Boyce was one of these physicians. Dr Matheson, subsequently Professor and Chairman of Anatomy, was another medical superintendent to be responsible for the hospital x-ray machine. Meanwhile, Third carried on his radiological practice in his private office.

Some mention must be made of certain documentary evidence of Third's work. His writings give an insight into early thoughts regarding x-rays. Partly they reveal to us a man who was ahead of his time. For example, the *Kingston Medical Quarterly* published in October 1899 a paper by Third, "The Roentgen Ray—Early Diagnosis of Tubercular and Other lesions."[1] [It is noted in the article that it had been "[r]ead before the Kingston Medical Society November, 1899"—editor's note.]

He also noted that "radiology as an aid to surgical diagnosis was no longer questioned: fractures and dislocations had become easily diagnosed; foreign bodies and necrotic areas of bone readily located. Much too much we fear, has been claimed for radiographs as a means of diagnosis of biliary, renal and vesical calculi."

Third at that time did not place much faith in x-rays for therapy. "To the therapeutic value of the x-ray we have given comparatively little attention believing, as we did, that it was to the field of diagnosis that its operations largely belonged and that any therapeutic effects were merely incidental."

His observations on the use of x-rays in obstetrics are as follows:

> *In the field of obstetrics the results are interesting, but so far of little practical value. We have diagnosed the position of the viable foetus in utero by fluoroscopic examination. This method, however, possesses no distinct advantage over the older and tried methods, and until better results are obtainable, its use cannot be seriously encouraged.*

The author goes on to state the accuracy with which the diagnosis and the extent of disease of a tubercular joint can be determined. One skiagram* which is reproduced carries the legend "Joint lines not very well shown." This is certainly not an overstatement. It makes one realize that x-ray diagnosis in those days was, to some extent at least, an act of faith. (Even today, of course one believes that at times such diagnosis may be an act of faith and an expression of hope and that charity is required to accept it.) [This is Dr Jones writing nearly fifty years ago—editor's note.]

In his paper Third was a strong advocate of x-ray diagnosis of diseases of the lungs, particularly tuberculosis. He noted that x-rays "sounded a warning note when auscultation and percussion have indicated no departure from normal." One can see that he was in advance of his time. It was thirty years before it was generally accepted that a radiographic diagnosis of pulmonary tuberculosis could show the lesions in advance of physical examination.

Third placed his faith in fluoroscopy as the method of choice and thought skiagrams unlikely to replace fluoroscopy in thoracic work. From his point of view at that time, how right he seems. Even the most advanced of his contemporaries, using the first attempts at intensifying screens in 1898, were unable to obtain a "radiograph of the thorax" in less than 30 seconds.

Again, in the *Kingston Medical Quarterly* he contributed an article entitled, "Some of the Diagnostic and Therapeutic Uses of the Roentgen Rays" in April 1902.

Three years after his scepticism about the value of x-ray therapy, Third had become an advocate of x-ray therapy and he lists cancer of the lip, rodent ulcer, lupus vulgaris, psoriasis and cancer of the breast as amenable to treatment. He says, however, "one word of caution in conclusion." (He uses more than one word but what he says is apt.) "As a therapeutic agent the outlook is hopeful, but let us 'make haste slowly.' As a diagnostic agent the great value of the ray cannot be questioned, but we must not lose sight of the fact that it is a powerful weapon, a double-edged sword. For the present, at least, let us consider it a valuable adjunct to other means of diagnosis rather than a keen competitor for supremacy." He goes on to say, "There are three things that never should be placed in the hands of the patient: the hypodermic syringe, the thermometer and the x-ray photograph". Any objections?

In *Queen's Medical Quarterly* of July 1905 Dr WH Rankin (a visiting New York surgeon) writes in an article on "Abscess of the Lung," "As an aid in clearing up the diagnosis in the lung empyema, we may use the x-ray, but

Queen's University

Queen's University has an esteemed place in Canadian scholarship out of proportion to its size. In radiology this has been especially true. As early as the 1930s, at a time when specialization was usually achieved in an unstructured way, the innovations there in creating a formal university-based educational program presaged much that was to happen later in Canadian medicine. It will be apparent from the stories in this volume both of radiology at Queen's and of the Canadian Association of Radiologists that Dr WA Jones was central to these developments locally and nationally. It is fortunate, therefore, that Dr Jones has left us an account in his own words. His account is complemented by a description of more recent events by Dr Robert Nolan, his successor twice removed.

At first Dr Jones comes across from the written record as a consummate diplomat and someone of vision and insight but a somewhat austere individual. And then I found a letter of his signed with the inevitable "WA Jones" but with a line added which read "Jonesey to you." This, and the devotion of his residents who called themselves collectively "The Jones boys," suggests that we should not mistake the formality of correspondance in the early years of this century for evidence of a lack of human warmth. That is a mistake I almost made.

— Brian Lentle

it is not entirely to be depended upon, for, unless the tube is directly over the abscess, the shadow on the plate may be misleading. Should the abscess have ruptured and the cavity contracted and the heart drawn over, the x-ray could be of little service and it would be quite misleading in the case of an aneurysm of the aorta." This excerpt leads one to suspect that even in those early days radiologists were having trouble with their clinical colleagues.

In 1918 Dr JP Quigley, having returned from army service overseas, became radiologist of the Kingston General Hospital, Hôtel Dieu Hospital and Sydenham Military Hospital. He gave excellent service to these institutions.

In 1925 it was decided to give control of the Department of Radiology to a specialist confining his practice to radiology. Dr Quigley was offered the position, but he was too fond of general practice and did not wish to give up his patients. To confine himself to radiology exclusively was something he could not bring himself to do.

In December 1925, therefore, the present writer Dr WA Jones, who practiced his first radiology in England under Major AH Pirie in 1919, took over the control of the Department of Radiology of the Kingston General Hospital. He became the Lecturer in Radiology of the medical faculty. In 1930 he became professor in charge of the department.

This was a period of rapid change in radiology, with new techniques and new interpretations appearing in rapid sequence. The department expanded rapidly, and in 1932 the Ontario Institute of Radiotherapy (Kingston Division) was added to it. This expansion brought modern deep x-ray therapy to Kingston. Dr Frederick Etherington, who had been carrying on radium therapy privately for several years, turned his radium over to the clinic. The Ontario government brought the amount of radium up to over 400 mg giving a quite adequate amount for treatment purposes. (This amount was later increased to 700 mg, and a cobalt-60 beam unit was later installed). The institute filled a great need. In 1935 Dr RC Burr joined the department enlivening the hospital with his buoyant optimism.

Between 1925 and 1954 about 35 young men have been trained in radiology and half of them have stayed in radiological practice full time. Undergraduate teaching of radiology is given more stress at Queen's than in most Canadian universities. A paper covering this matter was published in the March 1954 issue of the *Canadian Medical Association Journal*.[2]

In 1930 a course leading to the DMR (Diploma of Medical Radiology) was started at Queen's. The diploma has been awarded to only five graduate students to date.

In September 1939 Jones was granted leave of absence by the university for military service and for six years Burr, almost alone and under great handicap, competently carried on radiology at the hospital, as well as the teaching at Queen's.

On the return of Jones in September 1945 the work had so grown that it was decided to divide the department. Since then, diagnostic radiology has been under the control of Jones, and the therapeutic radiology under Burr.

For a short time Dr Eric E Johnson was associated with Jones and Burr; he has since moved into private radiological practice in London. Then Dr Bruce T Colwell became attached to the department. AF Holloway, MSc, was the physicist in the Division of Radiotherapy.

The history of radiology at Queen's would be incomplete without the story of the work of a beloved former professor of physics, Professor JK Robertson. Robertson took a great interest in radiology and in between 1910 and 1920 began to give the teaching of x-ray physics a prominent place in the medical curriculum, a development that has proven an incalculable advantage to Queen's students. Robertson also published text books on this subject, which, through a number of editions, have circulated far and wide over this continent and in Great Britain. Where graduate radiology is taught, Robertson's name is well known. Since Robertson's retirement in 1951, Professor BW Sargent has ably carried on this work.

Although not directly connected with the clinical department of radiology Professor JA Gray, Chown Research Professor of Physics at Queen's (1924–1952), has also influenced clinical radiology. Gray is probably best known for his work on x-rays and radium. Working before and after World War I, he showed experimentally that there was a change in the wave length of x- and gamma-rays produced by scattering in light elements. This change was later demonstrated spectroscopically and explained theoretically by AH Compton and is referred to as the Compton Effect.

Thus, radiology at Queen's has run the full gamut of development. Within a year of Röntgen's amazing discovery its implications had been appreciated by one of our clinical staff. Over the years the clinical department has attempted to keep abreast of the developments in diagnostic and therapeutic radiology and has been fortunate in having had associated with it two leaders in the field of radiological physics. Much more lies in the future.

Acknowledgements:
Reprinted with some editing and slight abbreviation from the *Queen's Alumnni Review*, Kingston, Ontario, May–June, 1954, and published with permission, as well as with the permission of Dr Jones' daughter Mrs Margaret Roberts of Manotick, Ontario.

Chapter XIII • *An Update on Radiology at*

Queen's University

Robert L Nolan

Dr William A Jones, who wrote the piece on the early history at Queen's which preceeds this, had been appointed Head of X-ray and Physical Therapy in 1930. He then had the rank of lecturer in the Faculty of Medicine at Queen's University. In that era the British system of university promotion was in effect. In this system there is a single professor (equivalent to the modern Canadian designation of professor-and-chairman), the successively lower ranks being senior lecturer, lecturer and junior lecturer. It is thus likely that Dr Jones' position was equivalent to that of assistant professor. In 1935 Dr RC Burr, a surgeon with an Edinburgh fellowship, joined Dr Jones.

Queen's had offered a Diploma in Medical Radiology (DMR) from 1930. The curriculum included one academic session at the university and two terms of clinical education mixed with service of 11 months each. The course fee was $150.00, the examination fee $100.00.

After the hiatus caused by the war, Drs Jones and Burr divided responsibilities in 1946 ; Dr Jones, as a full professor, was responsible for diagnostic services, Dr Burr, assistant professor, was in charge of "radiotherapy and physical therapy." By 1955 this divide was even greater with separate Diplomas in Medical Radiation Diagnosis (DMRD) and Therapy (DMRT).

Both Drs Jones and Burr later served as presidents of the Canadian Association of Radiologists. [Dr Burr is at the present time—1995 —retired in Kingston but has been able to supply the editors with valuable materials and contacts in the preparation of this volume].

Drs Jones and Burr can be credited not only for creating a golden age in radiology at Queen's but also for a considerable impact on the subsequent shape of Canadian radiology. That age gave way to change in 1960 with the appointment of Dr SL Fransman, a graduate of the University of Amsterdam, as Professor and Head of Radiology. Then Dr Burr was appointed Professor of Radiotherapy, and Dr Jones became the first Professor Emeritus of Radiology in 1961.

In 1966 Queen's agreed to the division of radiology into Departments of Diagnostic Radiology (head, Dr Fransman) and Therapeutic Radiology (first head, Dr Burr).

In 1977 the arrival of a General Electric large-aperture computed tomographic scanner signified the transition into a modern Department.

Ultrasonography followed in 1979. In that year the diploma courses were discontinued, and residents could seek certication as specialists by completion of the examinations of the Royal College of Physicians and Surgeons. In 1980 Dr TW (Tom) Challis was appointed Professor and Head of Diagnostic Radiology. He was succeeded by the writer in 1991 first as Acting Head, and later in 1992 as Professor and Head.

The arrival of a magnetic resonance imager in 1994 meant that a full range of diagnostic services was provided in the department; the faculty numbers 14, the residents 11. Dr Eric Sauerbrei, a professor serving as research director, provided national leadership in bringing together people in similar roles from programs across the country. In such ways the legacies of Drs Third and Jones live on.

A plaque made using a magnifying glass used by Dr WA Jones in his practice

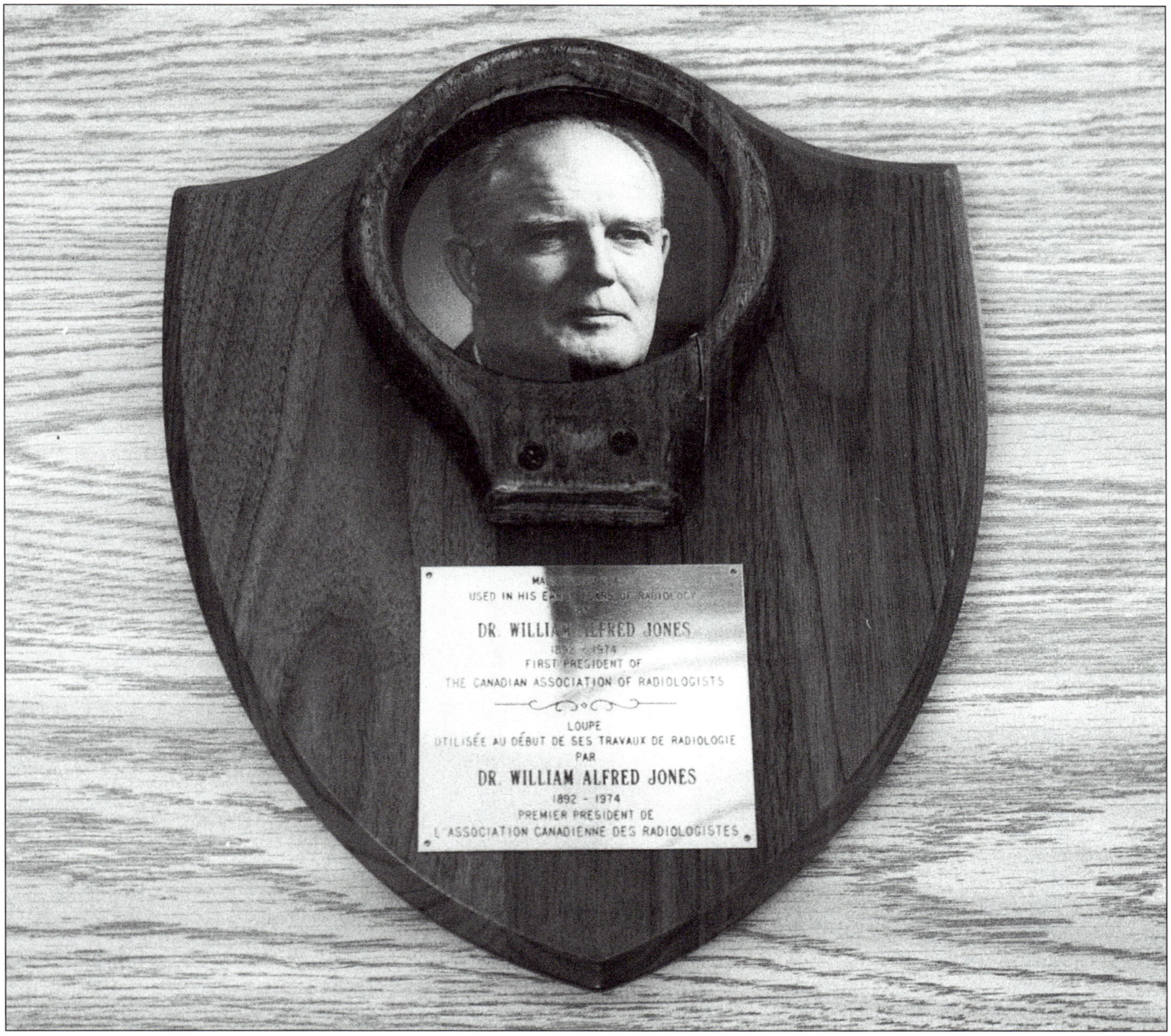

Chapter XIV • *Medical Imaging at*

Royal University Hospital

and the University of Saskatchewan

C Stuart Houston

DR EARLE WESTON SPENCER

The history of the radiology training program at the University Hospital is largely the history of two men, Dr Spencer and Dr Kent.

EW Spencer was born on August 15, 1906 at Port Huron, Michigan. He received his medical education at the University of Manitoba, graduating with his doctorate in medicine (MD) in 1931. After a period of general practice in Alberta, at Brandon and at Rivers, Manitoba, he took training in diagnostic radiology under the guidance of Dr Digby Wheeler at the St Boniface Hospital in Winnipeg. While still a resident in radiology in Winnipeg, Dr Spencer wrote "Simplified Planigraphy."[1] An article quoted in Glasser's *Medical Physics* (Vol 1, 1944, p1267) as the definitive mathematical proof of tomography.

Dr Spencer registered with the Saskatchewan College of Physicians and Surgeons on September 9, 1938. When Dr EE Shepley, the Chief of the Department of Radiology at Saskatoon City Hospital retired at the end of 1938, Dr E W Spencer took over his position, effective January 1939. Spencer also found time to obtain his diploma in diagnostic radiology from the American Board of Radiology in 1939.

In July 1940 he enlisted with the No 8 General Hospital. While overseas, he studied therapeutic radiology and obtained the diploma of medical radiology from the Royal College of Physicians and Surgeons of England in 1943. He was discharged from the Army on February 22, 1945 and shortly thereafter became the Acting Director and subsequently Director of the Saskatoon Cancer Clinic. The Cancer Clinic at that time was located in a small wing on the second floor of Saskatoon City Hospital.

As a radiotherapist with the Saskatchewan Cancer Commission,

Spencer developed a radium dosage calculator which he and physicist Dr Harold Johns described in the *American Journal of Roentgenology*.[2] One of these calculators is on display in the Spencer Memorial Library in Royal University Hospital, a gift from Dr Johns.

Dr Spencer's prime interest was diagnostic radiology. When Dr Richard DeLancey Johnson retired as the Director of the Department of Radiology at St Paul's Hospital, Saskatoon on July 25, 1946, Dr Spencer accepted the position. In addition to his position as chief of the department, he was also the consultant radiologist for the Saskatoon Sanatorium and for the Department of Veterans' Affairs, which, during the war and for some years afterward, maintained a hospital at the air force base in Saskatoon.

In March 1947 Spencer joined Dr AB MacDonell, Chief of the Department of Radiology at Saskatoon City Hospital, in his private practice in the Avenue Building, which had opened on February 4, 1946. In 1949 Dr Spencer was elected president of the Canadian Association of Radiologists. In 1950 he was president of the medical staff at St Paul's Hospital in Saskatoon.

Dr Spencer carried on in these various duties until the University Hospital opened in Saskatoon late in 1954. At that time Dr Spencer was appointed Professor of Radiology at the University of Saskatchewan as well as Chief of the Department of Diagnostic Radiology of the University Hospital.

Dr Spencer had one assistant, Dr Sidney P Traub, a neuroradiologist, who came in early 1955 and left in 1962 to be Professor and Head of Radiology at the University of Oklahoma. One of Spencer's first two residents, Dr Michael J Smart, went to Mount Auburn Hospital, Cambridge, Massachusetts for a year of fellowship training in GI radiology under Dr Richard Schatzki and then returned for two years as the third staff radiologist. Smart then left for a private radiology practice in Nanaimo, British Columbia. Other residents who trained under Dr Spencer were Joe Sungaila, Barney Reilly, Gordon Bray, Michael Kenny, Clarence Chouinard, Bob Little, Stuart Houston and Gerry Levell.

On November 15, 1962 Dr Spencer left the University Hospital in Saskatoon and moved to Ellsworth, Maine as Chief of the Department of Radiology at the Maine Coast Memorial Hospital. In 1965 he moved back to Canada to serve as Chief of the Department of Diagnostic Radiology at Digby General Hospital, Nova Scotia, until his retirement in 1974. Dr Spencer died at Halifax, Nova Scotia on March 11, 1976.

As Dr AW Becker said, at the dedication of the EW Spencer Memorial Library on 23 April 1979:

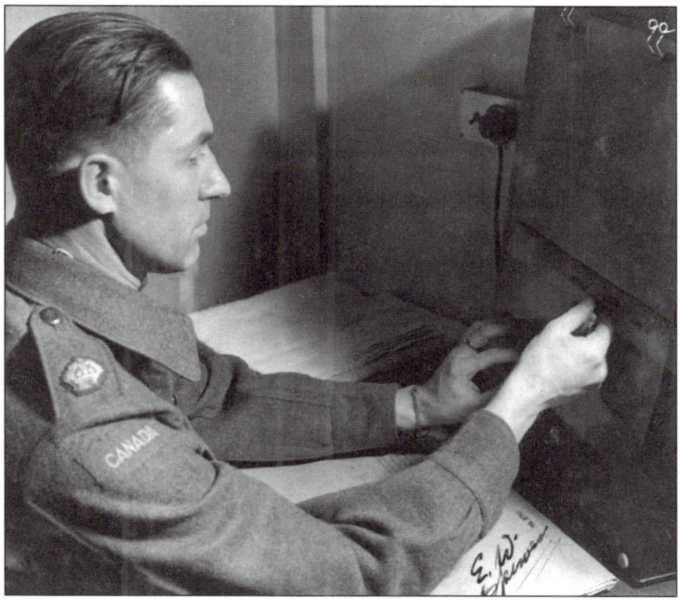

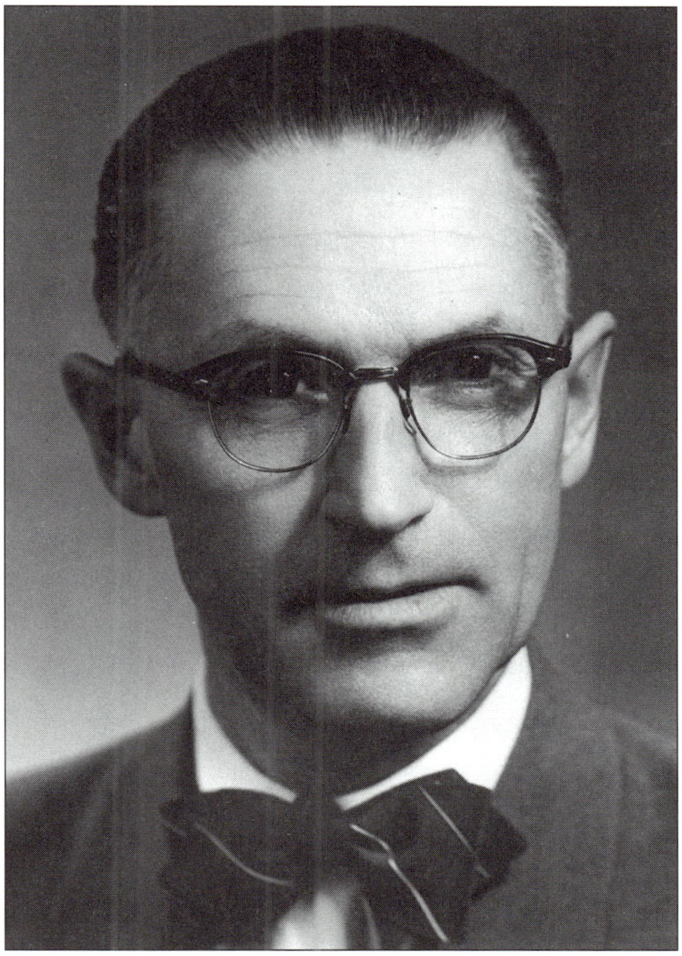

Top and above
Dr Earle Weston Spencer

Dr Spencer had an open mind and was quick to grasp new ideas. He is credited with designing and constructing one of the first tomograms in western Canada while still in training with Dr. Digby Wheeler at St Boniface Hospital in Winnipeg. As you may suspect, this was hand powered, a far cry from the push button computerized tomography which is in use today.

In therapeutic radiology, Dr Spencer designed a slide rule that could be used for calculating radium dosage. To my knowledge he had no special training in mathematics; thus, to produce a complicated slide rule he had to be some type of genius. One of the original rules is on display along with the article describing its use.

His hobbies were music, photography, travelling [particularly in his private plane]. Somewhere along the line he lost his directional beam, as we were forever getting lost when we flew with him. I am sure that this did not deter his path to Heaven. Those of us who knew him count ourselves fortunate for he was indeed a fine man. The irritations of medicare in 1962 forced him to locate elsewhere.

HENRY PETER KENT

It was a happy day for the University of Saskatchewan on April 1, 1963 when Dr HP Kent was appointed Professor and Head of the Department of Diagnostic Radiology, and a sad day when he died on July 27, 1990.

Dr Kent was born on April 30, 1915. He was a private person who rarely mentioned anything about his past, but he did tell me that his father at one time was director general of the giant Siemens Company for Spain, Portugal and Morocco, and was stationed in Madrid. Dr Kent obtained his BA and MA at Cambridge University in 1937 and 1941, respectively, and his batchelor of medicine (MB), and of surgery (BCh) from Cambridge in 1942. He was a regimental medical officer with the 17th LAA Regiment, Regular Army, 1943–1944, stationed in Naples, Italy and General Duty Officer, Malaria Officer and temporary Company Commander of the 10th Field Ambulance, Royal Army Medical Corps, 1944–1945, during the campaign in Greece. He took the Millbank Course in Radiology in London in 1945–46 and was a graded radiologist with the 94th British Military Hospital in Hamburg, Germany, 1946–47. In 1947 he demobilized with the rank of W/S Captain.

Dr Kent trained under Dr MH Jupe in the London Hospital from 1948–1950 and then was a consultant radiologist and secretary of the medical staff committee at the Hackney Hospital, London, 1951–52. At Hackney, with a single illuminator, he could view only one large film at a time, but films were scarce and used sparingly. Early in 1953, he moved to Canada to become the radiologist at the Medical Arts Clinic in Regina. Dr Kent was keenly interested in academic medicine and on April 1, 1963, a few months after Dr Spencer's departure, he happily accepted an appointment as the Professor and Head of Diagnostic Radiology at the University of Saskatchewan.

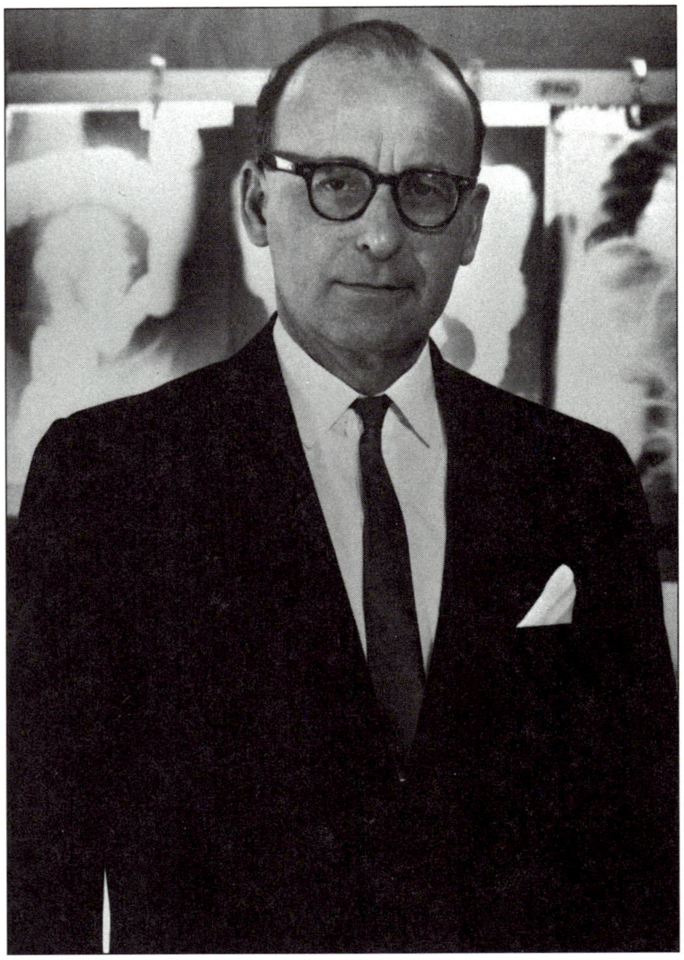

Dr Henry Peter Kent

A superb general radiologist, Peter Kent worked efficiently, rarely missing a significant observation or diagnosis. He enjoyed teaching radiology residents and was a disciplined, organized administrator. He lectured widely at meetings of the Canadian Association of Radiologists and as a visiting professor at other medical colleges. He was elected a Fellow of the Royal Society of Medicine, London in 1948, and a Fellow of the American College of Radiology in 1974. His publications included two scientific papers while a registrar, five as a private practitioner of radiology in Regina and two papers, one editorial and one memorial while department head. In later years he researched the early development of hospitals in Mexico and in Spain.

He was secretary of (and the only medical doctor on) the University Hospital Role Study, which reported in 1980. Keenly interested in continuing medical education

(CME), he served as Chairman of the Faculty and the Dean's Advisory Committee on CME from 1965 through 1971. He was the second person to receive the University of Saskatchewan CME Award of Merit, in 1975. He served on the executive of the Faculty of Medicine, 1971–1977. He was Chairman of the Medical Advisory Committee, University Hospital, 1969–1972 and served as a member and chairman of many hospital committees throughout his tenure. As part of these duties, he wrote a number of administrative documents entitled "Rules and Procedures for the College of Medicine," "Radiological Referral Centres," "CT Scanner," "Anaesthetic Practices in Saskatchewan," "Division of Oncology" and "Proposals for Bed Allocations at University Hospital." Interested in maintaining standards in non-academic and rural hospitals, he was Chairman of the Saskatchewan College of Physicians and Surgeons' Advisory Committee on Medical Imaging, 1982–1985. He was President of the Section of Radiology of the Saskatchewan Medical Association, 1965–66 and was Commissioner and Vice-Chairman of the Saskatchewan Cancer Commission, 1973–76. He relinquished the headship on June 30, 1982 at the age of 67, but continued to work full time (at half pay) for another two years, and then half-time for another three years as professor emeritus. His retirement party was held on May 12, 1989.

It will be evident from the above that Dr Kent was a conscientious worker who took delight in onerous jobs, while allowing his younger assistant to do the fun things in radiology such as serving on the test committees and examining boards of the Royal College and for five years editing the *Journal of the Canadian Association of Radiologists*. Dr Kent was a skillful critic of manuscripts and a tremendous help in preparing my early book reviews and scientific papers. He translated papers from French, Spanish and German, encouraging and helping junior staff in every way possible.

He ran a good department, working long hours. Almost every night and on weekends he took a briefcase full of documents for further study at home. He belonged to the old school.

It was typical of his modesty that Dr Kent left a specific request that there be no funeral or memorial service of any kind for him. He is remembered through the HP Kent Teaching Room in the new MRI wing of the Royal University Hospital.

Dr Kent's logic was inexorable. When one of the technologists came to him and suggested that female radiology technicians should be allowed to wear pantsuits and different colored uniforms, he immediately pointed out the inconsistency in giving the name of "uniform" to something that was non-uniform—but nevertheless gave his consent. Although he was a smoker, and the rest of us had many health problems, he seemed indestructible throughout his working years. An ardent upland game hunter, he could keep up with hunters much younger than himself. His garden was another favourite extracurricular activity. Dr Kent's longstanding interest in art and history led to an interest in genealogy. This interest, centered primarily on Mrs Kent's family, became his passion in his retirement.

He is survived by his wife, Judith; his daughter, Ariane E Phillips and her husband, David, of Edmonton; his son, Richard S Kent and his wife, Celeste, of Ottawa; his granddaughter, Sarah C Phillips; his grandsons, Graham and Stephen Kent; and his sister-in-law, Dr BR Salz of Saskatoon.

RECENT HISTORY

Dr CS Houston became department head on July 1, 1982 for a five-year term. He soon obtained approval to change the name of the university department, which included the hospital departments of Diagnostic Radiology and Nuclear Medicine, to the Department of Medical Imaging. When Houston stepped down, he was succeeded by Dr Stanley Tchang who took three successive one-year temporary appointments as head. Dr Kenneth C Chow then took one year as acting head, 1990–91. Dr Tchang then accepted a three-year term as head from 1991 through 1994.

Over the years, the department has had a close involvement with teaching of medical students at all levels. A higher percentage of Saskatchewan graduates chose diagnostic radiology than any other specialty except internal medicine. More radiology trainees have stayed in Saskatchewan than trainees for most other specialties.

Chapter XV • A Century of Radiology at the

University of Toronto

Edward Shorter

The University of Toronto occupies a somewhat distinctive position in the history of radiology. In few other medical centres is a single university department responsible for such a large population and such a variety of teaching hospitals. In the beginning the radiology department of the University of Toronto was mainly situated in a single hospital, Toronto General Hospital. The hospital controlled the academic department and not the other way around as was so often the case elsewhere. Because the Toronto General Hospital provided the seedling from which radiology in Toronto and in much of English-speaking Canada grew, the story of a century of radiology at the University of Toronto is a story predominantly situated at Toronto General Hospital.

EARLY DAYS: 1896–1917

The story began on the streets. Early in 1896, just weeks after Wilhelm Conrad Röntgen on New Year's Day had sent out prints of an article describing his new discovery, "A man appeared in the entrance hall of a Yonge Street [main street] theatre with a small coil-type X-ray machine and a hand fluoroscope, through which, for a small charge, people were allowed to look at the bones of their extremities." To drum up business the operator frequently demonstrated the device on his own hand, ending up with "a rather severe X-ray burn."

This otherwise unknown man sought treatment at the office of Dr Edmund King. A former military surgeon with an interest in pathology who was then on the staff of St Michael's Hospital, King was curious about the burn. After learning how the patient had received it, King ordered an x-ray outfit built for himself.[1] On

February 10, 1896 he demonstrated it to members of the Toronto Camera Club.[2] In 1896 and 1897 King appeared at meetings of the Toronto Clinical Society, fluoroscope in hand, letting members "examine their own and their fellows' osseous framework."[3] It was apparently in these February days of 1896 (and at the latest by April) that King started using the primitive fluoroscope in his practice,[4,5] and the credit for introducing clinical radiology to Toronto goes to him.

Meanwhile, radiology was arriving with equal rapidity in the Toronto hospitals. First to use the new technology, in February 1896, was the Toronto Grace Hospital, a homeopathic institution.[6] This coincided with the introduction of radiology at McGill University in Montréal, the institution with which the University of Toronto was then having a friendly competition.[7]

In February 1896 the University of Toronto also saw great interest in radiology. A Toronto graduate student in chemistry studying in Heidelberg had sent home an offprint of Röntgen's article. This stimulated a group of physicists and chemists, led by JC McLennan, a demonstrator in physics at the university to come together on February 6 and take pictures of various objects, including a human hand, with a Crookes' tube.[8] The group included at least one medical member, Dr Charles Sheard of Trinity Medical College, who was quoted in the *Toronto Evening Star* as saying that x-ray experiments were underway.[9] It is to McLennan, however, that credit properly goes for introducing radiology to the university. One week later, other university experimenters took the first "skiagraph" (from the Greek word for "shadow") to have survived from this era, showing the skeleton of one of the group members'

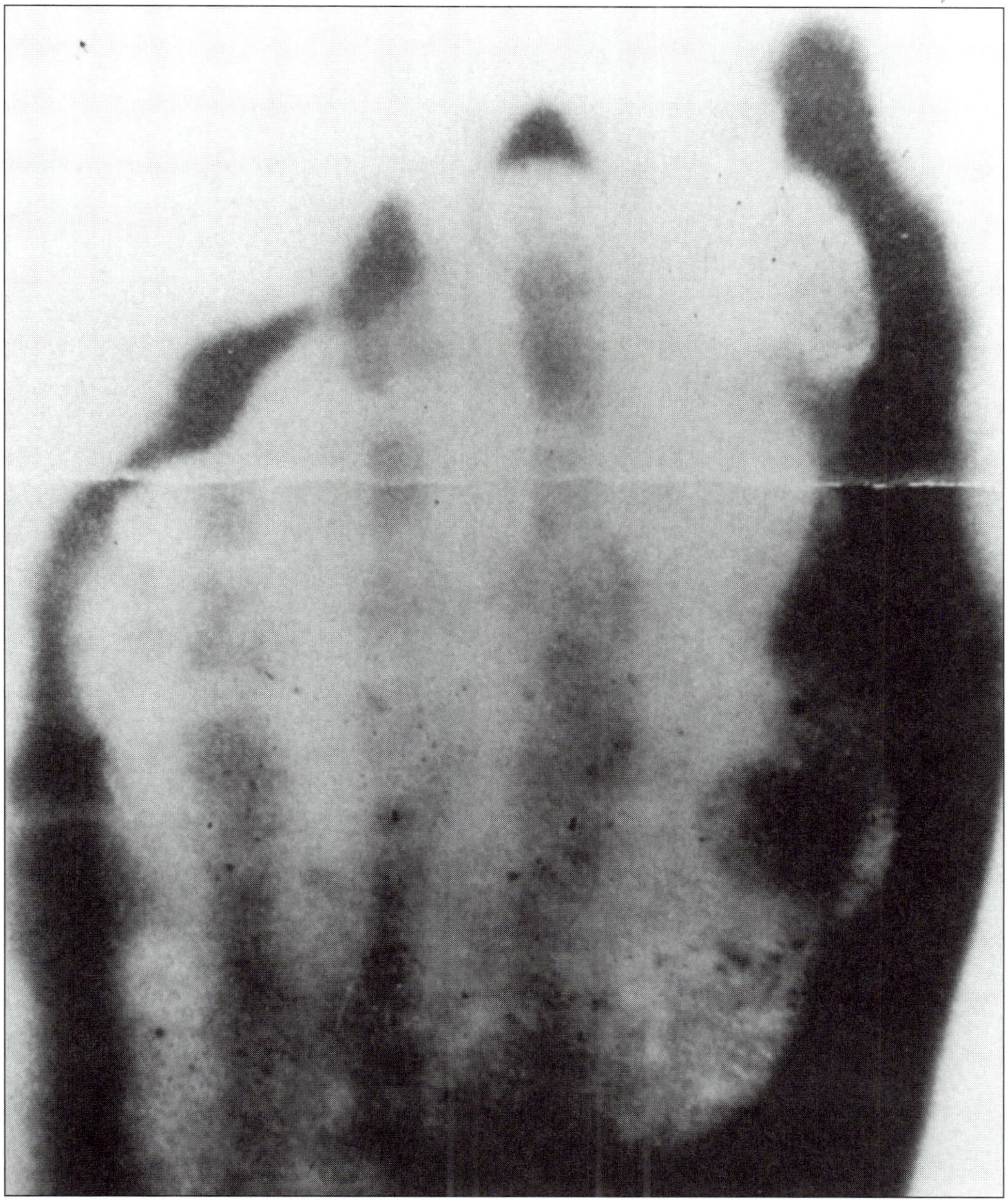

An early radiograph of a foot with a bunion, taken February 1896 at the University of Toronto feet (obtained after a 30-min exposure). The *Evening Telegram* published a line drawing of the photograph of the foot, showing a bunion.[10] Given such enthusiasm, the medical press gloated in March that Toronto and Montréal would take back seats to none in "what is incorrectly called 'the new photography.'"[11] And the lay press lauded "the absolute safety of the much-prized vacuum tubes."[12]

Toronto's two big teaching hospitals—the Toronto General Hospital and the Hospital for Sick Children—also adopted Röntgen's new invention in 1896. The Hospital for Sick Children acquired its apparatus sometime before September 1896. Their annual report for 1896 displayed their enthusiasm for the new apparatus: "To show that the trustees are keenly alive to the progress of science, as applied to the healing art, our X-ray equipment has just been imported from Europe, and this wonderful evolution of the scientific genius of the 19th century is added to the fine mechanical appliances on hand."[13] The surgeons of that hospital put the new apparatus to work immediately in setting fractures. Eager donors contributed ever more pieces of equipment. Charles R Dickson, who had two medical degrees (Queen's University in 1880 and New York University Medical College in 1881), had already been appointed as "electrician on staff" at the Hospital for Sick Children and thus in 1896 became, practically speaking, the first academic radiologist in Toronto.

Exactly when Dickson left the hospital is unknown. But we do know that in 1906 Samuel Cummings became the hospital's radiologist. Cummings, who like Dickson had medical degrees from both Canadian and American universities, cut Toronto's first scientific profile in radiology. As with many physicians of his day, Cummings was oriented toward Central Europe, having taken postgraduate courses in yearly visits to Germany before World War I. He also owned a large German medical library and spoke the language fluently.[14,15]

Cummings, like Dickson, remained at the Hospital for Sick Children only a short time. On his departure a change occurred that was not atypical of early radiology departments. The service was turned over, not to another physician, but to a radiographer, B Frank Fenner, who ran the radiology service at the hospital until he was lured away by the rival Toronto General Hospital. In those days radiology was not considered an exacting enough subject to require a medical specialist.

Radiology arrived at the Toronto General Hospital slightly later than at the Hospital for Sick Children. In November 1896 the board of trustees of Toronto General Hospital authorized "on recommendation of the Medical Superintendent, apparatus for the Röntgen Rays for use in surgery, comprising coil, tubes, cells etc."[16] The device did not arrive until 1897. The minutes of the board of trustees from 1900 onward detail the purchase of large amounts of equipment, but all of it was commissioned under the aegis of radiographer Fenner, who apparently conducted the investigations himself, interpreted them, and received a portion of the fees. (A certain Dr Todd mysteriously appeared in April 1911, resigning in November of that year to hand the reins back to Fenner.[17])

BUILDING A DEPARTMENT: 1917–1949

A new chapter was opened in the history of academic radiology in Toronto in 1917 with the arrival of Gordon Earle Richards at the Toronto General Hospital. Richards dominated the history of radiology in Toronto from 1917 until his death in 1949. Born in 1885 in Lyn, Ontario, Richards had been a gold medalist at the University of Toronto as a medical student, graduating in 1908. He first practiced in British Columbia as the medical officer at a mining camp.[18] A colleague whom he met there, Dr CW Prowd, directed his attention to radiology, and when Richards served overseas in the First World War with the Royal Army Medical Corps, he wrote an interesting note for the *British Medical Journal* on the radiologic localization of foreign bodies. Reflecting on the pressures of combat surgery Richards commented, "One of the chief virtues of this method is speed, which is important when a large amount of work is at hand."[19] It is unknown why Richards was able to leave the army during the war or why Toronto General Hospital singled him out as the physician who should end the Fenner era.

Richards came to Toronto under the same financial arrangements that prevailed at several Canadian radiology departments in those years: the service was to be run essentially as a private business. The hospital would buy the equipment and provide space, and the radiologists would receive a portion of the fees (which the hospital took charge of collecting from patients), pay support-staff salaries, and retain the residual. As also was common at the time, the radiologists were additionally charged with running the "hydrotherapeutic department" and the "electrocardiograph."[20] Fenner shortly left the hospital, and Richards was faced with the task of building a department.

Richards had a certain administrative style, exemplified perhaps by his bookplate, which shows a Crookes' tube and attributes to WC Röntgen the probably apocryphal remark, "I didn't think, I tried" (*tentando non cogitando*).[21] Richards was a restless tinkerer and fabricated, with the helpful technical staff of Toronto General Hospital, numerous devices useful in radiotherapy, a field in which he developed a growing interest. Reflecting perhaps the spirit of the British Columbia mining camp, Richards also demonstrated an ability to inspire leadership. Wrote one biographer, "He had the ability to stimulate an *esprit de corps* in his department, built on a feeling of intense personal loyalty to the chief."[22]

In the explosive growth of radiology after World War I, Richards needed more staff, especially to help on the diagnostic side while he busied himself with radiotherapy. (Both the diagnostic and the therapeutic services were located in the Dunlap Building of Toronto General Hospital.) In 1919, he took on William Howard Dickson, a McGill graduate of 1904 who, like Richards, had worked at mining camps in British Columbia. But unlike Richards, Dickson had sought systematic training in radiology in the United States, studying gastrointestinal disease with well-known radiologist Lewis Gregory Cole of New York City. (Dickson later helped to pioneer the use of thorium dioxide for radiography of the alimentary tract.) Said to possess an "almost oracular" diagnostic ability in gastro-intestinal radiology,[23,24] Dickson soon made a name for himself in Toronto and was perhaps prevented from becoming an international figure only by his premature death of long-standing heart disease in 1933 at age 55.

As Dickson fell ill in February 1932, Richards took on two young men, Arthur Singleton and Malcolm Hall, to replace him. The three of them would provide the leadership core in radiology for the next 30 years. The secret of the radiology department's extraordinary success with budgets, space, and the procuring of new equipment over the years is that these men developed the stability required for exercising influence. They were, for example, easily able to achieve an audience with the premier of the province when some particularly costly item was required. It was virtually unknown for the hospital's board of trustees to refuse a request from the radiology department.

With Richards' death in 1949, Singleton became acting director (later chief) of diagnostic radiology at Toronto General Hospital. Hall became chief in 1962 when Singleton retired, and Hall stepped down in 1965. Unlike the founding generation's orientation toward Europe, Hall and Singleton turned toward the United States. Singleton had graduated in 1923 from the University of Toronto and had trained in radiology with Douglas Quick, head of the radiotherapy department at Memorial Hospital in New York, before returning to Toronto in 1925. Singleton was a Chancellor of the American College of Radiology from 1952 to 1956 (president in 1957) and presided over the international Congress of Radiology in Montreal in 1962. Hall also was a medical graduate (in 1928) from the University of Toronto and took postgraduate training at St Francis Hospital in Pittsburgh, returning to Toronto two years later to join the radiologic staff of the Toronto General Hospital.

These 30 years represented a time of considerable innovation. On arriving at Toronto General Hospital, Richards established an outpatient service that soon handled close to 1000 patients per year.[25] The kind of "tinkering" that characterized radiology departments everywhere went steadily apace. For example, in the early 1920s, Richards combined roll photographic film with the single intensifying screen that had just come into use; he and Dickson later designed a complete serial gastric unit that was motor-driven and used 30 cassettes.[18]

On the academic side, in 1923 Richards and JC McLennan, by now professor of physics at the University of Toronto, established a structured postgraduate course in radiology leading to a university diploma.[26] Dr Eugene Shannon, later the chief of the radiology department at St Michael's Hospital, was one of the first two graduates. The diploma program continued through the years and gave its graduates formal recognition as specialists in radiology.

In re-forming the relations of the hospital to the university, it was agreed in 1920 that the chief of each service in the Toronto General Hospital would also function as the head of the university department. Thus, Richards served in that role, initially with the rank of associate (after 1933 associate professor), while other members of the hospital service also had such academic appointments as senior demonstrator. In 1925, the Toronto General Hospital appointed interns (housemen) in radiology for the first time. Later called senior interns, they actually served as residents.

With Richards' death from leukemia in 1949, the result of his decades of involvement with radiotherapy, an era in the history of radiology in Toronto came to an end.

GENERATIONAL CHANGE AFTER 1949

In the postwar period, Richards, Singleton, and Hall were the first three chairpeople, a nucleus of historical continuity reaching back to 1 917. When Hall retired in 1965—simultaneously as chief at Toronto General Hospital and chairperson of the university department—the baton passed to a much younger generation, individuals who identified with a subspecialty within diagnostic radiology and who were oriented toward research in addition to service. In Richards' heyday the Toronto General Hospital had three diagnostic radiologists. By 1991, The Toronto Hospital (the new name for the Toronto General Hospital, which merged in 1986 with the Toronto Western Hospital) had 31 diagnostic radiologists. By 1991 the number of diagnostic radiologists with university appointments in the city as a whole had grown from a handful to 107, spread over eight teaching hospitals.

The big generational change in the history of Toronto radiology occurred in 1965 when Brian Holmes, almost 20 years Hall's junior, became chairperson of the University of Toronto Department of Radiology and radiologist-in-chief at Toronto General Hospital. Holmes received his medical degree from the University of Western Ontario in 1943. Having attended in 1944 a crash course for the military in radiology organized by Richards at Toronto General Hospital (Richards put on five such courses), Holmes became a radiologist in the Royal Canadian Army Medical Corps. After discharge from the army he took three years of postgraduate training with Larry Robbins at the Massachussetts General Hospital, then joined the radiology department at Toronto General Hospital in 1950 as assistant radiologist. In the late 1940s the Royal College of Physicians and Surgeons (RCPS) of Canada had created a fellowship in medicine with emphasis on radiology, and in 1951 Holmes became the first radiologist to gain that fellowship by examination.

Holmes played an important part in introducing Sven Ivar Seldinger's technique of percutaneous catheter arteriography to Toronto and also worked to develop precise cine-venography methods for localizing incompetent communicating veins in patients with varicose veins and ulcers.

EMPHASIZING RESEARCH: POST–1965

When Holmes came in, he saw his major challenge as orienting the department toward systematic research. This was an era in which it was uncommon for radiologists to do research. As Holmes explained his plans to an associate dean, the dean remarked, "I never thought of research in connection with radiology."

To make available suitable research space, in 1968 Holmes established the Radiological Research Laboratory, which later was named after him. His original plan was to send away a member of the university department for a year of work, who would then come home and become a kind of research spark plug for the department as a whole. But when no one suitable could be found, in 1968 the radiology department brought Eric Milne, a radiologist interested in pulmonary physiology, from Harvard to become the laboratory's first director. Situated in the Medical Sciences Building, the laboratory was funded partly from the clinical earnings of the university wide radiologists (who agreed to surrender most of their annual honorariums of $200 to the university) and partly by a development grant from the Medical Research Council.

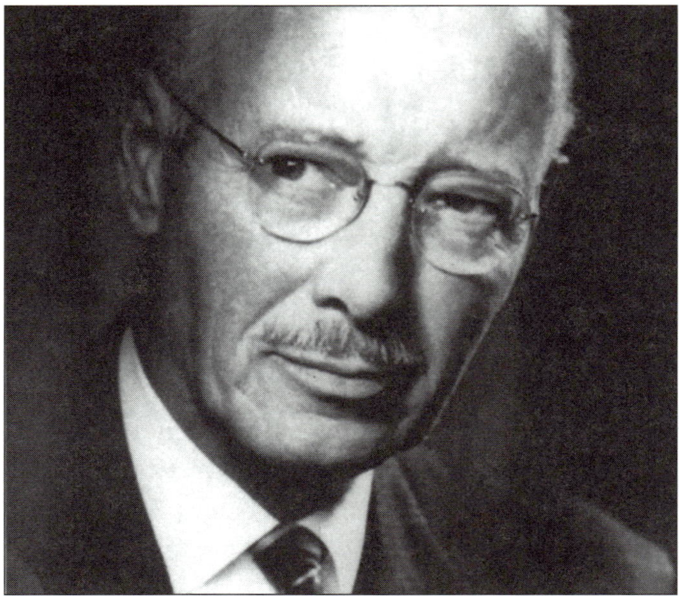

When Holmes stepped down in 1973 to become dean of the Faculty of Medicine, the task of providing research leadership passed to the new chairperson, Edward Lansdown. Lansdown, who had done his residency under Singleton and Holmes, had gone to Winnipeg in 1968, serving as chief at St Boniface General Hospital from 1969 until his return to Toronto in 1974. Lansdown arrived amid the revolution of imaging technology of the 1970s, shortly after the first computed tomography head scanner had been installed at the Toronto General Hospital. His 10-year term coincided with some remarkable advances in imaging: sonography, single-photon emission computed tomography, and magnetic resonance (MR) imaging. Although the installation of these new diagnostic and research tools in the teaching hospitals took place more slowly than in most of the major United States centres, by the end of 1984 Toronto had adequate imaging technology, with the exception of MR imaging. (At that time there was only one unit in the city, at Princess Margaret Hospital.) During his term as university chairperson, Lansdown recommended the purchase of a positron-emission tomography scanner, although this was not finally installed until 1993 at the Clarke Institute of Psychiatry.

When Eric Milne left Toronto in 1975, it was not possible to recruit another experienced radiologic researcher to succeed him as director of the Holmes Laboratory. Lansdown therefore shifted the focus of activity at the laboratory from lung physiology to medical physics, recruiting as director Harold Johns, who had just retired as the founding chairperson of the faculty's department of medical biophysics.

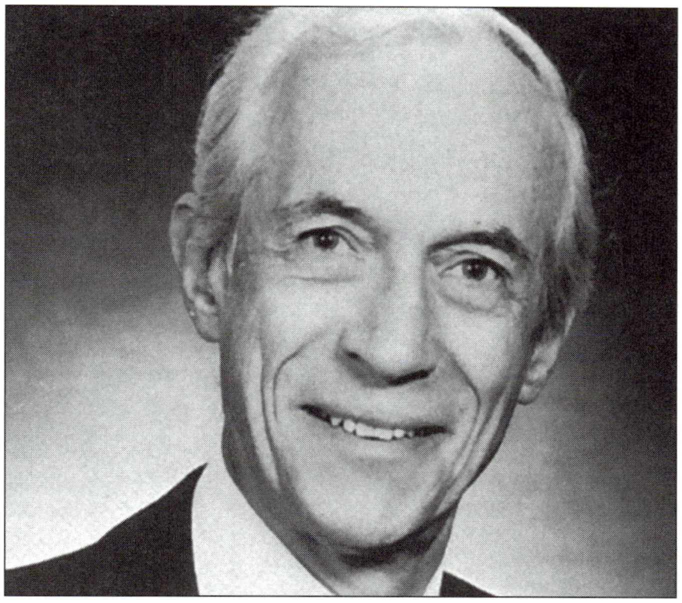

Far left
Dr Arthur C Singleton

Left
Dr R Brian Holmes

FROM HOSPITAL- TO UNIVERSITY-BASED PROGRAM: THE 1970s AND AFTER

When Holmes became chairperson in 1965, three hospitals in Toronto had teaching programs in general radiology: Toronto General Hospital, Toronto Western Hospital and St Michael's Hospital. Even though Holmes had created a senior advisory committee in 1965, naming to it the chiefs at each of the affiliated hospitals, each hospital still admitted students independently and trained them as it saw fit. The only common feature was a pediatrics rotation at the Hospital for Sick Children, through which all residents had to pass. This fragmentation of postgraduate training posed a problem, because graduates of the program had different kinds of experiences as they attempted their qualifying examinations for the Royal College of Physicians and Surgeons. From the outset of the new regime, it was clear that the hospital-based programs should be converted into a single, comprehensive university-based program. Yet achieving this was a task of 20 years.

Holmes began by creating a senior advisory committee for the university department and naming to it the chiefs at each of the affiliated hospitals: Louis Harnick at Toronto Western Hospital, Bruce Bird at St Michael's Hospital, and John Munn at the Hospital for Sick Children. Other hospitals in turn would acquire their own teaching programs so that the city would have five separate hospital-based training programs only loosely affiliated with the university.

In 1971 Holmes look the next step, setting up a small radiology office on the University of Toronto campus, with a tiny budget, in order to gain "the full recognition of the truly academic aspects of departmental function as opposed to hospital service function," as Holmes put it.[27] The office was to provide space for the new coordinator of the university program (and room for staff to administer the radiology research laboratory, which had just opened). Soon after, however, plans for effecting the transition from a hospital-based to a university-based program came to a temporary end. Holmes later said he had been reluctant to tread too much on the feet of the other chiefs—people like Louis Harnick—who were also close personal friends of his.

In the 1970s changes in specialty certification forced the issue of university control onto the agenda again. After the Second World War the RCPS became increasingly involved in graduate education in radiology. In Toronto the RCPS began accrediting the freestanding hospital-based training programs, which put the chairperson of the radiology department in the position of being responsible for program quality in hospitals other than Toronto General Hospital, where he was chief. This responsibility led to some uncomfortable moments when RCPS inspection teams identified weaknesses in certain hospital programs.

In 1984 matters came to a head when, as a matter of university policy, the department of radiology was subject to a periodic five-year review. This time the external reviewers, Richard Greenspan from Yale and Joachim Burhenne from the University of British Columbia, pressed emphatically for a move to a comprehensive university based program. Extensive consultation ensued with Lansdown, with Dean Fred Lowy, and with the chairpeople of other departments and members of the department of radiology itself. From these discussions it was clear that the five separate hospital programs for training residents should be combined under the university into a single program with 48 trainees.

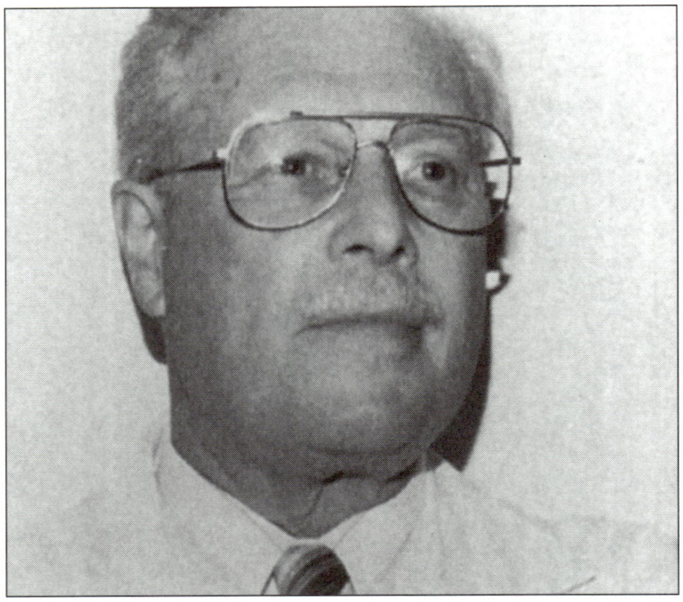

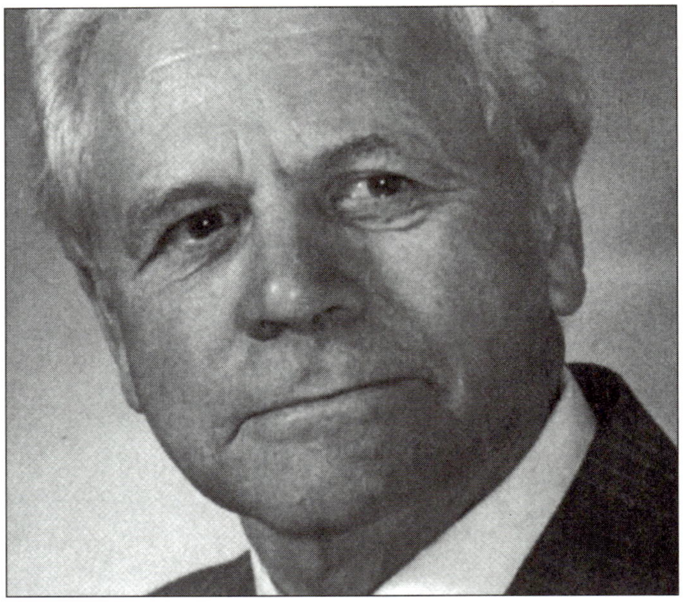

Left
Dr Edward Lansdown

Right
Dr Gordon Potts

NEW DEPARTURES AFTER 1985

In 1985, Gordon Potts was appointed chairperson of the university department of radiology. He intended to push forward both research and the move to a university-based program. Born in New Zealand, Potts had trained in neuroradiology at the Atkinson Morley Hospital and the National Hospital for Nervous Diseases (Queen Square) in London with James Bull. After seven years at the Neurological Institute in New York with Juan Taveras, Potts was recruited to the New York Hospital–Cornell Medical Center by John Evans. Here he became involved in research on the formation and absorption of cerebro-spinal fluid.

As Potts was appointed chairperson in Toronto, he undertook extensive discussion with Dean Lowy and the hospital radiology chiefs about the ideal administrative relationship between the university chairperson and the nine affiliated hospitals. Until then the university chairperson always had been radiologist-in-chief at Toronto General Hospital, which tended to identify that hospital as the university hospital and the other hospitals as lesser academic participants. Potts therefore decided to separate the posts of departmental head and hospital radiology chief. Rather than taking responsibility for the day-to-day operation of a busy clinical department, he would concentrate on the teaching and research programs of all the affiliated hospitals. This measure introduced the concept of a neutral university chairperson, one with a similar relationship to all the hospitals.

When Potts arrived in Toronto in 1985, 99 diagnostic radiologists were employed in the nine teaching hospitals (five of which had resident training programs in radiology), whose 5000 beds and associated outpatient clinics provided tertiary care for a population of almost 4 million persons in and around the city. Two hundred fifty students entered the medical school every year. The integration of this sprawling program was therefore a major challenge.

With the help of the radiologists-in-chief, Potts started to unify the five hospital programs. The residents were to be appointed to a base hospital (one of the large general hospitals) but rotate about the strongest teaching divisions of the other affiliated hospitals. Both faculty and residents soon started to see advantages in this new combined program. Previously, the teaching hospitals had diverse kinds of divisional structures. Some divisions were organized around a single technique (e.g., CT, MR imaging, sonography, nuclear medicine, and angiography), others around organ systems (cardiovascular, respiratory, gastrointestinal, genito-urinary, musculoskeletal, and neurologic). Ultimately, the new program would push all affiliated hospitals toward structuring themselves around organ systems.

On the research side, Potts tried to put into action the initiatives that Holmes and Lansdown had already adumbrated. Although the radiologic physicists had initiated a strong program of funded research, there had been relatively little ongoing, funded, hypothesis-driven research by clinical radiologists. Potts attempted to steer research in this direction. He persuaded the residents to become involved in research, presenting their findings at an annual residents' research day. Although the residents had originally been resistant to the notion of research, they went on to become proud of their work.

In the late 1980s, the medical physicists moved from the Holmes laboratory to a new research facility at Sunnybrook Medical Centre. The Holmes laboratory itself found a new home at Toronto Western Hospital, where in 1986 a small-bore 2-T research MR imaging unit had been installed for small animal studies.

In 1991 Walter Kucharczyk followed Potts as university chairperson. After a residency in Toronto, Kucharczyk had moved to San Francisco for neuroradiology training with Hans Newton. He soon became recognized as an authority on MR imaging of the CNS. Like Potts, Kucharczyk chose to take a neutral chairperson's position. He declined the post of hospital radiologist-in-chief and instead concentrated on the university, with the goal of building on the strengths of the existing radiology residency and fellowship programs under the centralized leadership of the university program directors. To encourage hypothesis-driven research, Kucharczyk also increased the amount of research funding. Thus, despite the growing crisis in the funding of hospitals and universities in Ontario, Kucharczyk was able to accelerate the pace of research and bring the department together.

The history of this large radiology department, spread out over a number of hospitals, shows the importance of leadership skills in forging a comprehensive training program and program of research. By the mid-1990s much had changed in academic radiology in Toronto from a century previously. The discipline itself had become a demanding medical specialty rather than a craft for radiographers. Diagnostic radiology and radiotherapy had divorced completely. In 1994, one year before the 100th anniversary, the Department of Radiology of the University of Toronto officially changed its name to the Department of Medical Imaging to reflect more accurately a century of progress in which Dr King's simple x-ray machine had grown to include nuclear medicine, sonography, MR imaging, positron-emission tomography, and a huge variety of imaging-guided therapeutic techniques.

Acknowledgements:

The author gratefully acknowledges comments on earlier drafts from Michael Bliss, James Connor, R Brian Holmes, Walter Kucharczyk, Edward Lansdown, Gordon Potts, Anne Marie Shorter, and from two anonymous reviewers and the editorial staff of the *AJR*. Michhael Langevin, Suzanne Keppler, and Erika Stefler helped with the research.

Editorial Acknowledgements:

This article has been published in the *American Journal of Roentgenology*[28] and is published with the kind permission of both the author and the *Journal*. The illustrations are reproduced with the permission of the Canadian Museum of Health and Medicine at the Toronto Hospital, Canada.

London, Ontario

EE Johnston

VICTORIA HOSPITAL

Dr George McNeil was the pioneer Radiologist in Western Ontario. He was a member of the Medical Staff at Victoria Hospital from 1902 to 1940. Until 1934 this appointment was part-time and from 1934 to 1940 it was full-time and Dr McNeil served as head of the Department of Radiology.

Dr Ivan Smith joined Dr McNeil in 1938 as his assistant in therapeutic radiology. In 1942 Radiology was split into Diagnostic and Therapeutic arms, with Dr Smith becoming head of therapeutic radiology, a position he occupied until his death on April 7, 1962.

Dr WF Bryan succeeded Dr McNeil in 1940 but left to join the American Army in 1942, when he was succeeded by Dr HS Wismer. When Dr Wismer resigned in March 1948 he was briefly—March and April—succeeded by Dr A Bernstein and then Dr A Bartelink assumed the post as head of Radiology from May 1948 until June 1953. Dr Paul New, a member of his staff, succeeded him in 1953 until he in turn resigned in 1958. A longer period of stability and leadership followed under Dr Gerald Copestake, already a member of staff, from 1958 until his resignation in 1968.

Dr Stewart Lott was acting head of the Department of Therapeutic Radiology from Dr Smith's death in April 1962 until May 1963, when Dr TA Watson became head of therapeutic radiology. Members of his staff in 1968, were Drs I Thomson, John Fetterly, G Miller, F Heagy and P Bannerjee.

Dr Fred Heagy went on to pioneer a nuclear medicine service and was an early president and archivist of the Canadian Association of Nuclear Medicine. He was succeeded as head of nuclear medicine by Dr Albert A (Al) Driedger. These physicians, with Dr Michael Chamberlain at the University Hospital, Dr Lionel Reese, Dr Trevor Cradduck a physicist, and later Ms Pamela Zabel, a radiopharmaceutical scientist, were to form the nucleus of the strong nuclear medicine group at the University of Western Ontario.

Dr EE Johnston succeeded Dr G Copestake as Chief of Diagnostic Radiology in July 1968. His associates at that time were Drs DS Rajic, J Allcock, RB Treleaven, Craig MacDonald, A Reid-Smith and Robert Coates. Dr AC MacDonald succeeded Dr E Johnston in July, 1978 and remains as chief to the present date. His associates were Drs R Coates, W Pexman, M Lefcoe, J McCallum, R Baker, R Haddad, K Sparrow, J Elliott and J Shewchum.

Dr AC MacDonald succeeded Dr Johnson in July, 1978, and remained Chief until July 1, 1988, with the partnership otherwise being unchanged.

Dr Michael S Lefcoe succeeded Dr MacDonald in July 1988, and remains Chief of the Department of Radiology of Victoria Hospital to the present. His associates are Drs AC MacDonald, W Pexman, J McCallum, R Baker, R Haddad, K Sparrow, J Elliott, C Yoshy, L Harker, and D Moote.

Dr TA Watson resigned as Director of the London Clinic, Ontario Cancer Foundation, in 1980 and was succeeded by Dr H Bush. Dr Bush served in the position for some five years and was then succeeded by Dr L Levine. Therapeutic radiologists associated with the clinic over those years were Drs P Bannerjee, A Hammond, A Dar, A Cheung, P Corbett, L Gaspar, and C Ago.

ST JOSEPH'S HOSPITAL

From an uncertain date until 1922, a Dr Thompson was the hospital's only Radiologist. Dr HE Schaef succeeded him in 1922 and served the hospital until his death in 1937. Dr M Morrison was his successor until his death in 1949. Dr K Faulkner, who was associated with Dr Morrison, succeeded him in 1949 until his death in 1951 when Dr MB Hill became Head of radiology until his resignation in 1968. He was succeeded by Dr WW Wilkins. Other members of the department in 1968 were Drs MB Hill, DA Nicol, F Linsdell, Hugh Edgar, Thomas Brown and Paul Greenhow.

Dr J Black served as Head from July 1976 until September 1983, and Dr C Coates from then until December 31, 1983. Dr S Eakins became Chief in March 1984 and remains in that position. Associated with him are Drs. J Black, F Linsdell, H Edgar, T Brown, P Greenhow, C Coates, L McCurdy, R Kozak and D Mowbray.

WESTMINSTER HOSPITAL

This hospital was at first served by part-time radiologists: Dr HE Schaef from 1931 until his death in 1937, Dr Ivan Wilson from 1931 until 1942, Dr HS Wismer from 1942 until 1947. Dr Paul Andras was named Chief of Service in radiology in 1943 until 1947. Dr Paul Hauch, who was also part-time, was named Chief in 1947 and served until 1951. Dr BJ Shapiro was named Chief of Service in 1951 until his resignation in 1955. Dr MF Bennett succeeded him (1955 to 1958) and in turn Dr WL Teskey succeeded him (1958 to 1968). Dr John Agnos was named Chief of Service in 1969 and had Drs W Teskey and N Dare associated with him. Later he was joined by Drs G Hamilton and R Cable.

Finally the Department at Westminster Hospital was disbanded when Victoria Hospital took over Westminster Hospital in 1977. At that time, Dr Agnos went into private practice in radiology and Dr Gavin Hamilton opened a private office in London.

The Westminster Hospital Department of Radiology then became part of the Victoria Hospital Radiology Department, and the Department was closed and replaced by a new department constructed in the new Tower building at the Westminster site as the Westminster Campus of Victoria Hospital.

PRIVATE OFFICES

Drs George McNeil, HS Wismer, HE Schaef and I Wilson all had offices for the private practice of Radiology. Drs M Morrison and Paul Hauch also established their own private offices. Dr M Gilmore succeeded Dr Ivan Wilson for one year in 1953 before going to Stratford General Hospital.

In 1968 there were three private offices belonging to: 1) Dr Paul Hauch, 2) the radiology group at St Joseph's Hospital and 3) Drs MA Bloomfield and WC Trusler. Dr Gavin Hamilton opened a private office in 1974. Subsequently the Victoria Hospital Radiologists also opened a private office.

UNIVERSITY HOSPITAL

University Hospital opened in 1972 with Dr L Carey as Chief Radiologist. His associates were Drs J Allcock and R Gold. Drs L Hutton and T Munro were recruited in 1974.

Dr Barry Hobbs succeeded Dr L Carey on July 1, 1986. His associates in 1994 are Drs L Carey, L Hutton, T Munro, A Fox, R Rankin, F Viñuela, D Pelz and D Boch.

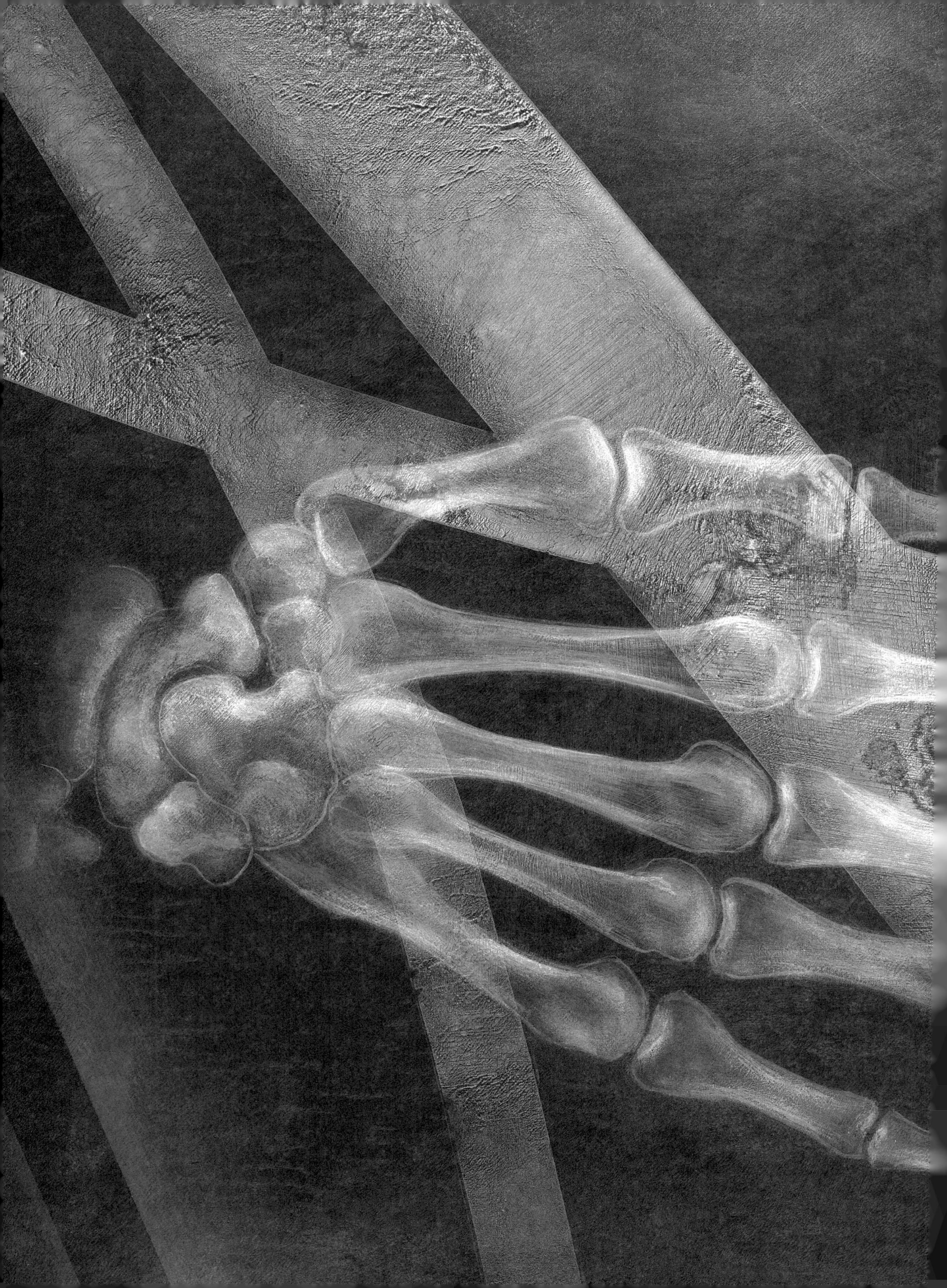

Part Five: People

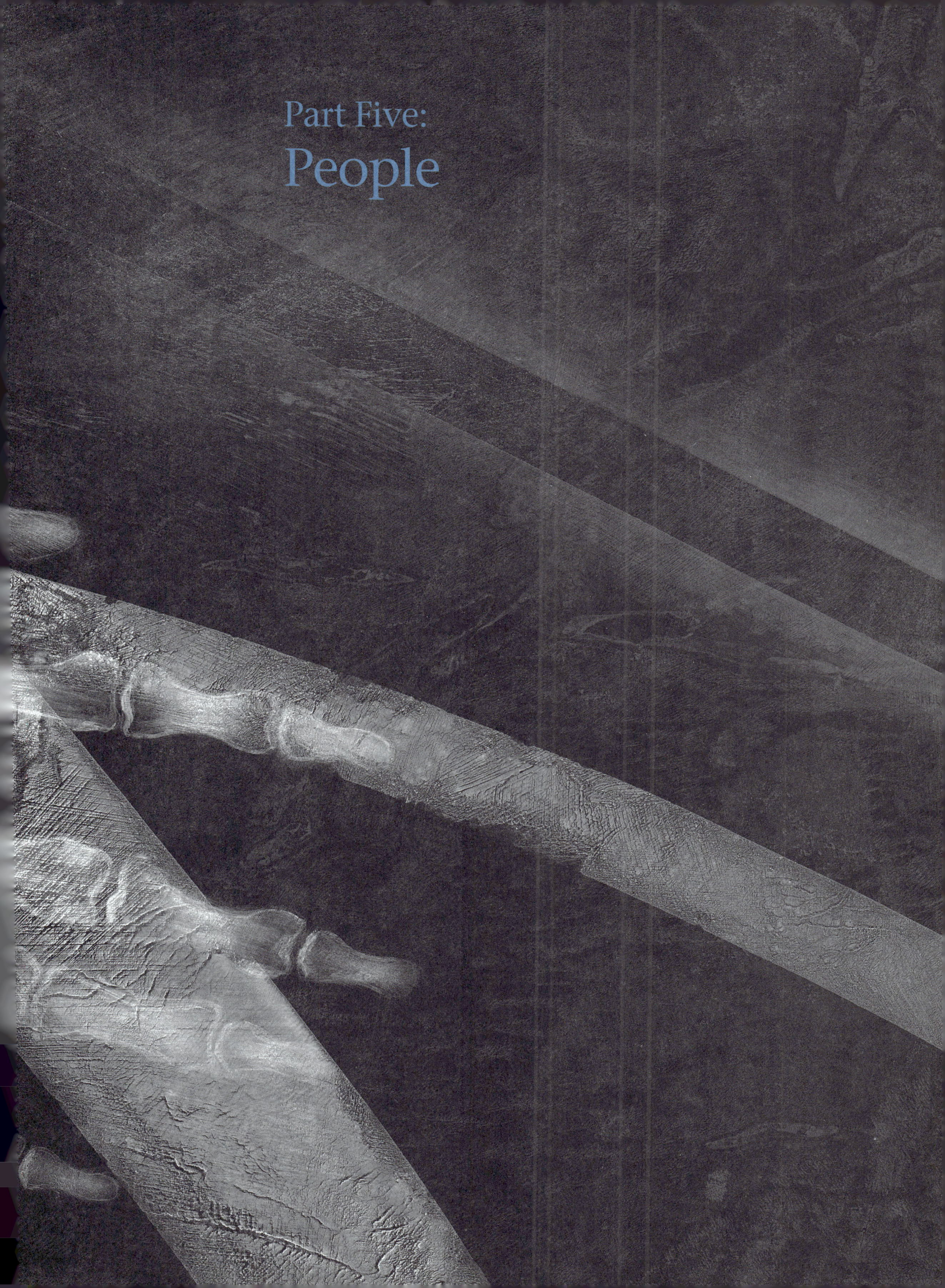

(a) The Founders

"Who knows whether the best of men be known, or whether there be not more remarkable persons forgot than any that stand remembered in the known account of time."
— Sir Thomas Browne

It is impossible to look back at events in the radiological sciences in Canada without a sense of being dwarfed by the individuals who have contributed so much in the past . Equally it is a daunting task to select those particular individuals about whom to include some words, from among so many who might qualify. In the final analysis the guide used has been to choose individuals from differing eras and backgrounds in the hope that their lives speak not only for themselves but for a multitude of others who might be described here. In reading material to prepare this section I have also been very conscious of the insight of Emerson who wrote: "There is properly no history, only biography." That view seems particularly true of the people described here. They seem to have had unusual degrees of foresight and patience, but also great wisdom and perseverance. Their biographies are our collective history.

— Brian Lentle

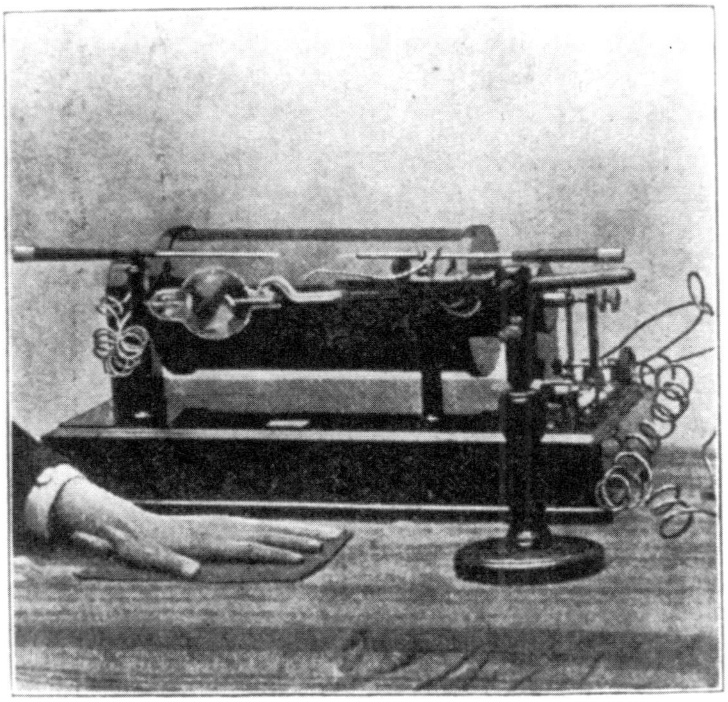

FIG. 1.—INDUCTION COIL AND TUBE ARRANGED TO PHOTOGRAPH A HAND.

I *Dr James Third*

William A Jones

Kingston's earliest radiologist was Dr James Third, and in the unhurried days at the close of the last century he contributed his quota of early radiological observations.

Within a few months of Röntgen's discovery of an invisible light, a "light that was never on land or sea," Third persuaded the board of the Kingston General Hospital to install an "x-ray machine," but no record exists of what kind of a machine was installed. One of Third's contemporaries, Dr GW Mylks Sr, recalled that in the summer or autumn of 1896 Third painted a piece of cardboard with a fluorescent medium which had been recommended and made his own fluoroscope. Mylks was a medical student acting as an undergraduate intern. Came a day when he was used as the guinea pig for the demonstration of the new apparatus, and, wonder of wonders, he saw the bones inside his hand and watched their movements. Third was the Medical Superintendent of the Kingston General Hospital. He retired from this position in 1897 and then carried on x-ray work along with his private medical practice. Later, he became professor of medicine at Queen's University.

It is very difficult to get a great deal of information regarding the radiology of those days, but a few documents exist. On reading these documents the writer was impressed by two things. The first was that Third's writing gave an insight into his early thoughts regarding x-rays, showing us a man who was thinking ahead of his time. Second, if new members of medical faculties were required to read some of the papers contributed by their predecessors in the faculty, they might know something about the kind of man who went before them. When the writer knew him, Third was an old man and his day was largely done, and the younger men of the Faculty of Medicine who had not known Third in his youth had no conception of the contribution he had made to medicine.

The writings of that period seem rather odd to us in these days [circa 1960], dealing as they did with problems that were then unsolved but which are now understood as a matter of course. To those oldsters of us who had experienced similar things they do not seem as odd as they do to the later generation of radiologists. Simple though many of these things were, they were nevertheless unsolved problems. One reflects that as late as 1927 at a meeting of the American Roentgen Ray Society held in Montréal, some of our revered seniors, most of them since deceased, discussed very seriously the meaning of an odd shadow sometimes found at the hip joint. The meaning of this shadow has since become common knowledge: it is the acetabular bone. At about this time radiologists and other clinicians were just becoming aware of atelectasis of the lung as something apart from either atelectasis of the newborn or post-operative pneumonia. Nowadays, of course, any third year medical student can talk learnedly about even segmental atelectasis.

Third was a strong advocate of x-ray diagnosis of diseases of the lungs, particularly of tuberculosis. He noted that the x-ray "sounded a warning note when auscultation and percussion have indicated no departure from normal." One can see that he was in advance of his time. It was 30 years before it was generally accepted that the radiological diagnosis of pulmonary tuberculosis will often show the lesion in advance of ordinary physical examination. Third placed his faith in fluoroscopy as the method of choice for diagnosis and thought that skiagrams were unlikely to replace fluoroscopy in thoracic work. From his point of view at that time, how right he seems. Even the most advanced of his contemporaries using the first attempts at intensifying screens (1891) were unable to obtain a "radiograph of the thorax" in less than 30 seconds.

Third used to say, "There are three things that never should be placed in the hands of the patient: the hypodermic syringe, the thermometer, and the X-ray photograph." Any objections?

All this was in the days of static machines, large primary and secondary coils encased in wax, mercury interrupters, and glass photographic plates.

Acknowledgement:
This was probably published in *Illuminator* in the late 1950s. It was found in the CAR archives. Permission to republish it has been graciously given by Dr Jones' daughter, Mrs Margaret Roberts of Manotick, Ontario.

AND YOU THOUGHT THINGS WERE BAD AT THE END OF THE TWENTIETH CENTURY...?

Margaret Angus

Dr James Third is Recruited to Kingston General Hospital...

There were also to be special economies in the operation of the Hospital: a single dining room had to serve the Superintendent and his family, the House Surgeons, the Superintendent of Nurses, and all the nurses. Only candles *were to be used after eight pm. The Superintendent was instructed to submit weekly, detailed financial statements to the Board. The committee also recommended that the graduate nurse in the Doran Building be given three month's notice, and that the nurses in training not be paid after September 1896. They said that one medical graduate at no salary should replace the two undergraduate House Surgeons (a saving on board, room, and laundry), and that the Medical Superintendent's salary should be reduced by $100 to $900. The penny-pinching and constant scrutiny of expenditures were bad enough, but a cut in salary was too much. Dr Kilborn submitted his resignation in January 1896, saying that although he had been given excellent cooperation he felt that his position had "not been as cordially acceptable as in former years." He asked to be relieved at the earliest convenience so that he might engage in private practice. The Board commended his work, accepted his resignation and decided to advertise for a new Medical Superintendent at $600 a year. Fifty-eight men applied for the job. On 17 February 1896, the Board appointed Dr James Third of Trenton, a Queen's graduate, to become Superintendent of the Kingston Hospital in June…*

Dr James Third arrived in June [1896] to take over his duties as Medical Superintendent. Greatly excited by the implications of x-ray, he persuaded the Board to acquire the materials so that one could be built for the Hospital. Although Dr Third was quickly convinced of its value as a diagnostic agent he was slower to recommend it in therapy. He became a strong advocate of x-ray in diagnosing tubercular lesions in the lung when auscultation and percussion indicated no departure from the normal. While he was Superintendent of the Hospital he was in charge of, and made good use of, the x-ray machine. By some experimental work he also improved the fluoroscope then available and exhibited its work at a meeting of the Kingston Medical and Surgical Society.

The annual report of the Kingston General Hospital, as of 30 September 1896, showed improvement in the financial situation. The City of Kingston grant had been increased to $1000 and there had been a saving of $870 in salaries and household expenses. The Board of Governors complimented Superintendent Third who had "discovered and stopped leaks in the expenses," and Superintendent of Nurses Miss MacMillan who had surmounted the many difficulties with sick nurses during the typhoid epidemic. They noted that "the machinery of the Hospital is running without friction or trouble of any kind." The staff at that time included nine Attending Physicians, the two Superintendents, a Housekeeper, two House Surgeons, twenty nurses, and twelve servants.[1]

…And Dr William A Jones Becomes the First Full-Time Radiologist

With increased and improved accommodation some of the part-time services had to be made full-time. For example, Dr RJ Gardiner and WE McNeill of Queen's, serving on the Management Committee, gave strong support to the Medical Staff request for a full-time radiologist. Dr WA Jones, who did his first x-ray work in England in 1919, had been practicing his profession as a radiologist in the city. He offered to set up a Radiological and Radio Therapy Department at the Hospital and to take charge of it, provided certain conditions were agreed upon. The Hospital would purchase his office equipment, supply accommodation, light, heat, and laundry free; for these he would give free service to the public ward cases and be available for paid work on a shared fee arrangement. The first charge on fees would be for depreciation of equipment, cost of supplies, repairs, salaries of extra staff, and equipment valuation. The balance was to be divided ninety per cent to the Director of the Department, Dr Jones, and ten per cent to the Hospital. The service began in January 1926. By March, X-ray began to show a profit and by the end of the year the 1926 receipts had doubled those of 1925. It was a profitable arrangement for both of the partners in the plan.[1]

II *Gordon Earle Richards*

— A Little About His Life and Times

William A Jones

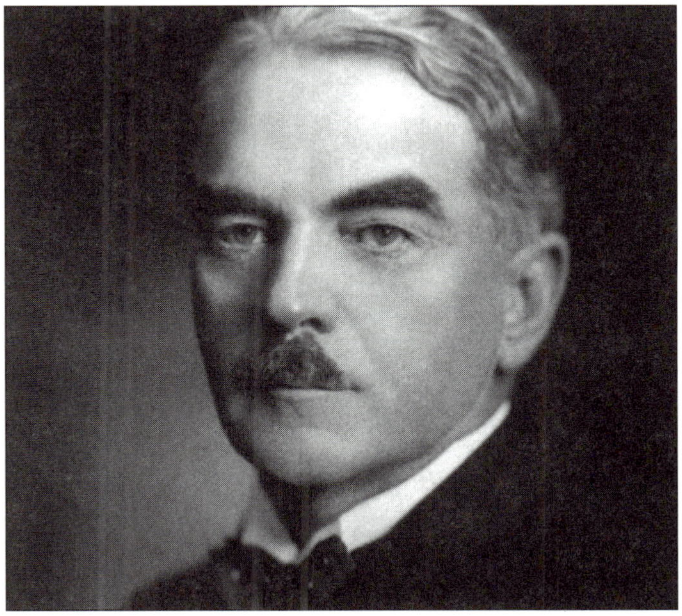

INTRODUCTION

I want to try and write something about Richards as I knew him. I cannot hope to give a really adequate picture of him but I do want to describe some of my own recollections of him and a little about some of his friends and his work. This will be the sort of recollection that makes a great deal of use of the first personal pronoun. That, unfortunately, is necessary in the context in which I now venture.

Richards, a stranger to most of you, and too soon, already, quite unknown to a few of you, I have known and highly esteemed. He had an inner warmth that at times would burst through his natural reserve and show itself in genuine friendliness. I felt that he was my friend. He and one of his contemporaries, that genial Scotsman, Howard Pirie, have influenced my own radiological career more than other men, for they were my teachers.

THE CONTEXT

It is helpful to compare contemporary events and figures in order to place an individual in his proper setting. So I will mention these things while trying to show part of the background of the changing picture of a man's life.

The North West Rebellion occurred in 1885. This same year Gordon Earle Richards was born at Lyn, a little place in Ontario, lying about four miles north of the St Lawrence River, not far from the heart of the Thousand Islands. I made a special trip to Lyn to see what kind of a place such a man came from. I'll write about that presently.

Let us now back track for the moment. A few years before Richards' birth, there were born two men who, like Richards, were destined to make their marks upon early Canadian radiology. On Christmas Day in the year 1875 at Dundee in Scotland, Alexander Howard Pirie first saw the light of day and a little later at Grenville, Quebec, in May, 1882, Léo E Pariseau was ushered into a rapidly changing world. In later years Richards came to know these men rather well. The dry Scot's wit of Pirie and the rather volcanic, irrepressible, keen, cultured mind of Pariseau were much appreciated by Richards. Many a time have I heard him chuckle over their outstanding and very human qualities. Richards was also able to appreciate their worth and their contributions to early Canadian radiology. Both Pariseau and Pirie were justly recognized as "characters" in their own right. Besides their very worthy efforts professionally, they were known and well liked because of their interesting and colourful personalities, which, once known, were thoroughly appreciated.

In 1891, Sir John A MacDonald, first Premier of Canada, died. Four years later, 1895, when Richards was ten years old, there was discovered something new, something which, in the language of this day and age, if such language had been in use then, would have been described as "out of this world." About three months later, in January, 1896, a distinguished, black-whiskered scientific gentleman, dressed in a Prince Albert frock coat (the very essence of that sartorial dignity which, along with policemen's helmets, vanished at about the time of the First Great War), delivered his famous preliminary communication on a new kind of ray—the x-ray. Röntgen had launched the rocket which may some day either take us to the stars or finish our civilization.

The South African War commenced in 1899 when Richards was just fourteen years of age and attending High School in Athens, Ontario. One can imagine him asking his father, as boys did ask their fathers in those days, whether, if the war lasted another year or two, he could go as a bugler. Buglers were heroes to young lads then, as space-fighters are to the boys of today.

EARLY YEARS

In 1908 Richards graduated from the University of Toronto as the Gold Medallist of his year. He practiced first in British Columbia and was the medical officer at a mining camp in the northern part of the province. In British Columbia he became associated with Dr CW Prowd, a charming, well-liked man, who afterwards became the radiologist at St Paul's Hospital in Vancouver. In later years Dr Prowd preferred to do all his travelling by air, while Dr Whitelaw, another radiologist in Vancouver, was allergic to air travel and always used the train. Richards used to like to tell about a convention some of us attended in Chicago in 1937. He met Prowd as he got on the elevator in the Palmer House Hotel. Says Richards, "Hello, Prowd, did you fly down?" "Hell, yes," says Prowd. As he got off the elevator he met Whitelaw. Says Richards, "Hello, Whitelaw, did you fly down?" "Hell, no", says Whitelaw. I can still hear Richards tell that anecdote and hear his not too infrequent chuckle as he told it. Richards was a very serious man, but he did have his moments of humour.

I well remember a quip that he made in an address of welcome to the members of the Radiological Society of North America, meeting in Toronto in 1928. This was in the days of prohibition in the United States. In those days it was the lucrative and kindly custom to smuggle thousands and thousands of bottles of excellent Canadian whiskey across that invisible line that bounds our country to the south. In his inimitable way, parodying a famous phrase of Kipling's, Richards referred to it as "our far-flung bottle line." This was a rather typical example of his dry sense of humour.

WORLD WAR I

On August the fourth, 1914, came the First Great War. Soon Richards was a lieutenant in the Royal Army Medical Corps. There is a story that he and Prowd flipped a coin as to which would have the privilege of army service. Richards won. He was stationed in the Near East during the Dardanelles Campaign. He saw service as a radiologist with 21 General Hospital Royal Army Medical Corps (RAMC) with duty on the Isle of Lemnos and at Alexandria in Egypt. Pariseau and Pirie also found themselves overseas in army service. The July, 1916, number of the *British Medical Journal* published an article, "Localization of Foreign Bodies," by Lieut GE Richards, RAMC. This would appear to be Richards' first essay into the medical literature. He describes a simple method of fluoroscopic localization of a foreign body by means of shifting a flat piece of wood in which is embedded a flat piece of metal, having the diameter of a shrapnel bullet.

That same year, 1916, the *British Medical Journal* published:

- Notes on an intensifying screen for use with x-ray plates.
- An article on "The Soldier's Heart," by Sir James Mackenzie.
- An article, "From the Visible to the Gamma Ray Spectrum." with a long paragraph stressing the dangers of x-rays.
- An article on the "Physics of a Surgical Dressing," by Lt Col A Primrose, CAMC. (Of note Primrose had been one of Richards' teachers.)

Later in August, 1917, Richards published an article on "X-ray Reports" in the *Journal of the Royal Army Medical Corps*. He described a method of making a miniature print of the x-ray plate so that a finished reproduction could accompany the x-ray report to the surgical wards. This brings to mind that during the First World War it became routine to make prints of x-ray plates. The x-ray report was typed or written upon the backs of these prints and so passed on to the surgeon. I well remember doing this and reporting plates in such a way. I still have in my possession the print of an injured foot with the report typed on the back and signed by Pirie. Richards' method was to make a reduced-size print by means of a special field-made apparatus which he used. He recommended it not only for use in making a report, but also as a convenient method of keeping x-ray records in small space, instead of the storage of bulky glass x-ray plates. This, of course, was the forerunner of the 1955 method of copying x-ray films for preservation and storage onto roll films.

TORONTO

Richards returned to Canada in 1917 to become the first radiologist at the Toronto General Hospital. To this position he brought an indefatigable store of energy and the gift of originality. At thirty-two years of age he took over this charge. For thirty-two years he was the guiding genius of the department of radiology of that great institution.

Pariseau returned from the war, going to l'Hôtel Dieu de Montréal and later Pirie returned to the Royal Victoria Hospital. These three men, Richards, Pariseau and Pirie, exercised a profound effect upon Canadian radiology for years.

In addition to his marked success as director of the department, Richards also instructed many aspiring young medical men in the art of radiology. Many radiologists practicing today owe their start in their chosen life work to the kindness and encouragement so readily given to them by Richards. Also, during the late war, from 1940 to 1945, he gave freely of his time and energy to instruct young radiologists for the defense forces. To his very great sorrow, his son Stuart was killed in action, serving with the Air Force.

In a paper published in 1925 on "Radiation Treatment of Benign Disease of the Female Pelvis," Richards discusses the actions of both x-rays and radium in these conditions. It is quite interesting to note that in describing the method of treating fibrosis uteri, the single x-ray dose is described as follows:

Spark Gap, 9 inches; milliamperes, 5; filters, 6mm aluminum; time, 15 minutes; distance, 10 inches.

In these days of accurately measured high kilovoltages, long target–skin distances, heavy filtration and dosimeters so conveniently measuring dose, the above factors seem to belong to an almost prehistoric past. Yet they were still in use in 1925.

Today [Jones was writing in 1955—Ed] it seems a long way from the days of primary and secondary coils, gas tubes, mercury interrupters and glass x-ray plates to the streamlined, shock-proof, automatically relayed gadgets and precision x-ray machines and films of today. Yet Richards, like some other few of us, started his x-ray work with these machines.

Pirie at 69 and Pariseau at 62 both died in 1944 and left a distinct sense of loss. Two outstanding pioneers had become memories.

One of Richards' earliest papers was on "Physiotherapy or Treatment by Physical Agents." This reminds us that, in the earlier days of radiology in Canada, nearly all radiologists practiced physiotherapy in addition to radiology. Indeed, many of our French-Canadian colleagues still do. The paper is undated but almost certainly was published in the early twenties. In a short paper he covers what was even then the wide field of physiotherapy in a lucid, informative manner. In rereading the paper one is impressed with Richards' "down-to-earthness" in the common-sense, logical and modest way in which he handles his subject. His tolerant and fair summing up of results of treatment were typical of him. One feels that a quotation from this paper will serve to introduce the present generation of radiologists to one facet of Richards' character well worthy of emulation. I wish that it were possible for me to imitate Richards' rather crisp but intimate method of speech and delivery in order that you might appreciate what I mean by the phrase, "down-to-earthness."

In describing the results of treatment of pneumonia with diathermy, a procedure which had been highly recommended by Dr H E Stewart, he says in part as follows:

> *The method and technique described by Dr Stewart were followed carefully and during the winter each alternate pneumonia patient received this treatment in addition to the usual routine, while the other alternate patients did not receive diathermy. At the end of the period our group of cases had one death more to record than those who had not received diathermy. The only conclusion we felt justified in drawing from this work was that diathermy did not materially affect the death rate of lobar pneumonia in the type of case met with in the Public Wards of a General Hospital. The reason is probably found in the fact that the average day of admission of these patients was the fifth day of the disease. The patients, therefore, were very seriously ill and some were almost moribund. A few felt benefit from the treatment in the sense of added comfort, relief of dysnoea, etc, but in others we concluded that this was more than offset by the inconvenience and consequent fatigue of arranging the electrodes and giving the rather prolonged treatment. But since Dr Stewart specifically states that the treatment must be given during the first 48 hours and since in our cases it was not possible to start treatment until the fifth day we do not feel in a position to make any statement on the merits of the method other than the above. This will have to come from those who have an opportunity of using it in the early stage of the disease.*

Those of you who have been schooled in the sulpha drug and antimicrobic treatment of pneumonia may reflect that a patient with pneumonia is more fortunate nowadays.

Richards' paper "The Systematic Study and Classification of Stereograms of the Chest" was published in the *Canadian Medical Association Journal* in 1927. In this article there is an insistence on careful review, in sequence, of the different main landmarks of the chest when examining a film. This is a common enough procedure today but it was not so then. It was characteristic of Richards to be painstaking, logical and analytical in his examination of any matter.

In this paper Richards mentions "massive collapse." Today the word "collapse" or "atelectasis" is on every medical tongue. It is somewhat difficult to realize that just previous to, and indeed for some time later than, this paper of Richards' in 1927, this was not so. In those days almost anything that happened in the chest after an operative procedure, if it escaped being labelled "pneumonia," was almost certainly called an "embolus." Atelectasis was something that occurred in the newborn.

Curiously enough in his paper, under infections, the matter of fungus infection of the lung is not mentioned. One recollects, however, that fungus infections, which now interest so many people, were little known in those days.

Richards published an article on "Osteochondritis Dissecans" in the *American Journal of Roentgenology* of March, 1928. This was a little-known condition at that time. However, Richards pointed out that König had described it in 1887 and Freiberg and Woolley again in 1910. Several other papers on the subject had been published later. Richards illustrated four examples of osteochondritis dissecans of the knee, described one of the elbow and illustrated a case of this condition in the hip joint.

It is interesting to note that in the discussion that followed this paper of Richards' at the American Roentgen Ray Society meeting in Montréal in 1927, one of our old and respected confreres from Philadelphia stated: "On several occasions I have found a small, round body, about the size of the end of a lead pencil, in the region of the tip of the acetabulum and the upper surface of the head of the femur. I don't know what this is. It may be something which is well known, with which I am not familiar." Our own old friend of those days, Howard Pirie, in referring to the above "small, round body" stated: "I have been very much interested in it myself. I have at least eight cases of it. Sometimes it is on one side only but most frequently it is on both sides. At the present time we are calling it a sesamoid bone in the reflected head of the rectus femoris." Others present also mentioned this curious bone.

How strange to the ears of most of you that the many studious and knowledgeable men who attended this meeting should have devoted so much time to the discussion of such a common extra ossicle as the acetabular bone. Today the occurrence of this bone is such common knowledge that its presence is ignored, except that when seen it is classified subconsciously as non-pathological.

I mention it as one illustration of the, at first, slow build-up of radiological knowledge. That which was a mystery in the early days is now often commonplace. That which is a mystery today may be commonplace tomorrow. Many of us might be a good deal more humble today if we could foretell what our successors of twenty-five years hence will think of some of our present ideas.

In one of his earlier papers Richards discusses the "Co-Relation of Results of Goitre Treatment by Surgical and x-ray Methods." This paper was given in Vancouver at the Canadian Medical Association meeting of June 23, 1920.

Richards published a very scholarly description of the histological characteristics of the thyroid gland and its pathological modifications. The physiological properties of x-rays are discussed. A statement which most of you will find curious but which was widely held for many years is included "It is a well known fact to all by this time that when any living tissue is exposed to x-rays or radium the first effect is stimulation." The destructive effect is then mentioned and a series of 300 cases treated by x-rays is presented. The summary is captioned in eight points, bearing on the marked improvement or temporary improvement of a large percentage of patients having hyperthyroidism.

Again, later, in a paper entitled "Radium—Its Proven Uses and Limitation in Therapy," published in 1931, Richards argues the case for radiation treatment of hyperthyroidism. He says in part: "Hyperthyroidism is a disease in which treatment by x-rays and radium has not received the degree of acceptance by the profession at large which the results warrant."

I recall that some years before the last war, Richards said to me, "The truth of the matter is, that in these days about the only patients that are being referred for radiation treatment of toxic goitre are medical men, their wives, sweethearts, children and close relations."

Nowadays, of course, the physician at least supports the beneficent effect of radiation. This is possibly because radiation has now been parcelled up into a neat little medicine called radioactive iodine which can be given, with all the rites of orthodox medicine, as ministered to by the internist.

In his later years most of the papers published by Dr Richards dealt with the matter of radiotherapy. However, as late as January, 1938, in conjunction with Dr AC Singleton, he published a paper on diagnosis with the title "Giant Cell Tumours of the Spine," and again in January, 1942, a paper, "A Discussion on Surveys of the Chest; with Comments on the 14 x 17" film used in the Canadian Army."

His last publication was on radiotherapy and was published in two parts in the *British Journal of Radiology*. This paper was the Skinner Lecture given at the Faculty of Radiologists meeting in England in May, 1947. The title of the paper was "Mammary Cancer; The Place of Surgery and Radiotherapy in Its Management." This was a masterly piece of work, the result of many years of investigation, treatment and compilation of matters of infinite detail.

One aspect of Richards' attitude toward treatment was his willingness to change and modify treatment as experience led him to adopt new ideas. By this I would not have you think that his mind did readily flit from one idea to another. He did, however, readily adapt himself to new thought when such was logically acceptable. He was of an inventive and original turn of mind and made his own innovations.

About the end of the First Great War, at a time when the single intensifying screen had just come into use, he experimented with it and with roll photographic film, for serial gastric work. In the early twenties he designed a gastric couch upon which the patient could be moved centred and localized over a metal ring, for serial radiography of the stomach. A little later, in collaboration with his associate, Dr WH Dickson, they designed a complete serial gastric unit, motor driven, using thirty cassettes.

He was the Canadian pioneer in deep x-ray therapy. In the early twenties, in association with Mr TB Hurst, he built his own "homemade" 160 kV transformer with a 48-inch rectifying disc. In the late twenties he designed and had installed a filter indicator, on the control of a more modern therapy unit.

When one hears talk nowadays about low temperature surgery, it is interesting to recall that Richards, following the lead of Chamberlain, experimented with low temperature (85°F) treatment of cancer patients, during the early days of the Second Great War. This method was, of course, the precursor of the "hibernation method" of performing heart surgery.

In a paper published in June, 1925, he described a method for the treatment of local recurrences in the skin in the management of breast carcinoma. It involved making a mould of the chest wall, using dental modelling compound, to hold radium needles on the skin of the chest. Eight years later in a paper presented in Chicago, in September, 1933, he described a method of treating larger areas of the chest wall by means of a cotton jacket embroidered with staggered rows of radium needles. This performed a similar function to the dental wax mould, but was more comfortable and was designed to give a more even distribution of radiation.

AT THE PEAK OF HIS CAREER

All in all Richards published over fifty papers on radiological subjects. Some few of these were published in collaboration with his faithful associates, but nearly all of them were his own work. The publication of papers, however, is only part of the work of a man. Papers are that part of his work that bubbles over, above and beyond the call of enthusiasm. To really know a man you must see him on his daily round and watch him at his work. It was well worthwhile to follow Richards and watch him in his contact with patients and his fellows.

He was a man to admire for his tremendous capacity for work and detail, his thoroughness and scientific intensity and, with it all, a warm kindness for his patients and a tolerant attitude to his medical confrères. Singleton, his friend and associate for many years, records that some years before his death, "He was the guest of honour at a dinner where one hundred women, all former cancer patients with no recurrence in periods from five to seventeen years, celebrated most happily."

Dr Richards' official positions included: Attending Radiologist-in-Chief, Toronto General Hospital; Director of Ontario Institute of Radiotherapy; Managing Director, Ontario Cancer Treatment and Research Foundation; and Professor of Radiology, University of Toronto.

He was the founder of the Canadian Association of Radiologists. His was the thought that brought us together in Toronto and sparked the formation of the national organization which has honoured him by instituting this Memorial Lecture in his memory.

At the peak of his professional career, far too young, he passed away. He died on the thirteenth of January, 1949, at the age of 64 years, following an illness due to aplastic anaemia, the result of exposure to the radium used by him in the treatment of literally thousands of patients.

RICHARDS THE MAN

Richards always looked forward to his one month of summer vacation on the Rideau Lakes. Here he secluded himself for four weeks and quite cut himself off from professional associations. He read the books he had wanted to read all year. He built boats, fished and did those other things he had wanted to do. Then, refreshed, he plunged back into his work with all the vim and vigor which so characterized him.

Richards designed a very interesting and effective bookplate for the books of his library. The plate symbolized the legend of Röntgen's discovery of x-rays by use of the symbols of the key, the book and the photographic plate. This brings out another facet of Richards' character. Despite his scientific attitude and his insistence upon proof and accuracy, he had a feeling for the quasi-romantic aspect of science, the imaginary limbus that adds mystery to facts. He denied the truth of the key and book tale but he was nevertheless mightily interested in it as an intriguing sidelight.

He was much interested in a book to which I drew his attention. It was *The Lost Continent of Mu*, a rather imaginary, or at least, a far fetched, yet seemingly credible account of a lost continent of the Pacific. In return he referred me to Donnely's *Atlantis*, a book supporting Solon's and Plato's tale of the lost continent of Atlantis in the Atlantic.

That was one of the things I liked about Richards. He was the type of medical scientist who could be critical and realistic professionally but who was also enough of a mystic to harbour a liking for unreal and unproven things. He liked to let fancy linger, at least occasionally and temporarily, on life's possibilities.

Once in a while , Richards allowed himself a degree of relaxation during the working months of his year. He lived in a delightful house on the edge of a golf course. Of his actual prowess as a golfer, I have no knowledge. I played only one game with him. This was in the days when the name of Bobby Jones, of golfing fame, was a household word and babbled on the lips of even the young fry of the land. Richards was good enough to invite me to dinner, to be preceded by eighteen holes of golf. We spent a delightful afternoon on the links but I regret to record that neither of us covered himself with glory. At the end of the game we wended our way disconsolately to the Richards' door. There, to one of Richards' young hopefuls, I was introduced as Dr Jones. "Are you Bobby Jones?" says the young one. Richards, gravely and very sternly said, "No, indeed, he is not Bobby Jones."

A RETURN TO LYN

Now for a trip into yesterday—to Lyn.

Have you ever gone into a little village to inquire into the happenings of more than half a century ago? I recommend it as an adventure into improbability. It gives rise to rather interesting reflections upon the transience of human affairs. My quest was for someone about 70 years of age who could tell me about the life of Richards as a boy. I hoped to find an old schoolmate. An easy task, one would think. I did not find one. I found a native of the village, an old gentleman of eighty, the surviving oldster of his generation still residing in the village, who remembered him and knew his father well. The school that Richards attended still serves as a school. It is an old four-room building of brown stone, strangely time defaced, and too soon falling into ruin; yet it was built only eighty seven years ago, in 1867, the year of the Confederation of Canada, and had only been standing twenty-three years when the boy Richards entered it as a student. A block away is the solid and interesting grey limestone house where Richards was born. Up a side street (on the road to Athens, no less) is the quaint old stone church which he attended and of which his father was the minister for many long years. A region of curious names—nearby are the hamlets of Lillies and Tincap and not far away are Oakleaf, and Plum Hollow where the witch lived. Round about is a country of rolling hills, creeks, ponds, lakes and woodland. South is the great St Lawrence and the Thousand Islands; an interesting country, filled with hollows and ravines, farmlands, rocky hills and hills of rocks. At one point near Lyn, the farmland is so vastly irregular that the farm there has been called "Crazy Acres."

The village skirts the bank of a stream known to the village simply as the "Creek" and I strongly suspect that in Richards' boyhood it was called the "Crick." This stream meanders along through deep twisting ravines to join with a couple of similar streams, just short of the St Lawrence which, immediately beyond their confluence, the waters enter near Butternut Bay. Butternut Bay! This name alone is sufficient to stir up nostalgic memories of boyhood and helps us to place Richards amongst the surroundings of his youth.

All in all, it was a great country for a boy to grow up in, with all the fishing and hunting territory that the heart could desire. How Richards' heart must have gone back to it; how pleasant to have spent, as Singleton has put it, "A serene old age, in rural surroundings of which he had dreamed."

VALEDICTORY

On Friday evening, the 28th of March, 1947, Queens University, at a special Convocation held in Grant Hall in Kingston, Ontario, honoured Dr Richards by conferring on him the honorary degree of Doctor of Laws. The citation which immediately preceded the conferring of this well-merited dignity, coming as it did so close to the end of his career, makes a fitting conclusion.

Vice-Principal McNeill, in presenting Dr Richards to Principal Wallace, spoke as follows:

> *Mr. Vice-Chancellor, in the name of the Senate of this University, I have the honour to present to you for the Degree of Doctor of Laws, honoris causa, Gordon Earle Richards, Doctor of Medicine, professor of radiology at the University of Toronto; director of the department of radiology at Toronto General Hospital; managing director of the Ontario Cancer Treatment and Research Foundation; a foremost Canadian scientist in cancer radiotherapy, internationally known as teacher, researcher, administrator, greatly serving mankind.*

Editorial Acknowledgement:

Dr Jones based this article on the Gordon Richards Memorial Lecture which he presented at the Annual Meeting of the Canadian Association of Radiologists on January 11, 1955 in Ottawa. It was subsequently published[1] and is reproduced, with some minor editorial changes, with the permission of both the *Canadian Association of Radiologists Journal* and Dr Jones' daughter, Mrs Margaret Roberts of Manotick, Ontario.

Dr AC Singleton wrote of Dr Richards in an editorial following Dr Richards' death.[1] Part of that editorial reads as follows:

> *That he did greatly serve suffering mankind in one of its most grievous afflictions, the record of his more than thirty years of unremitting fight against cancer bears tribute. It was the grand aim and purpose of his life. Into that fight he threw all the zest of a crusader. All the knowledge, skill, originality and persistence with which he was so richly blessed, were devoted to that cause. It was the concentration of these qualities into his technique for the treatment of malignant disease that brought results of outstanding excellence and carried his fame abroad. He had an infinite capacity for detail and thoroughness. One example of this alone, the records of progress in countless numbers of cases treated, and illustrated with superb color photography, won admiration which was wide and sincere. His originality shone forth in the many special methods and devices he developed for the more efficient application of radium and röntgen rays in cancer treatment. In 1920, following studies in Britain and Germany, he established Canada's first high voltage center for cancer therapy, and every year the number of his patients extended into thousands. Some years ago he was the guest of honor at a dinner where one hundred women, all former cancer patients with no recurrence in periods from five to seventeen years, celebrated most happily. But the price Dr Richards paid for those years of service to others was the sacrifice of a serene old age in rural surroundings of which he had dreamed. In a confidential letter to a friend written in October, 1948 he spoke of the aplastic anemia due to radium from which he suffered, and he intimated that his remaining days on earth would be few. His death, three months later, removed a figure of*

world renown in the profession of Radiology, and he will be sadly missed by his co-workers in that field. In 1947 Dr Richards was selected to deliver the Skinner Lecture of the Faculty of Radiologists of London, on cancer of the breast. It was the first occasion since the lectureship was inaugurated that any authority on cancer outside Europe was so honored. He was Founder of the Canadian Association of Radiologists, Fellow of the Toronto Academy of Medicine, member of the Ontario and Canadian Medical Associations, member of the American Roentgen Ray Society and of the Radiological Society of North America, and also Councillor of the American College of Radiology. He will be sadly missed by his fellow Radiologists, the profession at large and by a host of patients he has benefited.

III *Dr William Alfred Jones*

First President of the Canadian Association of Radiologists

RONALD BURR

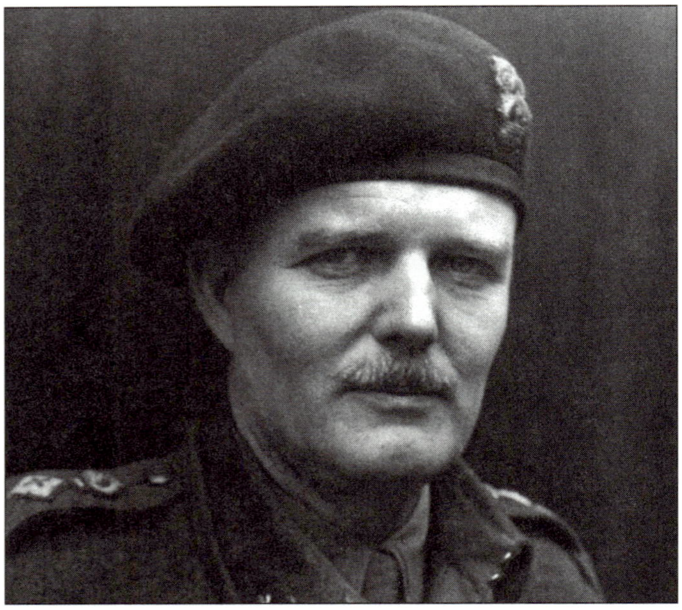

Dr William Jones was born near Ailsa Craig in Ontario on March 29, 1892. He graduated from the University of Western Ontario in medicine in 1914 at the beginning of the First World War and served with the Canadian Expeditionary Force in Canada and England with the rank of Captain from 1915 to 1919. While in Europe he trained in radiology with Dr Alexander Howard Pirie and this resulted in his specializing in radiology throughout his medical career until he retired in 1965. He obtained further education under Dr Gordon Richards in Toronto.

He was professor of radiology at Queen's University for 32 years, and known to all as the "Chief." Dr Jones retired from Queen's staff in 1960.

In the Second World War he enlisted in 1939 and rose to the rank of full Colonel in command of 22 and 10 Canadian General Hospitals in Normandy and Belgium. At the beginning of the war he established, with the support of the Department of Pensions and National Health, the policy of x-raying the chests of all recruits for the Armed Forces. He was very pleased that this procedure was adopted. Service with the Princess of Wales Own Regiment in Kingston as RMO for twenty years between the wars led to his becoming Honorary Colonel in 1968.

He was a leader in medicine as shown by the many senior positions he held. These included the presidencies of the Canadian Association of Radiologists, the Ontario Medical Association and the Kingston and Frontenac Medical Society. He was a member of the Council of the Ontario College of Physicians and Surgeons. The Ontario Medical Association honoured him with Life Membership and the Canadian Medical Association with Senior Membership.

He had long and valued service with the St John Ambulance Association of which he was a generous supporter, commencing in 1916. He was instrumental, with Dr LJ Austin, in training first year Medical students at Queen's in First Aid. In 1963 he was made Knight of the Order of St John. He was also a life long Mason and was a Past Deputy for Ontario.

Dr Jones was the first physician to describe the disease he called familial multilocular disease of the jaws, sometimes called cherubism.[1-4] It was briefly called Jones' disease. Thus Taybi and Lachman reference Jones' 1933 article as the earliest publication in this context.[5] The disease itself is familial and hereditary and has the pathological appearance of giant cell granuloma. Jones also published on histoplasmosis, among other diseases.

My own association with Dr Jones began in 1931 when he approached me to become a junior interne in his Department of Radiology in the Kingston General Hospital and to receive in return free room and board in the internes' quarters. This made me one of a group named the "Jones Boys" and began an association which lasted for the remainder of his life and most of mine. During that time he has been teacher, advisor, benefactor, associate and business partner as well as all around good companion.

No act of his, in my mind, better demonstrates his qualities of generosity and desire to reward excellence in young people than his support of a young man who after graduating from high school attracted Dr Jones' attention. He took him into the X-ray Department as a technician and later encouraged him to enter Queen's Medical School. Unfortunately, he did not succeed at this, but later found his niche proceeding to a doctorate of philosophy degree in English. He ultimately became a Professor of English in an Eastern Canadian University. He wrote to Mrs Jones, after Dr Jones died, and said, in part: "I should have so much liked to tell him how much I had learned from him and what a solid basis of ideals he gave me to build upon—he used always to emphasize concepts of being methodical, meticulous, thorough, painstaking..." He spoke also of "his high professional excellence and as well of his goodness, compassion and great generosity, whose memory I will try to honour." With these thoughts the many students and associates of Dr Jones will heartily agree.

Dr Bruce Colwell, another associate, speaking at a testimonial dinner for Dr Jones, quoted Mr Norman Fisher as having written some remarks which were true of Dr Jones:

> *[T]he problem is not just more education, not just more science and how are we to provide this—it is essentially the problem of how we are going to produce young people who are educated in both science and the humanities, who are trained in the skills of the modern world and yet have some acquaintance with the wisdom of the ages, who have the knowledge of techniques but also an understanding of the significance of human life. Technology is easy, education is difficult—our task for the 1960s is to combine the two.*

Colwell went on to remark that the Chief had done this for all of his life, and that he was a man ahead of his time.

Dr Jones was made an officer of the Order of the British Empire in 1945 by George VI and Commander of the Order of St John of Jerusalem in 1957 by Queen Elizabeth II.

In 1961 Dr Jones travelled to the Canadian Arctic and afterward he wrote a most beautifully descriptive narrative of his trip. He marvelled at the great ice floes and days with 24 hours of sun light, but he said the sight that impressed him most was the sky as he stepped off the plane on returning from Frobisher Bay. He looked up into the dark velvety night sky studded with brilliant stars that made him feel a strange peace. He felt grateful for daylight and dark, quiet and restfulness, the beauty of the night and that Canada was his home. At the end of the trip he said "For me the voyage had come to an end."

Dr William Jones died in Ottawa after a short illness on September 29, 1974.

IV *Léo-E Pariseau, Radiologiste*

Albert Jutras

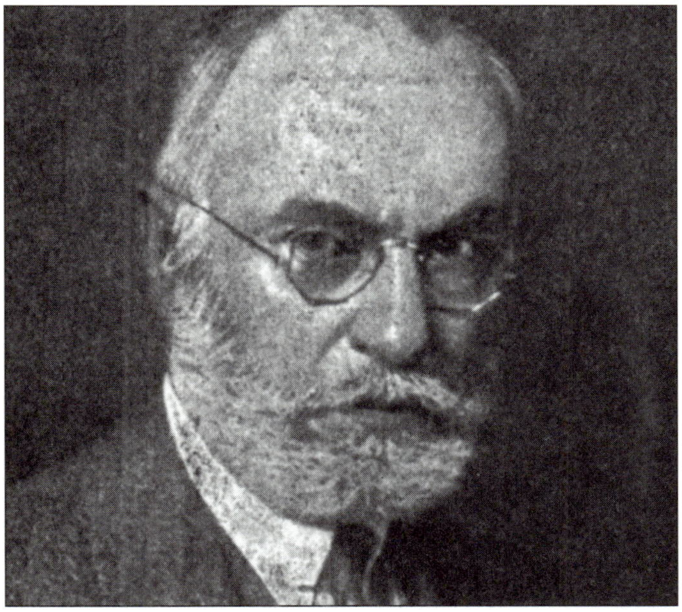

La radiologie ne remplissait pas toute seule l'existence très active, comme on sait, du Docteur Léo-E. Pariseau; il accordait une bonne part de son temps à d'autres sciences et à d'autres oeuvres. Néanmoins, c'est son titre d'électroradiologiste que ce grand médecin et ce savant préférait et c'est celui-là qui lui servait d'identité.

Dès l'obtention de son doctorat en médecine, à l'âge de vingt-quatre ans, Léo Pariseau commence et poursuit ses études de radiologie à l'Hôpital Notre-Dame de Montréal, de 1906 à 1909. Durant ce stage, il est aussi professeur d'électricité à l'École Polytechnique.

Il consacre les années qui suivent à l'étude de l'hygiène publique; mais, en 1913, nous le retrouvons à l'Hôpital St-Vincent de Sherbrooke où il conduit le service de radiologie en même temps qu'il remplit les fonctions d'hygiéniste de la ville. En 1915, son tempérament et ses convictions le poussent à s'enrôler et jusqu'à la fin de la guerre, il sera radiologiste à l'Hôpital Militaire Laval de St-Cloud, en France.

Le Docteur Pariseau n'était pas encore de retour au Canada que les autorités de l'Hôtel-Dieu de Montréal le sollicitaient de réorganiser et de diriger le Service d'Électro-radiologie. Durant vingt années près, de 1919 à 1938, il honora et porta loin le nom de cet hôpital. En outre d'une connaissance profonde de sa spécialité, Pariseau était un érudit, polyglotte, écrivain, naturaliste, physicien et chimiste. De telles qualités en faisaient un personnage dominant dans les sociétés et les congrès de radiologie.

Un des pionniers et des maîtres de l'électroradiologie

médicale, il reçut, à ces titres et à d'autres, beaucoup d'honneurs: Service médical; Officier de l'Instruction Publique de France; docteur ès-science Honoris causa de l'Université Laval; membre du Royal College of Physicians and Surgeons; Fellow of the American College of Radiology; vice-président de la Radiological Society of North America; membre de la Société de radiologie médicale de France; secrétaire et fondateur de la Société d'électroradiologie canadienne-française; membre honoraire de la Canadian Association of Radiologists; président de la Société médicale de Montréal; membre de la McGill Physical Society; membre de la Montréal Physiological Society; président de la Société de Biologie; premier président de l'ACFAS; rapporteur sur la physiothérapie au Congrès des Médecins de Langue Française de l'Amérique du Nord en 1930; etc...

Dans l'oeuvre écrite du Docteur Pariseau, l'électroradiologie occupe une place comparativement peu volumineuse. C'est que, par une forme de scrupule, un raffinement de sa conscience professionnelle, il craignait de donner l'impression de la réclame en publiant sur des sujets de sa profession. Toutefois, durant les dernières années de sa vie, il avait modifié son concept et il regrettait désormais de n'avoir diffusé davantage les trésors d'observations radio-cliniques qu'il avait entassés au cours de sa carrière. Au moment de sa retraite en 1938, nous avions esquissé un projet de travail en collaboration. Il s'agissait de recherches chimiques, physiques, biologiques et cliniques sur un procédé tout-à-fait inexploité pour l'opacification aux rayons X des cavités de l'organisme. La mise au point de la méthode promettait, croyions-nous, de grands progrès en physiologie et en médecine. Par malheur, les maladies de plus en plus sérieuses dont mon maître fut affligé ne lui permirent pas de donner suite à notre dessein commun. Dégagé de l'exténuante besogne journalière du radiologiste d'hôpital et de toutes les obligations accessoires auxquelles entraînent les soucis de la clientèle et les activités universitaires, il rêvait de pousser ces expériences et bien d'autres depuis longtemps conçues. Comme il aurait aimé, dans la paix de son foyer qui lui tenait aussi lieu de laboratoire et de bibliothèque et où les instruments scientifiques prenaient autant de place que les livres et les objets d'art, finir sa vie dans des oeuvres scientifiques de très longue haleine pour aider à l'avancement de la radiologie médicale. Il écrivit encore sur des sujets d'érudition, prépara quelques conférences, expérimenta sur les couleurs mais l'invalidité l'empêcha d'accomplir tout ce que son imagination créatrice lui proposait.

En analysant la longue bibliographie de Léo Pariseau, parue dans notre Journal en 1937, on se rend compte que si les travaux se rapportant à la médecine et à l'électroradiologie ne sont pas les plus nombreux, leur liste couvre quand même plus de trois pages imprimées, bien que ses innombrables communications et conférences devant les sociétés savantes de notre pays et de l'étranger n'entrent pas dans l'énumération.

Dans tout ceci, il importe de relever les travaux qui ont davantage répandu le nom du Dr. Pariseau hors de notre pays. Citons d'abord ses traductions de trois livres. C'est à lui en effet que fut confié le texte français de l'édition polyglotte dans Annals of Roentenology sur *les mastoïdes* (Law, 1920), *La vésicule biliaire pathologique* (A George, 1922) et *les troubles digestifs chez les nourrissons et les enfants* (Leon LeWald, 1923).

Je rappellerai aussi l'enthousiasme que Pariseau provoqua à la Société de Radiologie Médicale de France quand, en 1930, il exposa ses recherches sur la répartition des courants diathermiques. Jusqu'alors, la diathermie s'appliquait d'une façon empirique. Par de la gélose contenant du tétraiodo-mercurate l'argent en quantité suffisante pour teindre la masse en jaune serin et qui vire progressivement à l'orange puis au rouge entre 37° et 42°, Pariseau a pu observer *de visu* comment se distribue l'échauffement et donner les bases rationnelles de l'application des électrodes. La méthode calorimétrique de Pariseau est une acquisition pour la science.

L'usage que Pariseau fit des rayons X et du radium, de 1906 jusqu'à sa retraite en 1938, tant pour le diagnostic et le traitement des maladies que pour ses expériences de laboratoire, lui causèrent de graves ennuis notamment la perte d'un oeil et des ulcères chroniques de Röntgen aux mains. Quelques mois avant sa mort, il dut subir l'amputation de l'index gauche devenu néoplasique. Les métastases pulmonaires, auxquelles il succomba, ne dépendaient pas cependant des radiolésions digitales mais bien, d'un épithélioma du gros intestin opéré au cours de l'été 1939. La vérité exige cette précision; il n'en reste pas moins que la longue série des méfaits que les radiations lui infligèrent, mérite à Pariseau l'auréole des martyrs de la science.

Jusqu'au dernier jour, il demeura radiologiste. Quelques heures à peine avant d'expirer, il me demanda de le radiographier. Je reverrai toujours sa main décharnée me guidant pour le centrage de l'ampoule radiogène. Je me souviendrai aussi de la discussion du cliché. Suffoquant, cachectique, en partie aveuglé par l'ulcération de son bon oeil, mais avec une lucidité étonnante, le Docteur Pariseau recourait une dernière fois au procédé médical dont il conservait la maîtrise afin de connaître l'étendue des ravages dont sa poitrine était le théâtre et se procurer le renseignement pronostique dont il avait besoin pour décider du moment où exprimer ses suprêmes adieux à sa femme et aux siens.

L'humanité perd avec Léo-E Pariseau un type extraordinaire; la radiologie canadienne, son plus brillant chevalier.

L'EX-LIBRIS DE LÉO PARISEAU

Jadis, je ne sais plus quelle corporation de chirurgiens avait un sceau où figurait une main dont l'index portait à son extrémité un oeil grand ouvert.

Certes, les chirurgiens d'aujourd'hui n'ont point démérité; mais parfois les malades ont l'inscrutable physionomie du Sphinx. Si les chirurgiens n'appelaient alors certains spécialistes à leur secours, les positions respectives de l'oeil et du doigt pourraient bien être inversées!

Nos distingués confrères le savent et ils font de nombreux appels aux lumières des radiologistes et des autres aruspices du laboratoire. Il paraît qu'ils n'ont qu'à s'en féliciter.

En attendant le satisfecit qui consolera mes vieux jours, je me suis décerné...une image. Bien entendu, l'orgueilleuse devise qui la souligne s'applique aux seuls cas particuliers où j'y vois clair moi-même.

Ami des vieux livres, je ne pouvais pas ne pas donner une forme archaïque à mon ex-libris. Adonné au paradoxe et à l'antithèse, j'ai pris plaisir à confronter un chirurgien du moyen-âge avec notre moderne ampoule de Crookes. Ennemi de la pudidonderie, j'ai fait déshabiller la patiente. Respectueux des artistes, j'ai laissé le talentueux Jean Lébédeff développer à sa manière le thème que je lui assignais.

Remerciements:

Cet article, paru dans *Le Journal de l'Hôtel-Dieu de Montréal* est reproduit avec l'autorisation de la fille de Dr Jutras, Mimi, et de son gendre, le Dr Guy Duckett, lui-même un radiologiste de marque.

V *Dr Léo Pariseau*

ALBERT JUTRAS

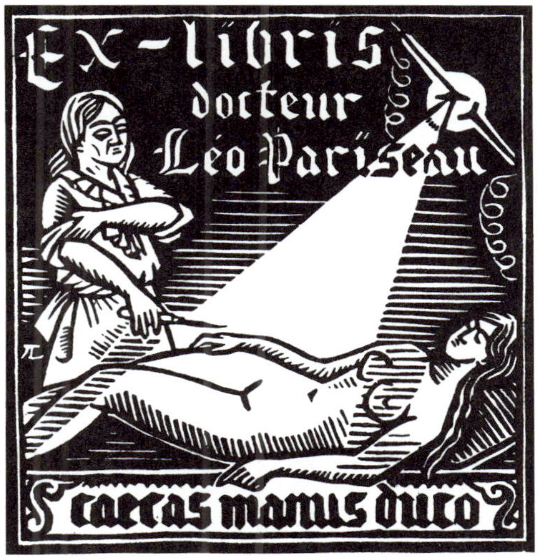

Born at Grenville on May 24, 1882, Dr Pariseau was the son of the late LS Pariseau, civil engineer, and Mrs Pariseau, formerly Miss Lawlor. As a professor in the École Polytechnique of Montréal Dr Pariseau was among the first Canadians to specialize in radiology. During the Great War he served as radiologist at the Laval Hospital at St Cloud from 1914 to 1918 and returning to Canada after the armistice he was appointed radiologist at the Hôtel-Dieu, holding that position until a few years ago when ill health forced him to retire. Founder of the *Hôtel-Dieu Journal*, Dr Pariseau was the author of many articles on scientific and historical subjects. He was an accomplished bilingual speaker. He possessed a large library on the history of medicine, which is to be installed in...the new University of Montréal.

Dr Pariseau married Yvonne Hebert, daughter of the sculptor, Louis Philippe Hebert.

A spirited character, and endowed with a high sense of honor and duty as well as an extensive knowledge in various fields of thought, he rightly earned a reputation as a colourful public speaker and a writer of note. Electroradiology was his special medical activity and he made numerous contributions to the subject. For these and for his qualities as a man, he acquired the admiration of the medical profession at large which has been highly justified. In the face of successive and long illnesses his resignation was dignified and noble. His daily contacts with x-rays and radium in diagnosis and treatment of diseases had cost him dearly and his unstinted devotion towards the sick was the cause of the loss of an eye and severe, painful chronic Röntgen ulcers of the fingers. In fact, a few months previous to his death he submitted to an amputation of the left index finger where already neoplastic changes had set in. The pulmonary metastases, nevertheless, to which he finally succumbed were in no way related to this lesion. His interest in radiology dates back to 1908 when as professor of electricity at L'École Polytechnique de Montréal he explored the technical and medical possibilities of this promising method. He may be considered as one of its foremost pioneers in Canada. At the outbreak of the last war, Dr Pariseau was established in Sherbrooke, Québec, where he also was acting in the capacity of public health officer. He relinquished his post and immediately volunteered for service in the army being assigned as radiologist to the Hôpital Laval de St Cloud throughout the whole period of hostilities. Demobilization followed and Major Pariseau assumed the position of radiologist in chief at the Hôtel-Dieu de Montréal. This post he occupied until 1938 when due to ill health he was forced to retire.

In 1932, in association with three colleagues of this hospital, he founded *Le Journal de l'Hôtel-Dieu*. For the greater part of twelve years he was its editor-in-chief, the body and soul of the publication. As a writer his activities were tremendous, for Dr Pariseau was the author of numerous topics of science, history, medical ethics, sociology, bibliography, etc. His literary works would easily make up many volumes. He was a translator of note. The French version of three volumes of *Annals of Röntgenology* was indeed a remarkable feat.

A consistent worker, as well as a brilliant lecturer, he made his influence felt by frequent public utterances before scientific and historical societies. His presentations were noted for their accurate documentation as well as the illuminating demonstrations which oftentimes embodied entirely new and convincing experiments. His make-up was that of a soldier; never a moment did he hesitate, whenever he deemed it necessary, to uphold the honour and dignity of the profession, to throw himself wholeheartedly and with vigour into the fight. He played an important role in many notable lawsuits, in the interest of medical ethics and in defense of the fraternity against the practice of quackery. 'Tis true, he swaggered along, elated by his lofty ideals, but he was neither a Cyrano nor a Don Quixote. One had only to listen to him in private conversation to realize that it was his serious outlook on things which was the basis of his inferences; and that at no time could one doubt that he was swayed by motives that were unselfish and chivalrous.

He maintained his opinions most forcibly and sometimes even violently, but would readily recognize in an opponent who knew how to put up a good fight the qualities of the man—and maybe then, the conversation would continue its course in a most friendly spirit, intermingled with anecdotes, followed up by frequent citations which would drive home his point. To him who considered time such a precious thing, he did not hesitate even when in physical pain to give himself entirely to his friends and enjoy their conversation during many long hours. It was customary for him to receive in his magnificent library, a great collection indeed of old and modern books, comprising all forms of human knowledge, chosen with much intelligence and loving care, where Dr Pariseau, without leaving his home, could verify the important facts of history and science from Aristotle to our times. At various meetings, by means of his own books, he would introduce the whole historical background of the feature topics which were up for discussion and study.

He saw to it before his death that this marvelous collection should not find its way into the hands of the dealers but would be handed on to become the property of the University of Montréal. This institution now is the proud possessor of the Pariseau Library, as McGill contains the Osler Library. A few hours before his death, in a soft and hesitant voice, he repeated to those about him how happy he was to have his wish finally realized. Such a sense of service, even after death, shows the greatness and loftiness of view of Dr Pariseau. The outcome of this generosity may well be the foundation of a chair of history of the sciences. Thus the great master, who was amongst us and whose loss we deeply feel, will continue in the mystery of eternity to stimulate the love of study and research for generations to come. Throughout his illness, by means of frequent radiograms, he himself attentively followed the progress of dissemination of neoplastic changes which had already reached his lungs. With much stoicism and a most edifying calmness he watched the various stages, knowing quite well the inevitable issue. Faced with death, dominating pain and partly suffocating, he husbanded his last bit of strength in preparing the catalogue for his library and in setting up the list of what constituted his laboratories of chemistry and physics which he also bequeathed to the University of Montréal. When this was finally attended to he laid himself down to die. Clear in mind and light of heart he waited, without fear, to be delivered from this earth and then, with much simplicity and dignity, he gladly passed to the great Beyond, grateful for the affection and care shown him.

There is no reason to despair, if of such men humanity is made.

Acknowledgement:
This article appeared in *Le Journal de L'Hôtel-Dieu de Montréal* and it is reprinted with permission and with the kind permission of Dr Jutras' daughter, Mimi, and son-in-law Dr Guy Duckett, himself a distinguished radiologist.

VI *From Szechuan to Saskatchewan*

A Profile of HE Johns and the Story of the Development of the "Cobalt Bomb"

Clive L Greenstock

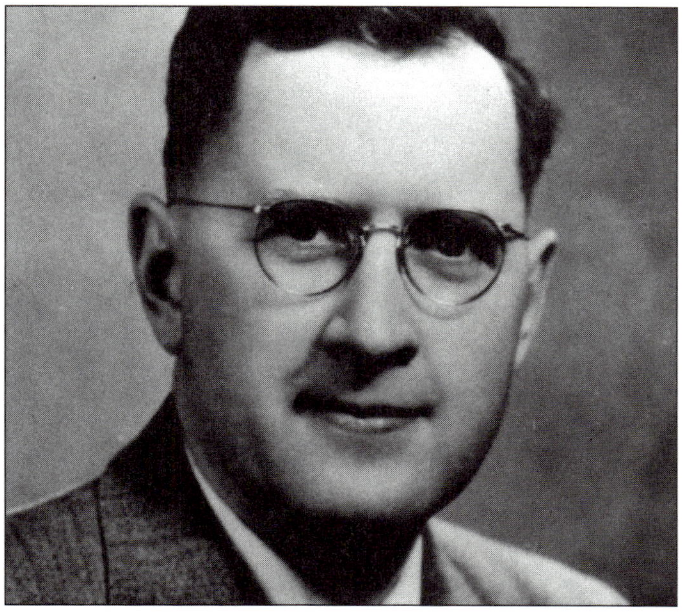

The first of HE Johns' ancestors to arrive in the New World from Devon, England in 1848 settled and established themselves in Exeter in southwestern Ontario. Harold's grandfather is said to have carried on his shoulders a hundredweight (112 lb) sack of seed grain from London, Ontario to Exeter. I think that this is a vivid demonstration of the energy and drive exhibited a century later by the grandson.

The first of the Johns' to leave the farm and attend university was Alfred (Harold's father), thus establishing a tradition followed wholeheartedly by HE Johns, his brothers and sister, and their subsequent offspring. Harold's father was a gold medallist at the University of Toronto in 1907, where he obtained his BSc (mathematics and physics). He received a masters degree in mathematics and a Bachelor of Divinity in 1908 and 1910, respectively. Alfred married his second cousin Myrtle Madge in Toronto, August 17, 1910 just before setting off for China.

Harold Elford Johns was born on July 4, 1915 in a Buddhist temple outside the city of Chengtu, in the province of Szechuan, West China. His mother and father pledged themselves and their lives to the church (Presbyterian and Methodist respectively) and went to China in 1910 on their honeymoon to become missionaries. Harold's mother taught English, and his father mathematics at West China University during the week; he preached on Sunday. This continued for 16 years before the rise of Chiang Kai-shek and the upheavals of the birth of Chinese communism forced him and his family to leave China to return to Canada. Harold and his brothers and sister acquired their academic and intellectual abilities, as well as their spiritual development, from their parents and family.

Harold's childhood in China was interesting and challenging. Because both parents were fully occupied with teaching and missionary activities, he and his brothers and sister were brought up by a Chinese nanny, Da Nyang, from whom they learned to speak Chinese. Unfortunately, all that remained fifty years later was his ability to sing "Jesus Loves Me" and say a few swear words in Chinese. He lived in a large two-storey faculty house on the campus of West China University, surrounded by a brick wall and guarded by a gateman. These were turbulent times in China, with feuds between rival warlords, with indiscriminate looting, rape, murder and mayhem. On his fifth birthday, in Kwan Shien where the family spent their summer holidays, he had all his birthday presents stolen in the night. Every summer was spent in Kwan Shien, but without motor cars and paved roads or even bicycles, the trek was arduous and dangerous. It meant travelling a distance of 40 miles by sedan chair over mountainous terrain. In 1924, when Harold was nine years old, he persuaded his father to allow him to join a two-week walking expedition to Tsao Go Lao, Tibet about 150 miles away. This required discipline, strength, endurance and determination. They were required to hike more than 20 miles per day through snow-capped mountains, reaching passes up to 10 000 feet in elevation and scrambling down the other side, trudging through river valleys, crossing gorges by rope bridges and other hazardous feats, with each member of the expedition carrying up to 80-pound loads on their backs! He successfully completed this epic challenge.

Harold's teenage years were spent briefly in Tacoma, Washington and then in Brandon, Manitoba during the Great Depression. Coming from China and behaving like a "Chinaman" meant that he was frequently teased and picked on or was the subject of discrimination, alienation and prejudice which forced him to develop ways to protect himself, deflect scorn, and hide humiliation. In so doing he developed a strong sense of independence, inner strength and self-discipline that would ultimately serve him well. The family later moved to Hamilton, Ontario where Harold attended McMaster University and obtained a BSc in mathematics and physics in 1936. He then received an MA and a PhD in physics at the University of Toronto in 1937 and 1939 respectively. A chance to hold a post-doctoral fellowship at the Cavendish Laboratory, Cambridge University with Dr John D Cockcroft was dashed by the advent of World War II. Instead, he accepted a position in the physics department at the University of Alberta in Edmonton.

The following year (1940) Harold married Sybil Hawkins, whom he had met at the University of Toronto. She provided the support and encouragement on which to build his scientific career and helped nurture his competitive instincts, steering them onto the dance floor, to the bridge table and into choral singing, only the latter of which activities would meet with the approval of his strict Methodist parents. During the war years HE Johns found himself in a backwater, scientifically, socially and intellectually. In true Johns fashion, however, he set about to do his bit for the war effort and enthusiastically threw himself into teaching air force pilots physics and mathematics and the practical aspects of radio and radar navigation within the Commonwealth Training Scheme. In addition, he became the official radiographer for western Canada, performing tests on aircraft castings using an obsolete x-ray tube obtained from Ottawa. This experience was invaluable and proved to be a critical turning point in his career.

At the end of the war Harold was invited by Dr EL Harrington to join the physics department of the University of Saskatchewan in Saskatoon and to spend half of his time starting the medical physics group at the newly created Saskatchewan Cancer Commission in Regina under Dr Alan Blair, Medical Director.

Here was a golden opportunity—being in the right place at the right time—with the freedom to make a name for himself, a supportive employer and sufficient funding to achieve progress in the pioneering field of medical physics. In typical Johns' fashion, he charged forward, embarking on a trip around North America to visit the leading institutions and talk to their scientific personnel. While in Toronto, *en route* back to Saskatchewan, he took advantage of the opportunity to hear Professor VM Mayneord of the Royal Cancer Hospital, London, England, who was giving a month-long series of lectures in physics to radiologists directing the various cancer clinics in Ontario. This fortuitous occasion helped initiate the ideas which were eventually to lead to the publication of the first edition of *The Physics of Radiology* in 1953.

Mayneord, like many leading scientists from Europe, had spent the war years in North America. Between 1940 and 1945 he and a small group of the nuclear science elite had worked secretly in Montréal and Chalk River to design and build a reactor to produce materials for the first atomic bomb. Ironically, these scientists were recruited by Dr JD Cockcroft under whom HE Johns had originally planned to do a post-doctoral fellowship at Cambridge. They were a part of the Atomic Energy Project, which was coordinated with the Manhattan Project and represented an allied scientific initiative to exploit nuclear fission and produce an atom bomb before Adolf Hitler's scientists in Germany were able to do so. These projects led to the development and production of many new radio-isotopes for medical research, radiopharmaceuticals for nuclear medicine and the invention by Harold Johns of a new treatment of cancer. The device was called the "cobalt bomb," by a writer for *MacLean's Magazine* in 1952 and was first used in Canada for the treatment of cancer in 1951.

Upon his return to Saskatchewan, Dr Johns reported on his trip, and in response to a request for recommendations from his boss, Dr Blair, he asked for a 25-MeV betatron and a cobalt-60 unit. The first betatron had been built in Urbana, Illinois by its inventor Dr Kersh, who had improved on work originally carried out by Dr Lester Skaggs. This design was then in production by Allis Chalmers, and the price tag was $80 000.

Undaunted, Dr Blair arranged for an appointment with then premier of Saskatchewan Mr TC Douglas. When introduced to HE Johns, the premier recollected that he had been taught mathematics by Harold's father, Alfred Johns. Douglas must have been favorably impressed, because the meeting resulted in a decision to approve the request to install a betatron in the Saskatchewan Cancer Clinic.

The Atomic Energy Control Board (AECB) provided $30 000, and the betatron was delivered and, after considerable testing and evaluation, installed in 1947. It provided reliable service until 1962. The first patient was treated by Dr TA Watson on March 29, 1949. In the meantime the NRX reactor at Chalk River had been started up in July 1947, and shortly after (1948–1950), Drs WV Mayneord and AJ Cipriani had loaded three samples of cobalt-59 into it. The resulting three 1000-curie cobalt-60 sources were originally selected for Saskatchewan, London, Ontario, and for Mayneord to take to the United Kingdom. However, because of uncertainties about ensuring safety and security

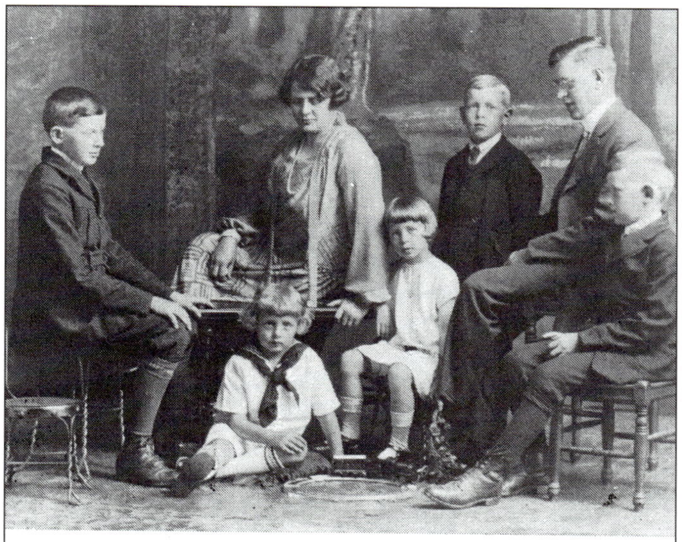

THE JOHNS FAMILY IN MAY OF 1925

Left
The Johns family in May 1925 about to return to Canada. Harold is in the sailor suit at the front

Left below
Dr Johns with colleagues, 1951

Left bottom
Dr Johns explains the operation of the radiation beam aperture to young Princess Margaret in 1967

Below
Lake Boshkung, Ontario after 1962 International Congress of Radiology in Montréal: (back row) Lloyd Kemp, John Greening, Frank Ellis, Harold Hewitt, Charlie Wilson, Gordon Whitmore, Jack Fowler; (front row) Jan Cederlund, Harold Johns, Sylvia Fedoruk, Maurice Tubiana, Doug Cormack

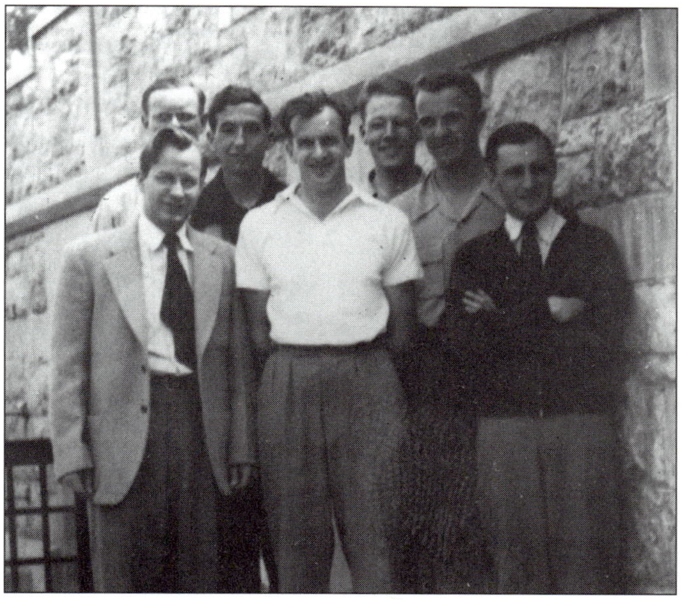

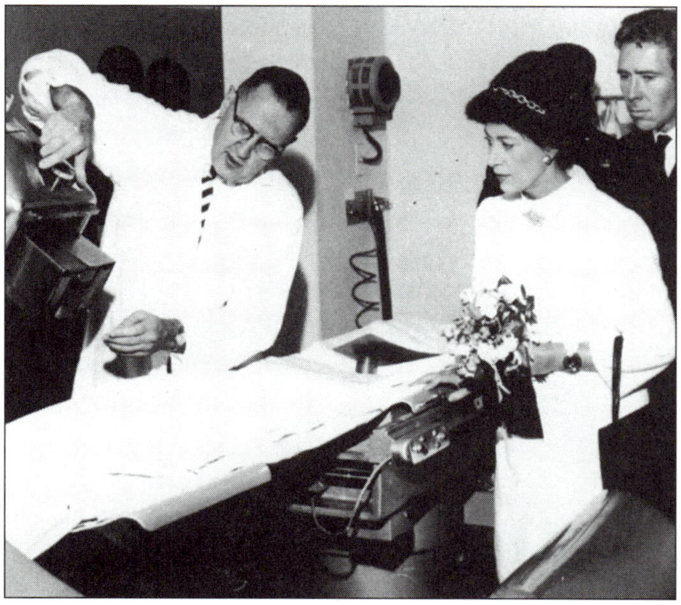

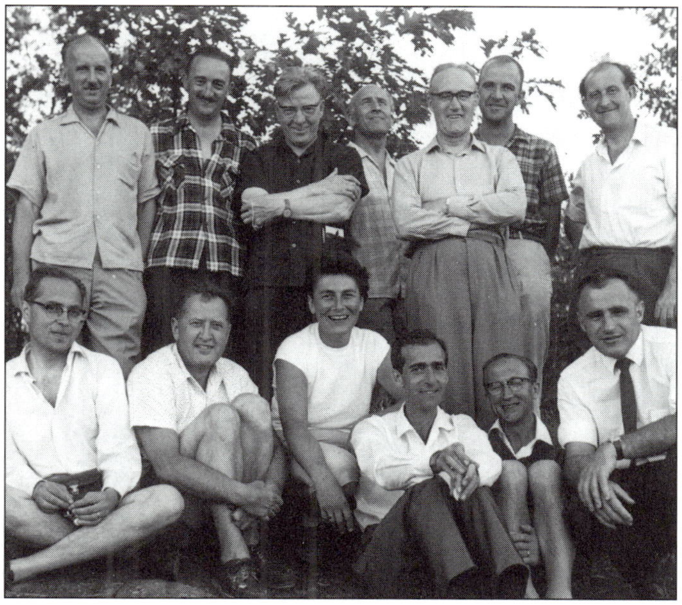

of radioactive materials in post-war Europe, Mayneord declined to accept the source for shipment to England; instead, it was sent to Dr Gilbert Fletcher at the MD Anderson Hospital, Houston, Texas. The first two Canadian cobalt-60 sources were delivered in the summer of 1951, and the first patients were treated by the fall.

Dr Johns' life in Saskatchewan centred around the university, and this was a very fruitful and creative period in his life. It was here that he trained the first Canadian medical physicists who were later to join him when he moved to Toronto. There were long days and long nights working on experiments, but there was still time for playful student pranks. An example was the time when HE Johns was late for his lecture and jumped in his car only to find that it would not move. After several attempts to figure out what had happened, he eventually discovered that the car had been put up on blocks so that all the wheels were off the ground! Another time he came out to the parking lot after a late session at the laboratory, and his car was nowhere to be found. Wondering if he was becoming absent-minded, he walked home. Next day everyone was talking about the whereabouts of his car. Somehow it had ended up on the roof-top of the betatron building!

HE Johns began to build a reputation in Saskatchewan. Many well-known scientists would visit and give guest lectures at the university. Travelling in those days usually meant taking the overnight train from Toronto or Vancouver. On one occasion, Dr WB Lewis visited the university but his departure was delayed six hours because of bad weather. It was just before Christmas and HE Johns was making a dollhouse for his daughters Gwen and Claire, so after supper HE Johns invited WB Lewis to help with the construction. By the time they were ready to leave for the train station, WB Lewis had wired up the doll's house with light bulbs in every room, connected through switches to a battery. It was not nuclear powered, but nevertheless was greatly treasured by the daughters on Christmas morning. Surely scientists are little boys at heart.

In 1956 Johns moved to Toronto where he became the Head of the Physics Division, Ontario Cancer Institute (OCI). He methodically started to build a strong research and development group in medical biophysics. After many battles with the University of Toronto, he eventually succeeded in creating the Graduate Department of Medical Biophysics in 1958. With his graduate students from Saskatchewan as key staff members, he built a team which was to become the most productive research group in medical physics and created a generation of energetic, keen and well-trained medical physicists.

Harold Johns was an incomparable teacher. His research career was built on his skill in motivating students, putting them at ease, instilling confidence, supporting and cajoling them to ensure that everyone produced to the limit of their capability. His office door was always open, and his favorite opening gambit was to say: "OK. Now what are you trying to say? Show me what you mean. Go to the blackboard. Explain what is going on here. How are you going to proceed? What is the plan? Let's get on with it!"

Everyone felt part of the team right from their first day because of the atmosphere of tolerance, understanding, acceptance and support. The sense of purpose, the work ethic and the challenging environment were shared by the workshop, library and secretarial staff, administrators, technologists, students and scientists. The feeling of being equal partners and part of an extended family was created and sustained by the active involvement and personal relationships shared with HE Johns. What was a typical day at the lab like? There was always time for work and time for play. Friendly (and not so friendly) celebration ranged from one-arm push-ups in the cafeteria, races up and down eight flights of stairs, and the famous squash ladder. Not least, every graduate student had to successfully pass all graduate and undergraduate courses, submit and defend a thesis, write a paper for publication in a peer-reviewed journal—and win at least one game of squash against the master!

Christmas and summer vacations were no exceptions. The annual Christmas party was legendary for the impromptu skits about "a day in the life of a grad student"—shades of "Second City," "Saturday Night Live," or a "Night at the Improv." The social gathering of the year was the traditional Christmas carol sing-song at the Johns' residence. The piano was hauled out to the middle of the living room, and staff, students, spouses, friends and family would gather round and sing with gusto, working their way through the song sheets, with short breaks to drink some punch, until every song had been sung. The singers were ably accompanied at the piano by HE Johns' eldest daughter Gwen, who performed this duty enthusiastically every year for 15 years, from the time she was 10 years old until she moved to England for a year in 1968. The Christmas sing-song subsequently became a tradition in her home.

Even the mandatory trips to the Johns' summer cottage at Lake Boshkung were a *tour de force:* days spent hauling rocks or pouring cement, water fights and other feats, from leaping off the roof of the boat-house to ski-jumping, jump-starts off the dock, star-gazing, canoe jousting and, after a hearty feast, evenings of charades.

Many conservative visiting professors from the UK, Europe and Scandinavia have been initiated into the challenges of water-skiing at the cottage. One non-swimmer mastered this skill while still puffing on his pipe!

Graduate students would perform endless hours of manual labor in the mistaken beliefs that a) the projects would be completed, b) there were signs of progress or an overall plan, and c) a good job would further one's career or facilitate getting one's PhD.

Every September, the whole department would take off to the cottage for a week. These Boshkung Conferences were an opportunity to indulge in an intensive retreat and workshop to bring everyone up to speed on all the latest research being performed at OCI and to introduce new staff and students and ensure that they all became imbued with the infectious spirit of friendly rivalry, fierce loyalty and pride in reaching new heights of scientific achievement. This remains as a living legacy of HE Johns—his humanity, generosity, humility, tremendous energy and hard work extending over a lifetime of scientific discovery.

HE Johns never was one to put on airs and graces but treated everyone with consideration and respect and showed genuine interest in every one of his staff. Many technologists, students and other staff can attest to his generosity and kindness. He reached out and touched all who worked with him—with a friendly greeting, a quiet word of support and encouragement, an invitation for supper or a weekend spent at the cottage. These have been the hallmarks of "the professor," the family man, the inquisitive mind, the competitive spirit, the indefatigable worker, the intrepid explorer and the boy-at-heart.

Science is universal and HE Johns always encouraged his staff to develop the exchange of ideas that is so essential to maintaining a viable scientific research program. In 1960 he moved his family to California and took a sabbatical year at California Institute of Technology with Dr Max Delbruck to explore the newly emerging field of molecular photobiology. One of the secrets of success is knowing when to change fields of endeavour and what fields to move into. This move led to a new direction in Canadian medical biophysics; exploring the underlying mechanisms of radiation damage to genetic material and its biological consequences. Being in the presence of a Nobel laureate such as Delbruck was inspirational, but his autocratic, awe-inspiring, elitist style was not ideally suited to a prairie boy with farming and missionary roots. Delbruck would personally select attendees at important seminars and scientific meetings, and one time he had the audacity to give someone else's seminar because he could do a better job!

The OCI operated in a more democratic, cooperative fashion. One day, a telegram arrived addressed to HE Johns from a graduate student attending a cancer conference in the United States. It said, "Sell cancer treatment machines stop Stop current research program stop Convert space to animal research and set up a molecular biology lab stop A cure for cancer is at hand." This give and take and the flexibility and opportunities to develop new directions without undue bureaucratic impediment allowed OCI to become Canada's premier cancer research institute.

In 1971, after ten years of pioneering work in photochemistry, HE Johns took another sabbatical with Dr Jack W Boag at the Royal Marsden Hospital, London, England to explore the important fields of computed tomographic scanning and diagnostic imaging, which were then emerging as key technologies in health care and diagnostic medicine around the world. With the foresight of HE Johns, Toronto scientists remain at the forefront of this promising activity.

On April 19, 1978 in Rideau Hall, Ottawa, the achievements of his illustrious career and his international reputation were recognized in a ceremony at which the Governor General of Canada appointed him an Officer of the Order of Canada. This represents the highest of many honours received throughout his career and is a fitting tribute at the culmination of a lifetime of devotion to scientific excellence in the cause of cancer research and improvements in diagnosis and treatment.

Harold Johns officially retired in 1980 after a rewarding and productive career in which he supervised 68 graduate students and was author or co-author of over 220 scientific publications in peer-reviewed journals. On the technical side, he obtained several patents, and his invention, the "cobalt bomb," is still being used to treat cancer in radiotherapy or oncology centres in over 70 countries around the world. It is estimated that more than seven million patients have benefited from treatments received from the over 3000 cobalt-60 teletherapy units in operation in 1995. The majority of these units have been designed and built by AECL in Canada, based on the original concepts developed in the late 1940s by HE Johns in collaboration with a mechanic friend Johnny MacKay of the Acme Machine & Electric Company in Saskatoon, Saskatchewan.

VII *Claude James Bodle* RT ASXT

1891–1980

William Doern

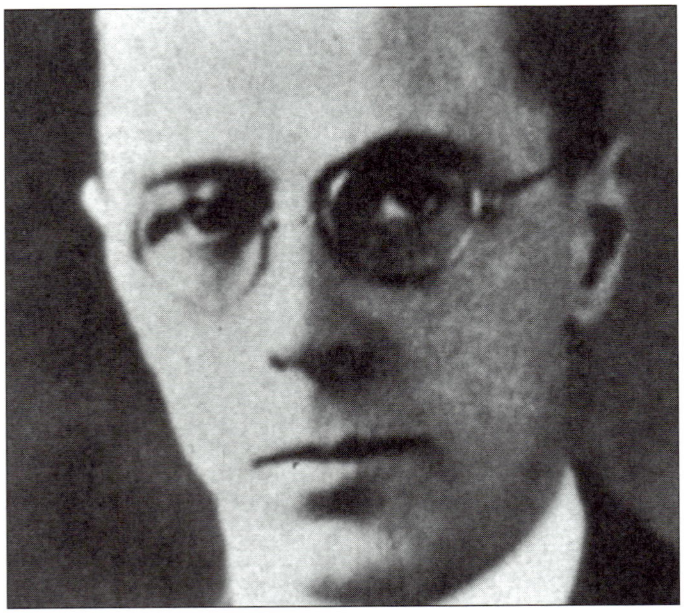

Claude James Bodle ART ASXT*, First President of the Canadian Society of Radiological Technologists, was a thin wiry individual with the potential energy of a high powered transformer, and the staying power of an English bulldog (probably a heritage from his English ancestors and upbringing).*[1]

CJ Bodle graduated in pharmacy from the University of Manitoba in 1916 and went directly into the Canadian Army Medical Corps, 11th Field Ambulance, Canadian Expeditionary Force, where he spent the next three years. In 1919 Dr Currie McMillan, a Winnipeg radiologist who had also been in the army, asked Mr Bodle to work with him as an x-ray technician. In those days there were no short courses in x-ray work, and few books. So Claude Bodle had to learn his new trade the hard way: from his employer, by experimentation, and later by travelling hither and yon in the United States and Canada to learn from other technicians and radiologists from knowledge they had acquired the same way.

In October 1920 he went to Chicago to a meeting organized by Dr Ed Jerman. There, the American Society of X-Ray Technicians was formed, and Claude Bodle became a registered charter member. In the late 1920s he had the honour of being elected President of the American Society of X-Ray Technicians. Claude James Bodle was the only member of the Canadian Society of Radiological Technicians (CSRT)—later the Canadian Association of Medical Radiation Technologists—who had the honour of being president of both the Canadian and American Societies.

In November 1929 the Manitoba Society of X-Ray Technicians was formed with a membership of two registered technicians, Claude Bodle RT and Bill Doern RT, and a small group of local x-ray operators as charter members. Claude Bodle RT was elected president, a position he held at intervals for a number of years. In 1942 Bodle was appointed to the board of directors, who were to organize a Canadian Society of Radiological Technicians. In 1944 the CSRT was formed. Claude James Bodle was its first *elected* president.

I became closely associated with Jim Bodle and had the greatest respect for his outstanding knowledge about every aspect of radiography. Those who were closely associated with him felt that he had forgotten more about radiography than most of us will ever know.

Bodle had a great sense of humour, which he gladly shared at meetings and especially during the many long train trips of the earlier years to eastern and western Canada. His hobby was artwork, which he studied late in life. His contributions were recognized in many ways including those that follow:

- Honorary Membership in the British Society of Radiographers, 1951.
- Life Membership in the Manitoba Society of X-Ray Technicians, 1954.
- Welch Memorial Lecturer CSRT, 1954.
- Life Membership, Canadian Society of X-Ray Technicians, 1967.

Acknowledgement:

This tribute, from CAMRT archives, was written by Bill Doern RT in January 1988 when Mr Doern was 88.

(b) The Builders

One machine can do the work of 50 ordinary men. No machine can do the work of one extraordinary man.
— Elbert Hubbard

To someone with a biologically based education, and without obvious historical prejudices, the evolution of the radiological sciences in Canada appears to take on the characteristics of an organic whole. I conclude that while the occasional Newton or Einstein, or in our case Röntgen, will arise to change the course of human destiny, most often history is made by men of insight and imagination who see a need or an opportunity to advance both their own and societal goals. And who do so without sacrifice of their integrity. It seems to me that that is a reasonable bargain. In the case of the people chronicled here it is also apparent that society got more than it gave: in the words of someone who proof-read this text "they were all compulsive over-achievers." And yet most if not all seem to have preserved the human touch. There is not one I wish I had not met.

— Brian Lentle

VIII *C Wesley Prowd* MD
FRCPC FACR

Anon

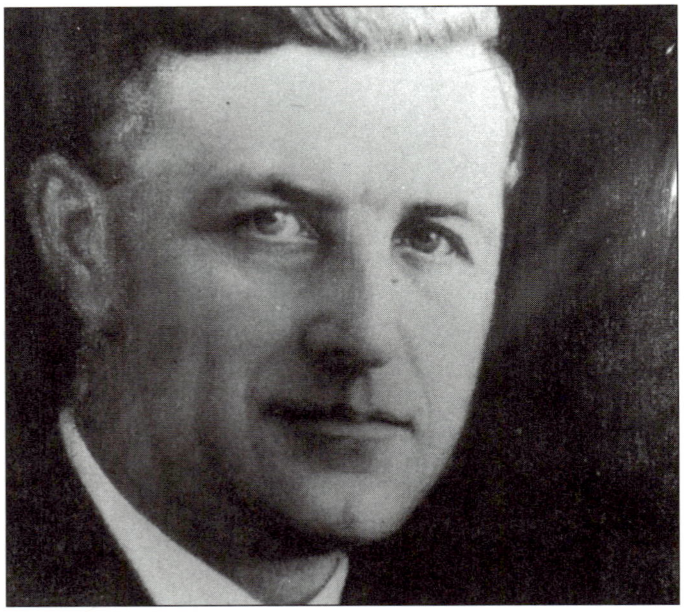

A short time after Dr Gordon Richards returned to Vancouver in 1919 from military service, he was offered the position of Head of the Department of Radiology in the Toronto General Hospital. Later, he was appointed Professor of Radiology at the University of Toronto. When Richards departed, Dr Prowd was appointed to take full charge of the radiology department of St Paul's Hospital in Vancouver. Until 1920 Dr Prowd remained in general practice, in partnership with Dr HB Gourlay, in the Bower Building on Granville Street. In 1920 Dr Prowd travelled to Germany, Stockholm and Paris for some months to study radium. He brought back some radium with him and began treatment with this new and powerful therapeutic agent. It became Dr Prowd's custom to visit the great European centres every three years, where progress was being made in Röntgen and Curie therapy. He also inspected and studied the recent developments at the plants of Siemens, near Berlin, and Phillips, at Eindhoven in Holland.

Consequently, Dr Prowd installed the first deep x-ray therapy machine in western Canada in St Paul's Hospital.

When the north wing of St Paul's Hospital was completed in 1931, the space set aside by the Sisters for the radiology department was complete with lead protection in some of the walls and with electrical connections made adequate, not only for that time, but also for future developments. St Paul's possessed the best equipped and laid out radiology department of any hospital of comparable size in Canada. Dr Prowd's advice and counsel played a considerable part in this achievement.

In 1933 the Sisters took over the diagnostic and therapeutic radiology equipment from Dr Prowd, placing the management of the department under Sister Charles Spinola, though Dr Prowd remained as Medical Director of Radiology. In 1947 the radium equipment was purchased from Dr Prowd by the Sisters of the hospital.

Dr Prowd worked hard, arriving at the hospital a little after 8 am and leaving at about 6 pm. These hours were adhered to for many years, though later, and particularly in the last two years of his service, his radiological activities became considerably curtailed.

Dr Prowd also became a member of the Trail Riders of the Rockies. Each year this organization met in Banff to make a trail-riding trip of some 250 miles. Dr Prowd continued these rides and became the proud possessor of a coveted enamel badge, achieved for riding 2500 miles through the mountains. Dr Prowd, it is hardly necessary to add, was very fond of the outdoors. Through his interest in riding, fishing and hunting, he explored the least known parts of British Columbia, and he developed an unusual knowledge of the province. He firmly believed that sunlight was the best antidote for the deleterious effects of exposure to x-rays. Nevertheless, he suffered for some years from a skin condition on one of his legs for which he thought amputation might eventually be necessary.

Of note Dr Prowd had a good memory and a fine thoughtful mind. He was particularly happy in giving a formal address or speech. Dr Prowd helped form the first medical representation at St Paul's Hospital, known as the Medical Advisory Board, and in April 1919 he was a founding member of the medical staff. He endeavoured by his leadership in his own department and by his unfailing loyalty to St Paul's Hospital to develop the services which this great hospital had been able to give to Vancouver.

Dr Prowd was particularly helpful to junior staff and made them feel at ease when discussing radiographs. Often some thought or word expressed by Dr Prowd was of great help in the care of a patient. He had excellent judgement and was not susceptible to the passing therapeutic enthusiasms for which x-rays were then being advocated.

Dr Prowd was extensively honored. He was president of the Canadian Association of Radiologists on two occasions; a member of the American Radiological Association; and a member of the Radiological Society of North America, which then had affiliations with the European Radiological Association. Dr Prowd also served as president of the Vancouver Medical Association in 1931.

Dr Prowd, the first doctor to advocate a free cancer clinic in British Columbia accessible to all its citizens, was a member of a committee which persuaded the provincial government to purchase $105 000 worth of radium, subsequently given to the Cancer Clinic in Vancouver.

In 1913 Dr Prowd married Mrs Eccles of Winnipeg, and they had two daughters, Barry and Patricia.

In 1947 Dr Prowd had a myocardial infarction from which he recovered, but he died of a second such attack in June 1949, aged 66 years and five days.

Acknowledgement:
This account, for which no provenance can be established, was found in the CAR archives.

IX *A Lady of Vision*

A Transcription of Part of the 28th Mary F Cameron Lecture

COLETTE GAZDIC

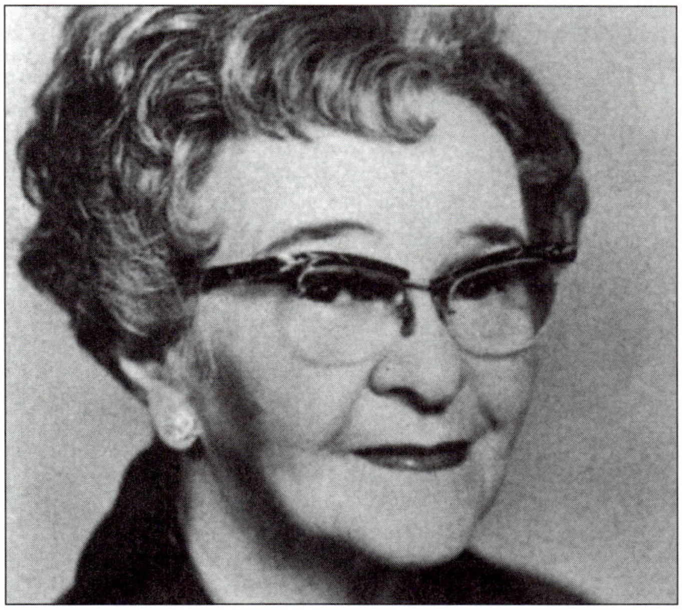

The Annual Mary F Cameron Lecture affords us the opportunity to become reacquainted with—or to introduce—a grand lady to a new generation of medical radiation technologists. Mary Cameron was a prime mover in the founding of both the Ontario and Canadian societies of radiological technicians.

Mrs Cameron was born shortly after the turn of the century. She was the granddaughter of Sir John Abbott, a prime minister of Canada, and received her early education at home in the province of Québec by private tutors. Her father, an Anglican minister, found time away from his ecclesiastical duties to teach Mary music. She shared her father's love for the arts and as a young woman spent time teaching music in turn.

Romance turned her interest toward x-rays. She married a young surgeon, Dr Keith W Cameron, from Perth, Ontario. Anxious to share her husband's interests, she decided that helping him with his x-ray work was the answer. However, shortly after their marriage, Dr Cameron became ill, and in 1922 the couple was forced to move to Texas. Dr Cameron recovered enough to become house surgeon at the Robert B Green Hospital in San Antonio, Texas. To be with him, his wife was further educated in x-ray technology by Dr MB Hamilton, one of the outstanding radiologists of the south western United States. Mary was appointed chief technologist at her husband's hospital. Eighteen months later, Dr Cameron died and, after six years in Texas, Mary returned to Canada. She took the post of chief technologist at the McGregor Clinic in Hamilton.

When Mary Frances first became interested in radiography, people installed their own equipment in small dark rooms and opened their doors to patients. Only large hospitals had the luxury of x-ray departments, which were often insufficiently staffed and equipped with primitive machinery. Wires were exposed and, if a visiting physician accidentally touched an unfamiliar lever or button and was thrown across the room by the electrical shock, what of it? Protection was not practiced in a methodical manner. Technologists trained for a while with a doctor who understood radiology, and no one asked potentially embarrassing questions about qualifications. They were, as you might guess, overworked and poorly paid. Some attempts in standardizing education had been made during World War I and a well-recognized textbook, *The United States Army X-Ray Manual,*[1] was published.

In June 1933 three technologists from Ontario attended the eighth annual meeting of the American Society of X-Ray Technicians. The American Society's president was a Winnipeg technologist, Claude Bodle. During the Rochester, New York convention Canadian technologists unsuccessfully attempted to organize a society in Canada. Upon his return home, Mr John Coones, affectionately known as "Jack," was encouraged by his radiologist to pursue the organizational possibilities, the start of a one man crusade!

Mr Coones gave unselfishly of his time, energy and money to gather together the first group of technologists. Jack was chief technologist at the Peterborough Civic

Hospital for 28 years and a commercial representative with the 3M Company for 14 years. He assisted the young association in its development and early maturation and cared greatly for the welfare of his fellow technologists. Jack had an interesting story about a certain letter received in response to his campaign request for establishing a technologists' society. "I have no objections to my technicians joining a society," wrote a radiologist, "so long as it has an all male membership," Mr Coones' incessant efforts culminated in an organizational meeting on February 13, 1935 at the office of Burke Electric & X-ray Corporation in Toronto.

A petite, brown-eyed woman, whom we would later come to know as Mary Cameron, was among the small group of enthusiasts who met in that Toronto firm's office. When the meeting ended, the Ontario Society of Radiological Technicians (OSRT) was off to a flying start. Mr JH Coones was elected president by acclamation, a post he would hold until 1937. Jack never ceased to encourage the membership to take an individual and collective interest in the affairs of the association. The OSRT honoured him with a life membership in 1970 and annually presents in his memory, the "Jack Coones Memorial RT Essay Award." The profession lost one of its staunchest supporters on April 15, 1974. Jack was 73 years old.

The newly organized society permitted technologists who were employed and who had completed the required training period of two years to become active members. Potential members were asked to remit to the OSRT secretary-treasurer an application for membership, a letter of recommendation from their chief, a $5.00 registration fee and the annual membership dues of $2.00. Technologists accepted for membership received the degree of Registered Radiological Technician, and after their name on the registry would appear RRT. Further recognition would be awarded to members who had done outstanding work in radiology by qualifying them as master radiological technicians. After December 31, 1936 candidates would be subject to examination set by the Ontario Medical Association.

On March 26, 1935, Mrs Cameron was granted a master degree in Radiological Technology.

Tommy Hurst was an outstanding and distinguished technologist who was well versed in the affairs and needs of a new organization. His support and leadership were greatly required during the formative years. Chief technologist at the Toronto General Hospital, he was regarded as a pioneer guide and teacher. He was among the first to organize classes for technical training in Ontario. In 1939 the society sadly accepted his resignation as president elect when enlisted for overseas service. He is remembered annually by our presentation of the " TB Hurst Memorial Academic Award" to the graduate technologist who has achieved the highest aggregate marks in the certification examination.

The year 1935 proved to be a time of tremendously hard work for those few involved individuals. Our first contact with the Ontario Hospital Association (OHA) took place on October 1, 1935 during the afternoon sessions of their twelfth annual conference. As OSRT President, Mr Coones presented a lecture entitled "The Work of the Radiological Technician." It is thanks to our early leaders that after 56 years we continue to benefit from our affiliation with the OHA. Successive meetings of the OSRT executive were held that year to formulate a constitution, to organize and plan the pursuit of a charter and to strike various committees. "On May 9, 1936 the Ontario Society of Radiological Technicians officially came into existence." Preparations for the first convention of the society were finalized, and members met at the King Edward Hotel in Toronto on May 22 and 23, 1936. The registration fee was $1.00.

Shortly after the society's formation, membership dues allowed the organization to reimburse its executive members for their travel on society business at a rate of five cents per mile and $2.00 a day for hotel accommodations.

By 1937 the OSRT Executive was planning area meetings in Ottawa and London for the purpose of acquainting the technologists with the aims of the society. The first groups of x-ray people to join were the western and eastern sections, with the northern section soon to follow. Our leaders were now empowered to attempt the formation of a dominion society. Mary Cameron was elected secretary-treasurer of the OSRT that year and invited to sit on the Dominion Organizational Committee.

In September 1938 the first examinations for registered radiological technicians were available. The society's treasury had grown to $1794.38. Mrs Cameron was the OSRT president-elect, and the first registrar, Ms Gwendolyn Wood, was appointed to the executive.

Supplementary letters patent, changing the name of the society to Ontario Society of Radiographers (OSR) and revising the objects and by-laws, were granted on May 17, 1939. The name change had been influenced by reports from the bank and commercial companies and by the difficulty in making oneself understood over the telephone. The new name was brief, more pleasing to the ear and distinctly easier to pronounce than the old title. It also conformed to the name of the British society with which affiliation was proposed. It was at that time that Mr Felix George Reason, OSR president, was asked to meet with the examining board to draw up a curriculum for student education. By October 29, 1939 a general outline of a syllabus and proposed examination covering all subjects were agreed upon and drafted. The syllabus consisted of studies in darkroom practice, physics, radiographic technique, anatomy, physiology and radiation therapy.

Born in London, England, George Reason came to Canada in his late teens with work experience as a darkroom technician. He became involved in radiography during World War I while serving as a Sergeant with the 4th Battalion. After the war, he found employment with the Christie Street Military Hospital, the Toronto General Hospital (as it was then called) and, lastly, the Toronto Medical Arts Building. Mr Reason was considered a born organizer, and for years the Ontario society's convention plans and national meeting arrangements fell on his able shoulders. He was one of the prime organizers of the provincial and national societies. Like many an x-ray pioneer, he carried scars of severe x-ray burns to his hands, which had necessitated several skin grafts. Mr Reason died on November 25, 1952 at the young age of 61 years.

By 1940, when Mrs Cameron was OSR President, there were 188 active members, 44 of whom were students. Two examinations were prepared that year and an Education Committee was created with George Reason and Mary Cameron as members. Their accomplishments included creating a contract for student technologists, the selection of textbooks upon which the examinations would be based and the finalization of a student curriculum. OSR certificates were printed in the new official colours of the society, purple and gold, symbolic of fidelity and quality. The first official registry was published, and the accounting firm of Martin & Weir was hired. With the help of well-wishers, the group established standards of work and saw its educational courses inaugurated. It adopted the medical code as its standard of ethics and even launched its own technical journal.

Being at the spearhead of this long battle might seem enough to absorb Mary Cameron's energies. But, as her contribution to the war effort, she was one of four technologists and two students to radiograph some 15 000 chests of airmen in the Hamilton district. This, at a rate of 90 per night, was accomplished in their spare time, of course. Mrs Cameron also managed to write papers on x-ray techniques and organize the Anglican Woman's Business and Professional Club. She was always actively involved in community and church affairs. The publication of the society's first official journal, *The Bulletin,* was undertaken with Percy Ghent as editor and Mary Cameron as business manager.

Born in England in 1888, Mr Ghent came to Canada in his teens and found employment with Toronto Sick Children's Hospital. In 1910 he moved to the Toronto General Hospital (TGH) where he worked closely with Mr BJ (Budgie) Fenner, who was considered to be a pioneer in radiography. Percy was an active participant in the amazing development of x-ray technology in Toronto. Many of his short stories were touched with his understanding of human nature and lightened by his whimsical humour. Affectionately known as "Pops," his verses and cartoons were given liberal circulation in the x-ray department as well as in the hospital. His book of poems, *Bits & Pieces,* was about the medical staff of the TGH. Another of his books, *Radiography has a Lighter Side,* he privately printed in 1936 and distributed, with his compliments, to members of the OSRT at their first meeting in Toronto. Unknown to many, he had a musical side and had composed the lyrics and music to a hymn for King George V. There was no limit to this man's talents; he also edited the "Canadian X-Ray News Letter" from its inception in 1945.

Ghent's *Toronto Telegram* column, *In The Spotlight,* lasted 21 years. He typed with painstaking accuracy in spite of his burned hands, another souvenir of the early years of radiography. Percy's trademark, a lively and constant reminder of his cheerful personality, was a yellow duck, Doodle-Duck-Dan, happily sketched on so many of his writings and alongside his signature on letters. He retired from the TGH's x-ray department in 1946. Tommy Hurst often told the story of Percy's biggest thrill, a discovery which made newspaper headlines: the existence of a certain radiograph of a canvas which revealed the bearded face of Sir George Ross, a former premier of Ontario, under the portrait of Laura Secord which hung in the Ontario Provincial Building in Toronto.

En route to Calgary where he was to present a paper and to gather material for his report on the national convention for the newsletter, Percy became very ill. In a Winnipeg hospital on September 21, 1952, with Mrs Ghent at his side and pen in hand, a great friend died. The first Percy Ghent Memorial Exhibit Award was presented in 1963 and continues today as an annual award for the best exhibit by an RT.

The OSR convention of 1941 found Mary Cameron delivering a lecture on the visualization of the placenta by soft tissue radiography. This pioneering research resulted in the development of the McGregor Clinic Placenta Cone, which found wide acceptance in both Canada and the United States. Mary would never lose sight of the importance of research and would go on to introduce the use of a plastic filter to improve pregnancy radiography. In his *Telegram* column Percy Ghent wrote, "Mary F. Cameron has specialized with such success on pre-natal radiography that her fame has spread across the continents. Articles she has written about the filter and other technical accessories used in producing x-rays of unborn babies have been widely reprinted. Ontario has some distinguished Radiographer!"

The Memorandum of Agreement forwarded to the Secretary of State requesting a charter for the Canadian Society of Radiological Technicians (CSRT) was dated July 1942 and signed by Mary Cameron, CSRT secretary-treasurer. It seems very natural that Mary would be elected vice-president in 1944, and president in 1945. It is thanks to the arduous labour and outstanding leadership of people like her and technologists of this provincial organization that the CSRT came into existence. The technologists of Canada owe a debt of gratitude to Ontario technologists for their untiring efforts to improve the status of their colleagues and the advancement of medical radiation technology.

By 1948 Mrs Cameron was prepared for her participation in the Sixth CSRT conference in Québec city. She demonstrated the importance of breath control in the taking of a radiograph. Technologists from across Canada were impressed by her new research in an old subject. Mary's technical skills had won her fame, and at the invitation of the American Society of X-ray Technicians she delivered a series of lectures in San Francisco. Her topic, "Structural Studies," embodied the results of over 20 years of experience at McGregor Clinic. She was the first Canadian x-ray technologist to be invited to lecture in the United States. Her refresher course was repeated in 1951 at the insistence of our southern neighbours.

During the early 1950s insurance companies had refused to insure x-ray technologists. X-ray workers were apparently placed in the same risk category as steeplejacks. It was rumoured that x-rays did not work themselves out of the body but continued to accumulate and every exposure increased the danger to the technologist. The mentality of the times no doubt created an expectation that x-ray workers might glow in the dark.

By 1950 the University of Toronto had in place an extension course for radiographers. The two-year program consisted of one year of university studies and one year of practical training in an x-ray department or equivalent practical work. Unfortunately, the classes were discontinued in 1954, and the Toronto hospitals established their own schools for x-ray technologists. There is an amusing story in the archives about six Hamilton women travelling back and forth to Toronto University in an old Ford. One stormy night, the ancient vehicle, reluctantly making its way back to Hamilton, went on strike. After many miles of walking in the cold of winter, the ladies safely made their way home in the early hours of the morning with the help of a good Samaritan. The fearless women continued their weekly jaunt to Toronto the rest of that winter, in the same old Ford. After all, one mulish Ford is no match for six women pioneer x-ray technologists attending Canada's first class for training in their craft. Moreover, one of the six was Mary Cameron, a leader in raising the status of x-ray technologists in this country.

Mrs Cameron became the first OSRT Life member on January 10, 1952 and received a CSRT life membership in 1953. She found herself eyebrow deep in the complex engineering feat of stage managing an international convention. The job involved setting up and working with committees all over the country. When asked why she would undertake such a tremendous challenge, she replied that the human element was what made her work absorbing and that no two persons were ever alike. From June 28 to July 2, 1953 the First International Convention of X-ray Technicians was held in Toronto at the Royal York Hotel. It was the American Society's 25th annual conference, and the twelfth conference for the CSRT. There were no less than 1022 delegates from every state in the United States and from every province in Canada. Mrs. Cameron, the general chairman, won a gold medal for her extensive research and was presented with a complete set of garden furniture for her Lakeshore Avenue home in Burlington. Not yet satisfied that she had done her share, she agreed to chair the CSRT Committee on Law.

In 1955 Mary Frances was invited to deliver the CSRT Welch Memorial Lecture. She was the Jerman Memorial Lecturer during the 1957 American Society of X-Ray Technicians' convention and that same year was awarded the CSRT George Reason Cup.

Mrs Cameron retired from the McGregor Clinic in 1958 but continued to devote her energies to her professional societies. She chaired the CSRT Committee on International Organization and was the delegate to the first meeting of the International Society of Registered Radiological Technicians in Munich, Germany in 1959. She was the ISRRT secretary for the Americas and the general chairman of the second international meeting in Montréal. She was the first paid full-time OSRT executive secretary, a position she held until 1962. In 1960 Mary was awarded an honorary life membership of the British Society of Radiographers.

On February 8, 1960 supplementary letters patent changed the society's name back to the Ontario Society of Radiological Technicians, with changes in objectives concerned with education and adding the technologies of radiotherapy and medical uses of isotopes to radiography. There would be three more supplementary letters patent before August 7, 1984 when the name change to Ontario Association of Medical Radiation Technologists (OAMRT) was finalized.

On February 7, 1966 we said goodbye to the *Bulletin* and welcomed *Filter*. The *Bulletin* had been established in 1953 when the OSRT membership numbered 425. A number of successive editors each gave of his or her personality and ideas for improvement, so that the *Bulletin* grew from a two-page to a twenty-page publication reaching into each of the eight sections, bringing together 1965 Ontario technologists.

It would be wrong not to acknowledge the work of another special lady from the McGregor Clinic. Her interest and participation in association affairs at local, provincial, national and international levels have made a lasting impression on the profession. Throughout her career, she has shared her knowledge in many papers, publications and exhibits. She has set an example for others to follow. In my opinion her greatest contribution is her 17 years of diligent service to the OAMRT archives. I only regret that we could not have made available to her that station wagon she so greatly deserved. I refer to the first Mary F Cameron Lecturer, Ms Jane Martin.

Mary Frances Cameron's numerous attributes have been praised by successive lecturers. Many have referred to her as a member with a keen mind, who was quick to action and as colourful a personality as one might seek in a friend. During the eighth annual lecture, Dr John Stapleton, Mary's radiologist colleague said, "Mary is a possessor of a keen, inquisitive mind backed up with a superhuman abundance of energy and a generosity of spirit and enthusiasm. She has been resolute in purpose, regardless of the task at hand."

Mrs Cameron would often write special little notes to people expressing her pride and joy in the continuing growth of her professional association. She died on April 17, 1989 at St. Joseph's Villa in Dundas, Ontario. Last year's lecturer , Brendan Corr, said, "Mary Cameron was a visionary of great passion who contributed in many ways to our profession. She had a vision of the role of the radiographer *long before that role was recognized* by physicians, government, the public or even the radiographer." A colleague, John Flanagan, expressed our sentiments best when he wrote, "The passing of Mary Cameron marks the end to an era in our society's history that will never be equalled."

The practice of honouring a leader like Mary F Cameron by means of an annual lecture bearing her name is one small way in which we can recognize her vision and accomplishments.

Editorial Acknowledgements:

This article has been reprinted in slightly edited form with the permission of Ms Colette Gazdic and the Ontario Association of Medical Radiation Technologists (OAMRT).[2] Ms Gazdic acknowledges her indebtedness to the OAMRT archives.

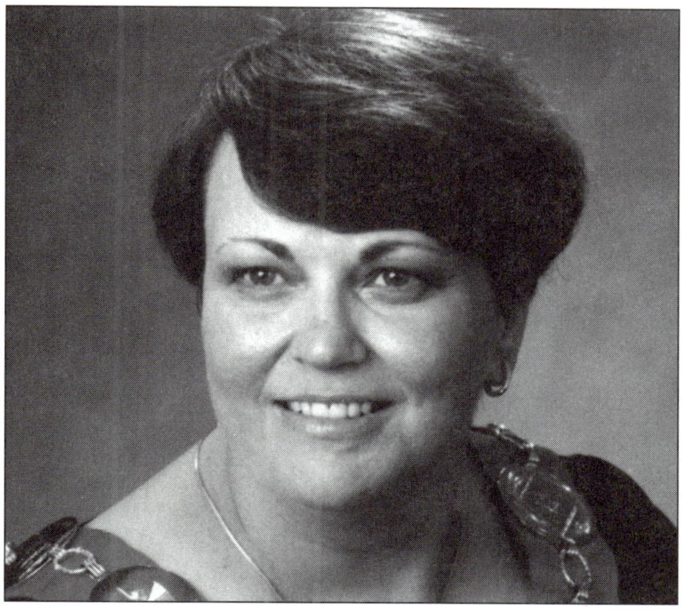

Ms Collete Gazdic

X *Dr William Herbert McGuffin*

(December 27,1886–October 25, 1949)

W B (Bill) Parsons

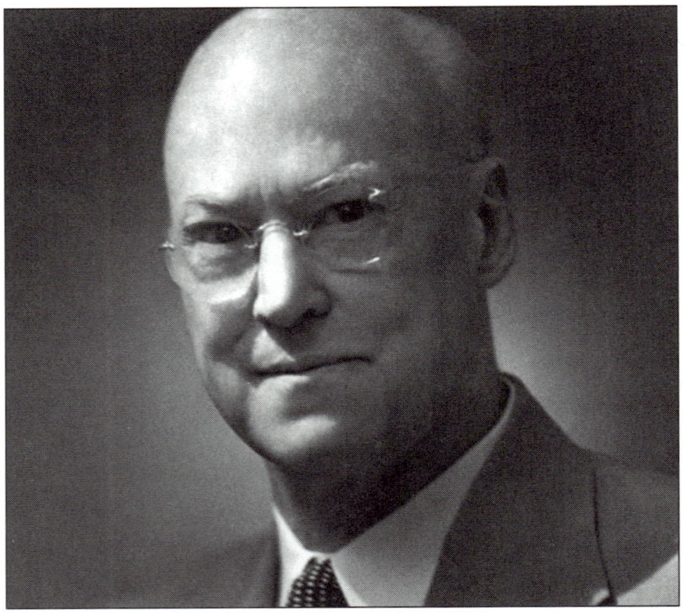

MD, Western University (London), 1910.
Fellow, American College of Radiologists, 1934.
Fellow, Faculty of Radiology, London, England, 1938.
LLD Honoris Causae, University of Western Ontario, 1946.
President, Canadian Radiological Society, 1925.
President, Radiological Society of North America, 1934–35.
President, Canadian Association of Radiologists, 1941–43.

This list gives only the partial measure of the man. His career in radiology began in 1912, though he did not specialize until 1918 after a vigorous period during World War I when he practiced both military and civilian radiology in Calgary. When he announced his intention to specialize, his confrères berated him for this ridiculous move. They said, "Why give up a busy, lucrative practice for this fad which might not continue to be a branch of medicine?" However, the doctor was interested and set up an office in his house doing only referred work. He had gained his understanding of radiology from the many visits to hospitals and radiological conventions which he had attended from 1912 on.

In 1929 Dr McGuffin started work on a building to house the Radium and X-ray Institute which he founded. Here he carried out both diagnosis and treatment, and for the latter he installed eight beds. Although this small, private hospital did not make money, Dr McGuffin continued to operate it. He did not have the heart to send people to the community hospitals where the rates were so much higher than in his institute. This applied particularly during the Dirty Thirties when so many of his patients had no money with which to pay their bills. As Dr McGuffin so often said, he liked people and liked to help them. He was a humanist, and the appeal of radiology was more in what he did for the individual than in the use of equipment.

It was this love of people that led Dr McGuffin to turn down the offer of the Chair in Radiology at the University of Western Ontario during the war. He was sorely tempted, but the thought of the amount of administration involved as well as the medical politics inherent in the position made him refuse it. His physical activities were somewhat limited: he appeared to have suffered some heart strain, and this led him to give up sports. His work became his major outlet, and much of his energy was directed toward the control of cancer. With the late Dr JS McEachren of Calgary, he founded the Alberta Cancer Society which later became the Alberta Division of the Canadian Cancer Society. In recognition of this work Dr McGuffin was made an honorary life member of the Canadian Society in 1949. Ten years later, the Calgary Medical Society set up the Dr WH McGuffin Memorial Lecture to commemorate what he had done for his community.

From the beginning Mrs McGuffin usually attended conventions with her husband. She reported that at many of the early ones it was sad to see the numbers who were suffering physically from exposure to radiation. In his later years her husband suffered greatly as well. He had many plastic operations on his hands and head. In 1949 the Calgary doctors were afraid to operate any more so they sent him to Dr Max Cuttler in Chicago, who in turn advised him to see Dr Mohn of Madison, Wisconsin, who had had considerable success with curettement of skin lesions. This procedure was carried out in Madison, and on his way home Dr McGuffin went to London, Ontario to visit a daughter. There he suffered a fatal heart attack.

Mrs McGuffin is reputed to have remarked that her husband liked teaching better than giving papers at conventions, though this he often did. It was a promise to give a paper in Havana that gave Dr McGuffin and his wife their first airplane flight. Because of some confusion over travel regulations, their departure was delayed past the time they could travel by rail and boat, so the doctor conquered his distaste for air travel and flew to Havana. He found he liked air travel, and from Cuba he and his wife flew down to Columbia to visit family.

Editor's note and acknowledgements:
This record was found in CAR Archives and is published posthumously with the permission of Dr Parson's estate. The illustration was kindly provided by the Glenbow Museum and Archives, Calgary.

XI *William Howard Dickson* MD

1878–1933

Canada's First Physician Specializing in Gastrointestinal Radiology

WALLACE ROY

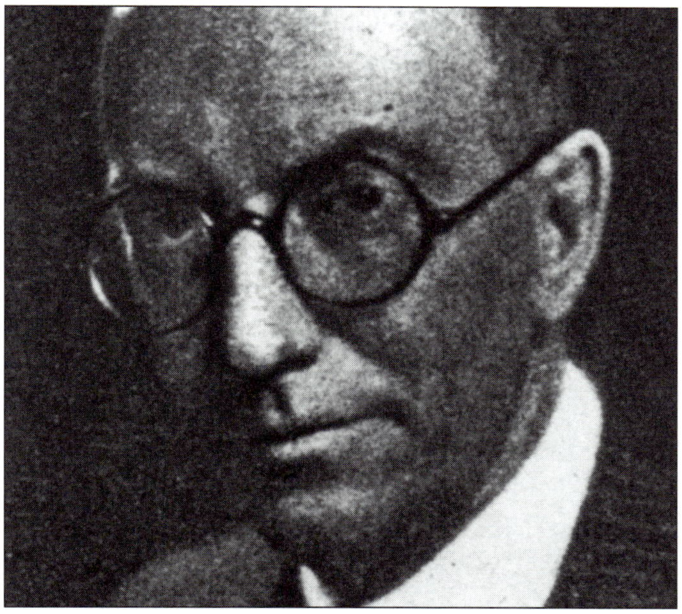

Dr Howard Dickson, one of the foremost diagnostic radiologists in the 1920s and early '30s, gained widespread recognition for his research concerning the use of contrast material in radiological diagnosis.

Dr Dickson, a native of Pembroke, Ontario, was the son of a practicing physician. After receiving his medical degree (CM MD) from McGill in 1904, he commenced practice in a small mining town in northern British Columbia where he became interested in the growing importance of x-rays in medical diagnosis.

In 1909 he moved his practice to Vancouver where he was able to investigate the use of x-rays in university physics laboratories and local hospitals.

Several years later Dr Dickson became associated with Dr Lewis Gregory Cole, an eminent, pioneer United States radiologist in New York City. Dr Cole invented the first radiographic fluoroscopic table with a spot film device, and in 1913 he was the first radiologist to use Coolidge's cathode vacuum x-ray tube, eliminating the use of the cumbersome gas tube.

Dr Dickson returned to Canada in late 1918 and en route to BC stopped in Toronto to visit his old colleague from Vancouver days, Dr Gordon Richards, who was in the process of establishing the radiology department at the Toronto General Hospital. Dr Richards convinced Dr Dickson to join him in Toronto where he remained until his early death in 1933. Dr Dickson quickly became a highly respected diagnostician in gastrointestinal radiology and an inspiring teacher at the University of Toronto.

In research he became intensely interested in the use of thorium dioxide (Thorotrast), a contrast medium which at the time was considered to be one of the great advances in medicine. Its use in diagnosis of diseases of the liver, spleen and brain was thought to be spectacular. Even though Thorotrast had a low level of radioactivity, it was believed to be a harmless and safe aide in the diagnosis of abnormalities, providing information previously unobtainable.

In an obituary note Mr Percy Ghent wrote:

> *"In his work," said Professor Goldie, "he was our leading light; with his simplicity and intellectual honesty, that clear-acting brain brushed aside the unessential to point out the way or face the fact with 'We do not know'."*
> *It was his frankness and honesty, indeed, together with an infectious enthusiasm for his chosen work that made him so inspiring a teacher. He was a tireless worker, a keen student, an original thinker. And of his many activities none was rewarded more earnestly, or more worthy of thorough preparation than his teaching. Yet Dr. Dickson never referred to his lectures to students —it was always his "talk to the boys".*[1]

Dr Dickson made many contributions to the medical and radiological literature and was in great demand as a lecturer in gastrointestinal radiology. He was a member of the Royal Society of Canada.

Dr W Howard Dickson was a diagnostician, researcher, and lecturer. He was one of the leading radiologists of his time when he died at age 55 of a heart attack in his office.

A daughter of Dr Dickson, Mrs Dorothy MacEachern, lives in Kleinberg, Ontario.

XII *William Doern* MSR

Anon

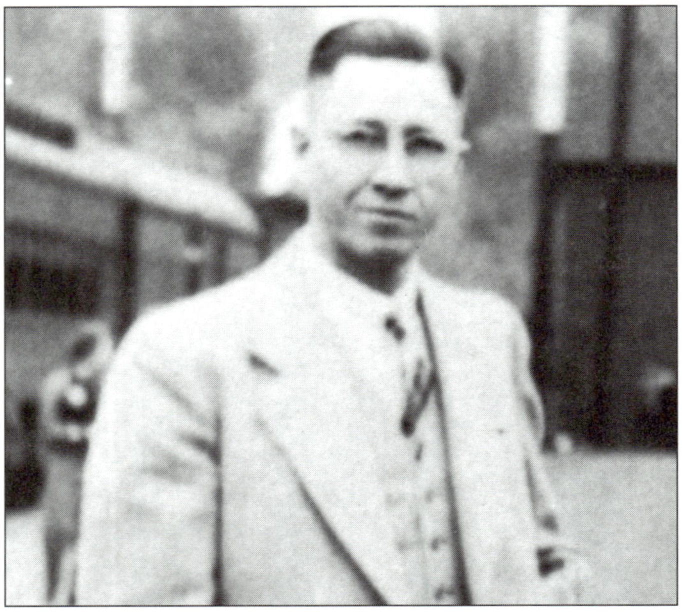

Mr William Doern is a technologist who has dedicated his considerable energies to furthering his profession.

Mr Doern served in committee and administrative roles at provincial, national and international technologist society levels. His appointments have been numerous, and the following list is given only as a limited example of the distinguished role he has played in the affairs of technologist organizations:

1929—1st Vice-president, Western Canadian Society of X-Ray Technicians.

1930–1931, 1935–1936—President, Western Canadian Society of X-Ray Technicians.

1943—President, Manitoba Division Canadian Society of Radiological Technicians.

1959—Welch Memorial Lecture.

Mr Doern was a member of the CSRT, has acted as a counsellor to the American Society, was an honorary life member of the Society of Radiographers (Great Britain) and is entitled to use MSR. His endeavours have been directed at improving the art and science of radiography and fostering the aims and objectives of the Canadian Society of Radiological Technicians.

In the year ending June 1967 his name appeared on the roster of the following committees:

- Committee on Technical Training
- Special Committee—Management
- Editorial Advisory Board
- The Advisory Board of The Manitoba Division, CSRT

Mr Doern married in 1935. Mr and Mrs Doern have four children: two sons, William and David, and two daughters, Catherine and Elsa. Bill, the eldest and Elsa, the youngest, have both trained at the Winnipeg General Hospital under their father and are registered technicians. Catherine maintains the family interest in the medical field, having graduated as a registered nurse. Dave served the radiological community as an employee of Canadian Kodak as an X-Omat specialist.

Mr Doern's interests outside the field of radiography were also quite numerous. He was an active worker in the United Church, an experienced traveller and camper, an accomplished photographer and—with his personal records collected over the years—an historian.

Mr Doern's dedication to radiography had been outstanding and certainly an inspiration for any experienced or aspiring radiographer.

XIII *Bede J Harrison* MB DMRE

From material provided by Philip Harrison, and written by him and his father Colin Harrison

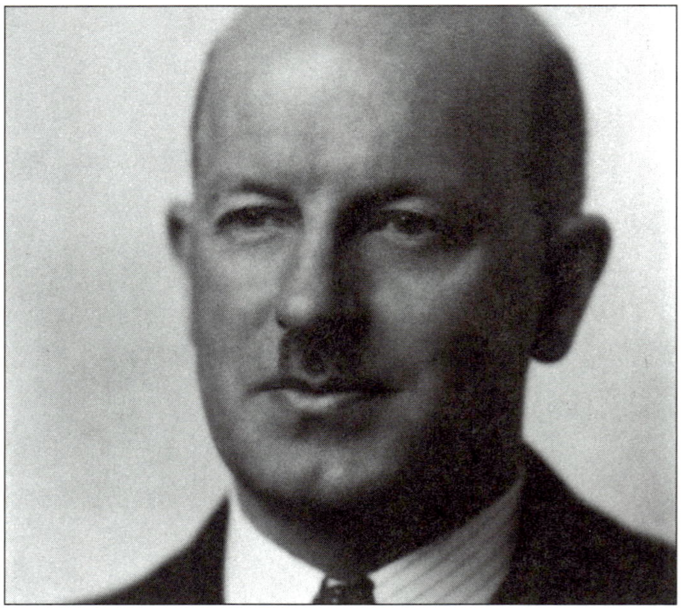

Dr Bede Harrison created the Department of Radiology at Vancouver General Hospital,and he published one of the earliest Canadian textbook of radiology.[1] He was born in Leichardt, Sydney, Australia in June 1887 of English and Welsh ancestry. He was to die in May 1979 in his 92nd year, at Richmond, BC.

After graduating as Gold Medalist from Sydney University and completing an internship at Sydney Hospital, he entered family practice in Dubbo, New South

Wales, where the practice he purchased include a "new-fangled" x-ray machine. The enthusiasm for radiology this initiated was later to be shared by his son and grandson, and his daughter was to be a radiographer. Soon Dr Harrison limited his professional activity to radiology and established a flourishing practice in both diagnostic and therapeutic radiology in Sydney, where he was on the honorary staff of St Vincent's and Lewisham Hospitals.

The Depression came and Dr Harrison moved with his family to England. However, there were no radiological opportunities available. As a locum family doctor he was paid sixpence (12¢) for a consultation, including the medicine prescribed (the patient was expected to bring his or her own bottle and cork). Disillusioned and disappointed, having faced destitution, the family decided to move back to Australia, though Marcella Bonnie, his wife, insisted that with "three lovely God-given children they could never consider themselves poor." [2]

While travelling across North America with his family en route to Australia in 1930, Dr Harrison learned of an opportunity at the Vancouver General Hospital. He soon settled into the hospital, but his arrival met with some opposition. There were those who thought that, because of the economic climate, the position should have been given to a Canadian. With charm, persuasion, enthusiasm, a great deal of knowledge and a bent for dialectics, Dr Harrison soon was accepted by the hospital staff.

Dr Harrison's wife died of pneumonia at a young age, six years after coming to Canada, and it is a reflection on his humanity that a daughter remembers Bede Harrison with gratitude, writing as follows:[2]

In a rather mysterious way my father gave me a great sense of worth, probably because of his warmth and affection. We shared the same sense of the ridiculous, chortling often at our own silliness.

His wife, Bonnie, wrote poetry. Some lines handed down in the family for domestic fun, however, tell us about the domestic habits of her husband:

But we laugh and we joke and we tease quite a bit,
At Daddy's occasional tidying fit.[3]

As early as 1933 Dr Harrison was speaking at the Radiological Society of North America conference on an accurate and reproducible method for describing the relationship between the x-ray tube and a patient part. In 1936 he published one of the earliest of the comprehensive radiological texts.[1]

Dr Harrison was a prime mover in the establishment of a cancer clinic in Vancouver. He developed the size and scope of the department at the Vancouver General Hospital and made it a centre for graduate education. His wide ranging skills and interests also resulted in the development of a special kind of pen adapted for use by those with arthritis.[3]

He retired from the hospital in 1951, and after five years in private practice from which he gradually withdrew, he retired completely. Dr Harrison died in 1979 in his 92nd year.

As the 1947 Osler lecturer ("Medicine and Some Orthodoxies") for the Vancouver Medical Association, Dr Bede Harrison concluded with a quotation from the Babylonian Talmud which seems to epitomize the man himself:

The day is short. The work is great. The reward is also great and the master praises. It is not incumbent on thee to complete the work but thou must not therefore cease from it.

Editor's note:

Dr Bede Harrison created one of the few radiological dynasties in Canada. His son and grandson, who have prepared this article, are radiologists. Dr Philip Harrison of St Paul's Hospital, Vancouver, has recently served as president of the British Columbia Radiological Association. His daughter, quoted above, was a radiographer.

XIV *Herbert M (Bert) Welch* RT

1888–1951

WQ Stirling

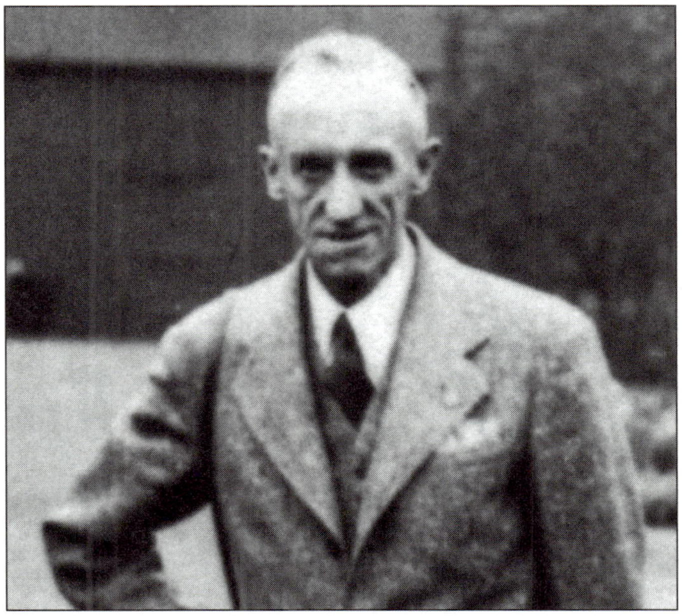

Bert Welch was one of the ablest officers and staunchest supporters of the Canadian Society of Radiological Technicians. His actions were always keyed to what he considered necessary and beneficial to the organization. There was no selfishness or thought of personal gain in his efforts to bring the society to a position of national importance and prestige. He fought the good fight in every way, and it is most gratifying to note that most of his suggestions have been adopted with resulting good for all the members. He was a familiar figure at conventions, always armed with facts, figures and a happy and charming smile. On the floor of the convention he was a hard hitter, a clean fighter and, above all, a generous loser. Away from the arena he was always surrounded by a host of admiring friends, all of whom can testify to his high standards.

Bert was born in Ashton-under-Lyme in 1888 and came to Canada in 1908. He took up ranching in the new land although he had been trained as an electrician in England. At the outbreak of war in 1914 he immediately joined up and went overseas with the engineers. His talents as an electrician were used in the installation of x-ray units for the army, and it was in this way that he became interested in what later proved to be his life's work. On returning to Canada after the war he took training in Toronto in x-ray methods and joined the staff of Colonel Belcher Hospital in Calgary where he remained until his death. His activities in Calgary were many. He served in the Amalgamated Civil Servants of Canada, and he took an active interest in the Overseas Association. He was instructor in First Aid to the Calgary Police, the RCMP and army teams and a member of the Board of Stewards of Hillcrest United Church.

He attended the Vimy Pilgrimage in 1938 and acted as standard bearer for Calgary. He was an ardent amateur gardener and won many prizes for his floral contributions at shows. When one notes that he was also an enthusiastic lawn bowler, a patron of the Caledonian Football Club and a supporter of the Calgary Stampeders and the Calgary hockey team, we can realize that he lived a full and happy life. His love for the CSRT made him beloved by all officers and members of the organization from coast to coast.

XV *Dr A Stanley Kirkland*

WB Stewart

Dr A Stanley Kirkland was born in 1890 in Independence, Oregon. In 1913 he received his MD CM from McGill and passed his licentiate of the Medical Council of Canada, one of the very early [physicians] so qualified.

He served in World War I overseas with No 1 Casualty Clearing Station and after the war served with the 14th Field Ambulance in the Canadian Militia.

From 1919 to 1922 he trained as a diagnostic and therapeutic radiologist in Montréal General Hospital. He was New Brunswick's first well-trained radiologist. He joined the Saint John General in 1922 and soon became consultant to other Saint John hospitals, particularly the Tuberculosis Hospital. He served as President of the New Brunswick Medical Society from 1929-1930.

In 1915 Dr Kirkland married Mary Elizabeth Roy and they had one daughter. Dr Kirkland enjoyed reading, fishing and playing "Auction 45's."

He wrote many articles for the *Canadian Medical Association Journal* as well as many tributes to his deceased friends, who were legion.

Acknowledgement:

This brief portrait from *Medicine in New Brunswick* is published with the permission both of the New Brunswick Medical Society and its author Dr WB Stewart.[1]

XVI *Albert J Jutras* MD

1900–1981

Guy Duckett

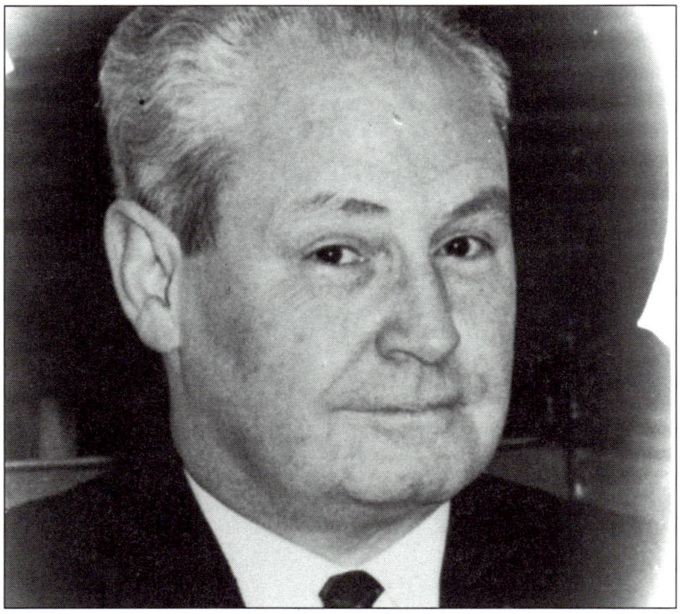

Throughout his career Dr Jutras's motivation, diagnostic acumen, and interest in his profession never wavered. He had been influenced to take up medicine as a youth by his uncle, a country doctor who took him on his rounds, and by his father, a dentist, who had graduated at the turn of the century.

Albert Jutras began the practice of medicine as a general practitioner in Northern Québec, and he retired as a radiologist in the same region, his career having covered a span of 55 years. He was a leading radiologist; he had been professor and Chairman of the Department of Radiology at the Université de Montréal; and for 30 years he was Radiologist-in-Chief at l'Hôtel-Dieu de Montréal.

Dr Jutras went to Paris in 1930 to study radiology at the Radium Institute, when Marie Curie was still chairman of the board and Caldius Regaud the chief. Dr Jutras was to work with Lacassagne, Coutard and Baclesse, all of whom were pioneers in international radiation therapy in France. Returning to Montréal in 1934, he began work as a radiation therapist at the Montréal Radium Institute, but he soon took a special interest in gastroenterology. His work in New York with Cole, who was involved with the early diagnosis of gastric cancer, was followed by work on gastric endoscopy with Schindler in Chicago. Dr Jutras later joined the staff of l'Hôtel-Dieu de Montréal where his interest in the esophagus, the stomach and the gall bladder continued.

His publications throughout his career numbered some 200. In 1949 he was guest lecturer at the Sorbonne in Paris, France, where he described his very extensive study of the function of the gastric cardia. Through these years he also wrote extensively about the superficial spreading of carcinoma of the stomach. His pioneer work on floating gallstones and, especially, the chronic cholecystoses is well known. In 1978 he was the guest speaker at a symposium in the Netherlands that was concerned with cholecystosis.

In the early 1950s Gershon Cohen, a good friend of Dr Jutras, had sent radiographs from Philadelphia to New York via television, and this impressed Dr Jutras very much. It led to what he considered to be his major contribution to radiological diagnosis: remote televised fluoroscopy. The remote-controlled tables that he conceived are still at the forefront of the practice of radiology.[1]

Dr Jutras had many interests. His collection of Canadian paintings was large and diverse. He painted very well, and he also transformed driftwood into graceful sculptures. His library was complete with French classics, and at one time he collected de luxe editions that he actually handled with white gloves. He and his wife Rachel, who died in 1977, often hosted visiting scientific, artistic, and literary celebrities from Europe, America or Canada in their home. Dr Jutras and his wife had a daughter, Mimi, and two sons, Claude and Michel, both of whom graduated in medicine.

Albert Jutras was past president of the Montréal Medical Society, the Association des Radiologistes de Langue Française du Canada, and the Québec Association of Radiologists. He was vice-president of the International Congress of Radiology held in Montréal in 1962. He lectured all over Europe and the Americas and was a visiting professor in many American cities, as well as a corresponding member of the Journal de Radiologie de France. In 1972 Dr Jutras was awarded the medal for scientific achievement by the Association des Médecins de Langue Française; in 1974 he received the Gold Medal of the American College of Radiology. In 1976 he was inducted into the Order of Canada. Albert Jutras trained many radiologists who now practice across Canada at the French-Canadian School of Radiology, where he was dean. In the 17th century Dr Jutras would have been known as a Renaissance man. Knowing his years were counted, he prepared a few last words that describe the man and his spirit:

"Du haut de l'infini, je lève mon verre et je vous dis... adieu."

I knew him well; he was my father-in-law.

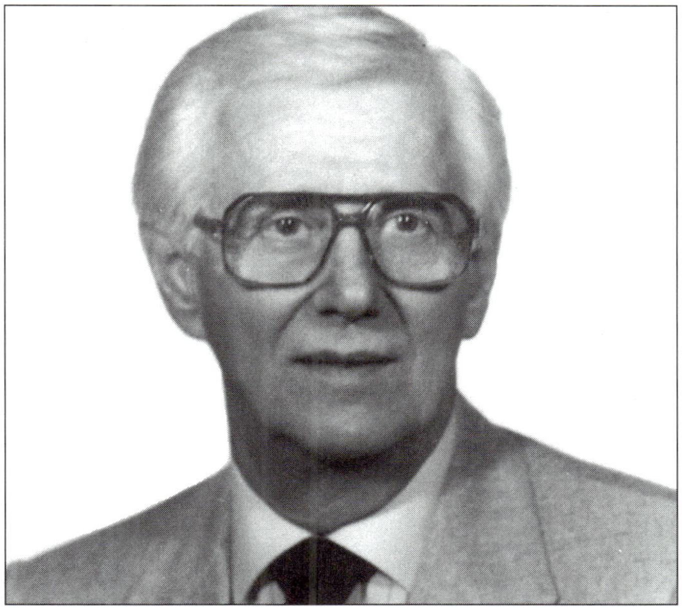

Guy Duckett

XVII *Le docteur Albert Jutras*

Jocelyne Lapointe

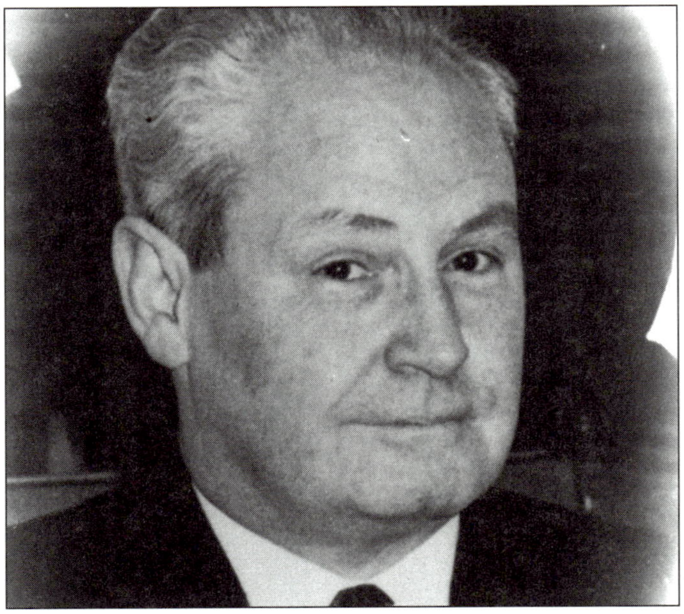

Né à Trois-Rivières en 1900, le jeune Albert Jutras suit son oncle, médecin de campagne, dans ses tournées. Il obtient son doctorat en médecine de l'Université de Montréal en 1925, et après cinq ans de médecine générale dans le nord du Québec, il entreprend en 1930 une spécialisation en radiologie à l'Institut du Radium à Paris, alors que Marie Curie y est encore.

Il revient à Montréal en 1934 pour travailler comme radiothérapeute à l'Institut du Radium mais s'intéresse en même temps à l'investigation du système digestif. Il fait des stages à New York et à Chicago, où il approfondit ses connaissances de la gastroscopie et de la détection précoce des cancers gastriques.

Il devient le directeur du service d'Electrologie de l'Hôtel-Dieu de Montréal en 1938, succédant à Léo Pariseau, poste qu'il gardera jusqu'en 1969. Il est le premier titulaire de la chaire d'Electroradiologie de l'Université de Montréal (1939) dont il demeurera à la tête jusqu'à la création formelle d'un département de Radiologie en 1964.

En 1969, il retourne à Amos, en Abitibi, pour travailler comme radiologiste jusqu'à peu avant sa mort en 1981.

Pendant 50 ans, il pratique la radiologie, d'abord comme radiothérapeute et ensuite comme radiologiste. Il étudie surtout le système digestif, la vésicule biliaire en particulier. Avec l'avènement de la télévision, il s'intéresse à la transmission d'images à distance. Selon lui, sa contribution majeure à la Radiologie est le dévelopment d'appareils de fluoroscopie controllés à distance, toujours en usage de nos jours. Par ailleurs, ses successeurs à l'Hôtel-Dieu poursuivent toujours les expériences de téléradiologie, pour desservir les communautés isolées.

Membre de nombreuses sociétés médicales, il a été particulièrement actif au Québec, servant comme président de la Société médicale de Montréal, l'Association des radiologistes de langue française du Canada et l'Association des radiologistes du Québec.

Bien que ses soixante-quinze publications scientifiques répertoriées à l'Index Medicus (1934-1964) soient surtout en français, il est reconnu par la communauté internationale et invité à parler en Europe et aux Etats-Unis. Il présente l'oraison Hickey en 1960 (mommé en l'honneur d'un fondateur et du premier éditeur du journal de l'American Roentgen Ray Society) sur les cholécystoses, est médaillé de l'Association des médecins de langue française en 1972, médaillé d'or de l'American College of Radiology en 1974, titulaire de l'Ordre du Canada en 1976 et l'invité d'honneur au Symposium sur les cholestéroses aux Pays-Bas en 1978.

L'Association canadienne-française de Radiologie, dont it fut un membre fondateur, honore sa mémoire lors de son congrès annuel en ayant un invité de marque présenter la conférence "Albert Jutras" et en octroyant le prix "Albert Jutras" pour souligner l'apport d'un individu à l'essor et au développement de la radiologie dans son milieu québecois.

Note de les éditeurs:

Notre intention initiale de publier simultanément des versions anglaise et française de ce volume ont dû se plier aux réalités économiques, avec comme résultat cette publication à contenu français et anglais différent. À cause de leur importance historique, nous célébrons la mémoire et l'oeuvre des docteurs Pariseau et Jutras dans les deux langues.

Editors' Note:

Our original intention had been to publish, simultaneously, both English and French editions of this volume. Alas, the cruel realities of the cost involved frustrated this intention, and we have had to resort, instead, to a publication with both French and English content. Because of the historical importance of Drs Pariseau and Jutras we are making an exception in their memory and here celebrate their lives and contributions in both languages. Similarly Sister Marie Flore Gagné is recognised in both languages for her immense contributions to Québec, and hence to our national life. Sister Gagné is fortunately alive and well at the age of 85 and is able to share this centennial year with us.

XVIII *Dr Andre Joseph Cipriani*

ANON

Dr AJ Cipriani was in his time the leading authority in Canada on the biological and medical aspects of atomic energy. He died at the tragically early age of 47. He was the first Director of the Biology Division of the Atomic Energy of Canada Limited plant at Chalk River. He became a scientist of international reputation in research related to the biological effects of radiation and he created a laboratory that was remarkable in the breadth of fundamental and applied investigations which its staff performed. The laboratory has contributed to the education of many national and international scientists who work in this field. From it have come major insights into radiation biology, for example the nature of the radiosensitivity of the tissues of persons with ataxia telangiectasia.

Cipriani supported and encouraged the development of the high specific activity cobalt-60 beam therapy units used for the treatment of cancer. These units were first made at Chalk River and have since been supplied to hospitals in Canada, the United States and world-wide. His unique education, combined with his native ability, popularity and striking personality, all contributed to the success he achieved in advancing a realistic understanding of the many problems associated with the use of radioisotopes, with radiation hazards, and with the lethal and other effects of irradiation on living cells.

He was a member of numerous national and international committees where his wide knowledge of the biological and medical field, as well as of basic physics and mathematical principles, was eagerly sought and his advice followed. He was Canada's representative on the International Commission on Radiological Protection and was chairman of that commission's sub-committee on the handling and disposal of radioisotopes. He was the Canadian representative on the United Nations Scientific Committee on the Effects of Atomic Radiation (UNSCEAR). He assisted in the organization and training of the army radiation detection units, and as a result of his firm control and administration of the health physics program, no employee at the Chalk River plant received excessive harmful radiation. He contributed many scientific papers to various international meetings, and to journals, as well as writing sections for British medical encyclopedias. He was a Fellow of the Royal Society of Canada.

Dr Cipriani was born in Port of Spain, Trinidad on April 2, 1908, the son of the late Leo P Cipriani and Helene Cipriani. He came to McGill University in 1928 with a scholarship, entering the Faculty of Applied Science with the intention of becoming an engineer. But his excellent ability in mathematics and physics led him to change in his third year to the honour course in mathematics and physics, from which he graduated with high first-class standing in 1932, receiving his Bachelor of Science degree. After a year of demonstrating in the physics department, during which period he completed some further engineering courses, he decided to study medicine and entered that faculty at McGill. He interrupted his course for two years to assist Dr Wilder Penfield and his staff with the design and construction of electronic equipment in connection with neurophysiological research. He received his medical degree in 1940. During World War II he served in the Canadian Army as a medical officer doing research on various problems, including that of motion sickness. On the conclusion of hostilities he joined the Atomic Energy Project when construction at Chalk River commenced.

Cipriani was a man of striking personality, and on meeting him one was immediately impressed with his ability, his genial interest in people and outdoor life. He was popular among scientists and local country inhabitants alike, and well known throughout the Ottawa Valley towns and villages as an enthusiastic fisherman with great skill. Many a visitor to the project has enjoyed a pleasant day of fishing with his guidance. He worked hard and was a man of action, and his sound judgement made him such a desirable member of any committee. He was fond of children and took special pleasure in interesting them in natural phenomena, whether insects of various kinds which he bred at the laboratory or flowers or geological specimens. Any weekend in the summer he could be seen in his open Model A Ford car, which he found useful for fishing expeditions, giving his own and other children a ride around the village, managing a huge load of active youngsters with kindly but firm discipline, which they respected. He was an active member of the Deep River Branch of the Canadian Legion and first president of the local chapter.

Acknowledgement:

This brief biography has been adapted from an obituary written on the death of Dr Cipriani by Dr David Keys, then of Deep River, Ontario.

XIX *Ruth M Duffey* FCSRT

ANON

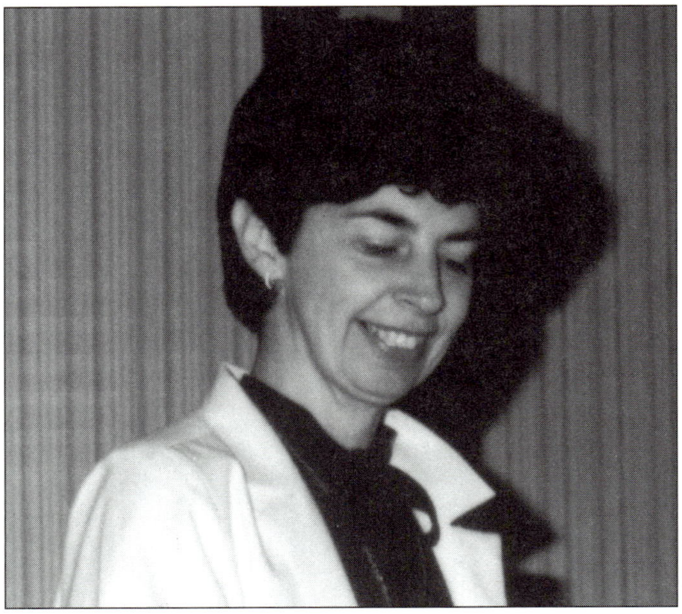

Ms Duffey was born and educated in Moncton, New Brunswick. Following graduation from high school, she chose radiologic technology as a career, graduating from the Moncton Hospital School of Radiologic Technology in 1958.

She continued her career at the Radiation Therapy Center, Hospital of St Raphael, New Haven, Connecticut for two years, following which she was appointed to the position of chief technician, Department of Diagnostic Radiology, the Moncton Hospital.

Her various opportunities for postgraduate work included one year spent in England, where part of the time she worked at the Middlesex Hospital in London. After Miss Duffey's return to Moncton, she attended several lectures in preparation for the fellowship examinations. As a result of this intense effort, Miss Ruth Duffey was awarded the first fellowship certificate presented by the Canadian Society of Radiological Technicians.

In 1973 Miss Duffey's administrative abilities were further recognized when she was appointed assistant to the administrator at the Moncton Hospital. From September 1973 to October 1974 she participated in an exchange of administrative personnel with the Royal Free Hospital in London, England, at the end of which time Ms Duffey returned to Moncton to the position of assistant administrator at the Moncton Hospital, the position she holds at the present time with the title of vice-president.

Ms Duffey has been a valuable member of the Canadian Society of Radiological Technicians (CSRT) since 1957, never sparing of her time or efforts particularly in the context of education. She served on the CSRT Standing Committee on Certification from 1971 until 1973, and during the latter part of 1972 acted as chairman of the radiography section of this committee. She has served one term as CSRT director and has been a member of the CSRT Resolutions Committee. She is a past president of the New Brunswick Division, CSRT and has been active at the international level, having served as a council member of the International Society of Radiographers and Radiological Technicians during 1968.

In 1974 Ms Duffey completed the Canadian Hospital Association extension course in hospital organization and management.

In 1962 she won the CSRT Essay Award for the best essay entered into competition by a radiological technician, entitled "Why a Fellowship?" In 1964 she shared the limelight with a fellow technician in winning the George Reason Cup for a scientific exhibit. In 1966 she won the Philips Rose Bowl for the best teaching exhibit entered in CSRT competition. In 1967 she was honoured by being invited to present the 16th Annual Welch Memorial Lecture. The subject chosen for this lecture was "Increasing Work-loads—a Challenge for X-ray Departments." In 1972 Ruth was the unanimous choice of the CSRT board of directors to receive the Mallett Award.

At the annual meeting of the New Brunswick Division of the CSRT held in Fredericton on September 27, 1975, Ruth was presented with a life membership in the New Brunswick Division.

With her busy day-to-day schedule, one wonders when Ruth has time to relax, but it is known that she enjoys painting, photography and travelling to faraway places.

(c) The Teachers

A teacher affects eternity;
he can never tell where his
influence stops.
— Henry Brooks Adams

The persons in this final section of brief biographies have in common with many others mentioned in this volume that they have had a passionate wish to teach; to share their excitement in the practice of their profession with others. Reflecting on my schooling, which has seen educational methods come and go and philosophies concerning pedagogy change, I am struck by the fact that what I remember is the people that have influenced me and not the tools they used. Those people were sometimes kind, sometimes demanding, sometimes articulate, sometimes blunt, sometimes rational and sometimes unreasonable—but never dull. To a person they were involved. I believe it was Lewis Thomas who pointed out that the word enthusiasm has its semantic origins in *en* and *theos*: that is God within. In that sense enthusiasm must be among the most beautiful words in the English language and the most desirable of traits in a teacher.

— Brian Lentle

XX *Robert G (Bob) Fraser*

Rosalind Aylmer

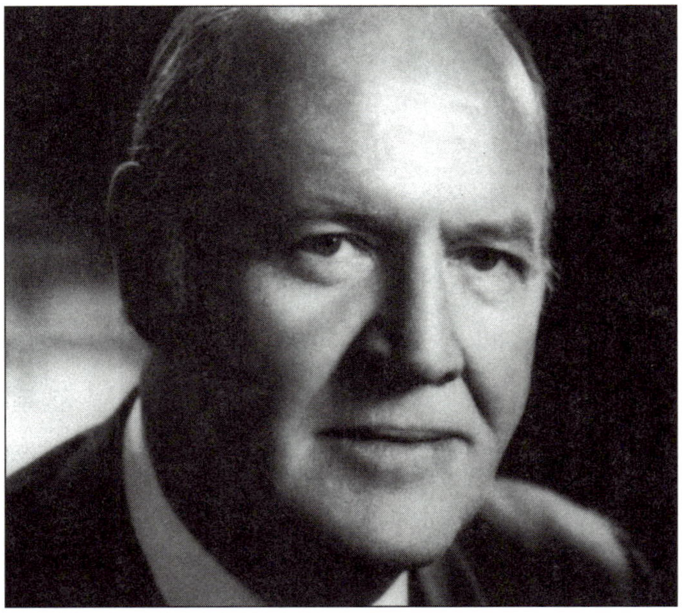

Robert Fraser was born in Winnipeg, Manitoba, in 1921. He attended the University of Toronto, from which he graduated in 1939, at the age of 18. He then went on to Medical School at the University of Manitoba at Winnipeg, and graduated from there in 1945.

He spent his internship at the Winnipeg General Hospital, a Pathology residence at the Washington University School of Medicine in St Louis, Missouri, and a residency in Radiology at the Royal Victoria Hospital in Montréal, Québec.

In 1951 he received his certificate in diagnostic and therapeutic radiology from the Royal College of Physicians and Surgeons of Canada, as well as from the American Board of Radiology.

Dr Fraser joined the McGill University Department of Radiology where he worked for 15 years. He became a full professor in 1968, and chairman of the department in 1971. Of those years he was to write:

> *During the second half of the 1960s, it occurred to some of those involved in chest radiology at the Royal Victoria Hospital in Montréal, that much time-consuming activity could be obviated if a device could be manufacteured that automatically fed exposed radiographs from a multifilm magazine into a screen-film changer and then directly into a film processor. This would not only take 14 x 17 cassettes out of the equation but would permit dry film viewing within two or three minutes. People intimately concerned in discussions regarding [the] feasability of such an apparatus included [myself], then Radiologist-in-Chief of the Royal Victoria Hospital, Mr Archie Wilkinson, Chief radiographic Technologist, and the late Mr Leslie Withers, then Vice-president of Picker (Canada) Ltd. On their recommendation, equipment was designed and constructed in the Picker plant near Toronto and was eventually installed in the Department of Radiology at the Royal Victoria Hospital in Montréal.*

The work and installation was completed in 1969. The unit incorporated features such as an air gap technique replacing a grid and a focus-to-film distance of ten feet with a special compensating filter mounted near the tube. For the next decade this became the standard against which all other chest radiographic systems were measured. Indeed other manufacturers built similar systems such that many thousands are now in use world-wide.

In 1976 he and his family moved to Birmingham, Alabama, where he joined the Department of Radiology at the University of Alabama. There he was made Professor Emeritus in 1988.

Dr Fraser has been very active in many radiology organizations, and is the founder of the Fleischer Society, an international and interdisciplinary group dedicated to the study of diseases of the chest.

Dr Fraser is also known for his interest in education in the field of radiology, but perhaps his most significant contribution to this field is the multi-volume work *Diagnosis of Diseases of the Chest* first published in 1970. This work has become the standard reference text in the field of pulmonary radiology.

A man of wide ranging interests, Dr Fraser's leisure activities include playing the bagpipes, a challenge successfully met by only a chosen few; and sports such as archery, fishing, golf and skiing. Dr Fraser has also had a life-long interest in working with his hands, the results of which include stone patios and walkways built at his vacation homes, as well as carefully crafted wooden board games, and intricate clock cases and other bibelots.

Dr Fraser and his wife currently make their home in Birmingham, Alabama.

XXI *Sister Marie-Flore Gagné*
FCSRT

ANON

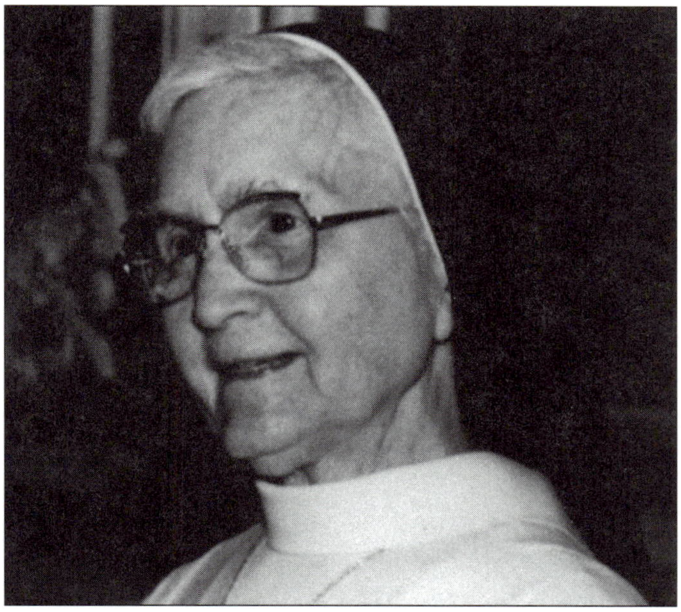

As quiet as the setting sun
As brilliant as its rising
Lighting the way for those
who follow...

When a person goes about her daily task with ease and silence, never seeking glory or praise, it is difficult to perceive her accomplishments. This became apparent when a decision to honour Sister Gagné was made. When finally a list of her accomplishments was compiled, it was impossible to imagine that one individual had done so many things and yet manage to remain so modest and unassuming.

Sister Gagné was born in St-Adrien de Ham, Québec and during her school years there became an accomplished organist. The parish church in St-Adrien de Ham lost its organist in 1929, however, when Marie-Flore Gagné decided to take up a religious life and entered the Augustine convent at L'Hôtel-Dieu de Québec.

Sister Gagné pursued a career in nursing, receiving her diploma from Université de Laval in 1936. Further studies led to a Bachelor of Hospital Science degree from Université de Laval in 1945. Some years later, her interests became directed toward radiological technology, and in 1956 she became registered in this profession.

In 1966 Sister received her fellowship in radiotherapy. A few years prior to her fellowship, Sister received the Gold Gaevert Medal for an excellent study and report entitled "Cobalt-60 in therapy." Never one to rest on her accomplishments, in 1967 she obtained her certificate in nuclear medicine.

How Sister found time for all of her achievements and studies, is beyond imagination.

As a nurse from 1936–1948 she was responsible for setting up a department of obstetrics at L'Hôtel-Dieu de Québec. She also organized the School for Radiotherapy Studies in 1957. In 1964 Sister became coordinator of the therapy and diagnostic programs, and in 1966 she served as therapy representative on the Canadian Society of Radiological Technicians (CSRT) Committee on Qualifications and became editor of the French edition of the CSRT *Journal*.

Having served her local society with the same unassuming vigour, Sister was honoured with a life membership in the Québec branch of the CSRT in 1972, and received the same honour from the CAMRT in 1979. In 1985, she received an Honorary Doctorate from Université de Laval.

XXII *Soeur Marie-Flore Gagné*
FSCTR

ANON (TRANS PAR JOCELYNE LAPOINTE)

Paisible comme le soleil couchant
Scintillante comme son lever
Illuminant le chemin pour ceux qui suivent...

Lorsqu'une personne accomplit ses taches quotidiennes avec facilité et en silence, ne cherchant ni gloire ni louange, il est difficile de reconnaître ses réalisations. Ceci devint évident lorsqu'on décida d'honorer Soeur Gagné. Quand la liste de ses succès fut enfin complétée, on trouva difficile d'imaginer qu'une personne ayant accompli tant de choses soit demeurée si modeste.

Soeur Gagné naquit à St-Adrien de Ham, Québec et, étudiante, elle devint une organiste accomplie, oeuvrant à l'église paroissiale. Elle quitta ce poste en 1929 pour prendre le voile et entrer au couvent des Augustines de l'Hôtel-Dieu de Québec.

Là, elle poursuivit une carrrière en nursing, recevant son diplôme de l'Université Laval en 1936. Continuant ses études, elle obtint un Baccalauréat en Sciences hospitalières de la même université en 1945. Quelques années plus tard, elle s'intéressa aux techniques radiographiques et fut certifiée en ce domaine en 1956.

En 1966, Soeur Gagné reçut son fellowship en radiothérapie (maintenant appelé Certificat d'agrément avancé). En 1962, on lui avait décerné la médaille d'or Gaevert pour une excellente étude intitulée "Le cobalt-60 en thérapie" et elle reçut une seconde médaille d'or Gaevert en 1972 pour "Le bétatron de 45 MV". En 1967, elle se qualifiait en techniques de médecine nucléaire.

Comment elle trouva le temps de combiner toutes ces études et ses nombreuses réalisations est stupéfiant et dépasse même l'imagination.

Comme infirmière de 1936 à 1948, elle fut responsable de la création d'un département d'obstétrique à l'Hôtel-Dieu de Québec. Elle organisa aussi l'École de Radiothérapie en 1957. En 1964, elle devint coordonatrice des programmes de Techniques de Radiodiagnostic et de Radiothérapie et en 1966 ele représenta la radiothérapie au Comité sur les compétences de la Société Canadienne des Techniciens en Radiologie (SCTR) (depuis 1979, connue comme l'Association Canadienne des Technologues en Radiation Médicale) et devint l'éditeur de la version française du journal de la SCTR (1965–1968).

Ayant servi la branche locale avec vigueur et sans prétension, la section québécoise de la SCTR la fit membre à vie en 1972 et l'ACTRM fit de même en 1979. En 1985, l'Université Laval lui décerna un Doctorat honoris causa.

XXIII *Sylvia O Fedoruk*

JOHN ALDRICH

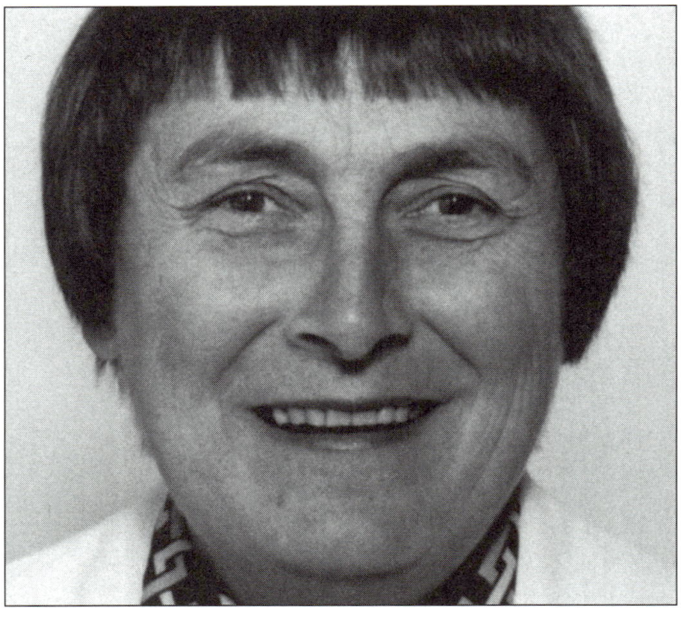

Sylvia has managed to combine in her life an outstanding career in medical physics, great contributions to public service and a full social life. It is possible only to touch upon such a wide range of activities.

Sylvia was born in Canora, Saskatchewan and has spent most of her life in that province. As an undergraduate she excelled in physics and graduated with high honours from the University of Saskatchewan. In 1950 Sylvia became Harold Johns' first female graduate student. By this time Dr Johns had already acquired quite a reputation as a keen investigator, and Sylvia became involved in several areas which were to have worldwide significance. In 1951 the first cobalt-60 machine was installed in Saskatoon, and she was to be involved in the very first calibration of such a device. Subsequently she turned to radioisotope scanners and worked with Johns on the dedicated neurological scanner which employed a unique curved trajectory for the detectors. In 1956 when Johns moved to the Ontario Cancer Institute, Sylvia stayed to develop medical physics in Saskatoon. There she continued her work on isotope scanners and worked with Trevor Cradduck on the design of Canada's first gamma camera. She became involved in all areas of medical physics, eventually becoming Director of Physics Services for the Saskatchewan Cancer Foundation. During her professional career she published numerous papers and gave many presentations.

The second Sylvia is the athlete. At the University of Saskatchewan she was a member of 12 intervarsity championship teams in basketball, track and field, volleyball, golf and hockey. After leaving university she distinguished herself in curling and was a member of the team which won the Canadian Ladies Curling Championship in 1961. She has been honoured by the University of Saskatchewan Sports Hall of Fame and the Canadian Curling Hall of Fame.

Perhaps even more impressive is Sylvia's career in public service. Her expertise was sought in numerous public bodies, notably the Rhodes Scholarship Trust, Saskatchewan Commission on Directions in Health Care, University of Saskatchewan Senate and the Atomic Energy Control Board, and she was appointed an Officer of the Order of Canada in 1986. Honorary doctorates have been bestowed upon her by four universities. In 1988 she became lieutenant-governor of the province of Saskatchewan.

Her friends and colleagues might also tell you of her warmth, her integrity and her willingness to help.

XXIV *Dr Peter Cockshott*

Giles Stevenson and Carl Zylak

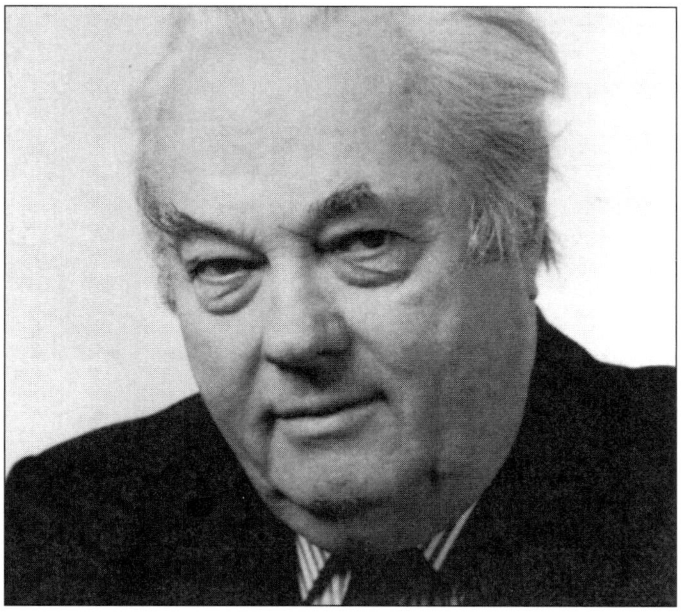

Peter Cockshott was born just outside Paris in June 1926, of English parents. He was educated initially in France and then in an English preparatory school before being sent to the United States in 1939. He spent one year at school in New Jersey studying American History before being accepted at Union College to read engineering at age 14, switching after two years to "premed." He was accepted to medical school by Edinburgh University and arranged passage as one of 25 civilian passengers on a troop-ship convoy from Halifax to Liverpool in 1943. In Edinburgh he joined the air squadron and learned to fly, developed a lifelong admiration for William Osler, and was an enthusiastic member of the Royal Medical Society, publishing his first paper as a medical student on the history of Colles' fracture.

He qualified in 1949, and spent eighteen months national service in the Royal Air Force as a member of the Aden Protectorate Levies. This time was one of his most vivid experiences and one that changed the direction of his life, awakening an interest in travel and in medical care for the underprivileged that characterized his later radiological career.

His radiological training in Edinburgh was completed in 1956, and he, his wife Una and the children left for University College Hospital in Ibadan, where in 1961 Peter was appointed Professor and Chairman of Radiology. He designed and built a department, collected (stamps, radiographs and friends), travelled widely, developed angiography and accumulated a vast knowledge of skeletal and tropical radiology.

In 1967 he was appointed Founding Chairman at McMaster University's new medical school in time to design the radiology department, which is still, 25 years later, a functional and esthetic masterpiece.

At McMaster, building on his international friendships, he served with WHO and the Radiological Society of North America. As visiting consultant he served all over the world but especially in the West Indies, Malaysia, Pakistan and Africa. He derived particular pleasure from his friends in the International Society of Radiology, the International Skeletal Society, the International Committee on Education in Radiology of the RSNA and the 1962 Club.

To those of us who have passed through or stayed at McMaster, he has been a friend, hero and rôle model. Erudite, witty and awesomely wide read, he encouraged and took under his wing generations of residents, fellows and young faculty. He and his second wife Colina have entertained and put up with the foibles of all of us. He seldom slept more than four hours a night, devouring the literature between 11 p.m. and 2 a.m.—*Lancet, New Scientist, British Medical Journal, Harpers, New England Journal, New Yorker.* A week never passed but that we would find on our desks by 7:30 a.m. some article in our own area of interest that Peter had torn out during his night's reading. From time to time, other typed or handwritten quotations would appear that had taken his fancy or seemed relevant to some issue of the moment. Examples of these are:

Pinned in the bone area:

We trained hard, but it seemed that every time we formed up into teams we would be reorganized. I was to learn later in life that we tend to meet any new situation by reorganizing, and a wonderful method it can be for creating the illusion of progress, while producing confusion, inefficiency and demoralization.

— Caius Petronius writing to his nephew in 64 AD.

On the chairman's desk at the beginning of contract negotiations:

I am satisfied myself that the present state of degradation and contempt into which the greater part of these [European and English universities] have fallen arises principally from the large salaries which in some universities are given to professors and which render them altogether independent of their diligence and success in their profession.

— Adam Smith, 1777

And in the week before his last illness:

History maketh a man to be old without either wrinkles or grey hairs; privileging him with the experiences of age without the infirmities thereof. Yea, it not only maketh things past present, but enableth one to make a rational conjecture of things to come. For this world affordeth no

new accidents, but in the same sense of things wherein we call it a new moon, which is the old one in another shape, yet no others thou hath seen formerly. Old actions return, furbished over with some new and different circumstances.
— Thomas Fuller, 1608–1661

Intellectual giants are rare; warm, friendly, inspiring and lovable ones even more so. Even when sick, Peter maintained an energy level and commitment that was an example to the rest of us. We rejoiced in his Radiological Society of North America gold medal and were amused by his characteristic response: "Why me?" He worked, taught at the view box, counselled, amused, encouraged and was productive until and, indeed, during his final brief illness.

XXV *C Stuart Houston*

A Radiologist for All Seasons

Brian Lentle

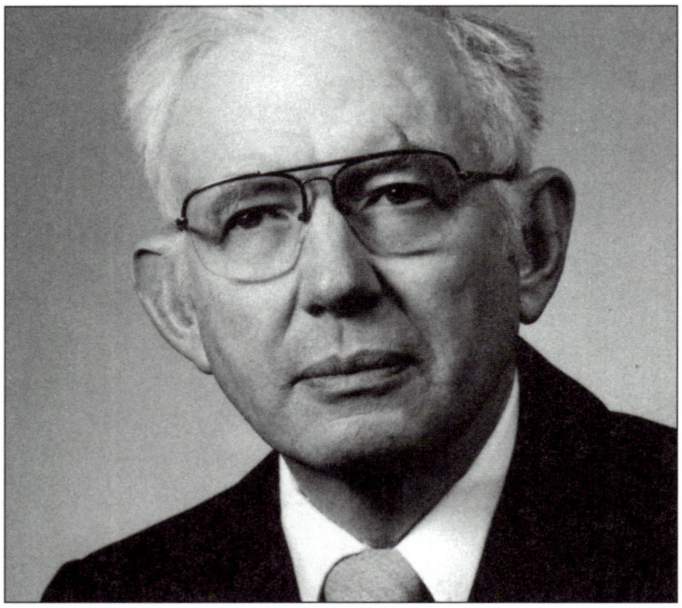

Dr Houston achieved so much in several endeavours that a brief biography risks trivializing his achievements.

Stuart Houston was born on September 26, 1927 in Williston, North Dakota. His family-practitioner parents moved to Yorkton, Saskatchewan one year later. Stuart was to become the quintessential Canadian and one of the renaissance individuals of Canadian radiology.

To begin at the beginning: Dr Houston graduated in medicine (MD) from the University of Manitoba in 1951. From 1951 to 1955, and again from 1956 to 1960, he was a family doctor with his parents in Yorkton, Saskatchewan. In 1960 Dr Houston began his formal radiology education at University Hospital Saskatchewan, spending one year at the Children's Hospital Medical Center at Harvard University where he was recipient of the George Von L Meyer Memorial Scholarship. Appointed lecturer in diagnostic radiology at the University of Saskatchewan in 1964, Dr Houston was promoted to become professor in 1969 and head of the department of medical imaging from 1982 to 1987.

The indefatigable Dr Houston has published an astonishing 231 works in medicine and its history, a number that includes three books, five chapters in books and 59 peer-reviewed scientific articles. There are, moreover, another 371 published works in ornithology and natural history, including three books and twelve book chapters.[1]

Up to the end of 1993 Stuart had also banded 105 490 birds of 201 species. The 2906 bandings recovered is the highest number of any private bander. A slight limp betrays the fact that this avocation is not without hazard.

For five years Dr Houston was editor of the *Canadian Association of Radiologists Journal*, a task he undertook with his customary energy and insight. I have a favourite piece of doggerel which always reminds me of Stuart:

The Editor's Passport[2]
The Editor stood 'fore the Heavenly Gate,
His features pinched and cold.
He bowed before the Man of Fate,
Seeking admission to the fold.
"What have you done," St Peter asked,
"To gain admission here?"
"I was the Journal's editor, Sir,
For many a weary year."
The Pearly Gates swung open wide
As Peter pressed the bell.
"Come in and choose your harp," he cried;
"You've had your share of hell!"

Except that I do not believe that Stuart's features were ever "pinched and cold." He taught me that the *Journal* was but a means to introduce to others his own sheer pleasure in scholarship for its own sake.

Dr Houston's passion for excellence has not gone unnoticed, although the awards it has brought have not changed the man. Dr Houston was awarded an honourary doctorate of literature (D Litt) by his university in 1987. He has been made a member of the Order of Canada, awarded the Saskatchewan Order of Merit, elected a life member of the American Ornithologists Union and elected president of the Canadian Society for the History of Medicine.

Stuart and his wife, Mary, are the kindest and most generous hosts. Their home reflects their scholarship and brings to mind words of the Rev Sydney Smith who wrote in *Lady Holland: a Memoir* that there is "no furniture so charming as books." The house is quite literally filled from wall-to-wall with books and records and this in every room, and I mean every room. They have entertained students and residents to dinner regularly to ensure that a sense of scholarship and humanity, and Stuart's own passionate commitment to his work, pervade their relations with those fortunate enough to study in the Faculty of Medicine at the University of Saskatchewan.[3] Now, in 1995 when contemplating partial retirement at age 67, Dr Houston has been elected honourary class president for the third time. Indeed, in residency programs in which I have taught or visited at numerous centres across Canada, it is common to find young physicians whose love of radiology was first prompted by Dr Houston. I suspect that these are the legacies by which he should be and might wish to be remembered, over and above the bulging curriculum vitae and the honours he wears so lightly.

XXVI *Dr Leonard Rosenthall*

Canada's Ambassador of Nuclear Medicine

Brian Lentle

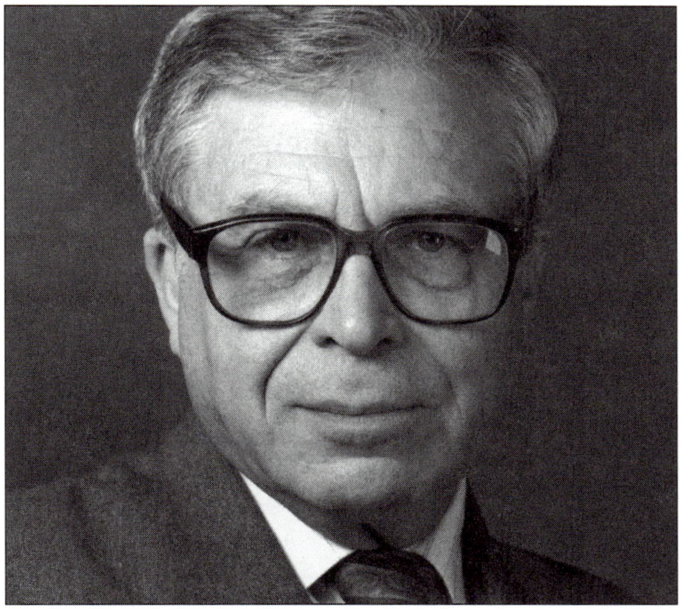

Dr Leonard Rosenthall is a formidable figure who has acted as a mentor for many of those who have gone on to be members of the early Canadian nuclear medicine establishment. His education provided a path from which his career has not wavered. After obtaining a Bachelor of Science degree at McGill in 1949, he spent time at the Massachusetts Institute of Technology studying biophysics, obtaining a master's degree in that subject at the University of Minnesota in 1952. Four years later Dr Rosenthall graduated in medicine (MD CM) from McGill University.

After Montréal internships, Leonard was a resident in radiology at the University of Chicago and in radiation therapy at the Princess Margaret Hospital in Toronto. He was immediately thereafter appointed to McGill University—where he had been a lecturer in mathematics from 1949–1950—in the Department of Radiology. He rapidly rose to be a full professor and Director of Nuclear Medicine at Montréal General Hospital.

He was faced, like many of us, with the choice of being a candidate or examiner in the first Royal College examination in nuclear medicine in 1976. Dr Rosenthall chose to be a candidate, already being certified as a specialist in Québec and the United States.

A fine and self-deprecating sense of humour characterizes the man. When I was in his laboratory, we would receive cards from wherever he happened to be lecturing signed "Himself." Despite his achievements Dr Rosenthall is never pompous and can again note in a self-deprecating way that he "loves to travel—with slides."

A *curriculum vitae* listing 204 papers, two books,[1,2] some 26 book chapters and a host of invited lectureships, risks missing the critical fact that much of this output has been at the forefront of developments in nuclear medicine. In particular he was an early investigator in recognizing the potential of gamma cameras to image dynamic events and not static tracer biodistributions. His scientific interests have been eclectic but are, perhaps, reflected most concisely in his two books on skeletal imaging (with another in preparation) and biliary disease.[1,2]

Dr Rosenthall is an excellent teacher and his clinical insights are highly valued in his hospital, as reflected by the physicians who come to consult. His aphorism on such occasions "sometimes wrong but never in doubt" reflects a determination to help in patient care and not retreat into equivocation or a listing of a long and not very meaningful differential diagnosis.

All of these talents have not, of course, gone unrecognized. In addition to consulting and lecturing all over the world, Dr Rosenthall has been president of the Canadian Association of Nuclear Medicine as well as the Eastern and the North Eastern Chapters of the Society of Nuclear Medicine. He was awarded a Special Certificate of Merit in "recognition of an outstanding contribution to the practice of radiological sciences in Canada and to this Association" by the Canadian Association of Radiologists as well as Certificate of Recognition from the Canadian Association of Nuclear Medicine "in recognition of his outstanding contribution as Secretary-General of the Fifth International Congress of the World Federation of Nuclear Medicine and Biology" in Montréal in 1990. Dr Rosenthall is listed in

"The Best Doctors in America" and serves on numerous editorial boards.

For recreation "Himself" plays tennis very combatively and, as noted, likes to travel "with slides." He is a keen gardener, both indoors and out, and is an "eclectic woodworker." He is devotedly married to Devorah (née Rabiner), who was born in Edmonton. They have three children. His letters are direct, dispensing with any "Dear ——" and come straight to the point with only one's name. His observation in a letter to me a few years back that "We all take ourselves too seriously" lives with me and characterizes someone who has done so much, but has never let that fact change the man. I had trouble extracting a photograph from him. When it came, "courtesy of the hospital medical illustrations department, who never [had] heard of an airbrush for portraiture," I learned that it was taken in a borrowed jacket and tie. Leonard is ever a man of substance but with no pretensions.

XXVII *Étienne LeBel*

Jocelyne Lapointe

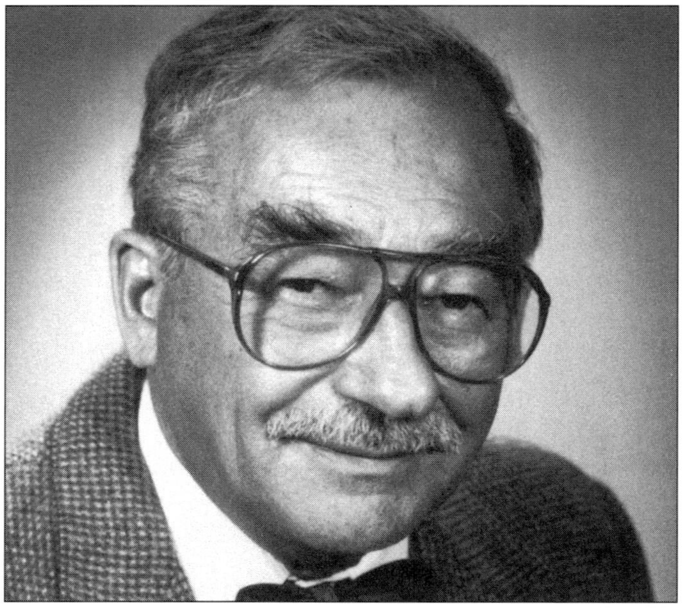

Originaire de Montréal (P.Q.), Étienne LeBel fit ses études à l'Université de Montréal où il obtint un BA en 1949, un MD en 1954, et un BSc en 1956; puis, la même année, à l'Université Columbia de New York, où il se familiarisa à l'utilization des radio-isotopes dans le laboratoire des hôpitaux universitaires Mount-Sinaï et Presbyterian de New York. Après avoir complété sa formation en radiologie thérapeutique à l'Hôtel-Dieu de Montréal, affilié à l'Université de Montréal, il obtient un certificat de spécialiste en 1958.

En 1959, il fonda et dirigea le premier laboratoire de radio-isotopes bien équipé à l'Hôpital Notre-Dame de la Merci, tout en oeuvrant à l'Hôtel-Dieu de Montréal.

En 1963, il devint le premier directeur du département de médecine nucléaire de l'Hôtel-Dieu, jusqu'à son départ en 1968.

Durant ces années à Montréal, il dirigea un groupe de radiologistes qui préparèrent un mémoire devant amener la création de la spécialité de médecine nucléaire en 1969, spécialité reconnue pour la première fois comme autonome dans le monde. Il est reconnu comme l'un des pères de la médecine nucléaire.

Fin 1968, il quitta Montréal pour se joindre au corps professoral de l'Université de Sherbrooke à la Faculté de Médecine où il devint le directeur-fondateur du Département de médecine nucléaire et de radiobiologie. Nommé professeur titulaire en 1969, il dirigea ce département jusqu'en 1985.

De 1983 à 1988, il fut le vice-doyen à la recherche et aux études avancées; de 1984 à 1993, directeur scientifique du Centre de recherche clinique du Centre Hospitalier Universitaire de Sherbrooke.

Ses activités, consacrées à la clinique, à l'enseignement et à la recherche, l'amenèrent à présenter ses travaux, plus de 80 publications et de 100 communications, dans plusieurs pays. Il oeuvra dans plusieurs organisations er associations professionelles, dont la Commission de Contrôle de l'Énergie Atomique du Canada, le Collège Royal des Médecins et Chirugiens du Canada, le Collège des Médecins du Québec, l'Association de Médecins Spécialistes en Médecine Nucléaire du Québec (dont il fut le président-fondateur [1974–1983]), la Society of Nuclear Medicine USA, comme président de l'Eastern chapter (1978–1992) et président du Québec chapter en 1992–93
et enfin, comme président de la Fédération mondiale de Médecine et de Biologie Nucléaire (1986–1990). Il fut arbitre externe de plusieurs organismes et fondations de recherche.

Son implication en médecine nucléaire l'a amené à présider plusieurs activités tant au Québec qu'ailleurs, dont le 19e Colloque de médecine nucléaire de langue française (internationale), à Québec, en 1978 et le Congrès mondial de médecine nucléaire et de biologie à Montréal en 1990.

Sa participation lui a valu de nombreux honneurs dont le Prix spécial du Président de la Society of Nuclear Medicine en juin 1987 pour sa contribution en tant que professeur, chercheur et médecin. Pour ces mêmes raison, en 1992 on lui décerna le prix Michel Sarazin, prix du Club de recherches cliniques du Québec et la médaille du 150e anniversaire de l'Université de Montréal.

XXVIII *Doubly Gifted*

BRIAN LENTLE

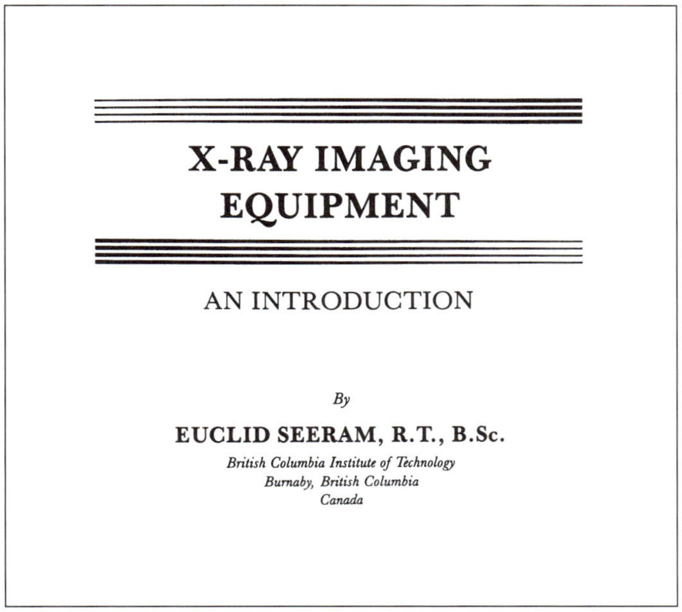
X-RAY IMAGING EQUIPMENT

AN INTRODUCTION

By

EUCLID SEERAM, R.T., B.Sc.

British Columbia Institute of Technology
Burnaby, British Columbia
Canada

Of making many books there is no end.
Ecclesiastes 12:12

Canadians have not been deterred by that biblical note of scepticism. Indeed, those working in the radiological sciences have contributed more than their share to the store of scientific literature. However, some notable few have also written or published in other contexts; hence the title.

An early and rare general textbook of radiology was written in Canada by Dr Bede Harrison and published in 1936.[1] Dr Harrison was then head of radiology at the Vancouver General Hospital.[2] Dr RG (Bob) Fraser of the Royal Victoria Hospital, Montréal, with his colleague Dr Peter Paré, has written several editions of the definitive *Diagnosis of Diseases of the Chest.*[3] Dr Fraser was sometime professor and head of radiology at McGill University. Similarly, Dr Joachim Burhenne has co-authored, with Dr Alex Margulis of the University of California at San Francisco, the equally monumental text *Alimentary Tract Radiology.*[4] Dr Burhenne at the time was head of radiology at both the University of British Columbia and Vancouver General Hospital. After several editions this editorial task has now been taken on by another Canadian, the talented chairman of radiology at McMaster University, Dr Giles Stevenson.

Equally widely known—if less loved—by generations of radiology residents, for whom mathematical equations are an anathema, is the volume *The Physics of Radiology,* first published in 1953 and written by Dr Harold Johns and Dr JR Cunningham.[5] Dr Johns' many contributions to the Canadian scene are celebrated elsewhere in this account.[6,7] In four editions and many reprintings, this text is used worldwide as a reference text in medical physics.

Dr Derek Harwood-Nash of the University of Toronto and a former director of the Department of Radiology at the Sick Children's Hospital in Toronto published a three volume textbook of pediatric neuroradiology which was definitive in its time.[8] Indeed pediatric radiology has been well represented among those putting pen to paper with monographs having been prepared by Drs Alan Daneman, David Gilday (an atlas)[9] and David Stringer (now at the BC Children's Hospital). Other pediatric radiologists contri-buting to their literature have been Dr Gordon Culham of Vancouver and Dr Martin Reed of Winnipeg. Diagnostic ultrasonography has always been strong in Canada with monographs coming from Drs Ted Lyons (including one on sectional anatomy) and Stephanie Wilson. In nuclear medicine Dr Leonard Rosenthall has been a prolific author, as noted elsewhere.[10] Last but far from least Dr Nestor Müller of Vancouver has written several monographs on the radiology of chest disease and stands poised to serve as one of the editors of Fraser's monumental work on *Diagnosis of Diseases of the Chest* in its next edition.

Mr Euclid Seeram, an instructor at the British Columbia Institute of Technology, has written the widely used text *X-ray Imaging Equipment.*[11]

Dr Stuart Houston, not content with a large number of papers and book chapters in his first vocation, might almost deserve a separate chapter for the trebly gifted. In addition to contributing two chapters to the present book, he has edited and seen the publication of some stylish volumes on early travel in, and exploration of, the Canadian north. Examples are *To the Arctic by Canoe, 1819–1821, The Journal and Paintings of Robert Hood;*[12] *Arctic Ordeal, The Journal of John Richardson, Surgeon–Naturalist with Franklin, 1820–1822;*[13] and *Arctic Artist: The journal and paintings of George Back, Midshipman with Franklin, 1819–1822.*[14] He has also published in the context of medical history (*RG Ferguson, Crusader Against Tuberculosis* and *Pioneer of Vision, the Memoirs of Dr TA Patrick.*) In addition, as a respected ornithologist and life member of the American Ornithologists Union, he has published extensively in this context, including the compilation *Birds of the Saskatchewan River.*[15]

Dr Joachim Burhenne, already celebrated above for his text on abdominal radiology, has found time to write *Sierra Spring Ski Touring.*[16] Dr Jocelyne Lapointe, from the same department, has proved to be the unlikely but skilled historian of the Naval Offi-cers Association of British Columbia, of which she is a member.[17]

Last but far from least and as noted elsewhere,[18] Dr Orest Semchishen has produced a volume of his photo-graphs of the prairies.[19] These spare and hauntingly beautiful silver prints are but part of his considerable artistic output.

The proper study of mankind is man.
— Alexander Pope

A TEXTBOOK

of

ROENTGENOLOGY

THE ROENTGEN RAY IN DIAGNOSIS AND TREATMENT

By

BEDE J. MICHAEL HARRISON, M.B., Ch.M.,
D.M.R.E. (Cantab), F.A.C.R.

DIRECTOR OF DEPARTMENT OF ROENTGENOLOGY, VANCOUVER GENERAL HOSPITAL,
ROENTGENOLOGIST TO VANCOUVER PUBLIC HEALTH INSTITUTE FOR
DISEASES OF THE CHEST

BALTIMORE
WILLIAM WOOD & COMPANY
1936

THE PHYSICS OF
RADIOLOGY

FOURTH EDITION

HAROLD ELFORD JOHNS, OC, Ph.D., F.R.S.C., LL.D., D.Sc., F.C.C.P.M.
University Professor Emeritus, University of Toronto
Professor Emeritus, Department of Medical Biophysics and Department of Radiology, University of Toronto
Former Head of, and now consultant to, the Physics Division, Ontario Cancer Institute and the Radiological Research Laboratories; University of Toronto

and

JOHN ROBERT CUNNINGHAM, B.Eng., M.Sc., Ph.D., F.C.C.P.M.
Senior Clinical Physicist, Ontario Cancer Institute
Professor, Department of Medical Biophysics
University of Toronto

Second Edition VOLUME IV

DIAGNOSIS OF
DISEASES OF
THE CHEST

ROBERT G. FRASER, M.D., F.R.C.P.(C)
Professor of Diagnostic Radiology, University of Alabama in Birmingham;
Formerly Professor of Diagnostic Radiology, McGill University;
and Diagnostic Radiologist-in-Chief, Royal Victoria Hospital, Montreal

J. A. PETER PARÉ, M.D., F.A.C.P.
Director, Respiratory Division,
Royal Victoria Hospital, Montreal

VOLUME ONE

NEURORADIOLOGY IN
INFANTS AND CHILDREN

DEREK C. HARWOOD-NASH, M.B., Ch.B., F.R.C.P.(C)
Head, Division of Paediatric Neuroradiology,
The Hospital for Sick Children;
Professor of Radiology, University of Toronto,
Toronto, Ontario, Canada

with the assistance of

CHARLES R. FITZ, M.D.
Paediatric Neuroradiologist,
Department of Radiology, The Hospital for Sick Children;
Assistant Professor of Radiology, University of Toronto,
Toronto, Ontario, Canada

with 3931 *illustrations*

THE C. V. MOSBY COMPANY
Saint Louis 1976

Inscribed for
Brian C. Lentle
Visiting Professor, University of Saskatchewan
22-23 February 1990

Arctic Ordeal

C. Stuart Houston

THE JOURNAL OF JOHN RICHARDSON

SURGEON-NATURALIST WITH FRANKLIN

1820–1822

Edited by C. Stuart Houston
Illustrated by H. Albert Hochbaum
Appendixes by John W. Thomson (Lichenology)
and Walter O. Kupsch (Geology)
Foreword by W. Gillies Ross

Orest Semchishen

In Plain View *Voir clair*

Martha Hanna

Canadian Museum of Contemporary Photography

Musée canadien de la photographie contemporaine

Volume 1

ALIMENTARY TRACT RADIOLOGY

Fourth Edition

Edited by

Alexander R. Margulis, M.D.
Professor and Chairman,
Department of Radiology,
University of California,
San Francisco,
School of Medicine,
San Francisco, California

H. Joachim Burhenne, M.D., F.R.C.P. (C)
Professor and Head,
Department of Radiology,
University of British Columbia,
Vancouver, British Columbia, Canada

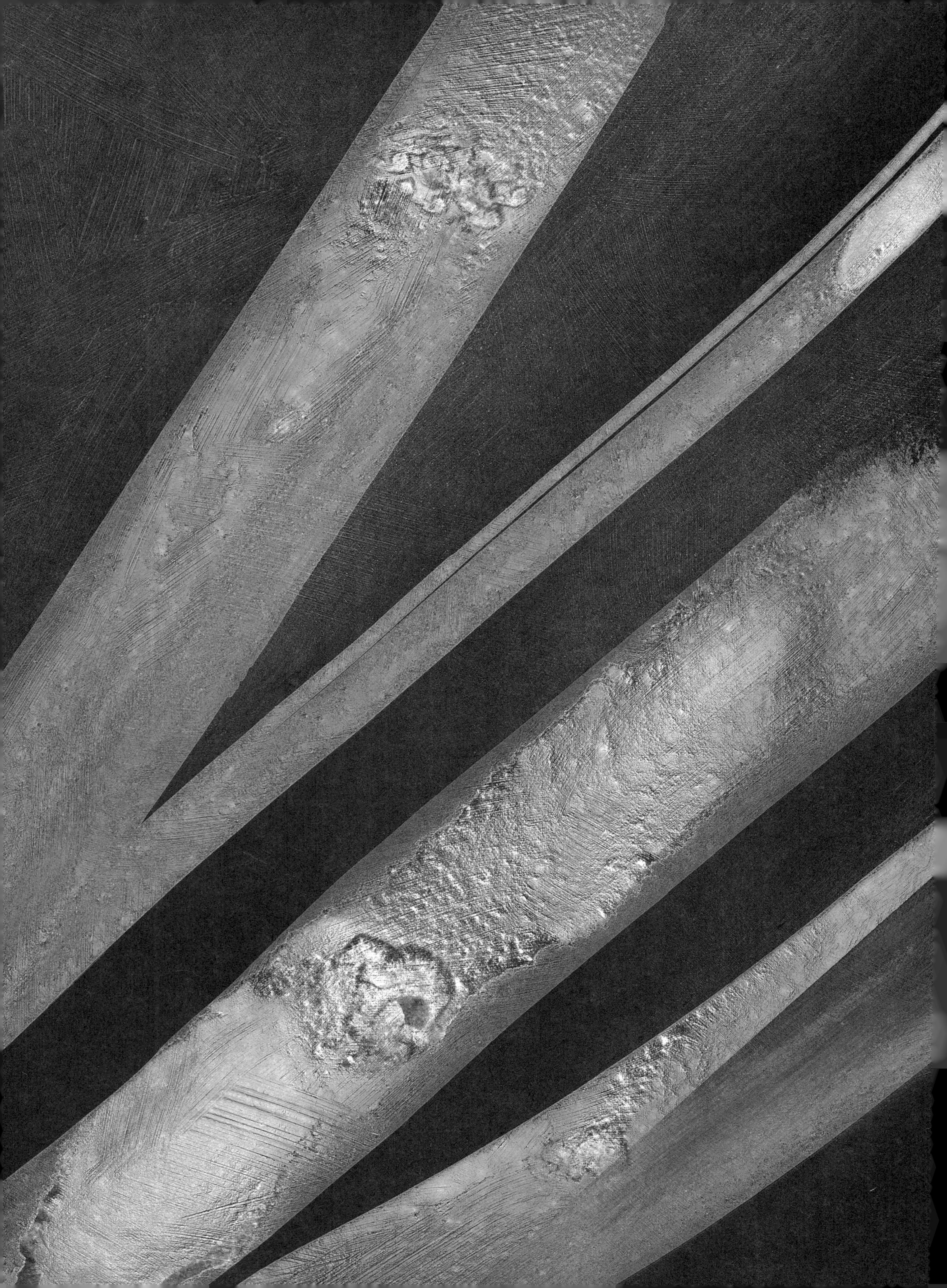

Part Six

Organizations of those Specialty Groups Working in the Radiological Sciences

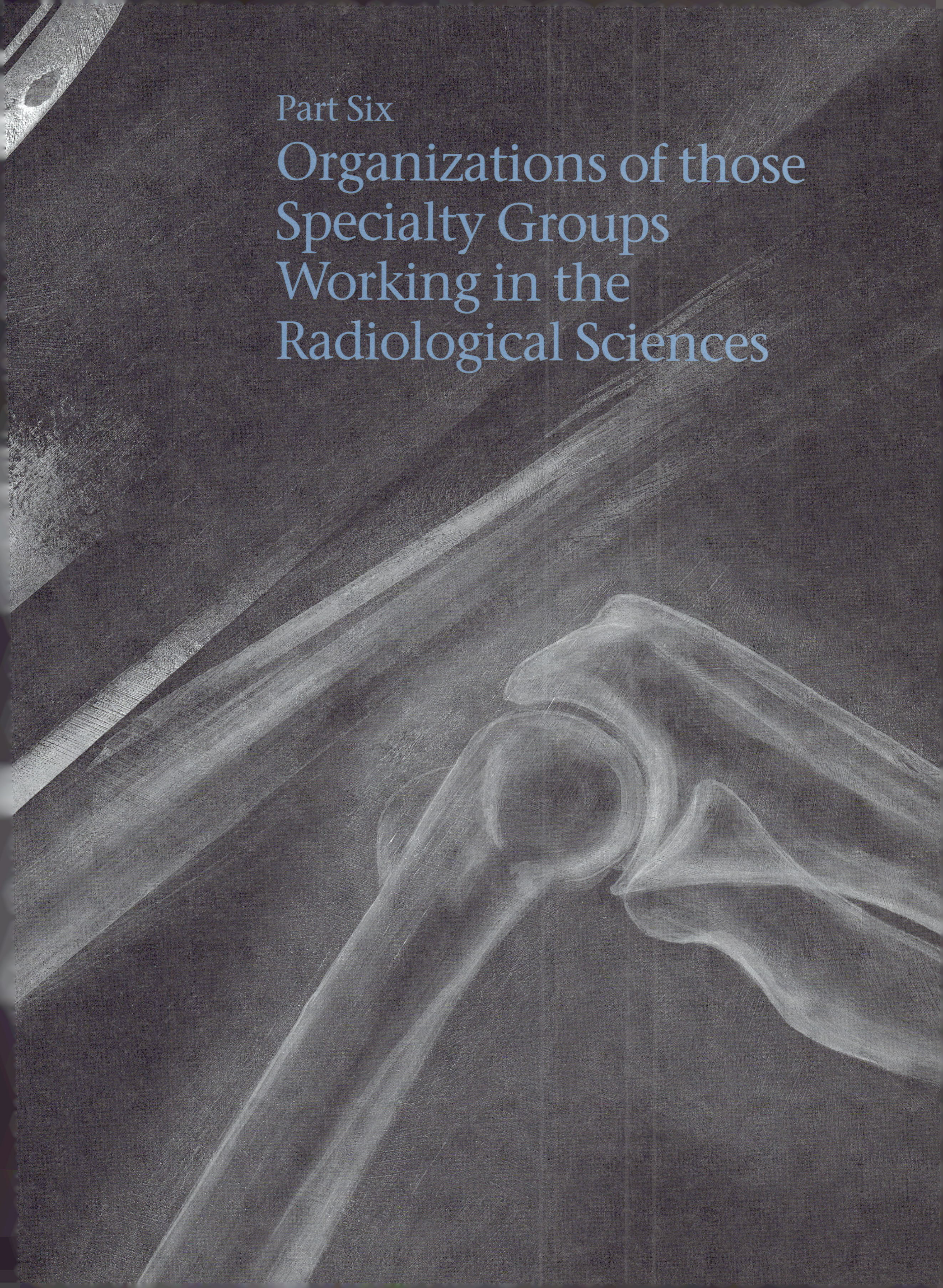

A wise nation preserves its records...

— Joseph Howe

Radiology departments have not needed to adjust to a multi-disciplinary culture: they began in that way. The first clinical radiographs worldwide were most often made by physicists. Within a typical department one may find administrators, clerks, computer scientists, engineers, medical physicists, nuclear medicine physicians, nuclear medicine technologists, nurses, porters, radiologists, radiographic technologists, radiopharmacists and secretaries, in addition to the patients. Many of these disciplines have organized themselves both provincially and nationally for the purposes of sharing experience, setting standards and arranging for continuing education.

At the outset there were no such disciplines. Such radiography as was possible was usually done by university physicists working in conjunction with physicians who had not specialized. Indeed, the whole edifice of medical specialty practice as it is found at the end of the 20th century was not in place in the early years of the century.

The first discipline to organize was that of radiographic technologists. In the best Canadian federalist tradition, their decision was to create provincial divisions, which came together under the umbrella of the Canadian Society of Radiological Technologists, later the Canadian Association of Medical Radiation Technologists. This association has remained strong and embraces radiographic, radiation oncologic and nuclear medical technologists. The first organization within the radiological sciences to be formed in Canada was the Manitoba Society of Radiological Technicians.

The Canadian Association of Radiologists (CAR) was created in 1937 in an era when radiologists practiced both diagnosis and therapy.

Subsequently, the knowledge base reached the point at which combined practice ceased to be a realistic proposition. As the specialties of diagnostic radiology and radiation oncology diverged, the oncologists came to separate from CAR and form their own organization named the Canadian Association of Radiation Oncologists. Before that schism CAR exerted a great influence on the evolution of Canadian medicine, introducing specialist certification by the Royal College of Physicians and Surgeons and sponsoring the first Canadian specialty journal.

Other organizations have addressed the issue of specialization and subspecialization differently. Medical physicists have remained unified while their certification process has recognized that individual expertise will usually embrace some aspect of the radiological sciences. Nuclear medicine physicians have had an organization, the Canadian Association of Nuclear Medicine (CANM), separate from CAR, and must weigh the advantages of affiliation with that larger organization against the disadvantages of remaining an autonomous, but small and poorly resourced, group. As the neuroradiologists, pediatric radiologists and other groups form their own organizations in the 1990s, they are choosing to remain under the umbrella of CAR.

At various times the idea of a confederation of these specialty groups has been proposed, most notably by Dr George Goodman. Perhaps in the future it will become clearer if size will effect a more powerful lobby, or if smaller more flexible organizations are more effective. Given the resource constraints imposed by maintaining a secretariat, the latter scenario is perhaps less likely.

The 1995 centennial celebrations bring many of these groups together in Montréal, to share in annual meetings. Perhaps this type of forum in which size is certainly an advantage, may serve as a catalyst for future joint meetings which may serve to optimize the scientific and social advantages of collegiality.

—Brian Lentle

Chapter I •

The Canadian Radiological Society

C Stuart Houston

During historical research into tuberculosis in Canada, I came across an account of the 1925 meeting of the Canadian Radiological Society (CRS). I had not realized that there had been a society in existence long before the formation of the Canadian Association of Radiologists in 1937.

In 1925 Dr RG Ferguson, Superintendent of the Tuberculosis Sanatorium at Fort Qu'Appelle, Saskatchewan gave an address, "Radiographic results in a recent survey of 500 school children," before the annual meeting of the Canadian Radiological Society. Dr Ferguson used slides to illustrate the significance of x-ray signs in these children. Ferguson stated that living and working conditions in the years to come would determine whether these children, most of whom had a positive tuberculin test, would eventually develop active tuberculosis or whether they had achieved some degree of immunity through their conversion to a positive tuberculin test.[1]

The CRS met that year with the annual meeting of the Canadian Medical Association in Regina.[2] The meeting had been advertised in the *American Journal of Roentgenology.* Delegates listed included a "Committee on Radiology" with Regina radiologist Dr Clarence Millwood Henry as chairman[3] and Dr James Victor Connell as secretary.[4] The secretary of the society was Dr EC Brooks of Montréal.

This was one of the largest meetings of the CMA ever held (June 22–26, 1925), with 363 registrants. The sessions were held in the Normal School on the outskirts of Regina. Twice as many new CMA memberships were sold as were ever secured at any previous annual meeting.[5] DA Stewart's editorial after the meeting had this comment:

Canadian Radiological Society Meeting (1922): Back row, left to right: CM Henry (Regina), HH Murphy (Victoria), EC Jerman (Chicago), W Brady (Chicago), Frank G Smith (Winnipeg), Frank S Bissell (Oakland), MacDonald (Winnipeg), R Michaud (Moose Jaw), and G Hettich (Chicago) Front row, left to right: CH Burger (Winnipeg), JC McMillan (Winnipeg), LK Poyntz (Portland), C Wesley Proud (Vancouver), LJ Carter (Brandon), Gordon E Richards (Toronto), BH Orndoff (Chicago), Rollin H Stevens (Detroit), AE Walkey (Hamilton), and WH Guffin (Calgary)

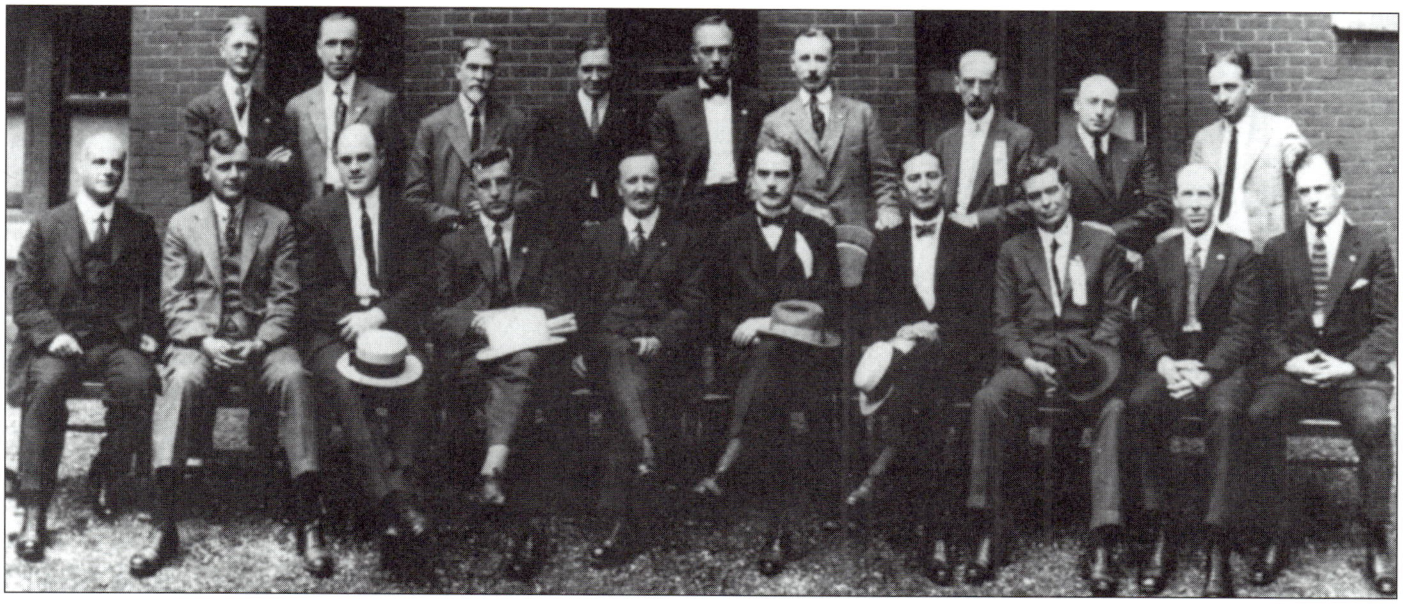

The Canadian X-ray Association did get off into a corner by itself occasionally but attended practically all of the main sessions also, and contributed useful papers of general interest.[5]

At the annual meeting of the Canadian Medical Association in Victoria, British Columbia in June 1926, Dr JC McMillan of Winnipeg gave a paper on "Lipiodol as an adjunct in x-ray diagnosis" before the general session.[6] WH Dickson, a radiologist at the Toronto General Hospital, contributed a paper to a symposium on duodenal ulcer.[7] WH McGuffin of Calgary discussed the "radiological aspect" in a symposium on goitre,[8] and Hugh MacKay read a paper on "Radium in Dermatology" before the combined meeting of the Pacific Coast and Canadian Radiological societies.[9]

In 1927 the Canadian Radiological Society held its meeting at the University of Toronto in conjunction with the Ontario Medical Association, the Canadian Public Health Association, the Canadian Tuberculosis Association, the Canadian Society of Anaesthetists and the Ontario Radiological Society.[10] At a joint session of all five groups, DA Stewart of the Ninette Sanatorium talked about bronchiectasis and other septic infections of the bronchii, Oscar Klotz of Toronto reported on primary tumors of the lung and WA Evans of Detroit discussed the then rare malignant neoplasms of the lung.[11]

The different organizations then had their individual meetings on the second day, Thursday, June 16. The Canadian Radiological Society and the Ontario Radiological Society heard RW Knight of Brantford discuss the relation of sinus infections to respiratory diseases; CG Brink of Toronto, röntgen-ray studies of dust inhalation; LR Hess of Hamilton, investigation of chest diseases by means of lipiodol; PM Andrus of London, the interpretation of the lesions of pulmonary tuberculosis; James T Case of Detroit, technique and results of cholecystography by the intravenous method; BR Mooney of Edmonton, anencephalus; WA Wilkins of Montréal, recurrent sarcoma; A Howard Pirie of Montréal, treatment of rodent ulcer; LK Poyntz of Chicago, investigations in physical therapy; WH Dickson of Toronto, unusual diseases of the colon; and WJ Cryderman of Toronto, duodenal diverticula.[12] The federal Department of Soldiers' Civil Re-establishment sent from each province those chest physicians who were responsible for the servicemen still in sanatoria after discharge from the forces. Reports were presented of the progress against tuberculosis made at Trois Rivières, Québec, and in the Maritimes, and of native studies undertaken by Dr Ferguson of Saskatchewan.

That year, an item by AHP (A Howard Pirie) in the July issue of the *Canadian Medical Association Journal* provided the following information:

> *The decision of the members of the Canadian Radiological Society to disband and continue their work as a section of the Canadian Medical Association will, it is hoped, prove mutually beneficial both to the radiologists themselves and to the members of the Canadian Medical Association who, while not specialists in this branch of medicine, are much interested in the results obtained. This Society was begun in 1912 as a section of the Canadian Medical Association and continued as such until 1919, when it decided to become a separate Association to be known as the Canadian Radiological Society. While much good work was done by the Society since it assumed its separate existence it was felt that better work could be accomplished by again merging with the Dominion Association. Every year the papers presented at its meeting have been becoming less technical but more interesting and valuable to the general profession. Among the subjects discussed this year were the value of skiagraphy in pulmonary tuberculosis, in diseases of the appendix, colon, and gall bladder, in diverticulitis, in sarcomatous conditions, and when associated with the use of lipiodol. As a result of this decision any member of the Canadian Medical Association in the future who may be interested in x-ray work, or in allied subjects, is at liberty to take part in the deliberations of this Section, which will function in a manner similar to the other Sections of the Canadian Medical Association.*[13]

This news item led to an editorial in the August issue, also by AHP, quoted in part as follows:

> *...We look forward to the future development of this Section of our Association as a valuable addition to the interest of our annual meetings. The four classical methods of student days: inspection, palpation, percussion and auscultation must to-day have a fifth added, namely, the employment and interpretation of the x-ray pictures. While radioscopy should in many cases be the last resort in forming our diagnosis, in others it should be the first. Doubtless, in the diagnosis of many forms of internal disease the other methods should be employed before having recourse to the use of x-rays; but for the diagnosis of many others, the information it gives is most valuable, and in the diagnosis of a case of fracture, it must be regarded as almost inhuman to attempt the old method of eliciting crepitus when it is possible to have a radiogram.*
>
> *We look forward to the transactions of this Section becoming the authority in Canada on radiography, and feel sure that radiologists will endeavour to maintain all their work at a high and strictly ethical standard. Already, unfortunately, there is evidence of the necessity of some regulation by law of those permitted to use x-rays, which in ignorant hands may be definitely dangerous. For some time past, numerous unqualified persons have been making use of x-rays for medical purposes, and such may become a real menace in our midst. Still more pregnant with danger is the establishment by commercial firms of so-called "beauty parlours" for the removal of hair by means of x-rays from face and arms and places where hair is not wanted, a method of treatment in which severe burns may be produced. The evil results, unfortunately, are slow in developing. It is quite possible that many of those who have been treated in this way may suffer in time from telangiectasis, a deformity which cosmetics can hide and no known treatment can remove.*
>
> *This method for the permanent removal of hair on a woman's face was employed some decades since but was given up ten years ago by those who had experience of the unfortunate results which may follow. When high voltage for x-rays was introduced some four years ago, it was hoped that with this increased strength success might be more assured. Unfortunately, although successful at first this new type of machine would appear to be more dangerous, and the law courts may yet be kept busy as the evil effects begin to become evident. Legislation to limit the use of this method of treatment to qualified persons is now called for and should be one of the early duties of this new Section of the Canadian Medical Association.*[14]

The radiology section faded into insignificance during the drought-stricken years of the Depression. The phoenix (the Canadian Association of Radiologists) did not arise from the ashes until 1937.

Chapter II • The Canadian Association of Radiologists

Brian Lentle

I hold every man a debtor to his profession
— Francis Bacon

Radiologists are often squeezed in a hospital or faculty between the more massive power blocks of internal medicine and surgery. The historical role of the Canadian Association of Radiologists (CAR) and of individual radiologists in Canadian medicine belies this image of radiologists as a small and unimportant specialty group. In reality, while acting through CAR, radiologists took the lead in introducing specialty certification in Canada. The journal that CAR sponsored was the first specialty medical publication in the country. The story of CAR is thus one which is central to the evolution of medicine in Canada as we know it today.

The association, moreover, has a proud record of national committment. It has been a bilingual organization from its inception, with its head office in Montréal, the birthplace of Canadian radiology. The greatest threat to the survival of CAR has been the high rate of enrollment of radiologists into military service during World War II.

Early radiologists were not physicians who were ready to play second fiddle to internists or surgeons. Rather, they had a keen sense of the future of their specialty and its central role in the care of the sick.

THE FOUNDING OF CAR

The Canadian Association of Radiologists (CAR) may not have been the first organization to represent Canadian radiologists, but it is the only one for which there is a consecutive record. There had been at least three earlier organizations representing some part of Canadian radiology. The Société Canadienne-Française d'Électrologie et de

Radiologie Médicales was founded in 1928[1] and continues to exist. The Canadian Radiological Society (see the article by Dr Stuart Houston above[2]) had also been active; the minutes of the meeting of 32 radiologists in Toronto in January 1937 which resulted in the formation of CAR. (appended as Annex A) noted that there had formerly been a Canadian Radiological Society. This society had been demobilized seven or eight years earlier and a Section on Radiology of the Canadian Medical Association (CMA) formed. There is anecdotal evidence that the Canadian Radiological Society (CRS) had been represented at the Stockholm International Congress of Radiology in 1920. Dr WA Jones recollected that CRS members Drs Currie MacMillan, Herbert McGuffin, CW Prowd and Gordon E Richards—as well as Jones himself—had attended.

Dr Gordon Richards invited all full-time radiologists in Canada to a meeting at the Toronto General Hospital on January 4 and 5, 1937. The minutes of that meeting are reproduced in Annex A. At that meeting CAR was created, with the following officers:

President:	Dr W A Jones (Kingston)
Vice-president:	Dr J E Gendreau (Montréal)
Secretary:	Dr A C Singleton (Toronto)

It is characteristic of Gordon Richards that he chose not to be elected first president, wanting it to be clear that he had no self-interest in promoting the idea of a national association of radiologists. He was acknowledged as founder and served as chairman of the Committee on Inter-relations. Nowadays, judging from the concerns it addressed, we should almost certainly call his committee one that deals with government relations.

From the outset there was broad representation by regional councillors.The first ones were Dr CW Prowd (Vancouver), Dr W H McGuffin (Calgary), Dr CM Henry (Regina), Dr Digby Wheeler (Winnipeg), Dr WM Gilmore (Stratford), Dr Paul Brodeur (Ottawa), Dr EH Shannon (Toronto), Drs Lloyd Ritchie and LA Gagnier (Montréal), Dr JE Perron (Québec), Dr SR Johnston (Halifax) and Dr AS Kirkland (Saint John). Already both the French and English speaking groups in Montréal were represented.

The minutes record that one advantage of a sectional affiliation with CMA was that that organization spoke for the profession and "not with the voice of the comparatively few [r]adiologists of the country." However, the radiologists of that era were addressing the need for some recognizable measures of radiological expertise as well as political action; one of the two recorded limitations of direct affiliation with the CMA was: "There is no standard of membership in the Section as at present constituted. Any member of the CMA may attend the meetings of the Section and presumably take part in the business and vote." The second limitation noted was that the CMA constitution limited a section to scientific activities, with all other professional issues to be addressed by the CMA as a whole. It is presumably from such concerns, especially those relating to standards of practice, that CAR in general, and Dr WA Jones in particular, became instrumental in the Royal College's coming to certify specialists, as recorded below.

Thus it was recognized that, while radiologists were urged to continue to belong to the CMA section, there was a need for the organization we now know as the Canadian Association of Radiologists (CAR). Indeed, this was the name proposed from the start for the nascent organization.

Under the heading of "Some Problems Facing the Proposed Organization" were the three following paragraphs (see the minutes appended[1]):

1. The education and qualification of Radiologists and along with this the training and controlling of radiological technicians. ("The training and controlling of radiological technicians had been met in Ontario by the formation of a Society of Radiological Technicians...")

2. The problem of x-ray fees with regard to the public, the Workmen's Compensation Boards and the Department of Pensions and National Health.

3. Other problems that may arise with regard to our inter-relationship with the general public and public bodies and with the rest of the medical profession.

Radiological practice in the first decades of the century was very different from that at present. As the publication list of Dr Gordon Richards (Appendix 2) makes clear, radiologists then performed both radiodiagnosis and radiotherapy. Egas Moniz in Portugal had made the first arteriogram only nine years earlier, while the first usable iodine containing contrast medium for intravascular use had been introduced in 1932, not quite five years before that first CAR meeting. Werner Forssman had, in a remarkable piece of self-experimentation which would be unthinkable in modern times, introduced a catheter into his own heart in 1929. That had equally been only six years earlier. He did get fired as a result.[4] One hopes that young investigators are treated more kindly in 1995.

Certainly, the modern explosion of acronym-laden radiology (CAT, PACS, DSA, PET, SPECT, MRI, etc.) which occurred after World War II was still decades in the future. This makes the foresight of Gordon Richards and his colleagues all the more important.

It reflects well on these early radiologists that their motivation in creating CAR clearly relates to their concern for maintaining standards of radiological practice. Radiographic technologists in Ontario (if not then known by that designation) were required to be admitted to practice by examination after three years' training. The education of radiologists had, however, not then been regularized. At the University of Toronto a Diploma in Medical Radiation Diagnosis (DMRD) was available after an eight-month course. At Queen's University a comprehensive course extending over three years had just been created. The first year included some clinical experience and university instruction in radiographic anatomy, pathology, radiobiology, radiophysics, radiographic technique, diagnostic radiology, radiotherapy and, last but not least, general medicine and surgery. After all this, the primary examination must have seemed an anticlimax. The first year was followed by two years of education at Kingston General Hospital. Remarkably, and presaging much later developments by which the Royal College would come to require all residency education to be university based, the hospital education was recognized by the university and successful completion of the final examination entitled radiologists to a Diploma in Medical Radiology (DMR). Those already in practice could arrange to take the diploma externally.

The minutes of that first CAR meeting relate that details concerning the requirements of the American Board of Radiology were to be obtained from Dr BR Kirklin at the Mayo Clinic and that the British Association of Radiologists, as it was then known, had established a fellowship examination, with details to be obtained from Dr S Cochrane Shanks at a Harley Street address.

A proposal to establish a Canadian College of Radiology was considered, while it was noted that the Committee on Specialists of the CMA had persuaded the Royal College of Physicians and Surgeons of Canada "to establish Boards for the purpose of overseeing the training, qualification and examination of specialists in Canada." The minutes add, "It is likely that the Radiologists will be asked shortly to form a Board for this purpose." It is thus evident that the pressure to create standards of practice and specialty certification was a grassroots expression of physicians determined to advance and regulate their profession and specialty. The role of CAR in this process is described below.

The resolutions of the inaugural meeting of CAR reveal a determination to have standards of training and examinations of radiologists in agreement with those standards prevailing in the United States of America and Great Britain. Perhaps even more unusually for those times, there was a concern that physicians undergoing training should not be exploited. Another concern was the legitimacy of short periods of education for those in remote areas practicing radiology part time. At that first meeting the possibility of the association publishing a journal was already being considered and minuted. The *Journal* when it appeared in 1950 was to be the first specialty journal in Canada.[3]

The outcome of the meeting was an organization called the Canadian Association of Radiologists with an organizational structure that was not to change in any fundamental way until the reforms advocated in the late 1980s by committees chaired by Drs JB (Ian) Sutherland of Winnipeg and Don Newman of Vancouver. An early concern in the business affairs of this newly created association was the inequities implicit in the survey of national fee schedules (see an attached Table). In ensuing correspondence it is recorded that the Ontario Workmen's Compensation Board had unilaterally reduced fees by amounts between 33 per cent and 50 per cent, a move resisted only by virtue of the radiologists being united in their stand.

Hand-written ledgers record that the annual membership fee in 1937 was $15. Membership numbered 91, including four women. A sum of $1080.10 was the cash balance carried forward from the previous year.

By 1938, *Rules, By-Laws and Regulations* were being published in revised form and in both languages. The object of the association was identified as being "to promote the interests of Radiology with special reference to the following aspects:

1—Clinical
2—Educational
3—Ethical
4—Economic.

Membership was classified as follows:

- Members: "(E)ngaged exclusively in the practice or study of Radiology in one or more of its branches...for a period of not less than five years."
- Members-elect: "Radiologists as described above of less than five years standing."
- Associate Members: "Medical practitioners duly registered in a Province of the Dominion of Canada, who are engaged in the practice of Radiology in one or more of its branches...who are not engaged exclusively in such practice, but who practise Radiology as the major part of their medical work...."
- Honorary: "(D)istinguished persons who have rendered services to radiology...."

It appears that this classification of members was based on one then in use in Great Britain. It is also stated that "If and when there is established a Canadian Board of Radiology, the examination of such a Board shall be the examination requirement for full membership...."

A published list of officers and members from 1939 lists the president as Dr JE Gendreau of Montréal, the vice-president as Dr WH McGuffin of Calgary, and the honorary secretary-treasurer as Dr AC Singleton of Toronto. Perhaps the most striking difference from 1995 is that there were then only three chairs of standing committees: Education and Qualification (Dr CW Prowd, Vancouver), Inter-relations (Dr WA Jones, Kingston), and Legislation and By-Laws (Dr AS Kirkland, Saint John, New Brunswick). Councillors had been appointed in Alberta, British Columbia, Manitoba, New Brunswick, Nova Scotia, Ontario (central, eastern, northern and western), Québec (English and French speaking Montréal, and Québec exclusive of Montréal), and Saskatchewan. There were three honorary members in the persons of Drs Léo Pariseau and A Howard Pirie (both from Québec) and Dr HM Tovell of Toronto. There were 102 full members of the association, 19 members-elect, and four associate members. One member had died in the previous year. Names of other members that are still fresh in memory included Drs Arthur Childe, Origène Dufresne, Albert Jutras, R Miller-Tait, W Ritchie and Arthur Singleton.

The initial pattern of annual meetings seems to have been a mid-winter meeting combining business and science, and a summer meeting in conjunction with the CMA annual meeting. However, in 1939 there were separate meetings, east and west. The latter took place in March in the Palliser Hotel and the Calgary General and Holy Cross hospitals. Dr Marshall Mallett reported a patient with Sudeck's atrophy, and Dr R Michaud described arthrokatadysis (a term which appears not to have survived into modern medicine), as well as films of Marie-Strumpell's disease.

Dr R Proctor discussed "The Situation with Regard to the X-ray in the Small Hospitals," a topic suggesting that some issues are perennial ones. This conclusion is reinforced by the fact that the dinner speaker was Mr Campbell McLaurin, KC, discussing "The Doctor in Court." On the lighter side, Dr and Mrs McGuffin entertained registrants at their home, while the annual dinner menu on the next evening lists fresh fruit supreme, essence of tomato au sherry, grilled chicken, ham and mushrooms with vegetables, a salad, and peach Melba.

The program records the presence of representatives in Canada of the Victoreen X-ray Corporation of Canada acting for General Electric and other electro-medical equipment suppliers. There is the promise that the Victor representative in one's area will "prove to be a worthy friend."

By the time of the midwinter session of January 1939 the current logo of the association was in use. That meeting was held in Kingston, Ontario, and the program was printed by courtesy of Dupont X-ray Film which was then, it appears, sold by Canadian Industries Ltd. The program was bilingual and so have been the affairs and activities of the association throughout its history. Perhaps that practice is why CAR has a better record of harmony between those from the founding nations than does its parent country. Canada as a whole was slower to embrace bilingualism.

Of sixteen presentations in 1939, ten concerned diagnosis and only one of these presentations was in the case-report format. Dr AB MacDonnell of Sarnia described patients with osteomyelitis of the skull and carcinoma of the jejunum. An invited speaker, Dr GB Lane of Timmins, spoke about tuberculosis in a mining town.

Some of the papers would not be out of place in 1995. Osteochondritis dissecans was discussed by Dr RC Burr of Kingston (later a president of the association), but I wish I could have also heard Dr WM Gilmore's talk entitled "The Horse and Buggy Radiologist." A paper on "The Application of a Method for Periodic Regeneration of Developer" by Dr Jean Bouchard of Québec suggests an early awareness of the need for economies.

The discussion of "A Preliminary Report Upon the Action of X-rays in Fractional Dosage on Staphlococci" by Drs WA Jones, GB Reed, JH Carr and Mr G Fiddes seems to be early evidence of a concern with basic science. However, it may have been a study less motivated by radiobiology than by the control of infectious disease because, in that pre-antibiotic era, there were reports on "X-ray Therapy for the Treatment of Acute Pneumonia" (Dr WR Scott, of Niagara Falls in both Canada and the US) and "A Few Considerations on the Actions of X-rays on Acute Infections" (Dr CG Campbell, Kingston). Dr Scott, who seems by implication to have practiced on both sides of the border at the same time, may have been the first United States registrant at a Canadian Association of Radiologists meeting. A paper on the "Treatment of Asthmatics by Roentgen Rays" (Dr R Veilleux, Trois Rivières) was the only other presentation that might be out of place in a modern session.

The predominance of local contributions to the meeting reflects, no doubt, the difficulties of travel in that era. There was a dinner and, on the final day, afternoon tea at the residence of Dr WA Jones who had just led a discussion of "Some of the Educational and Economic Problems of Radiology."

The eastern Canada midwinter session in 1940 was

held in Québec City on January 6, 7 and 8. There is no hint from the program to reflect those troubled times except one presentation by Dr E Perron (Québec) on "War Time Radiology."

The program was also completely bilingual and apparently printed by courtesy of Eastman, the Canadian Kodak Co Ltd. This program largely went beyond case reports although there was one paper by Dr MC Morrison of London on "Primary Tumours of Bone" which used "lantern slides." Of ten papers, eight addressed radio-diagnosis and only two treatment. Many of the titles might easily transpose into a contemporary program although the technologies used were no doubt separated from the present by an even greater distance than that between lantern slides and dual projection with video displays in a present-day lecture hall. Besides the papers alluded to, the program also included "Gall Stones and Medication" (Dr WL Minto, Montréal) "Controlled Compression in Stomach Exploration" (Dr A Jutras, Montréal) "Osteochondritis Dissecans" (Dr H Lachavite, Montréal) and "Treatment of Carcinoma of the Tongue" (Dr GE Richards, Toronto). There was a lively social program with two formal dinners, a lunch at Hôtel Dieu and a brief, final consideration of "professional matters." How times change. All registrants became members of the Québec Garrison Club for the duration of the meeting.

By 1943 CAR had published "Minimum acceptable standards for hospital radiologic departments or laboratories."[5] A membership list for the association was published in January 1945. It contains 148 members. By 1952 the membership had increased to 297 radiologists.

In 1948 the national headquarters of CAR was established in Montréal and the association incorporated. By 1959 there were 516 members in all categories and by 1968, 733. In 1950 the *Journal* had come into being (its evolution is documented elsewhere in this volume). The *Journal's* first editor was Dr JW McKay, who later also served as a president of the association.

In January 1948 the midwinter meeting was held in Kingston. It included one paper, subsequently published,[6] on the "Roentgentherapy of Pain." Dealing with the treatment of a wide variety of diseases, not only cancer, the paper brings to light one of the few examples of a major change in the way we practice, leaving aside the present schism between diagnostic radiologists and radiation oncologists.

The first women members of CAR were Drs Christina Fraser (Vancouver General Hospital), Helen Milburn (Women's College Hospital, Toronto), Elizabeth Stewart (Toronto) and Ethlyn Trapp (Vancouver), whose names appear on the 1937 membership roll. There is a note in the records, but no verification, that the first woman admitted to CAR was Dr Trapp. Another early member was Dr Vera Peters of Toronto, who was to achieve an international reputation as a radiation oncologist, particularly for her innovative work regarding the staging of lymphomas and treatment of breast cancer. However, in that era of suffragettes and the beginnings of the movement leading to political equality for women, the issue seems to have occasioned little comment and no debate. Nevertheless, it was to be another 56 years before a woman president of CAR was elected, in the person of Dr Stephanie Wilson. Photographs and records of council in the interval indicate that, despite the lack of overt sexism, CAR was a bastion of maleness, also apparent from the minutes of the first meeting of the association, which are appended.

THE ROLE OF CAR IN THE EMERGENCE OF SPECIALTY CERTIFICATION

Dr David Shephard, in a study of the development of the Royal College of Physicians and Surgeons of Canada, notes that "[t]he Canadian quest, par excellence, is unity" and that the college is a microcosm of the nation. One early crisis in the affairs of the college was the threat of physicians and surgeons to form two separate colleges.[7]

No sooner had this possibility been averted than a second crisis arose concerning the need to certify and, by implication, recognize specialists:

> *In the early 1930s Canadian radiologists expressed concern that no organization in Canada served their needs for a body that would lay down training requirements for, and examine and certify in, radiology. (At this time the College emphasized a broad education in medicine or surgery as the basis for specialist practice rather than a narrower training in a specific specialty such as radiology.) The College had, in fact, been engaged in discussions with the Canadian Medical Association (CMA) concerning a certification program, but progress was slow. The radiologists, impatient at an apparent impasse, threatened to establish their own college, and other specialties considered seeking specialty recognition by way of joining American specialty boards. The danger of separation was real and the College, as a result accelerated planning of the certification program.*[7]

In the minutes of CAR it is clear that what motivated the radiologists of that era to advocate specialty certification was a concern with standards of practice, as well as a need to maintain symmetry with postgraduate educational practices in Great Britain and the United States.

It is equally clear that CAR became the vehicle for these negotiations:

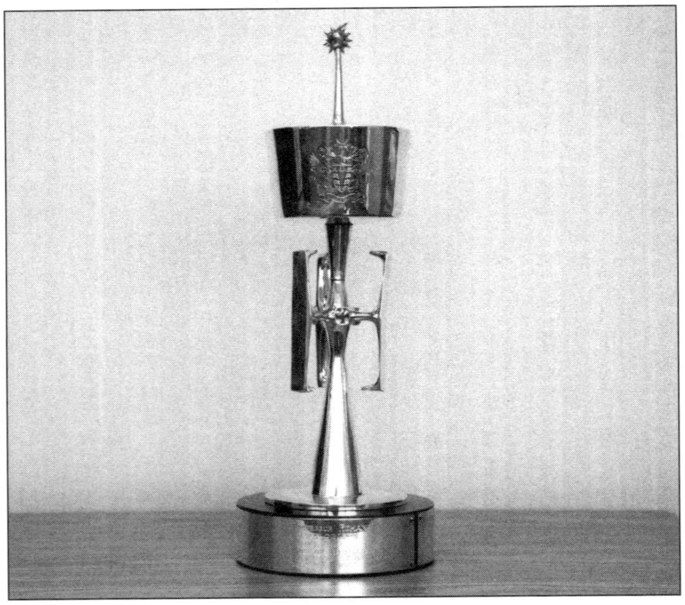

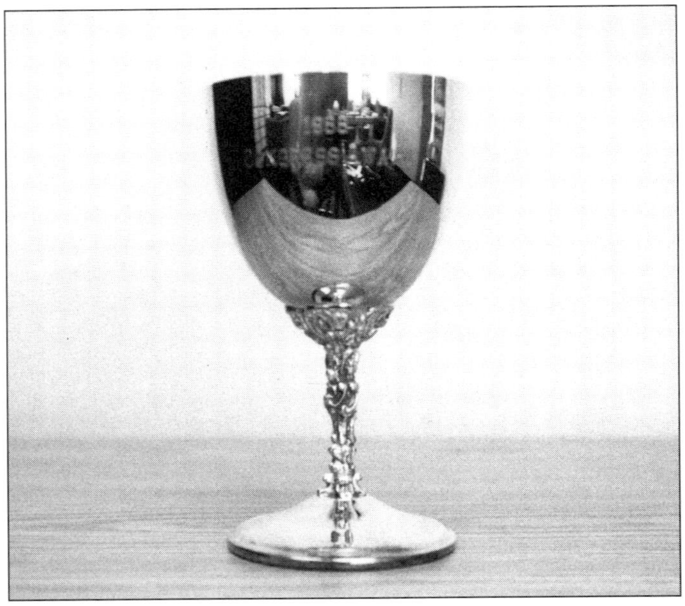

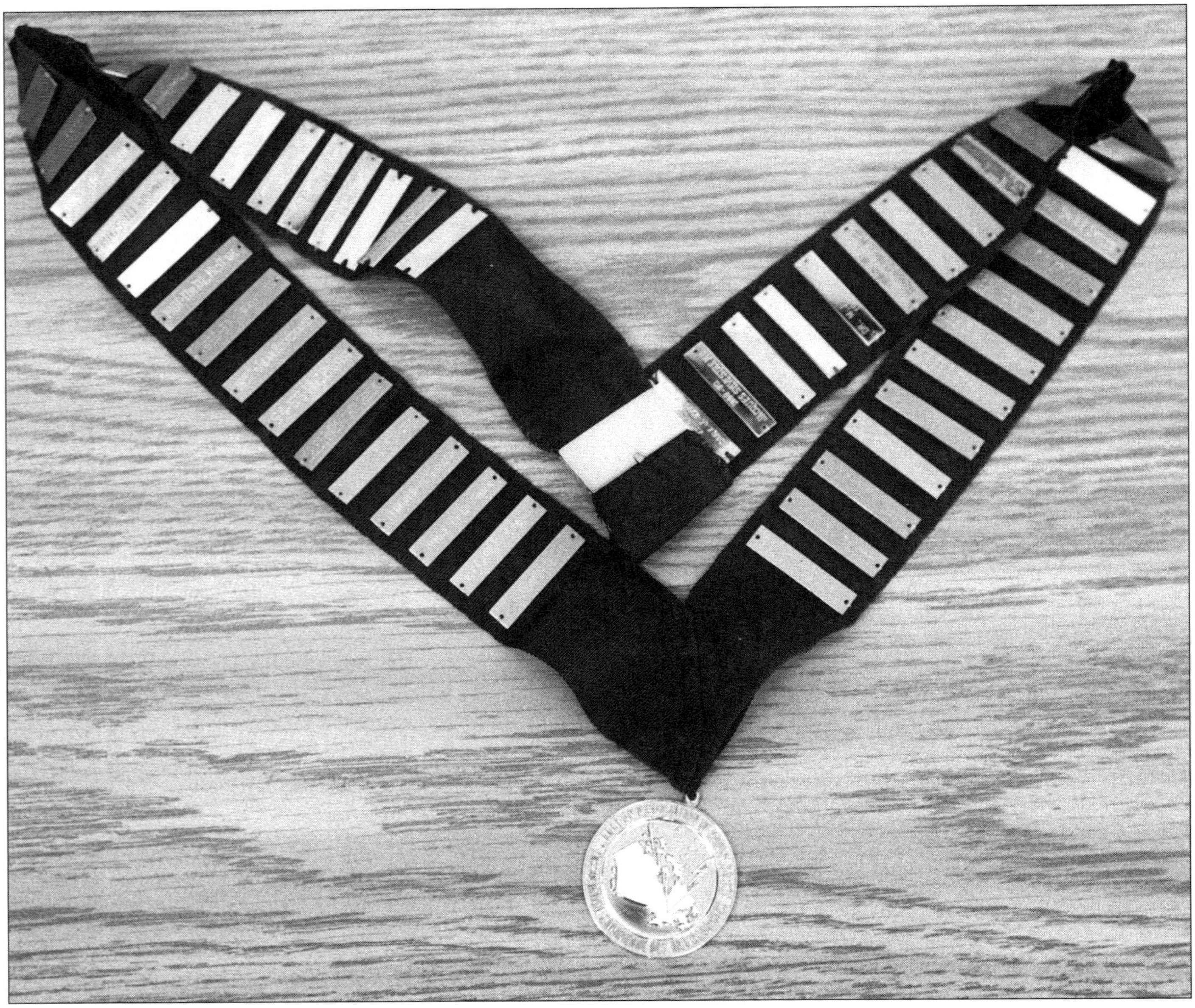

1895 - 1995

ROENTGEN

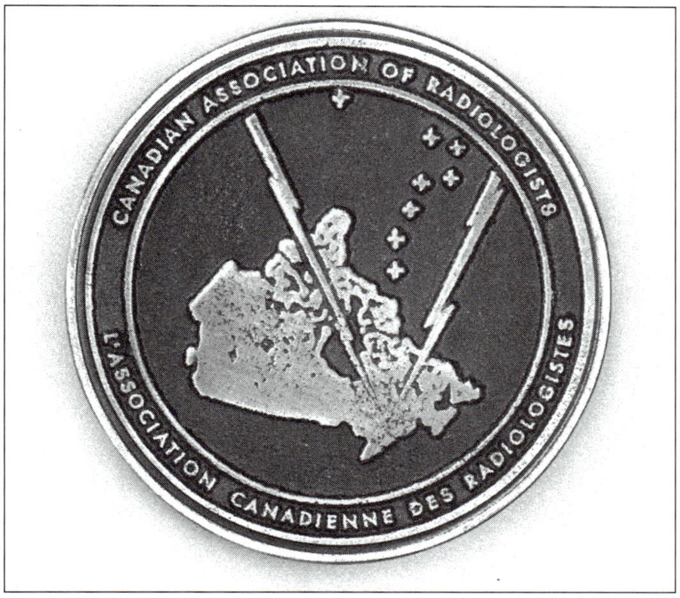

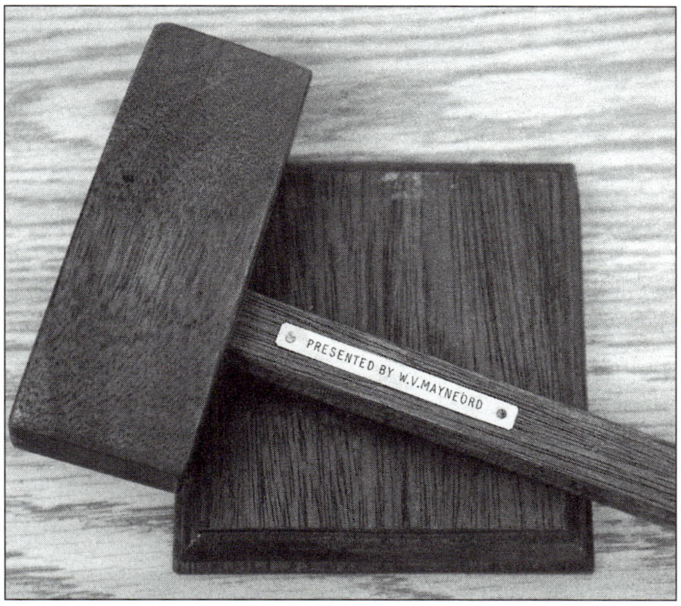

Opposite left
Loving Cup of the Canadian Association of Radiologists

Opposite right
Canadian Association of Radiologists—Congress Award Cup

Opposite below
Canadian Association of Radiologists—Presidential Collar

Left
Canadian Association of Radiologists—centennial logo

Left middle
Canadian Association of Radiologists' medal

Left bottom
Canadian Association of Radiologists—gavel and block presented by Professor WV Mayneord

It was now June 1936...and five years since the CMA's Section of Radiology had initiated a movement to establish a Canadian college of radiology. The radiologists were impatient: in Britain, standards of training for radiology were controlled by radiologists and in the United States, the independent Board of Radiology exerted similar control; but in Canada the CMA's discussions were stalled in an "impasse" and the Royal College offered "no standard of training nor examination [to] guide the candidate educationally or designate him as a radiologist.[7]

The sexist use of "him" is forgiveable since the first women members of CAR had not then joined.

The Canadian radiologists, who felt a need at that time to protect their interests and those of the public should a health insurance scheme be introduced into Canada, therefore resolved to press ahead with their plan to establish their own college. Dr. W. A. Jones, President of the Canadian Association of Radiologists, however, left room for negotiation. He reassured Dr. A.T. Bazin, President of the College, that, if the College's Committee on Specialists or the College itself could offer an alternative scheme that would meet the situation, the members of the Section of Radiology would be agreeable to work within that scheme.

The radiologists' action produced the desired effect. Neither for the first nor for the last time in its history, the College now hurriedly pursued the cause of unity. Dr. D. Graham, chairman of the College's Committee on Specialists, urged "prompt action" and recommended that the College take on the responsibility for certifying specialists.[8]

Dr WA Jones was the first president of CAR, and his wisdom, statesmanship and foresight are very evident in his handling of this and other matters. Needless to say, the college accepted the recommendation of its committee and the certification program was introduced in 1942; the first certification examinations were held in September and October 1946.

These events are also summarized by Dr HE MacDermot in *One Hundred Years of Medicine in Canada* as follows:

In 1937, after considerable discussion, the C.M.A. officially invited the Royal College to take over the certification of specialists in Canada. This move was precipitated by signs of unrest among the specialists, beginning with the Canadian Association of Radiologists. This body announced its intention to set up an independent College of Radiology to protect its own interests and those of the public unless the C.M.A. did something to settle the matter.[9]

Dr Jones' concern for consensus building is expressed in his three-page letter to all members of CAR, dated April 11, 1939. The letter (reproduced in full as Annex B) remains a penetrating analysis of the issues faced at that time, and it is of particular historical relevance since CAR served as a prime mover in the introduction of specialty certification in Canada.

However, by 1958 CAR was fighting a rearguard action in the Royal College in the debate following the recommendations of the Botterell committee. At that time there was a double standard for specialists consisting of certification and fellowship examinations. CAR briefly resisted this, arguing that "the Certification program was necessary in order to meet the country's need for radiologists."[10] In 1972 a single examination to assess specialist competence was introduced, and few would argue, from the perspective of over 20 years later that the result has been anything but positive both for Canadian medicine and the college.

The first examination papers for the specialist certificate in diagnostic radiology that I have found date from a year later, with the examination held on October 27 and 28, 1947. The papers read as follows:

Paper No. 1
THE PRINCIPLES AND PRACTICE OF DIAGNOSTIC RADIOLOGY

(Three hour paper—all questions of equal value)

1. Discuss the radiologic diagnosis of renal tuberculosis, including a consideration of the comparative value of excretory and retrograde pyelography.

2. A patient presents a tender mass in the right upper quadrant (of the abdomen). Discuss the diagnostic information which may be gained by means of the various Roentgenologic investigation measures which may be employed.

3. Discuss the Roentgenologic characteristics of bronchogenic carcinoma and the methods which may be used in a Roentgenologic investigation to establish the diagnosis.

4. Discuss the differential diagnosis of metastatic prostatic carcinoma, osteitis fibrosa deformans (Paget), polyostotic fibrous dysplasia.

Paper No. 2
THE APPLICATION OF THE BASIC SCIENCES NECESSARY TO THE PROPER UNDERSTANDING OF DIAGNOSTIC RADIOLOGY

(Three hour paper—all questions of equal value)

1. Compare the physical characteristics and the biologic effects of x-rays with those of the radiations from radon.

2. Using diagrams for illustration, discuss the anatomy of the lower respiratory tract with special reference to the pulmonary segments, showing by outline or diagram the

nomenclature you prefer for the bronchial tree.
3. Discuss the various functions of the liver, with particular attention to those that are radiologically important.
4. Describe the anatomic features of the temporal bone, and the various methods which must be used for proper roentgenologic examination of its various parts in disease.

A present-day candidate—if multiple choice questioning has not atrophied his or her ability to write essay-style answers—might well find that examination a leisurely exercise. Clearly, "discuss" meant just that, not list. It is unlikely that a modern candidate would know, however, the various projections which seem to be required to describe a radiographic examination of the temporal bone in that era (paper 2, question 4). In general it might be said that in 50 years technology seems to have changed far more quickly than the clinical problems it is used to solve.

MILITARY SERVICE

Dr Arthur Singleton provides some insight into the difficulties caused by World War II in his letter of September 6, addressed to Dr William A Jones at the Kingston General Hospital:

Dear Jones:
How are you getting on with the Medical Boarding, or are you still in that delightful occupation? I am writing to let you know that I have joined the Canadian Active Service Force in the capacity of radiologist to #15 Canadian General Hospital. This of course will necessitate my resignation as Secretary to the Canadian Association of Radiologists, and I have this morning written Gendreau to that effect. In my letter to him I stated that a new secretary should be appointed immediately, and that in my opinion the man should be of sufficient age or physically disabled to the point where he will not be liable for military service in order that our records may be kept complete and up-to-date, and that continuity may be maintained in the Association in spite of this bloody upheaval in Europe.
Drop me a line when you get a chance.
Yours sincerely,
(signed)
(Dr) Arthur Singleton

Medical Boarding was the examination of potential recruits to the armed forces. Dr Jones replied on September 11, 1939 as follows:

Dear Singleton:—
So, my son, you have beaten me to it and got yourself hooked up with the CASF [Canadian Active Service Force] ahead of me. Here I am still on Medical Boards and you've got into the the Active Service Force. However, I may beat you to it yet. I am wanting command of a Field Ambulance. Did you suggest any name to Gendreau as your possible successor? Is there anyone in Toronto medically unfit who could do the job properly?
Bless you my child and damn your hide.
Cordially yours,
(signed)
(Dr) WA Jones

Ten days later Dr Jones was writing a two-page letter, as Chairman of the Inter-relations Committee of CAR, in a more serious vein and addressed to Dr Gendreau. Part of the letter reads as follows:

The Department of Pensions and National Health have [sic] written to the hospitals asking them to do x-ray films of recruits' chests at fees ranging from $1.00 to $2.00. They emphasize the fact that they do not wish interpretation and simply want the films put away as a matter of record. The whole affair is so foreign to our way of doing things that I am sure the radiologists all over Canada are in rebellion at the moment…

A total of 89 radiologists from Canada served in the Royal Canadian Military Corps during this war, a number which included:

Dr Jean Bouchard	Montréal
Dr RW Boyd	Vancouver
Dr AE Childe	Winnipeg
Dr HE Duggan	Edmonton
Dr A Maxwell Evans	Vancouver
Dr DG Florendine	Calgary
Dr LR Harnick	Toronto
Dr RB Holmes	London
Dr Jean Pierre Jean	Montréal
Dr WA Jones	Kingston
Dr DL McRae	Montréal
Dr WB Parsons	Red Deer
Dr AC Singleton	Toronto
Dr KD Symington	Calgary
Dr GE Trueman	Kamloops

As might be anticipated from the accomplishments of such people, the war years were not idle times. Dr Jones sent out a questionnaire in September 1939 to 123 radiologists. Of the 81 who replied, 30 were serving abroad, six in Canada, 43 were still in practice in their home city and the balance had been found unfit.

At a 1940 meeting military radiologists decided to offer special radiological education for medical officers, amounting to 16 weeks of formal instruction followed by practical experience in hospitals. At least three Canadian radiologists used their time while stationed in Britain to obtain diplomas in Medical Radiodiagnosis (Drs HM Edmison, AE Turnbull and JA Ireland). The indefatigable

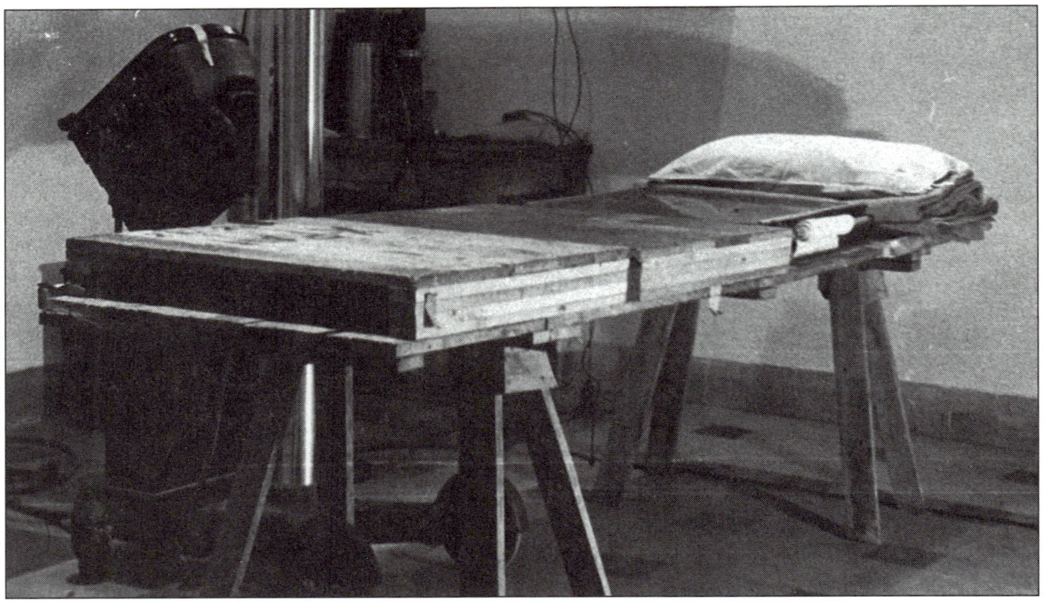

Radiographic table in a Canadian military hospital under canvas, Normandy, 1945

Colonel (Dr) WA Jones also arranged for an educational program for radiographers.

A scientific group (The Canadian Radiologists Overseas Group) also came into being and was chaired at various times by Drs Arthur Singleton, J Gosselin, D Eaglesham and Hector Duggan. The minutes record up to 17 attendees, with guest speakers such as Drs JF Brailsford, Peter Kerley and AE Barclay, and Miss KC (Kitty) Clark addressing the group. All are names still to be reckoned with in the annals of radiology. Scientific papers on military radiology during the war were contributed by Drs FH Bonnell, RW Boyd, AE Broome, HE Duggan, PP Hauch, WA Jones, RF Keevil, WB Parsons, AC Singleton, RL Smith, OT Steen and FG Stuart.[1]

While the spirit of CAR transplanted itself to Europe, these were difficult times for organized radiology. Of the 89 radiologists who served in the war only 27 had been discharged by October 1, 1945, and one had died while on active service.[1]

INTERNATIONAL RELATIONS

From the earliest times, and antedating CAR, Canadian radiologists have played a role in continental organizations. Dr GP Girdwood (1832–1917) of Montréal, referred to elsewhere in this volume as the father of radiology in Canada, was a founding member of the American Roentgen Ray Society (ARRS) and served as its president in 1902. He was mentor to Dr Howard Pirie, who also served as president of the ARRS in 1927. Dr Girdwood had been in the audience when Professor Owen Cox (1851–1923) showed the first clinical radiograph made in Canada in Montréal on February 8, 1896. He was to become the first radiologist at the Montréal General Hospital.

Dr William Henry Aikins had graduated from the University of Toronto in 1918, and he was for many years physician-in-chief at the Toronto General Hospital. The American Radium Society was founded in 1916, and he was appointed first president.

A page from the *Journal of the Canadian Association of Radiologists* in 1950 carries the following note:

> *MEETING OF EMPIRE RADIOLOGISTS WITH MEMBERS OF THE EXECUTIVE OF THE FACULTY OF RADIOLOGISTS*
>
> *June 29th, 1950*
>
> *On the Saturday following the Congress (International Congress of Radiology) there was held at the Faculty of Radiologists a meeting of Empire Radiologists with members of the Executive of the Faculty. There were in attendance, representing the Faculty, Professor B.W. Windeyer, the President of the Faculty, Dr. C.G. Teall, Dr. S. Cochrane Shanks and Dr. J.W. McLaren, all from the Faculty of Radiologists; from Australia—Drs. John O'Sullivan, D.G. Maitland and T.L. Tyrer; from Canada—Drs. A.C. Singleton, E.M. Crawford, O. Dufresne and Digby Wheeler; from New Zealand—Dr. R.E. Marshall; and from South Africa—Dr. S.F. Oosthuizen.*
>
> *It was the unanimous feeling of all present that some form of Empire liaison was most highly desirable. After very frank discussion it became clear that there was a very general desire for some form of link with the Faculty of Radiologists on the part of all overseas societies and it was felt that the* Journal *offered possibly the most suitable means. The suggestion was made that one number per year might be taken for papers by Canadian or Australian Radiologists or that an overseas number should be issued periodically…*

It is easy to be sceptical about the vision of "Empire"

then held, as well as of the faintly patronizing nature of the debate and the inability of the British of that era to adjust to their post-war status as a reduced world power. Nevertheless, credit must be given to those from Canada who were concerned that isolation must be avoided and standards measured in an international context. The reality, of course, has been that the US emerged from World War II as one of two super-powers, and, increasingly since then, Canadian radiology and radiologists have looked south as much as across the Atlantic Ocean for academic and political cross-fertilization. No doubt a large factor in this has been that Canadians were very much more seen as equals within organizations such as the Radiological Society of North America (RSNA). Indeed, Canadian radiologists have held many offices in such organizations: in recent years for example Dr Carl Zylak and Dr Douglas MacEwan have served as Presidents of RSNA, as well as of CAR at different times, and Dr David Fraser stands poised to so serve. Dr Arthur Singleton served as president of the American College of Radiology.

By August 1962 CAR found itself hosting the Tenth International Congress of Radiology in Montréal under the presidency of Dr Arthur Singleton. In a precedent taken up at the World Federation of Nuclear Medicine meeting in the same city in 1986, the events included an orchestral performance. The Montréal Pops Orchestra played the overture to *La Forza del Destino* by Verdi, Tchaikovsky's fantasy overture *Romeo and Juliet* and, after the interval, Sibelius' tone poem *Finlandia* and the overture to *Tannhauser* by Wagner. In between, Pierette Alarie sang arias from Mozart's *The Marriage of Figaro*, Donizetti's *Don Pasquale* and *Lakmé* by Delibes. The evening was sponsored by Atomic Energy of Canada Ltd, Dupont of Canada Ltd, General Electric X-Ray Corporation Ltd and Picker X-Ray Engineering Ltd, as these corporations were then known.

Fifty-five countries were represented at the Congress. "Essayists" (those presenting papers) came from 40 of these, with the largest numbers coming from the United States (175), Great Britain (60), and Germany (58) (no distinction seems to have been made between east and west in a country that was then divided). Canada had 51 speakers, but radiologists coming from as far afield as Argentina, India, Israel, Japan, Peru, Turkey, the USSR and Yugoslavia must have created a truly international sense. At this meeting the distinguished Canadian radiologist Dr Arthur Singleton received the American College of Radiology Gold Medal.[11]

CAR, through its representatives to the International Society of Radiology (ISR), has continued to play a role in world radiological affairs. Dr Peter Cockshott, in particular, had been a great servant of radiology in the developing nations before his untimely death in 1993. In articles and monographs he advanced knowledge of the radiological manifestations of tropical illnesses, and he contributed much to the development of a standard and easily serviced unit and darkroom for radiography in parts of the world where the infrastructure of power and running water is still being developed. Dr Joachim Burhenne has served on the scientific program of ISR, leading the transition of ISR meetings from conventional scientific forums into a means for continuing education in the less-well-developed nations.

ARTEFACTS

The medal of the Canadian Association of Radiologists, given to each person who delivers one of the major addresses at each annual meeting, is of a design already in use by 1939. It appears on the cover of the "Eastern Canada Mid-Winter Session" for that year. There is no record to indicate by whom it was designed, but it may be the work or inspiration of Dr Arthur Singleton, as will be apparent from what follows.

At the annual general meeting in Saskatoon in the summer of 1949 an idea and design for the presidential pendant and collar were offered by Dr Singleton and warmly received. He made the official presentation in both official languages to the Association in Montréal on Wednesday, January 4, 1950. A copy of the text of his speech survives and reads in part:

> *[I] see a number of the faces of those who were present at the organizational meeting of this Association, which was called at the instigation of the late Dr Richards and held in Toronto about this time of the year in 1937. I also see to-night many new faces and each year adds its number of new keen, younger men entering our specialty. It is a great pleasure to meet these men at our Annual and Mid-Winter Meetings. At the end of the first year the Canadian Association of Radiologists boasted almost one hundred members. Our Honorary Secretary-Treasurer tells me we now have in the neighbourhood of two hundred and forty, a very healthy growth.*
>
> *It has become a custom in this country that civic governmental bodies, scientific organizations and other established institutions have a Presidential Collar or other badge of office of President. This is not only a Canadian custom but is one which we have inherited from Britain, France and other European countries. It seemed to me that we had now become sufficiently grown up that such a collar of office was indicated.*
>
> *The Collar is of royal blue ribbon, carrying a medallion on*

which is inscribed the crest of our Association, with the map of our country including our latest and tenth province, Newfoundland, the lightning rays striking our Capital City, Ottawa, the North Star and the Great Dipper and bearing the inscription: "The Canadian Association of Radiologists —l'Association Canadienne des Radiologistes." On the ribbon are mounted bars on which are engraved the names of the Past Presidents of this Organization...
J'espère qu'il servira à trois fins: primo, à rehausser la dignité du poste de président; secundo, à raviver le souvenir de présidents eminents qui ne sont plus parmi nous et enfin—l'inscription étant en français et en anglais—à symbolisier cette amitié et cette comprehension qui ont été et qui sont une charactéristique si agréable de notre société. Il semble approprié que cette présentation se fasse à Montréal ou, depuis des années, existe une étroite coopération entre les radiologistes de langue française et leur collègues de langue anglaise.

A cup was given to the Canadian Association of Radiologists by the Faculty of Radiologists in 1962. It is used at each annual dinner, where traditionally, the incoming and outgoing presidents share a sip of some potent brew before the cup is passed from hand to hand. It carries the following inscription:

Presented to the Canadian Association of Radiologists by the Faculty of Radiologists 1962
This "Calix of Friendship" was presented by Professor Rohan Williams, President of the Faculty of Radiologists, and accepted by Dr Guillaume Gill, President of the Canadian Association of Radiologists, on the occasion of the Tenth International Congress of Radiology. Montréal, Quebec. August 29, 1962.

THE MODERN ERA

Perhaps one of the most decisive events in the recent history of CAR was the decision by the radiation oncologists in the mid–1980s to separate from the organization and form their own. The minutes of the meeting of the Executive Committee of CAR held at the 1986 annual meeting record that a letter from Dr David McGowan had been received in which he pointed out that there was a strong feeling among radiation oncologists that they should form their own political organization. It was proposed that independent organization (Canadian Association of Radiation Oncologists, or CARO), might meet with other oncologic specialties at the Royal College annual meeting. This separation did indeed take place in June 1986. Although clearly foreseen and perhaps inevitable, this parting of two groups with origins in common substantially reduced the size of the Association and the scope of its scientific meetings. A few radiation oncologists did maintain dual membership in CAR and CARO. Nevertheless, the oncologists saw a need both for an identity of their own and the opportunity to make linkages with other groups with whom they had an obvious affinity, such as the medical oncologists. Dr George Goodman had the distinction of being the last radiation oncologist to serve as president of CAR. He served with characteristic energy and insight, particularly in urging a national confederation of specialists in the radiological and imaging sciences. This idea is perhaps only now coming to be seen as possible, and in a sense will be realized with the multidisciplinary celebrations of the Röntgen Centennial in Montréal in 1995. Ironically, radiation oncology will be absent from this largest meeting ever of the radiation-related technologies and specialties.

After the separation of the radiation oncologists, CAR needed to reconsider its role and how it might best serve its members. The council had become very large and unwieldy and its midwinter meetings expensive, despite its members only being reimbursed for economy air travel and not accommodation. Cash reserves were shrinking, and common—if unsubstantiated—allegations were heard that CAR had become "an old-boys' club;" that it was an organization which was slow to respond and which did little for its general membership. Certainly, a shrinking fraction of Canada's radiologists were members. In this circumstance an *ad hoc* committee chaired by Dr JB Sutherland was created to re-examine CAR operations. As a direct result, a further *ad hoc* committee consisting of Drs Robert Campbell, Jean-Marc Dumas, and Keith Sparrow and chaired by Dr Donald Newman was asked to review the administrative structure of CAR. It reported to Council and the annual meeting of CAR in Québec City in October 1989. This committee recommended that:

Our Association requires structural re-organization at a "grass roots" level to ensure (that) the national body for radiology responds flexibly, quickly, and intelligently to our provincial and national educational, economic, medical, and political problems;
(that) [T]he affairs of the Association be conducted by "grass roots," elected division Councillors and [that this] ensures the elected Councillors always hold the balance of power in Council;
(that) Council becomes the governing body of the Association and the Annual Meeting of the Association a vehicle for information and discussion only.

Just when CAR lost most of the radiation oncologists who were members, *Journal* advertising revenue faltered

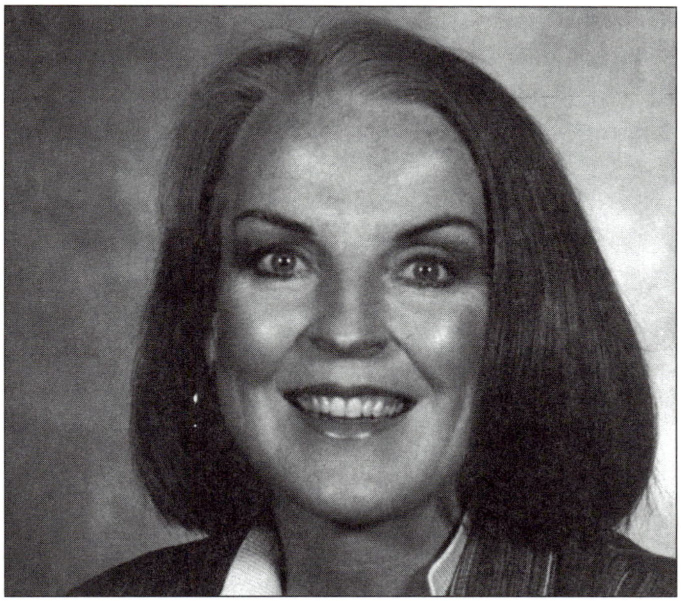

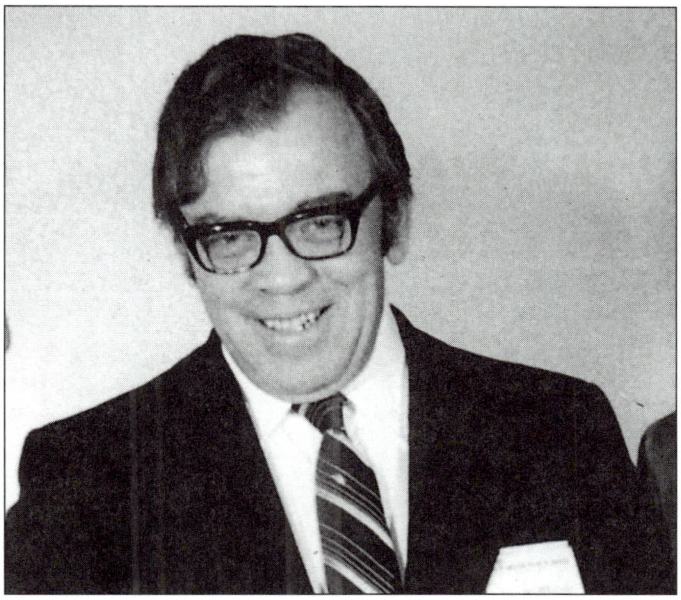

Above
Dr Stephanie Wilson, first woman president, Canadian Association of Radiologists

Right
Dr Ross Hill, former president of the CAR and moving force behind the creation of the Canadian Radiological Foundation.

with the economic down turn, and universities and hospitals, with their own fiscal woes, could no longer subsidize the editor and provide him or her with secretarial support. The *Journal* thus needed a greater fraction of the dues, to provide for payment of an honorarium to the editor and purchase of secretarial help. To its credit, Council considered but quickly and unanimously rejected discontinuing publication of the *Journal*.

The Sutherland–Newman reports were instrumental in effecting change within CAR. Their findings were widely accepted, and their recommendations implemented. The result was a streamlined council, a new approach to annual meetings and a number of comparable initiatives. Provincial councillors became represented on the executive committee of CAR by their chairman.

After many years of loyal and distinguished service to the association as its executive director, Ms Alva Pentecost retired in March 1989. In her place Ms Suzanne Charette was appointed in April 1989. Ms Charette has brought her own strengths to the association, including sound financial management, fluent bilingualism and a keen political sensibility. After many years at a classy Rue Sherbrooke address, the association's head office was moved to less expensive but equally commodious office space outside of downtown Montréal.

By 1994 membership in the association in all categories numbered 1255, and a surplus in excess of a year's budgeted spending meant that CAR was in a much sounder business position. However, it is ironic to observe that 1800 Canadians were by then members of the Chicago-based Radiological Society of North America (RSNA), while the total number of practicing radiologists in Canada was approximately 2000.

The association has been fortunate in its recent presidents who have left a legacy of initiatives to increase the relevance of CAR to modern medicine. Examples are Drs Guy Hébert, Barry Hobbs and Stephanie Wilson in pressing for CAR to develop positions on a variety of relevant issues, to embark upon guideline development and to redefine the format for Annual Meetings of the Association.

THE CANADIAN RADIOLOGICAL FOUNDATION

The first initiative, which in due course led to the establishment of this foundation was a bequest to CAR from Dr Carleton Pierce, formerly professor and chairman of radiology at McGill University, in the late 1970s. However, the force behind the realization of the foundation was Dr Ross Hill, whose efforts were the culmination of his contributions to the association as he stepped down from its presidency.

Dr Hill worked over several years to create the foundation and secure its tax-exempt status with Revenue Canada. The foundation was formally endorsed by a unanimous vote at the June 1981 annual general meeting of CAR.

The goals of the foundation have been to advance the art and science of radiology by education and research. The founding board of directors was chaired by then president of CAR Dr Bernard Reilly of Toronto. Dr Max Palayew served as chair of the Scientific Advisory Committee. A fund raising committee was to have been chaired by Mr Leslie Withers of Picker Canada whose untimely death prevented this further contribution to the national scene. Despite the lack of sustained fund raising activity outside CAR, individual radiologists have been generous: by the end of 1992 the foundation had raised $375 000, of which 80 per cent had been given by individual radiologists, including substantial donations from the President's Club, (comprised of ex-presidents) which was organized by Dr Ted Lansdown.

Beginning in 1986 the foundation has provided an annual fellowship for a young Canadian radiologist. The other objectives remain to endow research fellowships, bursaries for practicing radiologists and grants-in-aid awarded in peer-reviewed competition.

Much remains to be done, and the principle available for generating revenue from interest needs to be substantially increased. Nevertheless, those who have put the foundation in place have established a strong platform on which to build. It will almost certainly be seen as an important step in the association's coming-of-age as the years unfold into the second century of radiology.[12]

A PERSPECTIVE

It is always tempting to see the past as peopled by giants. Certainly CAR had its share of giants in the early years of its existence. While Dr David Fraser, who is very much of the present, is of a height which might have qualified him for a handsome basketball contract, he has been a giant of that other kind in his service on behalf of both CAR and RSNA. CAR's giants have been radiologists who were sensitive not only to the needs of their specialty but also to the greater perspective of medicine in Canada. It is instructive to remember that not only was the Canadian Association of Radiologists a prime mover in the introduction of specialty certification in Canada, but it also sponsored the first Canadian specialty journal, a record of which the association can be justifiably proud.

CAR, like many such organizations throughout medicine, is having to redefine itself in terms of the political challenges faced in 1995. Such change comes at a time when individual incomes shrink and physicians no longer belong and subscribe to specialty associations almost reflexively. To be sure, values have also changed, so it sometimes seems that the insistent question "What does CAR do for me?" will drown out the quiet dedication of physicians such as Dr David Gray, working in an unsung and unheralded way over many years to further the affairs of the association and his colleagues. CAR has a long record of contributions to Canadian medicine, to radiological education and to professional governance. These are accomplishments of the past, but they serve as the foundation for the present and future. Perhaps revisiting the history of the association and the role of those who have forged the specialty and contributed to the national scene will go some way to address the future relevance of CAR. History, after all, is of greatest interest and importance not in looking backward but when it serves as a beacon to guide our journey into the future.

Acknowledgement:
I am grateful to Dr Stuart Houston for constructive criticism.

Chapter III •

The Canadian Association of Medical Radiation Technologists:

Historical Aspects

Ron Wood and Brian Lentle, after Sister Mary DeLellis Crowley

INTRODUCTION

Very often technologists provide the important link between doctor and patient in a radiological service. Technologists have not been slow to recognize the advantages of a national association and have led physicians in creating such an organization and developing a journal.

The application of x-rays and other radiations to medical care has contributed greatly to the understanding and treatment of disease. However, the importance of medical radiation technologists in the remarkable progress of the radiological sciences has sometimes not been appreciated, even by technologists themselves.

In order for technologists to contribute in an orderly way to the care of patients, it has been necessary to establish educational standards. That need brought about the creation of a national organization in 1922, then named the Canadian Society of Radiological Technicians (CSRT) and now called the Canadian Association of Medical Radiation Technologists (CAMRT).

In this article we trace the historical development of the Dominion organization from the first provincial organizational meeting in Manitoba in 1929 to the mid–1940s. Since the history of the CAMRT is so closely interwoven with the education of radiologic technologists, tracing the history of the organization does in a large measure reflect the educational opportunities which were offered to technicians (as they were known in those years) and the manner in which they influenced the development of an incorporated society.

The discovery of x-rays was itself an event with immediate and international repercussions. There were a thousand articles on x-rays which appeared in scientific journals during the year 1896. Over 50 books on the same subject were published in the same year, not to mention innumerable commentaries.

In Canada Professor J Cox of McGill University was an early pioneer in the new science of radiology. As noted elsewhere in this volume and recorded by Evans[1] the first report of the medicolegal use of x-rays was in Canada. The examination of a leg for a gunshot injury was made by Professor Cox.

The radiological pioneers rapidly discovered how to perform many types of radiographic examinations. These examinations, of course, were sometimes experimental. The equipment, too, was extremely limited in capacity and efficiency compared with that available at the present time. Penetrometers—for measurement of the quality of radiation—were, for example, introduced as early as 1903.

Considerable confusion arose during this time due to the deleterious effects on many who were unduly exposed to x-rays.[2] Different degrees of dermatitis, anemia, epilation and skin cancers began to develop among the radiological pioneers. Fortunately, this state of ignorance was short-lived, and the necessity for protection was realized early. It was not until World War I, however, that methods of protection were carried out in a methodical manner.

During the war special training was given to roentgenologists, as they were often called then. In addition, short intensive courses were given to manipulators, army technicians, whose work consisted of the handling of films and the care of equipment. Their skills and the important role they played may be seen as the beginnings of the profession now identified as radiographic technology. A well-recognized textbook published at this time was the *United States Army X-Ray Manual,*[3] which was valuable for both roentgenologists and technicians.

The invention of the hot-cathode vacuum x-ray tube by Coolidge in 1913 revolutionized radiology. This tube enabled the operator to have more control of tube output than the gas tubes formerly in use. Other equipment which added to the progress of radiology included the devices to eliminate secondary radiation. Albers-Schonberg soon recognized the value of a compression diaphragm, the principle of which was later improved by Bucky, and in 1916 brought to greater perfection by Potter. Single-coated nitrate base x-ray film became available in 1914 and brought about great improvements in technique.

Amazing progress has continued to be made in the field of radiology since the day the world was startled by the report of an x-ray examination of a hand. With increasing knowledge, x-rays are now used universally in diagnosis, while in treatment their use has only latterly come to be replaced by more energetic gamma rays from cobalt-60 or accelerators. Since all specialties in medicine and surgery are making increasing demands on radiology, it is essential that provision be made for a satisfactorily equipped department and its staffing by well-trained personnel. According to MacEachern: "The department shall be under the supervision of a competent medical radiologist assisted by trained technicians."[4] This recommendation came to be one of the requirements for hospital accreditation by the American College of Surgeons, which was the forerunner of hospital accreditation now administered by the Joint Commission on Accreditation of Hospitals in the United States.

During World War II x-rays again played an important role in military radiology. Routine x-ray chest examination of all men inducted into the armed forces benefited individuals and helped control tuberculosis. To facilitate this examination, photo-röntgen [photo-fluorographic] units were installed in several centres in Canada.

Meanwhile, a new application of x-rays developed: to determine hidden defects in metals and other materials used in industry and in the military. This specialty of nondestructive testing, with its own technologist-practitioners, soon evolved.

A NEED FOR ADEQUATELY TRAINED TECHNICIANS

The beginning of the radiologic technicians' era dates back to World War I. Prior to this time radiographic examinations were made by physicists and physicians interested in this new field. With the rapid strides in the science of radiology and in its application to medicine, the need for trained technical assistants became evident. Most of the technical work at this time was disorganized and uncoordinated due to the inflexibility of technical factors and rather crude equipment. One of the first persons to initiate a systematic approach to the problem of teaching radiographic technique was Ed C Jerman, founder of the educational department of the General Electrical Corporation. A textbook published by Jerman in 1928, entitled *Modern X-Ray Technique,* was for its time a valuable guide to technicians, although earlier books such as those by Prince[5] and the United States Army[3] were already in use. Later, more complicated procedures demanded even higher degrees of skill on the part of radiologic technicians. Therefore, more didactic training was imperative so that the technician would be enabled to produce consistent diagnostic radiographs under all conditions.

ORGANIZATION OF THE AMERICAN REGISTRY OF X-RAY TECHNICIANS SPONSORED BY THE RADIOLOGICAL SOCIETY OF NORTH AMERICA

Members of the Radiological Society of North America appointed a committee in 1920 to study methods for the official recognition of radiologic technicians. This committee favoured the establishment of a Registry to enable technicians to become certified. Under the joint sponsorship of the Radiological Society of North America and the American Roentgen Ray Society, a plan was formulated in 1922 and was functioning as early as 1923. Appointed as examiner, Ed C Jerman did a great deal to further the education of technicians. Later, Alfred Greene in his office as executive Secretary also added to the success of this organization. The Council on Education and Registration, appointed in 1931, and composed of radiologists and technicians, succeeded in further raising the standards of the registry by making the requirements more stringent. The official title of the organization was changed from the American Registry of Radiological Technicians to the American Registry of X-ray Technicians in 1936. The Board of the Radiological Society of North America announced at their meeting in December 1942 their willingness to relinquish sponsorship of the registry provided the sponsorship was assumed by the American College of Radiology. This sponsorship became effective on May 6, 1943.

Through the untiring efforts of its members, the registry progressed remarkably: 4600 registrants were recorded in the first 20 years of its existence. In June 1943 the American Medical Association assumed the responsibility of accrediting schools which educated radiologic technicians. By 1948 the American Registry of X-ray Technicians stood on a strong foundation.

ORGANIZATION OF THE AMERICAN SOCIETY OF X-RAY TECHNICIANS

The first meeting of the American Association of X-ray Technicians was held October 25, 1920. At this meeting a group of 13 technicians, under the chairmanship of EC Jerman, met to discuss the organization of a society. The name of the society adopted by the group was the American Association of Radiological Technicians; this title was later changed to the American Society of Radiographers in order to lessen confusion with the American Registry of Radiological Technicians. In 1933 another change was made in the title of the society when it became the American Society of X-ray Technicians.

The chief object of this society was "to promote the science and art of radiography." Only registered x-ray technicians were eligible for membership in the society after 1925. At the annual meeting in 1929 the members present decided to publish an official journal of the organization, *The X-ray Technician*. Formerly, publications of the society had been published in *Radiology*.

From the original group of 13 members who organized the Society in 1920, membership steadily increased to 3000 members in 1947. The efforts of the organizers and leaders of the American Society of X-ray Technicians resulted in a well-developed, highly ethical professional organization which has attained international recognition.

ORGANIZATION OF THE BRITISH SOCIETY OF RADIOGRAPHERS

The Society of Radiographers of England was founded in 1920, and it is affiliated with the British Institute of Radiology. Candidates were required to pass the examinations conducted by the society and to have had "two years' experience in roentgenography" before they became eligible for membership. The qualifications for fellowship in the society were drawn up by its Council in 1936. Candidates may be certified by three different methods, depending upon the experience of the applicant: (a) by thesis, (b) by ordinary examination, and (c) by special examination. This arrangement went into effect in May 1937 when the ordinary examination for Fellowship was held in London.

On the recommendation of the Council of the Education Committee a special course of instruction was introduced into the curriculum in order to qualify candidates in the specialty of radiotherapy or—as it later became known—radiation oncology. A special certificate is issued for the successful completion of this course. An individual who passes the therapy examinations is entitled to use the letters SRCT (Society of Radiographers Certificate in Therapy); one who passes the membership examination is styled a Member of the Society of Radiographers (MSR). One who passes the membership examination as well as the special therapy examination uses the initials MSR and CT.

The membership of the society progressed until in 1948 it had reached almost 3000. The membership in this organization extended to South Africa and New Zealand but the examinations for these countries were controlled by the board of examiners in England. The objective of the British Society of Radiographers was: "To promote the science and regulate the practice of radiography and to consider and discuss all subjects affecting it."

The first publications for this society were printed in the *British Journal of Radiology*. As the membership increased, its members decided to assume the responsibility of an official journal of its own. Accordingly, the first issue of *Radiography* appeared in January 1935.

One of the outstanding early members of the Society of Radiographers was KC (Kitty) Clark, who became widely known through the publication of the definitive book which she wrote on x-ray technique, *Positioning in Radiography*.[6] A review of this book in *Radiography* states, "The contents are encyclopaedic, and the lavish array of radiographs and diagrams are invariably excellent; some of them are magnificent."[7]

RADIOLOGICAL TECHNOLOGISTS IN CANADA

The development of radiologic technicians—later described more properly as technologists—in Canada and elsewhere has been an evolutionary process. Supervised courses, adequate textbooks, and up-to-date, shockproof equipment were unknown to early technicians. Through methods of trial and error, as well as experimentation, these pioneers became proficient technical assistants to radiologists. Their spirit of leadership and constant endeavour accomplished much—and would benefit the radiologic technician's who followed—of later times in the science of radiographic technique and the formation of local and Dominion organizations.

The need for an organization to serve as the voice of technicians was recognized early. In the United States and in England national societies were organized in 1920, and these were sponsored by their respective societies of radiologists. In the formation of the American Association (later Society) of Radiological Technicians, Canada was represented in the person of Claude J Bodle of Winnipeg, Manitoba.

Since no organization for radiologic technicians existed in Canada before 1929, several sought and obtained membership in the American Society of X-ray Technicians when it began to function. In 1929 the Western Society of Radiographers was organized by Claude Bodle and William Doern of Manitoba. This society became affiliated with the American Society of X-ray Technicians (ASXRT) on March 5, 1930. Owing to a change in the constitutions and by-laws of the ASXRT, it was necessary for these societies to reaffiliate. Accordingly, the Western Society of Radiographers was reaffiliated with ASXRT on November 21, 1938. In September 1940, the name of this organization was changed to the Manitoba Society of X-ray Technicians. Following the organization of the Canadian Society of Radiological Technicians in 1943, the affiliation with ASXRT was discontinued.

The establishment of the American Registry of X-ray Technicians in 1922 aroused the interest of many Canadian technicians who became certified after passing the written examinations. The official roster of the American Registry of X-ray Technicians for 1947 listed 184 Canadian technicians.

ORGANIZATION OF SOCIETIES IN CANADA

In every nationwide profession there is the necessity for some means of unification and official recognition in order to fulfil the ideals of the profession. The recommendation, which follows, of the American College of Surgeons for the employment of registered technicians in approved hospitals is an example of this necessity for a national organization:

> *There are definite standards for the training of technicians and only those who are registered should be employed.*[4]

Canadian radiologic technicians recognized this need in their specialty. In order to qualify an adequate number of radiologic technicians, a resolve grew to organize a national society.

STEPS IN THE ORGANIZATION OF THE CANADIAN SOCIETY OF RADIOLOGICAL TECHNICIANS

The Provincial Societies

The Dominion of Canada in 1938 had 921 hospitals. The technicians of the province of Ontario, which had organized a provincial society in 1935, realized that there was a great need in Canada for the employment of radiologic technicians. They became interested in the formation of a Dominion-wide organization in 1938. Ethel Pugen of Toronto was appointed chairman of the Dominion organization committee. A proposed plan and constitution were drawn up by this committee and presented by Dr WH McGuffin to the Canadian Medical Association and the Canadian Association of Radiologists for approval at their joint meeting in 1938.[8] The plan was approved, and Dr McGuffin was appointed chairman of a Technician Committee for the Canadian Association of Radiologists. Dr McGuffin stated, "The Canadian radiological technicians can gain much by banding together for mutual benefits in addition to establishing desirable relationships with the radiologists."[9] It was felt that the first step toward a Dominion organization would be the establishment of provincial societies. Accordingly, letters were sent to all the provinces in 1939 by Ethel Pugen suggesting such a course of action. Details of the creation of provincial organizations are provided in Table 1.

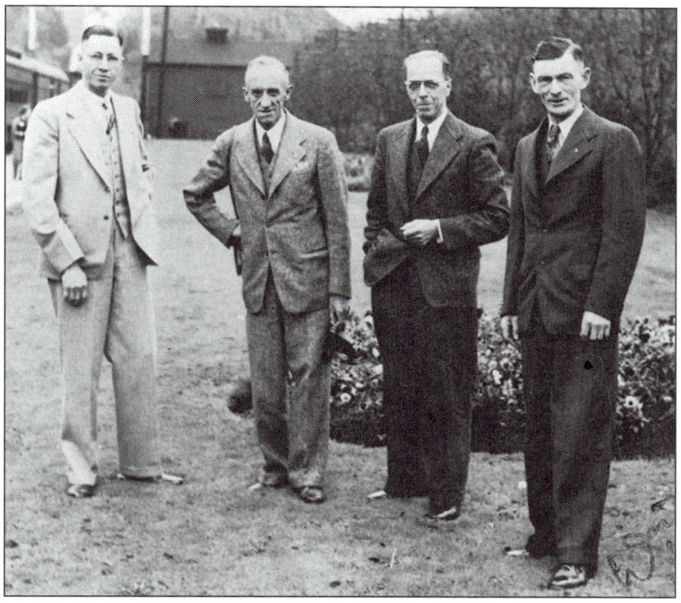

Left
CAMRT past presidents, Banff 1951. Left to right: Bill Doern, Bert Welch, Claude Bodle, Percy Hunt

Middle
CSRT board and delegates 1953 convention

Bottom left
CSRT logo

Bottom right
CAMRT shields

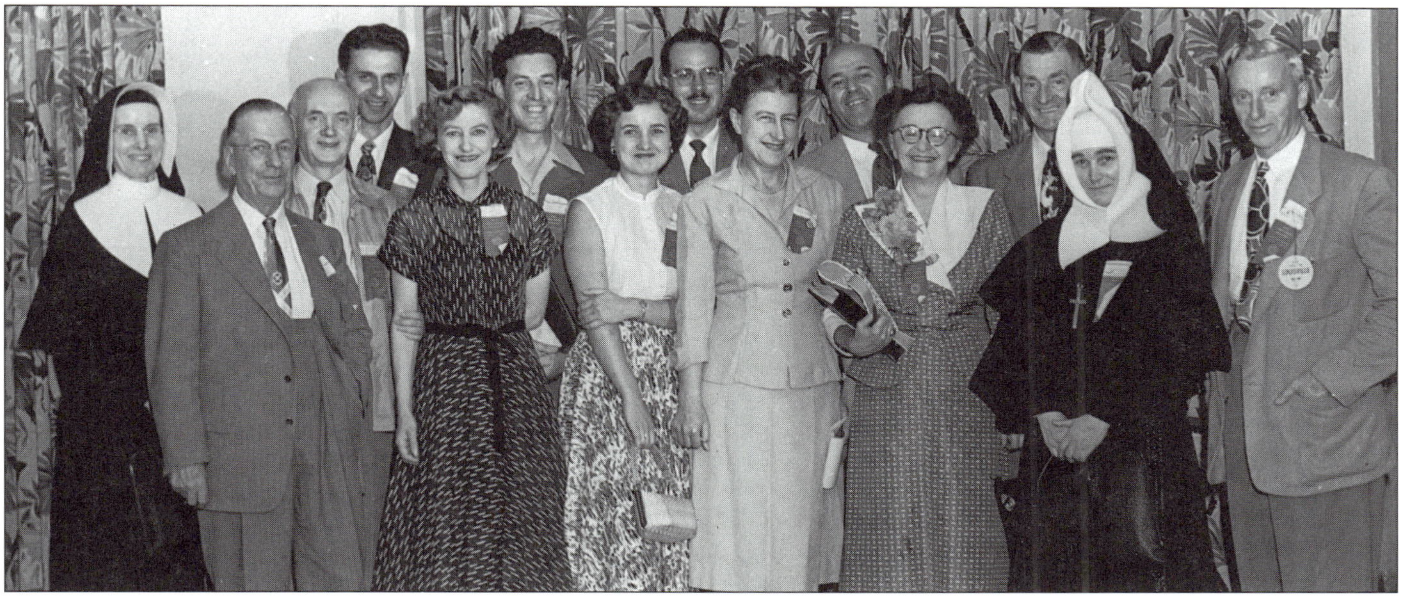

technique before they are eligible for membership.

Alberta

The organizational meeting for the province of Alberta in 1940 was chaired by Edward S Hoare of Calgary. Because of the great distances members would have to travel to attend central meetings, the organization divided into two parts: one group to be organized in Calgary, the other in Edmonton. The initial membership was between 60 and 70. At the first annual meeting in July, 1941, both the Calgary and Edmonton sections met to form the Alberta Society of X-ray Technicians. The official publication of this group was the *Alberta Technician*.[11]

In spite of transportation difficulties the membership of this Society increased to 80 members by 1948, 41 of whom were registered.

Table 1a

PROVINCIAL SOCIETIES

Province	*Year organized*	*Initial Membership*	*Total 1948 Membership*
Alberta	1941	60–70	80
British Columbia	1943	40	140
Manitoba	1929	25	152
New Brunswick	1940	16	49
Nova Scotia	1940	22	44
Ontario	1935	14	275
P.E.I.	not created		—
Saskatchewan	1940	38	90
Québec	1940	60	178

Table 1b

PROVINCIAL SOCIETIES (CONT.)

Province	*Full 1948 Members*	*Student Members*	*Educational Requirement*	*Education*
Alberta	41*	39*	Grade 11	2 years
British Col.	75	50	Jun matric.	2 years
Manitoba	70	59	Jun matric.	2 years
New Brun.	31	18	Jun matric.	2 years
Nova Scotia	38	6	Grade 11	2 years
Ontario	183	71	Grade 12	3 years
P.E.I.	–	–	–	–
Saskatchewan	34	56	Grade 11 (12 preferred)	2 years of radiologist supervision
Québec	112	38	High school matric.	2 consec. yrs.

* This table is taken from Sister Crowley's thesis. It is not clear why these two columns do not always add up to the total membership.

Manitoba

When plans for a Dominion organization were made the Manitoba Society of X-ray Technicians was already well established. This society was organized in 1929, with Claude J Bodle of Winnipeg as its first president. For several years this organization enjoyed affiliation with the American Society of X-ray Technicians. At the time of its organization the Manitoba society had an enrollment of 25 members, 10 of whom were registered technicians. By 1948 the membership had increased to 152 members.

Ontario

The Ontario Society of Radiographers was organized in 1935 with a membership of 14. JH Coones was its first president.[9] This organization grew rapidly, and in 1948 the membership numbered 275. Through the outstanding leadership of the technicians of this organization, CSRT came into existence. In 1939 the first provincial examinations were held for student technicians.[10] Students in this province are required to have three years training in radiologic

New Brunswick

The New Brunswick Society of X-ray Technicians was organized in March, 1940. Sister DeLellis of Saint John, the organizing committee chair, was elected the first president. Keen interest was shown by all the New Brunswick members in the formation of both provincial and Canadian societies for radiologic technicians. The membership in the New Brunswick Society, in 1948, had increased from the initial membership of 16 to 49. Much of the progress in this organization has been due to the whole-hearted cooperation of radiologists in the province, notably Dr EA Petrie, representative of the New Brunswick Medical Society to this organization, and Dr AS Kirkland, who gave valuable advice and assistance in its creation. The motto chosen for this Society was: *Non nobis sed omnibus* (Not for ourselves, but for others).

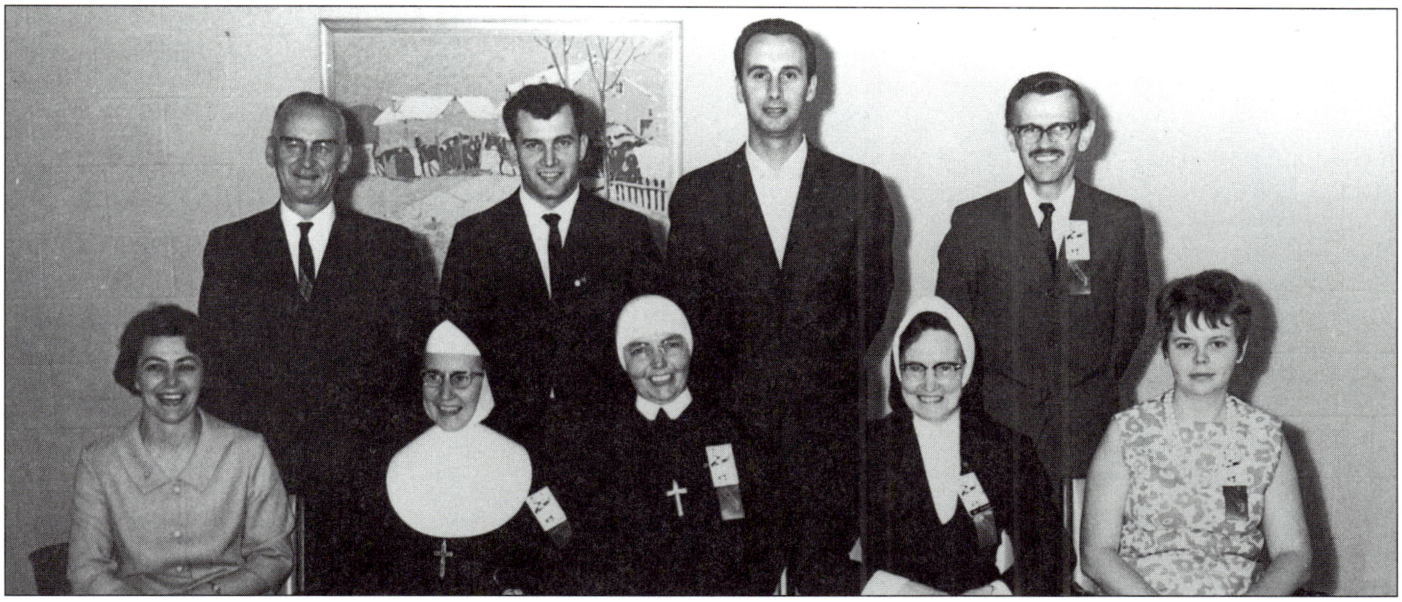

Official delegates 25th anniversary CSRT (1967)
Back, left to right: JP Connell, E Zemianski, B Price, PH Poitras
Front, left to right: PM Rogers, Sr M Eucharia, Sr M Roselina, Sr G Crowley, H King

Nova Scotia

In May 1940, the Nova Scotia Society of Radiographers was organized, with Albert Perry of Halifax as its first president. The annual three-day refresher course proved to be an excellent means for stimulating interest of both students and experienced technicians.

The co-founders of the Nova Scotia Society of Radiographers were Albert Perry and George Harrison,[12] who have been awarded life membership in recognition of their leadership and initiative. From 1940 to 1948 the membership increased from 22 to 44.

Saskatchewan

The Saskatchewan Society of X-ray Technicians was organized in 1940 under the direction of Sidney Johnson of Moose Jaw, who was elected the first president. Membership at this time was 38. During World War II many technicians from this province enlisted, causing a considerable drop in membership. In May 1946 renewed activity and a membership drive brought the enrollment to 70. Through the efforts of their competent secretary, Marie Perron, the drive was continued in 1947, increasing the total membership to 90 at the end of that year.

To meet the urgent needs in this province for laboratory and radiographic technicians, a program was prepared for candidates to take short, intensive courses in both these fields. Through the efforts of Percy E Hunt and his committee a comprehensive program was presented to the directors of the Canadian Society of Radiological Technicians and the Canadian Society of Laboratory Technologists for approval outlining the proposed plan. This combined training scheme was designed for the benefit of small hospitals, particularly in rural areas where one technician might carry out the duties of both technologies.

Québec

The Québec Society of X-ray Technicians came into existence in 1940 under the direction of Rosemary O'Hagen of Montréal, who was also its first president. The enrollment at that time was 60 members. By 1948 the membership had increased to 178. In addition to the active members there were 38 students, 28 associate and four honorary members. A syllabus for training student technicians was created by this society and sent to the various hospitals and radiologists throughout the province, as well as to the Executive of the Canadian Society. Because of the bilingual nature of this province, activities were from carried out in both English and French from the beginning.

British Columbia

British Columbia technicians did not create a provincial organization until May 1943, when William Q Stirling was elected as its first president. There was an enrollment of 40 members. Rapid progress resulted in 140 members in 1948, 50 of whom are student members.

Prince Edward Island

Although no provincial organization existed before 1948, six hospitals in the province employed radiographic technicians.

Below
CAMRT pre-fellowship lecture participants October 1963

Bottom
CAMRT board of directors 1967. Back, left to right: James G Williams, Alex Noseworthy, Robert Masse, Dr WM Little, John S Flanagan, W Ray Hansen, Colin JA Maxwell, Austin Singer. Front, left to right: PE Godley, Mrs El Hood, George C Hall, MA McMillan, AM Escaf

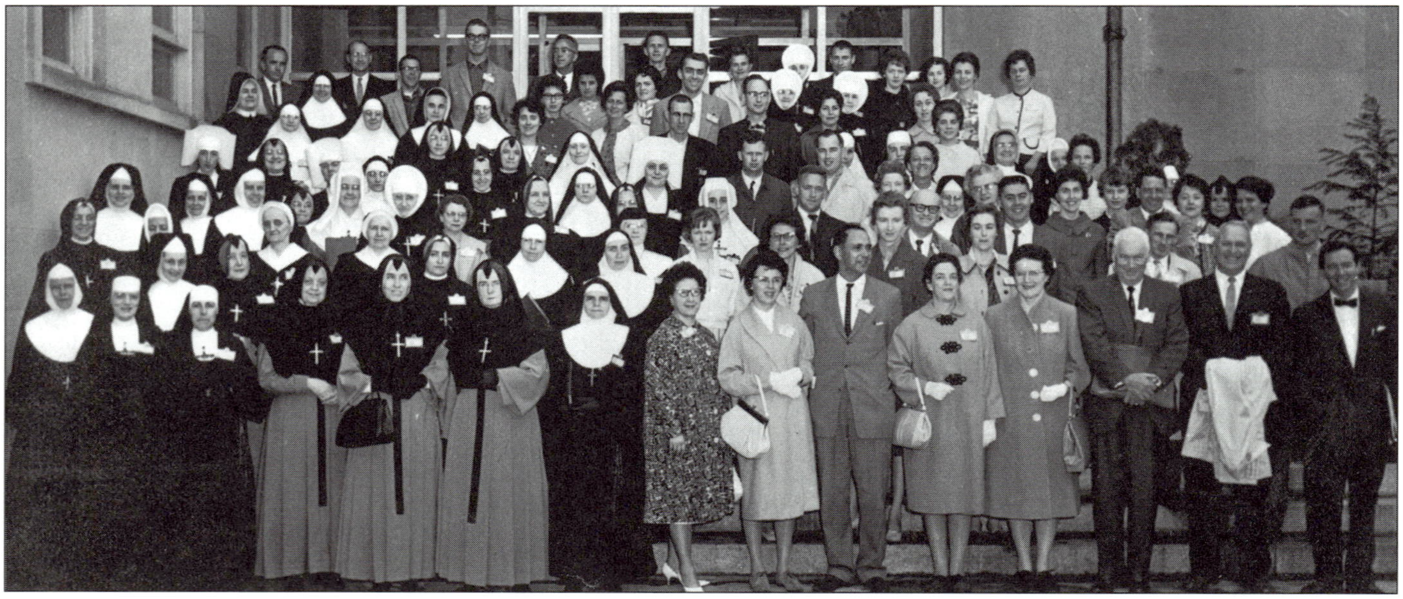

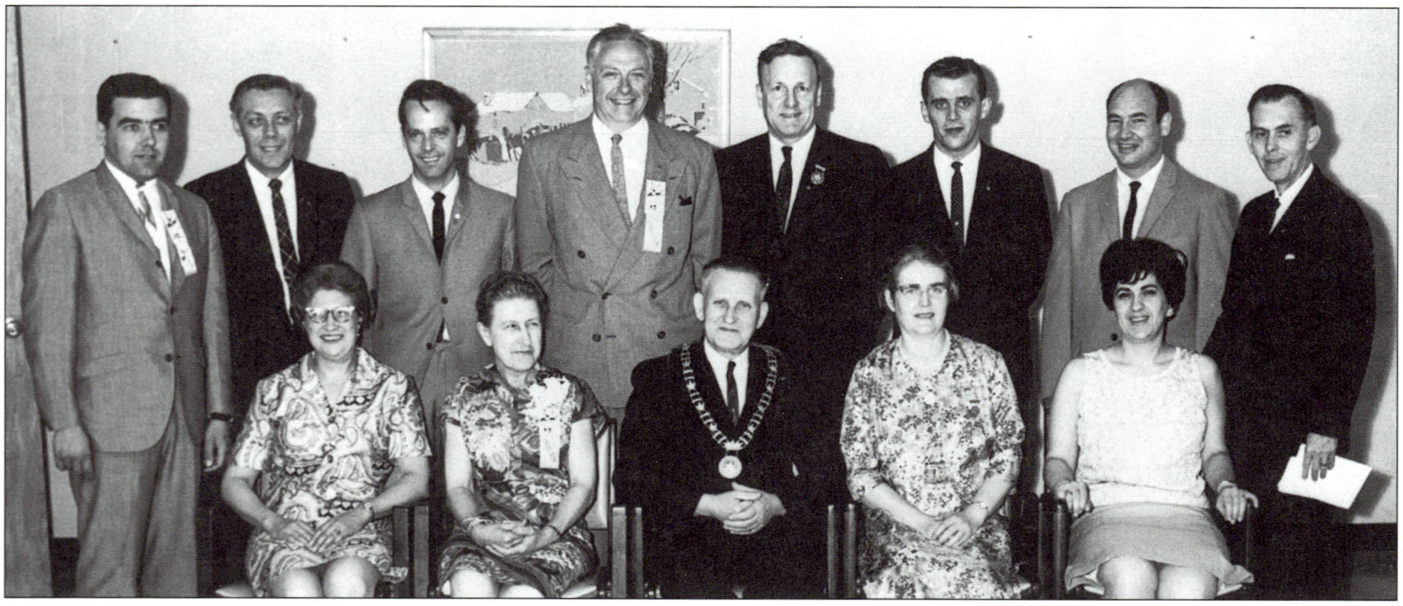

Below
CAMRT president George Hall cuts silver anniversary cake

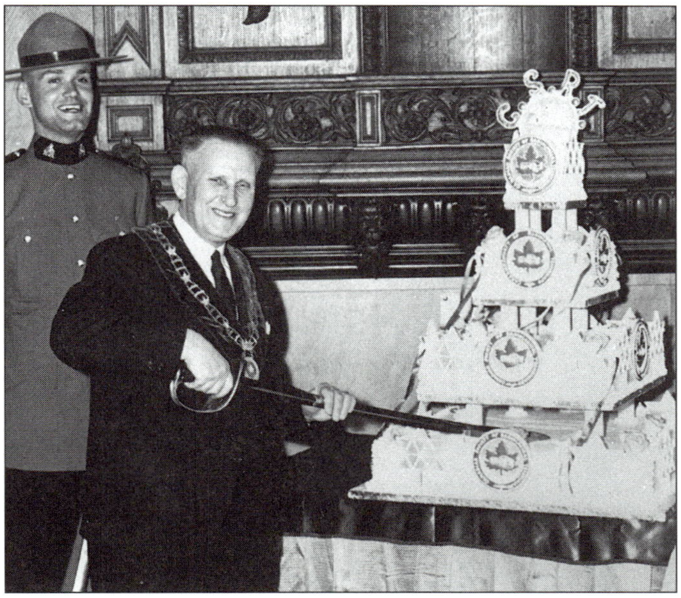

OBJECTIVES OF PROVINCIAL SOCIETIES

The organization of the provincial societies was the first step toward the formation of CSRT. Each provincial society had its own constitution and by-laws. These had, however, to conform to the standards adopted by CSRT. The main objective of the provincial societies was to promote the science of radiological technique. The occupation of the radiologic technician demands a comprehensive and painstaking technique. The radiologist can only interpret what is evident on the radiographs. Therefore, the technician must be aware of his or her obligation to produce consistently good radiographs of diagnostic quality.

One of the means of advancing radiographic technology was regular attendance at meetings, where technicians profit by the discussion of problems and techniques and the sharing of experience, both among themselves and with other health care workers.

In Canada the educational requirements adopted by the provincial societies were fairly uniform (Table 1b). One province requires their candidates to have a Grade 12 education before entry, four require junior matriculation, and the remaining three, grade 11. The advantage of matriculation certification—either junior or senior—is that it qualifies the student for university entrance should he or she later decide on such a course of action.

ORGANIZATION OF THE CANADIAN SOCIETY OF RADIOLOGICAL TECHNICIANS

The affairs of the Canadian Society of Radiological Technicians were and are controlled by a board of directors. The first board of directors consisted of seven members (Table 2). This board prepared the memorandum of agreement for the creation of the organization. These seven members held office until September 30, 1943 as specified by the constitution. After October 1943 the Society was to be governed by a board of five directors whose term of office was to be two years. As listed in the memorandum of agreement the directors were chosen as follows:[13]

1. One director nominated by the Canadian Medical Association.
2. One director nominated by the Canadian Association of Radiologists.
3. One director nominated by each of the member societies.
4. Two directors nominated by the members-at-large.

The directors nominated by the membership held other offices in the society: one was the president of the Canadian Society of Radiological Technicians and the other held the offices of vice-president and secretary-treasurer. In addition to the directors there were nine associate directors who served as a connecting link between the board of directors and their own provincial societies.

PERIOD FROM ORGANIZATION TO INCORPORATION

Following the organization of the provincial societies, plans were made for a Dominion organization. The constitution which had been drawn up for the Dominion society received the approval of the Canadian Medical Association and the Canadian Association of Radiologists as well as that of representatives from the various provinces. There followed an application for a Dominion charter. The foundation for the Dominion Society was laid by the Ontario Society of Radiographers, and the loan to defray the expenses of the Dominion organization was made by the Ontario society.[14] To pay for the cost of incorporation of CSRT, the Canadian Association of Radiologists generously donated two hundred dollars.

According to the memorandum of agreement, the name of the Dominion organization was to be the Canadian Society of Radiological Technicians. The first meeting of the board of directors of the Canadian Society of Radiological Technicians was held in September 1942 in Toronto. It was decided at this meeting that all technicians who were active members in a provincial society before July 1, 1942 were eligible for membership in the Canadian Society of Radiological Technicians. After this date all new candidates for membership in Canadian or provincial societies were required to pass an examination and to have completed two years' training.[15] At this meeting the following decision was made regarding examinations:

> *That the examining boards of the provincial societies will compile the examination papers for the students of their society, these papers to be submitted to the examiners of the Canadian Society of Radiological Technicians. This central board of examiners will review and approve these papers, returning them to be written by the students. Upon completion, examination papers will be returned to the central board to be marked. The student passing his examinations will thus become a member of his own provincial society and a member of the Canadian Society.*[15]

The provincial societies in relation to the Canadian Society of Radiological Technicians are called member societies. It was agreed at this same meeting that a fee of ten dollars be paid by each member society annually; also a one dollar fee for each active or associate member was levied.

At the second meeting of the board of directors in November 1942 the question of membership by British subjects not living in Canada was discussed. It was decided that membership in the Canadian Society of Radiological Technicians would be extended to all British technicians living in the western hemisphere.

PERIOD FROM INCORPORATION TO 1948

After an unavoidable delay, the charter for CSRT was granted in 1943. During the interval, however, the society had continued to make rapid progress. Measures were taken to adopt uniform educational standards and examinations. In 1943 the total active membership in the Society had reached 386.

The first annual meeting of CSRT was held in Toronto in September 1943. At this meeting the crest and motto for the society were adopted. The motto read, *Scientia et Mores* (Knowledge and Ethics).

In order to meet requests for a greater representation of member societies on the board of directors, ballots for nominations were sent to the various members. Ballots were also distributed to each member society for the election of an associate member from each province. The first associate directors elected were Dr A Comtois, French-speaking member; Herbert Welch, Alberta; William Doern, Manitoba; Sister St Stanislaus, New Brunswick; Albert Perry, Nova Scotia; Sister Mary Mooney, Ontario; Sidney Johnson, Saskatchewan; and Donalda Campbell, Québec.

At the first annual meeting life memberships were awarded to Percy Ghent of Toronto, Edward Hoare of Calgary and Henry Simkins of Montréal, in recognition of their many years' outstanding service in the field of radiographic technique.

In 1945 at the third annual meeting of CSRT in Montréal a decision was reached to prepare a curriculum which would indicate the subjects to be studied. In order to facilitate the marking of examinations, a resolution was made to reduce the examining board from five to three members. The 1946 annual meeting of CSRT in Niagara Falls dealt with many vital problems relevant to the progress of the society and the education of technicians. A committee was appointed at this meeting to investigate existing methods of education for technicians throughout Canada and to catalogue the possibilities for advanced training. The members of this committee were Drs AC Singleton, EA Petrie and Hill Cheney. At this meeting in 1946, several minor changes were made in the constitution of the society.

Of importance to technicians who wish to transfer to other provinces was the resolution regarding transfer of membership. Members in good standing in their own provinces are eligible for membership without payment of additional fees for that year when for occupational reasons they become members in another province.

Two new offices created in the Canadian Society of Radiological Technicians in 1946 were a secretary to the board of examiners and a registrar. Sister Rose Agnes of Saint John was appointed secretary to the chair of the board of examiners. Katherine Creelman of Moncton accepted the office of registrar. At this time membership in CSRT had reached 452.

The April 1947 issue of *Focal Spot* gives the revisions and regulations of CSRT board of examiners, prepared under the chairmanship of Dr EA Petrie with the assistance of Percy Hunt and Henry Simkins.[16] A few of these revisions were as follows:

1. *The board of examiners shall consist of two radiologists and one technician.*
2. *At least one of the radiologists shall be bilingual.*
3. *The technician shall be a member of CSRT.*

4. *Appointments to the board of examiners shall be made by the board of directors of CSRT from the nominations received in such a manner as the board of directors shall from time to time direct.*
5. *The chairman of the board of examiners shall appoint a regular member of CSRT resident or working in his district to act as secretary for the board of examiners.*

Further constitutional changes were made at the 1947 meeting in Saskatoon regarding the appointment of the board of directors, an increase in membership fees and the admission of persons engaged in the commercial sale of x-ray equipment as associate members of CSRT. A change was also made in the office of president: Up to that time the president of CSRT held the office of vice-president and secretary the year previously; thereafter the office of president might be accepted without the president-elect first serving as secretary-treasurer.

HISTORIAN

The need for an historian of CSRT was considered at the 1943 meeting in Toronto. Anne Hayward was appointed to this office and held it until her resignation in 1945. Sister Rose Agnes of Saint John was then appointed to this office in 1945. In 1947, after her appointment as secretary to the board of examiners, she relinquished the office of historian. The appointment of Percy Ghent of Toronto to the office of permanent historian in 1947 assured the members of excellent and complete records of CSRT. Percy Ghent's wide experience and unusual executive ability were well known to Canadian technicians of that era. He had been editor of *Ontario Radiographer* during the four years of its existence; he also edited *Focal Spot* until his position was taken over in 1944 by Leslie Cartwright.

OBJECTIVES OF THE SOCIETY

Then, as today, hospital governing bodies and administrators realized the need for continuing education for their staff. They were aware that growth in all branches of medical science required continuing education. The objectives of CSRT had been to establish standards and educational facilities to meet the needs of radiologic technologists. Professional education for the radiologic technician can be carried out in the following two ways:

1. By formal study at a college or university.
2. By a directed two-year course of study in a department of radiology. Unfortunately, in the past most of the emphasis has been on the clinical work of the student in the department and too little on theoretical considerations.

One of the main objectives of CSRT has been to promote the science and art of radiological technique. As a science it is a subject of systematized knowledge which has gradually evolved. As an art it deals with people, sick and well, under all conditions; the work thus calls for skill and ingenuity on the part of the technician. In order to attain these objectives CSRT has set academic standards for those who wish to enter this profession, and it also requires a standardized length of training in radiologic technique.

Some of the further objectives as listed in the memorandum of agreement[17] of CSRT were as follows:

- To organize a national association to guide local associations;
- To promote and carry out research and experimental work;
- To establish and maintain libraries;
- To administer and support charitable funds for the benefit of persons engaged in the science and practice of radiography and allied subjects, and their dependents.

CANADIAN NATIONAL REGISTRATION

At the 1944 annual meeting of the Canadian Society of Radiological Technicians agreed to have standard examinations throughout Canada, and the following resolution was adopted:

That a standard examination for membership in the Canadian Society of Radiological Technicians be set by the Dominion examining board, the examination to be held under the direction of the various member societies. Having passed this examination, a member shall be entitled to be addressed as "Registered Technician" (RT).[18]

Previously, each provincial society had prepared the examinations for its members and submitted them for the approval of the Dominion examining board. The examinations, held in May and November of each year, consisted of two parts, one written, one practical. The written examination included five subjects: anatomy, processing room technique, physics and apparatus, radiographic technique and therapy. For the practical examination, films taken by the applicant were submitted. To be successful in the examinations the candidates were required to have an average of 60 per cent or more in all subjects and a minimum of 50 per cent in each subject.

In 1947, 150 candidates wrote the examinations of CSRT. The yearly increase in the number of applicants for examination indicates the value of certification.

EDUCATIONAL REQUIREMENTS

At the first meeting in 1942 the board of directors of CSRT decided in principle to accept for national use the educational standards and curriculum of the Ontario Society of Radiographers; they also established that the length of the training period be two years. Slight variations in the educational requirements of candidates existed in each province before this uniform standard was required by the National society. At the annual meeting of CSRT in 1946, a resolution was made that junior matriculation—or its equivalent—be required for admission to examination. Two years continued to be the required length of education.

As early as 1943 the subject of university education for radiologic technicians had been discussed at the annual meetings of CSRT. The members attending the meeting passed unanimously a resolution to contact the deans of the various universities throughout Canada to inaugurate a course in radiologic technique as part of the university curriculum.

In 1946 Percy Hunt and Sidney Johnson were appointed to open negotiations with the Canadian Medical Association concerning the establishment of approved training centres for technicians.[19] At the annual meeting of CSRT that year a committee was appointed to obtain information on the education of technicians and to study the means whereby improved training and higher education for radiologic technicians might be obtained.

EDUCATION COMMITTEE

The committee appointed to study education for radiologic technologists consisted of Drs AC Singleton (Chair), EA Petrie and Bill Cheney. At the annual meeting of the Canadian Association of Radiologists in June 1947 a standing committee was appointed on the training of radiologic technicians. The members of this committee were: Drs Bill Cheney (Chair), Vancouver; Arthur Singleton, Toronto; Edward A Petrie, Saint John; and Jean Bouchard, Montréal.

At the 1947 meeting of CSRT in Saskatoon Dr Singleton gave a report on the replies to questionnaires sent out by Dr EA Petrie on training programs. In consideration of the work accomplished by Dr Desmond Burke of Toronto and Dr AE Perry of Regina in educating technicians, CSRT decided to invite *these* radiologists to join the committee and to continue this study for another year.

PUBLICATION OF A PROFESSIONAL JOURNAL

In order to maintain contacts and to disseminate scientific and professional information in an organization, the publication of a journal is essential. *The Ontario Radiographer,* the official journal of the Ontario Society of Radiographers in circulation from 1939 to 1943, was the first such publication for radiologic technicians in Canada. Percy Ghent of Toronto was its editor-in-chief.

After the incorporation of CSRT in 1943 members agreed on the need for an authoritative journal for the society. A suggestion was made that the *Ontario Radiographer* might transform itself into the publication for the Canadian society. This proposition was agreeable to the Ontario Society of Radiographers, and the Canadian journal came into existence in January 1944. Percy Ghent continued as editor, assisted by Leslie Cartwright as associate editor and WH Osborne as business manager. The title of the journal, selected by the editorial board, was *Focal Spot*. Much of the credit for the high standard which this journal attained belongs to the competent leadership of its editors. Percy Ghent relinquished his office in 1944, and Leslie Cartwright became editor-in-chief. The membership at the 1944 annual meeting of CSRT decided to appoint a board of directors for *Focal Spot,* to consist of an honorary president, president, business manager and secretary. The following officers were appointed at this meeting:

Honorary President	President of CSRT
President	Leslie J Cartwright
Business Manager	WH Osborne
Secretary	Ms G Cassidy

In 1945 Hugh J Menagh accepted the office of circulation manager. After the resignation of WH Osborne in 1946, Hugh Menagh performed the duties of both business manager and circulation manager until 1947 when George Ross was appointed business manager.

The increasing number of subscriptions to the journal of the Canadian Society of Radiological Technicians is a tribute to the excellence of this publication. The 1947 report of the journal shows that the circulation of *Focal Spot* includes "practically all countries of the English speaking world."[19]

SUMMARY

By 1948 membership in CSRT numbered nearly 600 technologists. Such growth pointed to a bright future for the organization.

Acknowledgment:

This material was prepared by Sister Mary DeLellis Crowley as a thesis presented to the Faculty of the School of Nursing of Saint Louis University in partial fulfillment of the requirements for the degree of Bachelor of Science in Radiologic Technology. It was in possession of CAMRT, to whom we are indebted for the material and for permission to edit it in this form.

Chapter IV •

The Canadian Association of Medical Radiation Technologists:

Later Years

RITA HUDEC AND LEWIS EDWARDS

THE 1950s

By the mid–1950s the Canadian Society of Radiological Technicians (CSRT)—later the Canadian Association of Medical Radiation Technologists (CAMRT)—had yet to emerge into its modern form. A name change lay ahead, as did the successful and not divisive creation of the discipline of nuclear medicine to join radiographic and radiation treatment technologies under the one umbrella of CAMRT. These developments challenged the wisdom and foresight of the Association's leadership, yet what emerged was the strong and vigorous institution of the mid 1990s.

The 14th annual convention in 1956 was held at the Empress Hotel in Victoria, British Columbia. Single room rates with bath were from $10.00 per night, and doubles with bath from $11.00 per night. Those prices are a measure of the distance that separates 1956 from 1995.

During the business sessions, chaired by President David C Sage Sr, the Board of Directors stated it would continue to do all that was possible to assist member societies to obtain provincial recognition. The matter of reciprocity with the Australian Institute of Radiography was discussed and accepted with the proviso that the views of the Australian Society of X-ray Technologists (ASXT) and the British Society be obtained. Members agreed that practicing therapy technicians with more than five years' experience would be admitted to membership without examination, and they decided to hold four-day-long annual meetings in June.

The registrar's report listed membership figures as follows: active, 876; non-active, 106; associate, 25; and radiologist, five. The society's budget was $4727.37 for that year.

Volume 13, number 2, published early in 1956, was *Focal Spot*'s 50th issue, and it carried a retrospective review of events related to the profession dating from 1924. Among the advertisements carried was one for a new publication—*Basic Principles of Radiation Safety* by Ray Fujimoto, BSc, R.T—which sold for $0.50, and one for Johnson-Hutchinson Ltd, Jewellers, listing "Gent's Style Rings, 10 karat heavy yellow gold, at $18.75."

In 1957 the second international joint meeting between the American Society of X-ray Technicians (ASXT) and CSRT was held in Washington, DC. A single room with bath at the Sheraton Park Hotel headquarters was listed at "from $7.50," and a "large parlour with two bedrooms" cost $30.00. Round-trip air fare from Vancouver to Washington was $336.20, and the same round trip by bus was $101.45. At the convention, registration was $3.00, and 11 refresher courses were offered, each consisting of four two-hour sessions, for $5.00 each.

At the society's annual general meeting, minimal standards of training were hotly debated, and an inconclusive report was received from a committee formed to investigate the cost of a permanent, paid secretary. It was announced that formal reciprocity had been concluded with the Australian Institute of Radiography.

The issue of liability insurance was the subject of some impassioned speeches, and the membership was advised that in 1958 separate examinations would be held for registration in either diagnosis or therapy but that technicians would have the option of writing the old "combined" examination for the last time in that year. It was then announced that the examination fee would be increased from $5.00 to $15.00.

A felt table cover with the society's logo was presented by the Nova Scotia, New Brunswick and Newfoundland divisions, and this adorned the head table at the annual general meeting for the first time. It was also announced that a design for the presidential chain of office and for the past president's pin had been approved.

Concern was growing among technicians about radiation protection, and "Reduction of gonadal dose in radiographic examinations," by MR Brown, RT, of the Saskatchewan Department of Public Health was published in *Focal Spot*. And reflecting things to come, the first restrictive legislative act in Canada with reference to radiography was enacted on April 10, 1957 in Saskatchewan.

At the 16th Annual CSRT Convention, held at the Fort Garry Hotel in Winnipeg, concerns included educational standards and a fellowship degree. A five-day, forty-hour week for radiographers was approved, and the society's crest was registered. During the convention's opening luncheon, Dr AE Childe presented President William Doern with a presidential chain of office, given to the society through the generosity of Dr EA Petrie, who unfortunately was unable to be present. The links of the chain were engraved with the names of the society's sixteen past presidents.

By this time, membership had grown to a total of 1241, and the budget was $10 619.68. As a result Mrs EI Hood was appointed permanent executive secretary at a starting salary of $4200.00 per annum. (The suggested starting salary for a junior technologist was $2700.00, and for a chief technician—first class—$5000.00 per annum.)

The 17th annual convention was held in 1959 at Queen's University, Kingston. The lecturers, among the "greats" of the profession, were Sister M de Lellis ("Meeting the Requirements of the New Curriculum"), Arthur W Fuchs ("Principles of Radiographic Exposure"), K Ray Fujimoto ("Fundamentals of X-Ray Protection"), and A Nanette Plowman ("Radiological and Physical Aspects of Radiation Therapy").

Focal Spot, as usual, carried all committee and special reports, together with the minutes of the annual meeting. There was one contribution by John S Flanagan, RT, entitled "Report on Wearing of Caps by Female X-ray Technicians." The report concludes, "While it is not essential that students' caps be standardized, it is felt there would be an advantage in RT's all wearing the same colour bands and that a uniform policy be adopted about wearing them." A resolution that would have required second-year students to present a thesis as part of the examination process was deferred "until such time as we are in a better position to handle its ramifications." Another resolution, requiring CSRT to publish in medical journals a policy statement asserting the professional status of radiological technicians, was approved.

On March 31st, 1959, one of the outstanding personalities in the history of radiography was honoured at a gathering in Toronto. The occasion was to mark the retirement of Mr TB "Tommy" Hurst from the post of chief technician at Toronto General Hospital.

A 1959 issue of *Focal Spot* contained the document "Accreditation of Training Schools for Radiological Technicians." It had sections on "The evolution of the training of radiological technicians in Canada 1929–1959," "The establishment of the Canadian Medical Association Committee on Approval," and an "Official list of interim approved schools." It was published by the Joint Council on Technical Training, Canadian Society of Radiological Technicians (CSRT) and Canadian Association of

Radiologists (CAR). This initiative was to result in the Conjoint Committee on the Accreditation of Technologist Education.

THE 1960s

The 18th Annual CSRT Convention was held in 1960 at the MacDonald Hotel, Edmonton where single rooms without bath went for $6.00, and twin beds without bath for $10.00. One of the most far-reaching items of business dealt with at this annual meeting was the approval of a Québec resolution that the society set up a course of training for radioactive isotope technicians within the framework of the existing training program and conjointly with the Canadian Association of Radiologists. Logbooks were to be used for the first time in the November 1960 examination.

For the first time in many years, the price of the Gent's Style Ring, 14 karat heavy yellow gold, was increased from $18.75 to $26.00, as advertised in *Focal Spot*.

In another initiative, a pre-fellowship lecture course was provided in French at the University of Montréal in June. At the same time the English language lectures took place at McGill University. These summer courses were provided in different centres for a number of years.

Successive annual meetings were held in Montréal, Saskatoon, Ottawa, Hamilton, Halifax, Chicago, Winnipeg, Banff, Saint John and Toronto.

The Montréal and Chicago meetings were international conventions of x-ray technicians, incorporating the ASXT and CSRT. The Montréal convention offered a choice of nine refresher courses, six of which had American or Canadian technicians as instructors.

In 1961 *Focal Spot* carried advertisements for technicians. A hospital department offered a starting salary of $300.00 per month, and a private office stated a range of $240.00 to 280.00 a month.

In 1962 the Nova Scotia society proposed two versions of a new x-ray technician pledge. Other suggestions came from Alberta, Manitoba and British Columbia, with the latter's chosen. (It was also agreed that sponsorship of cocktail parties should not be sought from radiologists.)

The first fellowship examinations were to be held in 1965, and this announcement created a considerable stir. In light of future events, it was significant that the paper which won the CSRT award was "Why a Fellowship?" by Ruth Duffey, RT. Membership had now increased to 2112 members, and the price of the gold ring had reached $30.00.

In provincial affairs, the WQ Stirling Award was inaugurated in British Columbia, and in Ontario, Mary F Cameron resigned from her position of executive director of the Ontario society although she was to continue to give her time and talent in other volunteer capacities.

A summary of the minutes of the the 21st annual convention, held at McMaster University, Hamilton, was carried in the September 1963 edition of *Focal Spot*. The following reports were dealt with: auditor, registrar, historian, awards, fellowship, joint council, personnel practices, publications, law, resolutions, qualifications, brochure, insurance, ISRRT, Advisory Committee for Development of X-ray Safety Standards, Advisory Committee to *Focal Spot*, Advisory Committee to CSRT, and the Scientific Research Committee. All committee reports, as always, were debated by the board of directors, by the delegates and by members at the annual meeting.

During discussion of the Fellowship Committee report an examining board was established, with the first fellowship examinations to be held in the spring of 1965. Debate on the Joint Council report resulted in, among other decisions, the raising of the entrance qualification to senior matriculation or its equivalent, effective January 1, 1965.

One resolution which was approved following some amendments read, "Be it resolved that the Advisory Committee of the CSRT be instructed to look into the possibility of investing in real estate with the thought of establishing a centrally located Head Office as stated in the Constitution in the not too distant future."

The Brochure Committee planned to change the format and the colour of the brochure and to equalize the male and female elements in the photographs. This task was to be handled by the Public Relations Committee.

Through this decade items related to undergraduate and postgraduate education continued to dominate the annual meeting. It was announced that a syllabus for isotope technicians' training would be completed by June 1965, and a target date of November 1966 was established for the first examination. Negotiations between the Joint Council and the Canadian Association of Laboratory Technicians had not ended successfully. It was decided to proceed without further input from either organization.

The name of the Fellowship Committee was changed to that of Post-Graduate Education Committee. This change was appropriate since the 1964 presidential message by Frank J Callaway introduced the possibility of an "Advanced RT" and of "Teaching Certificates." A committee of three was established to write a code of ethics for the society in the same year.

One edition of *Focal Spot* in 1964 carried five help wanted advertisements. Two of those specified "males," one specified "females," and two made no reference to gender. One of the latter two quoted a starting monthly salary of $290.00.

The Québec society was leading the way in education. A series of lectures was held on Saturday afternoons from October through May in French; the same lectures, given by the same lecturers, were provided in English on Wednesday evenings during the same period. At the same time, the University of Montréal provided a teacher-training course for registered technicians.

Alberta introduced the "Welch Memorial Trophy," to be presented annually for outstanding service during the past year. The first recipient fittingly was Mrs Bert Welch. The Manitoba division celebrated its 35th anniversary.

By 1965 five provinces had accepted Grade 13 or senior matriculation as essential for student enrollment.

At the annual meeting a curriculum for training of isotope technicians was announced; first examination would be held in November 1966 for students who had received two years of approved training. At the convention's closing banquet, President John Leatherdale presented a Diploma of Fellowship to Miss Ruth Duffey, the society's first fellow.

Legislation regulating radiographic technology was enacted in Saskatchewan in 1957, New Brunswick in 1958, Nova Scotia in 1960, Québec in 1961, and in Ontario and Alberta in 1963. The isotope section came into being in 1966.

In 1966 the editor of *Focal Spot* reported receiving six provincial journals on a regular basis, namely, *Gridlines* (British Columbia), *Scatter* (Saskatchewan), *KVP News* (Manitoba), *Filter* (Ontario), *Echo-X* (Québec), and *Back Scatter* (Newfoundland).

At the 1966 convention Soeur St Charles-Garnier of Québec City become the society's second fellow.

The 1966 annual report described a total membership of 3156—of whom 2526 were active members—and listed the budget as $47 658.10. The presidential address for 1966 gave some comparative figures relatedto the growth in numbers and in costs. In 1955 the pro rata cost per member to operate the society was $4.84. By 1959 the figure was $11.57. In 1965 it was $10.77, and for the fiscal year 1965–66 it was $11.22. The ring then sold for $31.50.

In that year the wording on appropriate certificates read, "Registered Technician in Nuclear Medicine Technology."

Announcements included one to the effect that reciprocity with the Dutch society had been approved. Another regrettably advised that joint CSRT-ASXT conventions had been discontinued. On a more pleasant note, members were advised that Agfa-Gevaert was sponsoring an award of a trip from anywhere in Canada to Brussels, plus $200.00, to a technician winning any combination of the current major awards. The first winner was Mrs Judith Gill of Fort William, Ontario. Mrs Gill had won the Gevaert Bronze Medal in 1960, the Gevaert Gold Medal in 1966 and the CSRT Essay Award, also in 1966.

In 1968 the official colours of the society became royal blue and gold. Bill Doern and George Hall were awarded Centennial Medals by the Government of Canada.

The society's 27th Convention in Toronto registered the record number of 566.

The Alberta division had decided some time earlier to proceed with their own advanced certification (AC) program, and at the annual meeting, members voted in favour of accepting the Alberta "ART" for the National "AC" under a grandfather clause.

THE ROSS REPORT

The annual meeting of 1967 set the association agenda for some years. The report from PS Ross & Partners recommended substantial changes in process and organization.

The Ross Report, "A Plan to Reorganize the Canadian Society of Radiological Technicians," was the culmination of a great deal of research and interviews with numerous technicians from all member societies. It encompassed all aspects of the society's affairs and made recommendations for administrative improvement, with long-term, interim, and short-term organizational plans. Following extensive and often emotional debate on the floor of the 1967 annual meeting, a Finance Committee was appointed to review all aspects of income and expenditures, and steps were taken to hire an executive director. The search for an executive director was given top priority since the successful candidate would assume office on or before June 1, 1968. At the 1968 convention, Mr. Arbo Mattila was introduced to members as the society's first executive director.

One part of the report dealt with committee restructuring. The board of directors acted on this matter, and with particular reference to the Committee on Qualifications, the effect was dramatic: this committee's total membership had been 35, and it was reduced to 22, a strategy endorsed by the membership at the annual meeting.

The board of directors also implemented a modified version of the short-term plan. An additional meeting of the board was introduced so more time could be spent on discussion. One immediate decision was to relocate the central office in eastern Canada by late 1969 or early 1970. The relocation to Ottawa, where office space of 680 square feet had been leased in downtown Ottawa at a cost of $200.00 per month, took place in 1969. The newest staff member, appointed to the position of registrar, was Miss Rita Hudec. This period also ended many years of service to the society by Mrs EI Hood, but Mrs Hood continued to serve as a consultant.

A further result of the Ross Report—a proposal to make changes to the society's major publication—was approved in 1970. *The Canadian Journal of Radiography, Radiotherapy and Nucleography* was published in September of that year in a new format, replacing *Focal Spot*. It was agreed that separate English and French editions of the *Journal* would be printed until it became financially feasible to combine them into one edition. Members stood to show their appreciation at the 1970 annual meeting with lengthy applause for Mr Les Cartwright's years of service as editor of *Focal Spot*.

At the 1972 annual meeting the Ross Report was again dominant as the society continued its restructuring. Miss Rita Hudec had been promoted to the position of certification secretary. Other issues given close scrutiny were the report recommendations that the proxy vote be discontinued and that official delegates were no longer necessary.

THE CSRT BECOMES THE CAMRT

A resolution submitted in 1965 by the Alberta division to change the society's name to the Canadian Society of Medical Radiological Technologists was tabled for one year to allow member societies time for discussion. Readers of the May edition of *Focal Spot* had had the opportunity to read a summary of the debate by student technicians of the Moncton Hospital on this proposal.

In 1966 the tabled resolution regarding the proposed name change was dealt with quickly by the annual meeting: it was tabled for one more year. Shortly thereafter, a resolution to change the name to the Canadian Society of Radiographers was also tabled "until the next annual meeting for study by the Committee on By-laws and for recommendations to be brought forward on the value of this name and any other name describing radiological technicians."

The committee struck to deal with the proposed name change reported to the annual meeting in 1967 that the majority of members did not favour any such change, and the committee recommended no change. Their resolution was approved. The report of the committee that had been appointed to study the effects of adding "medical" to the society's name was received, and the proposal was defeated in 1970.

The society's name, or what some members thought it should be, continued to provide the opportunity for endless debate. A motion to table a proposal changing "technician" to "technologist" was defeated. However, the addition of "medical" to the name came up again, and it was agreed on motion that a committee of three be appointed to study the question and return with a recommendation in 1970.

In 1972 a proposal to change the name again led to a great deal of procedural posturing and to some complicated amendments. The final amendment proposed, to change the name to the Canadian Society of Medical Radiological Technicians, was defeated. Following numerous other suggestions, the matter was again referred to a committee which was to report back in one year. Ultimately, this story came to an end in 1977 when a proposal to change the society's name to the Canadian Association of Medical Radiation Technologists (CAMRT) was approved.

THE 1970s

In 1970 the 28th annual convention was held in Vancouver. At the annual meeting a proposal to amalgamate the Committee on Qualifications, the Committee on Technical Training, and the Post Graduate Education Committee into a Certification Committee was approved. Subsequent annual conventions were held in St. John's, Montréal, Toronto, Saskatoon, Halifax, Winnipeg, Edmonton, Hamilton, Moncton and Vancouver.

By the early 1970s hospital-based training schools had been largely replaced throughout the country by community college programs. The CMA–CSRT Committee on Accreditation, under the chairmanship of Dr EA Rodko was hard at work, and the results of years of planning yielded a comprehensive network of schools which produced technicians educated to national standards.

With respect to educational programs in nuclear medicine technology, a resolution was approved at the 1970 annual meeting "that the CSRT not carry on the association with the Canadian Society of Laboratory Technicians but, in conjunction with the Canadian Association of Radiologists, approve education in nucleography."

At the convention's awards luncheon in 1970, Miss Linda Demkiw, an employee of Toronto Western Hospital, was announced as the 10 000th member to be registered with the society.

A national survey found that annual salaries for general duty ranged from $5559.50 to $7009.25, and those for chief technicians from $7244.42 to $9125.28.

The *Journal* in 1972 celebrated the society's 30th anniversary with a special commemorative edition issued in July. It brought greetings from Prime Minister Pierre Trudeau, Governor General Roland Michener and the Minister of National Health and Welfare John Munro. In addition congratulations were received from each provincial division and from those countries with which the Society enjoys reciprocity: Great Britain, the United States of America, Australia, Holland and Switzerland. Colleagues at the Canadian Medical Association, the Canadian Association of Radiologists and the Canadian Hospital Association sent greetings, as did numerous other organizations and friends. One anonymous member wrote the following: "CELEBRATION. Together we consider the merit of thirty elongated years. Accept my gift. An unseen cake and miles of roses to celebrate this day."

In October 1972, the First International Society of Radiographers and Radiological Technologists' (ISRRT) Congress of the Americas was hosted by CSRT in Toronto. Among the 500 registered delegates were representatives from 12 countries, and all were impressed with the educational programs and hospitality provided. At the closing banquet CSRT President Lewis Edwards presented ISRRT President Merv Allen with a gavel and board to commemorate the occasion, and guests gave congress chairman Terry West a standing ovation for his contribution to both Societies.

During the year the society became a recognized leader in many areas. A request was received from the California Society of Radiologic Technologists asking for permission to use the CSRT career brochure as a guide for a proposed brochure of their own. The South Africa Society of Radiographers asked for information on AC and fellowship examinations.

At the 1973 meeting the term "nucleography" was changed to "nuclear medicine." At the banquet it was announced that the society's latest award, the President's Medal, instituted by President Edwards, had been awarded to two distinguished and deserving members: Ed R Bailey and Arbo A Mattila.

Education at all levels continued to dominate society affairs in 1974, and an ad hoc committee was struck to consider such issues as that of radiologist's assistant programs as they might develop in Canada and the preparation and printing of a course of studies for candidates for advanced certification.

At the 1974 annual meeting, it was established in response to a question that the Committee on Medical Radiological Technician Training was a committee of the Canadian Medical Association, and this fact excluded technicians from serving as head of a survey team.

The *Journal* had been criticized for a year or two, but despite some reverses it continued to flourish. Advertisements showed some increasingly sophisticated equipment, and judged by their publications, technicians kept pace. Long-time contributors such as Cameron, Martin, Flanagan, Hall and Duffey were gradually giving way to Wilson, Mumford, Soni, Scott and Seeram.

A motion was approved at the 1975 annual meeting to allow nuclear medicine candidates, under a grandfather clause, to have one more opportunity to write the certification examination in 1976 under specified conditions.

At central office Norma Saunders had been promoted from membership services secretary to registrar. The board of directors considered the position of a director of education, and 1975 Welch Memorial Lecturer Lewis Edwards was asked to draft a job description, expected qualifications and salary range for the position.

Due to provincial government requirements and directives, the education of students, their examination and the accreditation of training schools was coming under the scrutiny of the Order of Radiology Technicians of Québec (ORTQ). Lengthy discussions ensued at various levels in an attempt to satisfy both parties while maintaining a national standard.

Ultrasound was assuming greater importance, and consideration was given to establishing a syllabus of training and subsequent examinations for certification. This might eventually lead to the formation of another section or discipline within the society.

A proposal received earlier from Holland College, Prince Edward Island was the subject of much discussion at board level. The proposal, supported by Health and Welfare Canada, would result in the production of syllabi using the *dacum* system. This system deals with educational objectives. Subsequently, the offer of federal funding was withdrawn.

A 1976 resolution designed to add one representative from each of the three disciplines to the board of directors was hotly debated but eventually tabled. However, it was decided that it was no longer necessary to have representatives from the Canadian Medical Association and the Canadian Association of Radiologists on the society's board of directors.

At the banquet a special presentation of a grandfather clock was made to Dr and Mrs Marshall Mallett for their many contributions, over many years, to radiography in Canada and the world.

Members were pleased to hear in 1978 that Mr TJD West had been appointed president of ISRRT and that, among other honours, Her Majesty Queen Elizabeth graciously recognized four well-respected association members with Silver Jubilee Medals: Sr MT Gauthier and Messrs George Hall, Ed Bailey and Arbo Mattila.

Also at the 1978 annual meeting a resolution was approved to fully investigate the means by which the association could ensure adequate and responsible representation in the field of labour relations for its members. The matter was referred for investigation to the Personnel Practices Committee, whose recommendations were endorsed in 1970.

In 1979 the Manitoba division—the oldest radiological organization in Canada—celebrated its 50th Anniversary. In the same year it was resolved to hire a director of education, and in 1981 Mr. Robert Broderick, RT(R), BSc, MA(Ed) of Sudbury, Ontario was appointed full time Director of Education.

THE EARLY 1980s

The 38th annual conference took place at Memorial University in St John's, Newfoundland in 1980, and subsequent meetings were held in Regina, Halifax, Toronto and Winnipeg. Head office staff in 1980 were Arbo Mattila, Rita Hudec, Norma Saunders, Anne-Marie Leduc and Judy Verch. The *Journal* advised that the ring was then selling for $238.00.

Negotiations continued with Order of Radiology Technicians of Québec concerning recognition of qualifications, and by 1977 a satisfactory resolution appeared imminent. However, a proposal submitted by OTRQ late in 1977 received a great deal of debate at board of directors' meetings, with representation from all parties involved. A review of the OTRQ examination by the association's experts suggested that the examination was not acceptable, and the association felt OTRQ had not met the terms of the 1977 agreement. The board put forward various proposals whereby successful candidates in Québec could attain association membership. At the 1978 annual general meeting, members formally approved all actions taken by the board in this matter.

The board struck an *ad hoc* committee to deal with CAMRT/OTRQ rapport in the area of certification. The committee, chaired by the association's translator, Mr Ferry de Kerckhove, presented a seven-page report in the *Journal*, and members were given the opportunity to vote by mail-in ballot on the report's very comprehensive recommendations.

The results of the poll reported at the 1981 annual meeting showed that 60 per cent of voters supported the report and the recommendations contained therein; only 400 of over 8500 members voted.

The executive director noted in 1981 that central office had moved into the computer age. He announced changes to the *Journal*, which in 1983 was to be published quarterly supplemented by six issues of a newsletter. The executive director also reported that during the year he had accepted with regret the resignation of Mr Broderick from his position as director of education. Shortly thereafter it was announced that Mr Earl P Rooney, BA, MEd, had been appointed to the position.

In 1982, following years of negotiation, Prince Edward Island was admitted to CAMRT as a division.

Continuing education flourished. The association offered a total of eight correspondence courses ranging from Pathology I, II and III, through Sectional Anatomy I and II, to "Polishing Your Written Communications," "Report Writing for Managers and Supervisors" and "Measuring Student Achievement." All courses were available in English, and Pathology I and II were also available in French. Total enrollment for the year was approximately 450.

In June 1982 the board struck the *Ad Hoc* Committee on Long- and Short-term Planning, with initial emphasis to be on public relations. The company hired to examine the association's image had produced a report which was not in keeping with the instructions given, and it was requested to revise its report accordingly. The new committee would be working closely with the company during the process.

The report of the Conjoint Committees on Accreditation was accepted with enthusiasm. Technologists had paid particular note to one sentence in the report: "He made his chairmanship the subject of a formal review as it is now possible for a technology representative to serve as the committee chairman and the terms of reference do not specify a set length of service for the chairman."

The financial statement of activity showed that total income for the year ended December 31, 1982 was $530 948.00, and that members' equity at the end of the year was $77 308.00. The registrar's report showed that, at the end of 1982 total membership had decreased to 8354 from the 1981 figure of 8614. The ring in 1983 cost $285.00.

The theme for the 1984 annual conference was "Imaging in the '80s." It was the first time central office administered such a conference.

Reflecting the changing technology available, the president in his message said that the board of directors had asked the appropriate committees to re-evaluate training syllabi to take into account nuclear magnetic resonance, digital radiography, computed tomography and positron emission tomography. The association announced the beginning of a joint venture with the Toronto Institute of Medical Technology whereby technologists could obtain advanced certification credits. Cambrian College in Sudbury announced that the first students from their completely bilingual training program would be graduating in 1985.

By 1984 technologist salaries ranged from $16 000.00 to $29 000, and those for chief technologists from $27 000.00 to $39 000.00.

CAMRT had successfully evolved to meet the challenges of another three decades and in 1992 met in Ottawa for an annual meeting that celebrated 50 years of contributions to its members and the people of Canada.

Chapter V • Les débuts de

la société des techniciens en rayons X du Québec

MARIE-FLORE GAGNÉ

C'est dans un cahier aux feuilles jaunies par le temps, précieusement conservé dans un coffre-fort au bureau de l'Ordre des techniciens en radiologie du Québec, que nous pouvons lire les quelques lignes suivantes qui témoignent de la première réunion au cours de laquelle fut créé notre groupement provincial.

"Une réunion fut tenue, mercredi le 10 avril 1940 à 8.00 pm dans la salle 310 du Medical Arts Building, dont le but est de discuter de la formation d'une société des techniciens en rayons X au Québec".

Rosemary O'Hagan du Montréal General Hospital, principale instigatrice de cette réunion de fondation avait été approchée à cet effet par la société ontarienne des techniciens en radiologie (Ontario Society of Radiographers). Elle avait fait parvenir des lettres d'invitation à tous les travailleurs en radiologie de la région montréalaise. Des religieuses des hôpitaux catholiques n'avaient pu, à regret, participer à cette réunion. Les techniciens présents, au nombre de vingt-cinq (25) sont en majorité d'expression anglaise. Au cours de la réunion, Rosemary O'Hagan agit comme présidente et Miss G. Morris de l'Hôpital Général de Lachine, comme secrétaire .

Le conférencier invité, le docteur William L Ritchie, du Montréal General Hospital, traite de l'importance du travail technique bien fait et donne son appui à la création, au Québec, d'une société des techniciens en radiologie à l'instar des autres provinces canadiennes. Le but de cette société sera double: premièrement, améliorer les standards du travail technique au moyen de cours et de démonstrations et deuxièmement, pourvoir la protection des techniciens.

La création d'une société nommément The Montreal X-Ray

Technician Society, est donc proposée et adoptée à l'unanimité. Le docteur Ritchie propose ensuite les initiatives suivantes: la nomination d'un président temporaire de la société, le choix d'officiers pour la prochaine réunion et la mise sur pied de trois comités. Le premier, celui des constitutions et règlements, devra établir des standards professionnels similaires à ceux des autres sociétés; le comité des membres verra à dresser la liste des travailleurs en radiologie et le comité des finances préparera le budget du groupe naissant. Leurs rapports devront être soumis à la prochaine réunion prévue pour les semaines suivantes. il y est également question d'accélérer les procédures afin de doter la société d'une charte.

PREMIÈRES ASSEMBLÉES

Le 23 avril 1940, une assemblée spéciale est tenue à l'Homeopath Hospital pour les religieuses techniciennes des hôpitaux catholiques qui n'avaient pu prendre part à la réunion du 10 avril. Soeur Camille-de-Jésus de l'Hôpital Saint-Jean-de-Dieu y est élue membre du comité exécutif.

Durant cette réunion, il est proposé: de contacter toutes les personnes qui travaillent en radiologie non seulement à Montréal, mais dans toute la province; d'établir un registre des membres, d'identifier les qualifications des candidats et de s'assurer qu'ils travaillent activement en technique de radiologie sous la surveillance d'un radiologiste.

Le 23 novembre suivant, une troisieme réunion a lieu au Montréal General Hospital. On y retrouve entre autres, Rosemary O'Hagan, le docteur Ritchie, le docteur Albert Comtois, radiologiste à l'Hôpital Sainte-Justine, le docteur Adams, radiologiste à l'Homeopathic Hospital et soeur Camille-de-Jésus, technicienne à l'Hôpital Saint-Jean-de-Dieu. Après le mot de bienvenue et la lecture des rapports des comités, le docteur Ritchie fait lecture des règlements en anglais et le docteur Comtois en donne ensuite la version française. On procède à l'élection d'un conseil provisoire dont les membres sont: Rosemary O'Hagan, présidente, soeur Camille-de-Jésus, vice-présidente, Jeanne Pigeon de l'Hôpital Sainte-Justine, secrétaire-trésorière, Agnès Muirhead du Montréal General Hospital archiviste.

Des réunions subséquentes ont lieu au cours de 1941; le 10 janvier, à l'Hôpital du Sacré-Coeur de Cartierville; le 8 février, à laquelle participent cinq hommes et cinquante-sept femmes dont vingt-trois religieuses; le 8 mars où l'on ne retrouve qu'un seul technicien et trente-cinq techniciennes et le 17 avril à l'Hôpital Notre-Dame de l'Espérance.

CHARTE D'INCORPORATION

Enfin, le 28 avril, a lieu la première assemblée générale des membres de la société des techniciens en rayons X de la province de Québec dûment incorporée. Cette assemblée se tient à l'Hôpital Général de Montréal. Y sont approuvés: la charte, les règlements, l'enregistrement et le sceau de la société. Le bureau des gouverneurs sera composé: d'un président honoraire, du président de la société, du vice-président, du secrétaire-trésorier et d'un comité de cinq membres dont trois seront membres actifs de la société et de deux radiologistes. La charte contient des articles concernant: les membres (leurs droits, leur représentation selon la langue, leur admission et expulsion); la régie des biens et fonds de la société; l'élection et les devoirs des officiers; les modalités d'amendement à la Charte; la formation de comités; la tenue des assemblées générales; le fonctionnement de l'exécutif; le quorum.

Les membres seront divisés selon deux catégories: les membres enregistrés et les membres affiliés. Les membres enregistrés sont des techniciens et se classifient de la façon suivante:

a) ceux qui ont satisfait à toutes les exigences de la société et qui travaillent sous la surveillance immédiate d'un radiologiste membre d'une société de radiologie;
b) ceux qui ont satisfait à toutes les exigences de la société, mais qui ne sont pas sous la surveillance immédiate d'un radiologiste tel que défini en (a), mais sous la surveillance immédiate d'un médecin ou chirurgien licencié, possédant un service de rayons X soit à son bureau ou à son hôpital d'attache.

Les membres *affiliés* sont ceux qui ont satisfait à toutes les exigences du bureau des gouverneurs, qui s'occupent en tout temps du travail des rayons X uniquement pour le compte d'un manufacturier distributeur d'appareillage à rayons X et de leurs accessoires. Par le biais des membres affiliés, plusieurs représentants de firmes commerciales pour appareils à rayons X se lient ainsi à la STRQ au cours des premières décennies. Ils rencontrent les techniciens dans leurs services respectifs et sont présents lors des assemblées ou congrès. Par le truchement de leurs représentants, plusieurs compagnies commanditent une réception, un voyage d'agrément ou offrent des prix aux auteurs des meilleurs travaux scientifiques.

Pourront devenir membres enregistrés:

1) tous ceux qui ont eu leur initiation dans la province de Québec, même ceux qui résident en dehors de la province; (ceux qui n'ont pas eu leur initiation dans la province et qui y sont maintenant résidents, sans tenir compte du nombre d'années d'expérience, seront sujets à un examen à moins qu'ils ne soient en mesure de répondre aux exigences de la régie de la société)
2) être de bonnes moeurs et avoir fait des études supérieures ou l'équivalent, tel que démontré par les

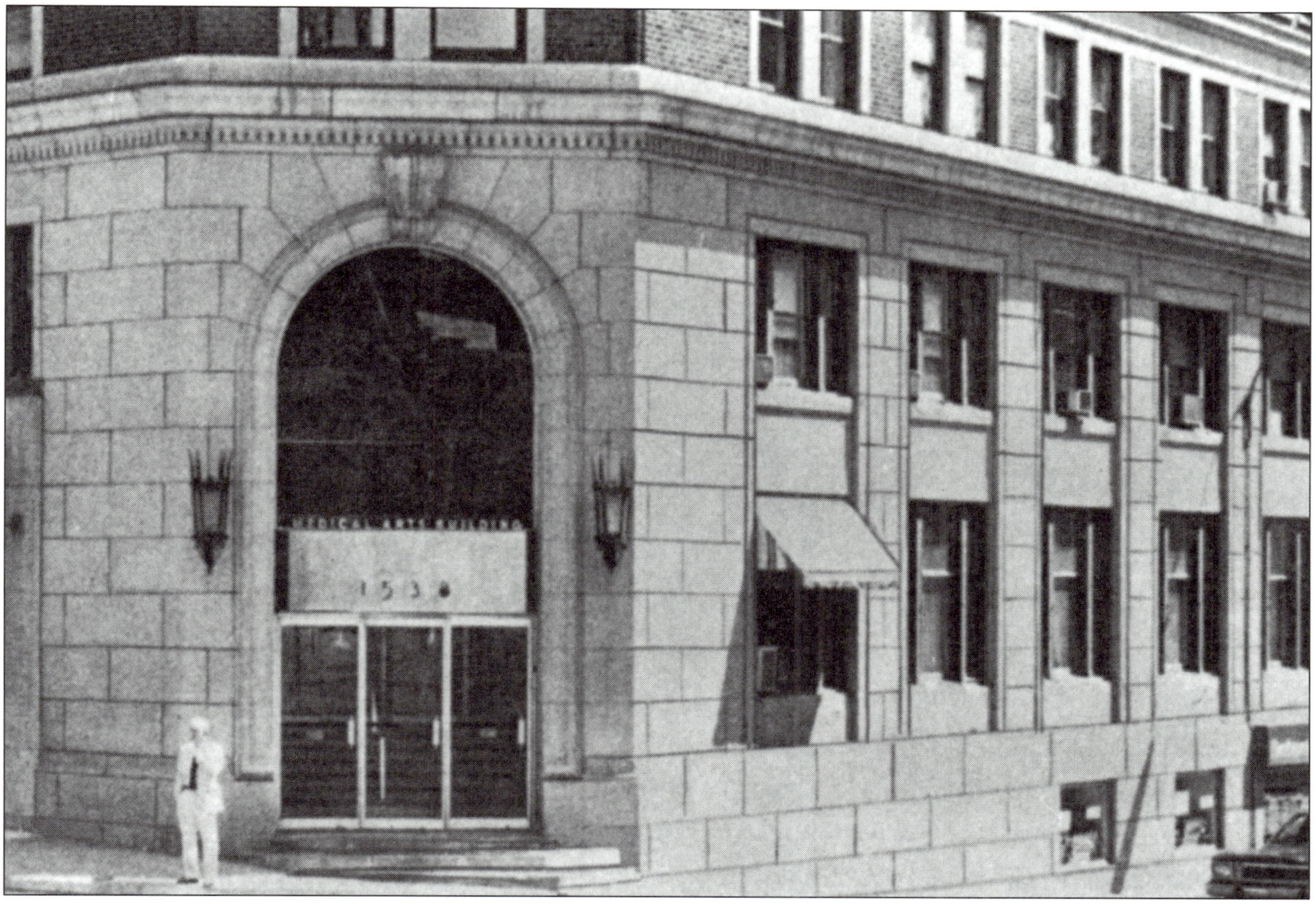

Le Medical Arts Building dont l'édifice existe encore aujourd'hui

certificats approuvés par le bureau des gouverneurs;
3) avoir au moins deux ans d'expérience y compris l'initiation dans les services de rayons X sous la surveillance d'un radiologiste ou surveillant médical;
4) fournir des références de l'employeur, du radiologiste ou du surveillant médical en charge du service et de deux radiologistes membres d'une société ou de deux docteurs en médecine.

La société pourra rejeter la candidature des techniciens employés dans une institution déclarée non conforme aux principes de l'éthique par les organismes médicaux. Le bureau des gouverneurs de la société sera habilité à adopter d'autres règlements et règles définissant plus spécifiquement les qualités requises des membres-aspirants.

Les membres devront se soumettre aux règles suivantes:
1) exécuter le travail et remplir les devoirs d'un technicien en rayons X strictement en conformité avec les règles et règlements du registre;
2) travailler seulement sous la direction et la surveillance d'un radiologiste compétent ou d'un docteur en médecine;
3) ne jamais donner ou écrire un diagnostic excepté sur la réquisition d'un praticien médical à qui la description de l'image vue au cours de l'examen aidera dans la formulation du diagnostic;
4) ne jamais s'occuper du travail des rayons X indépendamment, soit dans un hôpital privé ou bureau ou un service rattaché à une institution.

NORMES D'EXAMEN POUR LES ÉTUDIANTS (1942–44)

En 1942, il est décidé que la période de formation sera de deux années à l'issu desquelles chaque étudiant devra se soumettre à un examen composé de deux parties: l'une écrite, l'autre pratique. À cause de la difficulté d'évaluer les candidats quant à l'application pratique de la technique, les candidats devront présenter leurs pellicules radiographiques certifiées par leur chef comme ayant été réalisées par le candidat, sans assistance. On ne décerne un certificat qu'aux aspirants qui ont réussi l'examen avec une mention minimum de 70 % pour l'examen écrit et de 85 % pour le travail pratique.

Les examens se tiendront, en français et en anglais, le

dernier samedi d'avril et d'octobre de chaque année à un endroit déterminé par la société. En réussissant l'examen, le candidat devient à la fois membre de la société canadienne et de sa propre société provinciale. Il est convenu que tout technicien membre d'une société provinciale, le premier juillet 1942, est éligible pour la société canadienne. Mais qu'à partir de cette date, il sera obligatoire de passer les examens. Les questions d'examens seront préparées au niveau provincial, révisées et approuvées par la société canadienne, renvoyées aux différentes provinces pour être présentées aux étudiants et de nouveau, retournées à la SCTR pour correction.

Cette formule s'avère un échec. On mettra bientôt sur pied, un bureau provincial des examens qui s'ajoute au bureau central. Mais les examens préparés par le bureau provincial doivent toujours être approuvés au central. Et même si les corrections sont maintenant effectuées au bureau provincial, les résultats des examens sont encore soumis au bureau central. Cette méthode cause donc des retards et de la confusion.

Le premier examen officiel des étudiants se tient toutefois le 29 avril 1944, à l'Hôpital Saint-Jean-de-Dieu de Montréal. Les examinateurs sont les docteurs WL Ritchie et Albert Comtois. La collation des diplômes est présidée par le docteur Jean Bouchard qui remet aux gradués leur médaille et leur certificat de technicien en radiologie.

En raison des déficiences dans les procédures d'examens, on cherche une formule plus pratique. En 1944, lors du congrès tenu à Winnipeg, une résolution est adoptée à l'effet que la SCTR[7] en collaboration avec chaque province, prépare un examen uniforme pour tout le Canada. À partir de ce moment, la formation des étudiants s'achemine vers une formule plus précise et plus efficace.

PROJET D'UNE ÉCOLE DE FORMATION POUR LES ÉTUDIANTS

En 1946, la STRQ réfléchit sur la possibilité d'une école pour la formation des techniciens en radiologie. Déjà, une nouvelle série de cours est offerte aux étudiants à l'Hôpital Royal Victoria et un cours de physique est donné aux étudiants du Montréal General Hospital. On espère une école de formation affiliée à l'Université McGill. Mais, rien ne sera fait avant de recevoir le programme de la Société américaine des techniciens en radiologie qui existe depuis 1920 et qui possède des centres de formation pour ses étudiants.

Soeur Camille-de-Jésus commencera toutefois à donner un cours de formation de deux ans avec étudiants de langue francaise, à l'Hôpital Saint-Jean-de-Dieu. On espère que ce cours sera approuvé par l'Université de Montréal et celui des étudiants de langue anglaise par l'Université McGill.

C'est pourtant lentement que s'établit un programme de plus en plus perfectionné, pour la formation des étudiants. Au début de 1946, la STRQ demande à l'Association canadienne des radiologistes sa coopération pour l'établissement d'un cours de formation des techniciens en radiologie. De plus, la société s'intéresse à la situation des techniciens enregistrés et nonenregistrés, dans les différentes hôpitaux, en ce qui concerne: les salaires, le travail supplémentaire et la durée des vacances annuelles.

D'après le rapport de la société pour l'année 1946–1947, la province compte un total de quarante-sept membres étudiants. De ce nombre, quatorze se présentent aux examens de la société tenus le 2 mai 1946 à l'Homeopathic Hospital de Montréal. Le premier novembre suivant, treize étudiants se présentent aux examens de la société. De ce nombre, dix obtiennent leur certificat.

Lors des congrès annuels de la Société canadienne en 1945 et 1946, plusieurs questions relatives à la formation des étudiants sont soulevées. Elles se rapportent principalement à l'établissement d'un curriculum et aux méthodes de formation des étudiants à travers tout le Canada. Les politiques de formation établies par la STRQ seront, à partir de 1946, communiquées à tous les responsables des services de radiologie où l'on accepte des étudiants. Désormais, la STRQ n'acceptera que les étudiants qui pratiquent sous la surveillance d'un radiologiste reconnu et le temps de formation sera de deux années. La Société recommande que les radiologistes et les techniciens seniors organisent une série de conférences mensuelles, le soir, pour les étudiants de langue anglaise et d'autre pour les étudiants de langue française.

À la réunion de l'exécutif de la STRQ, en novembre 1946, Rosemary O'Hagan, présidente, presse le docteur BC Pierce, président honoraire de favoriser l'établissement d'un cours régulier pour la formation des étudiants-techniciens.

L'exécutif décide dès lors d'améliorer le curriculum pour les étudiants, lequel pourrait servir de guide pour l'enseignement. Un comité est formé à cette fin et les membres sont: Rosemary O'Hagan, présidente, EM Peterson, Rose Ducharme, JA MacLean et Rosina McHardy. Le 21 avril 1947, le comité soumet le curriculum au bureau des gouverneurs qui le présente ensuite à l'Assemblée générale annuelle de mai 1947 sous le titre: *Recommandations de la société des techniciens pour l'entrainement des radiographes*. Une fois approuvé par les membres, le nouveau curriculum est envoyé à tous les directeurs et radiologistes des hôpitaux où on forme des techniciens en radiologie. La société exige aussi que dorénavant, tous les clichés présentés par les étudiants, lors des examens, soient accompagnés d'un affidavit signé par le radiologiste ou le directeur en charge.

STATUTS ET RÈGLEMENTS DE LA S.C.T.R. POUR LA FORMATION DES ÉTUDIANTS

En avril 1947, le journal de la SCTR le *Focal Spot* publie les STATUTS ET RÈGLEMENTS révisés du bureau des examinateurs de la SCTR. Ceux-ci ont été préparés par le bureau des examinateurs, le bureau des directeurs et les directeurs associés de chaque province et ils représentent un accord général. Les principaux points sont:

1. Formation du bureau des examinateurs
   a) le bureau des examinateurs sera composé de deux radiologistes dont un bilingue et d'un technicien-membre enregistré de la SCTR;
   b) leur mandat sera de trois ans.
2. Qualifications des candidats
   a) les candidats devront posséder une immatriculation junior ou son équivalent et devront avoir participé à deux ans de formation sous la surveillance d'un radiologiste qualifié.
   b) le candidat ne possèdant pas les qualifications requises, devra soumettre sa demande au bureau des examinateurs de la SCTR par le biais d'un membre de la société provinciale concernée.
3. Demande pour examen
   a) les demandes pour examen seront faites par les candidats aux secrétaires des sociétés-membres. Après approbation par l'exécutif provincial, les demandes seront transmises au président du bureau des examinateurs;
   b) les demandes devront être présentées au bureau des examinateurs au moins un mois avant la date fixée pour l'examen;
   c) chaque candidat recevra un numéro de code qui accompagnera la lettre d'approbation envoyée au secrétaire de la société-membre;
   d) les candidats seront avertis par le secrétaire de leur société-membre de la date et du lieu de l'examen.
4. Détails concernant les examens
   a) l'examen se tiendra le premier vendredi de mai et de novembre de chaque année;
   b) le secrétaire de chaque société provinciale verra à la nomination de surveillants et choisira le lieu de l'examen. Les surveillants seront radiologistes, là où c'est possible, ou médecins ou surintendants d'hôpitaux ou membre exécutif de la société provinciale. Aucun candidat ne sera sous la surveillance de personnel de son hôpital ou de sa clinique d'attache. Les questions seront préparées par le bureau des examinateurs et seront traduites en français par une personne désignée à cet effet;
   c) les examens seront composés de deux parties: l'une écrite, l'autre pratique. L'examen écrit comprendra cinq sujets: anatomie, procédé de développement des films, physique et appareillage, techniques de radiographies, radiothérapie. L'examen pratique sera constitué d'un certain nombre de films réalisés par le technicien selon des techniques choisies par le bureau des examinateurs. Ces films, remis pas plus de quatre jours suivant l'examen écrit, seront appréciés au point de vue radiographique et technique de développement;
   d) le numéro de code du candidat devra apparaître clairement sur chaque page de l'examen écrit et sur les films. Ces derniers seront bien identifiés quant à la date et au lieu de leur réalisation;
   e) les feuilles de réponses et les films seront envoyés par le secrétaire de la société-membre au président du bureau des examinateurs.
5. Correction des examens
   a) le président du bureau des examinateurs distribuera les copies d'examens et les films aux deux autres membres du bureau. Après la correction, le résultat final sera envoyé au secrétaire des sociétés-membres et à l'éditeur du *Focal Spot;*
   b) pour réussir l'examen, le candidat devra obtenir un minimum de 60 % sur l'ensemble des sujets et un minimum de 50 % pour chacun des sujets;
   c) un échec dans plus de deux sujets nécessitera la reprise totale de l'examen. Les candidats ayant réussi l'examen recevront leur certificat de la société provinciale.
6. Reprise d'examens
   a) un étudiant qui a échoué à l'ensemble des sujets de l'examen peut se représenter à l'examen ultérieur;
   b) un étudiant qui a échoué à un ou deux sujets peut repasser l'examen seulement sur ces sujets à la prochaine période d'examens;
   c) un étudiant qui échoue à trois occasions, n'aura plus la permission de se présenter de nouveau;
   d) ces conditions peuvent être réexaminées par le bureau des examinateurs, en des circonstances spéciales.
7. Frais d'examens
   a) les frais d'examens sont fixés à 5 $ et devront accompagner la demande d'examen écrit ou encore les reprises;

b) les frais d'une reprise de un ou deux sujets seront de 3 $ et devront accompagner la demande de reprise;

c) le secrétaire des sociétés-membres fera parvenir 50 % de tous les frais d'examens au secrétaire-trésorier de la SCTR.

8. Contenu des examens
L'examen comporte, en 1946–1947, les matières suivantes: anatomie, physique et appareillage, chambre noire (procédé de développement des films), technique de radiographie (théorique et appliquée) et radiothérapie. Les questions sont de type traditionnel et requièrent des réponses élaborées. Les feuilles de questions présentées aux étudiants proviennent de la Société canadienne des techniciens en radiologie et portent le sceau de la société provinciale. Le temps alloué pour chaque matière est d'une heure et demie.

9. Amendements de 1948
L'assemblee annuelle de la SCTR, en juin 1948, tenue à Québec revise les STATUTS ET RÈGLEMENTS concernant les examens sur les points suivants:

a) le candidat en plus de posséder son immatriculation junior ou son équivalent et avoir complété sa formation sous la direction d'un radiologiste qualifié, sera âgé d'au moins 21 ans;

b) le candidat de 21 ans ne possédant pas les qualifications mentionnées ci-haut, verra sa candidature soumise au bureau des examinateurs de la SCTR par la société-membre impliquée.

L'examen régulier se tiendra toujours le premier vendredi de mai et de novembre de chaque année. Cependant, en cas d'urgence et à la discrétion des officiers et membres de l'exécutif de la société-membre concernée, il sera permis de tenir un examen le jour précédent ou le jour suivant la date fixée pour l'examen. Cette décision requiert la permission du bureau des examinateurs.

CONGRÈS ANNUELS

À partir de 1946, année qui suit la tenue du congrès annuel de la SCTR à Montréal, la STRQ donne plus d'envergure à ses assemblées générales annuelles, qu'elle nommera dorénavant CONGRÈS ANNUELS.

Le 18 mai 1946, une quarantaine de techniciens du Québec, sous la présidence de Jeanne Gagné, se réunissent en congrès à l'hôtel Windsor de Montréal. Les docteurs Albert Jutras et J-W McKay en sont les présidents d'honneur. Sept conférences y sont présentées: quatre par des techniciens et trois par des radiologistes. En 1947 et en 1949, le congrès annuel se tient également à l'hôtel Windsor. Toutefois, en 1948, l'assemblée générale de la société provinciale se tenant à l'Hôpital Saint-Jean-de-Dieu, décide de concentrer ses énergies, pour cette année, à sa participation au 6e congrès de la SCTR tenu au Château Frontenac de Québec, les 17 et 18 juin.

ÉTATS FINANCIERS

Durant sa première décennie d'existence, la STRQ voit ses finances progresser. À l'assemblée générale annuelle de la STRQ, le 8 mai 1942, à l'Hôpital Sainte-Justine, la trésorière donne le rapport financier suivant:

Recettes:	925,06 $
Dépenses:	435,78 $
En banque:	489,28 $

En 1943, l'état de compte est meilleur en raison de l'augmentation du nombre de techniciens enregistrés:

Recettes:	1 311,65 $
Dépenses:	594,81 $
En banque:	716,84 $

En 1946, le rapport financier se présente comme suit:

Recettes:	1 251,72 $
Dépenses:	1 183,74 $
En banque:	67,98 $

PREMIÈRE REVUE DE LA STRQ

À une assemblée tenue le 24 janvier 1942, Rosemary O'Hagan propose la publication d'une revue à l'intention des membres de la S.T.R.Q. pour les informer sur la société et autres sujets d'intérêt pour eux. Cette revue publiera aussi les textes des conférences données par les radiologistes lors des assemblées régulières et annuelles des techniciens.

Cette revue paraît en 1942, sous le titre: *Bulletin 1941–1942*. Elle est publiée en français et en anglais et donne la liste des membres enregistrés, étudiants et associés. À cette date, le nombre des membres enregistrés est de 74, (5 hommes et 69 femmes dont 41 religieuses); le nombre d'étudiants de 25 et celui des membres associés de 15, pour un total de 110 membres. Ce bulletin paraît de nouveau en 1943.

En cette même année, la SCTR est constituée et décide de publier sa propre revue, le *Focal Spot*. Les nouvelles et activités de chaque société provinciale y seront publiées à la condition que les responsables provinciaux[9] fassent parvenir les articles d'intérêt. Le tarif d'abonnement à cette revue est de 1$. Les articles sont publiés en français ou en anglais, selon la langue des auteurs. Une revue bilingue, *Écho-X*, sera en outre publiée au Québec en 1964 et deviendra la revue officielle des techniciens de la province[10].

Chapter VI • *The Canadian Organization of Medical Physics*

JOHN ALDRICH

From the very earliest use of radiation in medicine the medical profession turned to the universities for help. In Montréal, Professor John Cox of McGill helped in the production of the first Canadian clinical x-ray. In Halifax the first Canadian radon emanation plant was assembled by Dr Henderson, the professor of physics at Dalhousie University in 1925. The radium was purchased with monies left over from the relief fund for the Halifax Explosion of 1917. In Saskatchewan Professor EL Harrington used Henderson's design for his radon plant, built for the Saskatchewan Cancer Committee in 1931. This plant remained in operation until 1962. Harrington's involvement in cancer therapy led to the appointment in 1945 of Dr HE Johns to the physics department and as physicist to the Saskatchewan Cancer Commission. As is well known, Harold Johns initiated and actively developed world class medical physics programs, first in Saskatchewan (1945–1956) and later at the Ontario Cancer Institute in Toronto (1956–1980).

In the late 1940s and '50s medical physics groups were developing in other parts of Canada, notably British Columbia under Dr HF Batho and Québec under Dr LG Stephens-Newsham.

After graduating from McGill in 1948 Dr Stephens-Newsham went to Halifax, where he supervised the move of the radon plant—designed by Dr Henderson—to the new hospital. He also calibrated the new high energy x-ray tubes which had just been acquired. He then initiated a radioisotope laboratory for medical work. In 1951 he moved to the Royal Victoria Hospital in Montréal. Here he was involved in setting up a new therapy building and designing radioisotope laboratories and scanning facilities. With Dr Murray Telford and Dr John Crawford of the physics department of McGill he was involved in the design of an 8-MeV linear accelerator which became operative in 1965. In 1955 Dr René Beique was appointed physicist at Montréal General Hospital, Dr Roger Mathieu at Notre Dame. Later, Mr Jacques LaPalme was appointed to the staff of the Hôtel Dieu de Montréal, and Dr JL Wolfson to the Jewish General Hospital.

Dr Gordon E Richards, who was head of the Ontario Institute of Radiotherapy in Toronto in the 1930s, was an innovator in radiotherapy. He installed the first 400-kVp therapeutic unit, the only teleradium unit in Canada, and made the first attempts to employ low temperatures (i.e., liquid air) in conjunction with radiation in the treatment of cancer and for the control of pain. He recognized the need for physics assistance in his pioneering endeavours, and in the 1930s he enlisted the help of Professor JR MacLennan of the Department of Physics at the University of Toronto. For a short time in 1941 Dr JR Hines was the first physicist working full time in Ontario.

When the Ontario Cancer Treatment and Research Foundation (OCTRF) was formed in 1948 with Dr Richards as its medical director, Mr JG Brown was appointed as physicist. After a year's training at the Royal Cancer Hospital (now Royal Marsden) in London, England he returned to work at the Toronto General Hospital and later at the London clinic of the foundation, where he was joined by Mr PM Pfalzner.

In 1949 AF Holloway joined the foundation, and after receiving his PhD at the Royal Cancer Hospital in London, he returned to the Kingston clinic of OCTRF. In 1954 he succeeded Dr Pat MacDonald as Director of Physics at the Manitoba Cancer Foundation in Winnipeg. There he established an active medical physics group dealing with many aspects of medical physics: health physics, radiotherapy, imaging and biophysics. In 1980 he joined the Radiological Research Laboratories in Toronto, where he did research on radiation dosimetry as it related to medical imaging.

Dr JCF MacDonald was the third of these early OCTRF physicists, entering the field in 1951. After experience in the United Kingdom and Sweden he was appointed to the staff of the radiotherapy department of the Toronto General Hospital until 1957; Dr RG Baker came on staff in 1955. In 1957 Dr MacDonald became chief physicist at the London clinic of OCTRF. At the Centre for Chemical Physics at the University of Western Ontario, he participated in the design and construction of the AECL prototype racetrack microtron for radiotherapy in the 1970s, and pioneered work in the radiation sterilization of hospital linens. Many of his students are still active in Canadian medical physics. He retired in 1985.

Dr RJ Horsley, one of Dr Johns' earlier students, joined OCTRF at the Hamilton clinic in 1953 and was joined by RH Price in 1961. Dr Horsley later spent a sabbatical at the Gray Laboratories at Mount Vernon Hospital London, where he became interested in fundamental aspects of radiobiology. He returned to Hamilton, where he continued these interests and created an active physics group.

Following the development of the NRX reactor at Chalk River it was possible to produce high-specific-activity cobalt-60. The development of the cobalt teletherapy unit for cancer therapy in 1951 by Dr Johns' group, and independently by AECL, was probably the single most important step in the evolution of medical physics in Canada. The Atomic Energy Control Board has since insisted upon the presence of a trained medical physicist wherever such a unit was installed.

By 1954 the physicists employed in the seven centres of the Ontario Cancer Foundation had formed an association to advise the foundation and to "provide collective discussion and action for the advancement of the application of physics to radiation therapy." At its first meeting the secretary was instructed to communicate with other physicists working in the medical field across Canada with the intention of forming a Canadian Association of Medical Physicists (CAMP). Since the Canadian Association of Physicists (CAP) was concerned mainly with the interests of academic physicists and the Canadian Association of Radiology (CAR) was primarily a medical body with little interest by physicians in the problems of their non-medical colleagues, the recognition medical physicists required was not forthcoming from either of the two well-established organizations.

This situation led to the formation of CAMP in 1955. CAR—with whom the medical physicists worked closely—and CAP were concerned about this independent action on the part of a small group of medical physicists, and both actively worked to absorb this fledgling organization into the more well-established bodies. CAP, in an unprecedented step, decided to set up a division of medical physics, the first of many such limited interest groups in the physics community. This move was accepted by the members of CAMP and the Division of Medical and Biological Physics (DMBP) of CAP was established.

One of the first steps undertaken by DMBP was an attempt at certification of competency in medical physics, thus providing a basis for recognition by government agencies. This action was ill-conceived and premature and was not resolved for many years. However, for over 35 years DMBP was the official body representing physicists working in the fields of biological and medical research and application in Canada. Within the limitations imposed by a small population, a very large country and a variety of employment situations, DMBP did a creditable job, both as a scientific and a professional organization. Its most regular function was the organization of scientific meetings on a yearly basis. It has been the organization representing Canada at the International Organization of Medical Physics since about 1970. It organized the 4th International Conference on Medical Physics in Ottawa in 1976. In addition it provided many provincial and national committees—for example, Health and Welfare, the Atomic Energy Control Board and the Healing Arts and Radiation Protection Committee (Ontario)—with expert advice, especially on matters of radiation protection.

In 1979 the physicists working in a hospital environment in the fields of radiation therapy, nuclear medicine and medical imaging (most of whom were members of DMBP) recognized again the need for a peer review process to establish competency in the application of physics in the medical environment. To meet this need the Canadian College of Physicists in Medicine (CCPM) was legally established under a Canadian government charter.

Initially, a well-established medical physicist was admitted to fellowship in the college on the basis of his or her credentials (including years of experience, peer-reviewed publications, and recommendations from colleagues). The first board was composed of Ms SO Fedoruk, Dr AF Holloway, Dr HE Johns, Dr JCF MacDonald, Dr RM Mathieu and Mrs MEJ Young. Fellowship is now granted after passing a comprehensive written examination followed by an oral examination, both conducted by the examining board of the college. The written examination is in two parts, the second of which is based on a published bank of 110 questions which serve both as syllabus and examination format. The questions are revised regularly to reflect developments and changes in medical physics.

While the fellowship was designed to establish excellence in medical physics, by 1983 there arose a need to certify competence in the medical physics specialities. This need was met by the establishment of a membership category, which can be obtained after a shorter period of experience and by passing the written examinations only. A member is expected to attempt to attain the fellowship when his or her experience and publication record meet the required standards.

In recent years the college, following its original mandate, has established a coordinated series of symposia with a view to the continuing education of fellows and members. It is also involved in presenting the position of the medical physicist in discussions with governmental regulatory bodies and other professional organizations within and outside Canada.

In the mid–eighties the medical physicists once again reviewed their relationship with CAP. After much discussion it was decided to form a separate umbrella organization, the Canadian Organization of Medical Physics, combining the scientific and professional role of DMBP with that of the college. The new organization came into being in 1989.

The late seventies were a time of great expansion in medical physics. To try to plan for such expansion the executive of DMBP predicted in 1978 that the number of professional medical physicists would double in the following 10 years! Their prediction would prove to be correct. The main medical physicist groups in Canada have been associated with the major hospitals and cancer centres. Two exceptions are the research centres which have developed around the Robarts Centre in London and the Reichman Institute at Sunnybrook Hospital in Toronto.

Medical physicists in Canada have close ties with their medical colleagues in diagnostic imaging and radiation oncology as well as with their university counterparts. Annual meetings, reflecting this pluralistic interaction, have been held with the Canadian Association of Physicists, the Canadian Association of Radiologists, the American Association of Physicists in Medicine, the Canadian Association of Radiation Oncology, and the Canadian Medical and Biological Engineering Society.

Canadian physicists have been pleased to be involved with the organization of several important international conferences:

International Congress of Radiology, Montréal, 1962
International Congress of Medical Physics, Ottawa, 1976
Inter-American Meeting of Medical Physics, Chicago, 1984
International Organization of Medical Physics, San Antonio, 1988
International Radiation Research Conference, Toronto, 1991

Several Canadian medical physicists have been honoured with national and international recognition as follows:

The Coolidge Award (AAPM): HE Johns and JR Cunningham
Order of Canada: HE Johns
Lieutenant-Governor of Saskatchewan: Sylvia Fedoruk

In this centennial year Canadian medical physicists look forward with optimism to the future. From a slow and somewhat late beginning, medical physics in Canada has over the last 40 years grown to become a vital and active discipline employing nearly 250 full-time physicists. Despite reorganizations and budget restrictions the number of medical physicists continues to increase, and interest from undergraduate and graduate students is at an all-time high. The illustrious efforts of the pioneer physicists have made a solid foundation for future progress.

Acknowledgement:

This article is based upon historical material provided by many colleagues, especially John Macdonald, Jack Cunningham, Lloyd Stephens-Newsham and Doug Cormack.

Opposite right
Chairpersons 1975–1989

Opposite below
Chairpersons 1989–1994

Below
Chairpersons 1955–1974

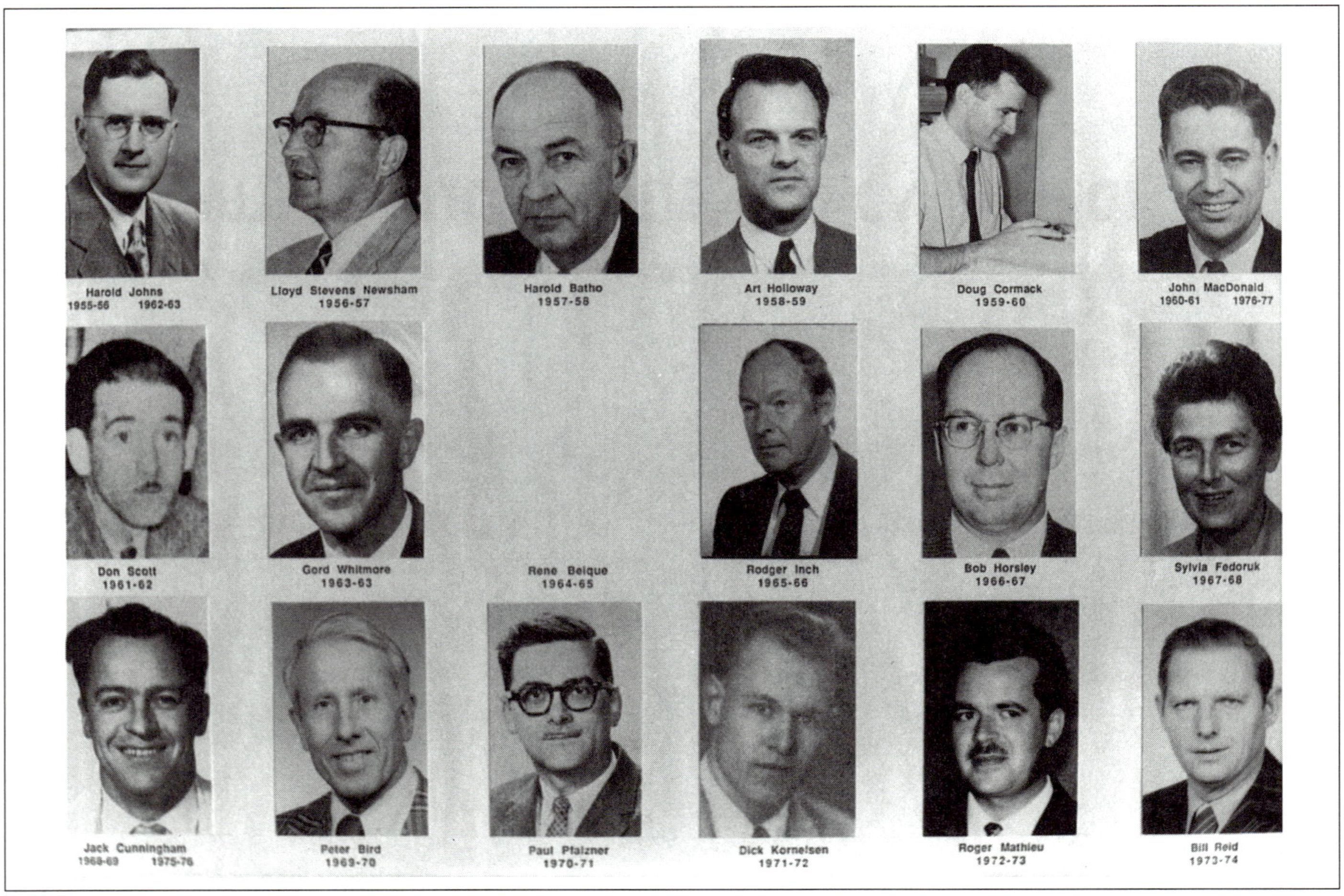

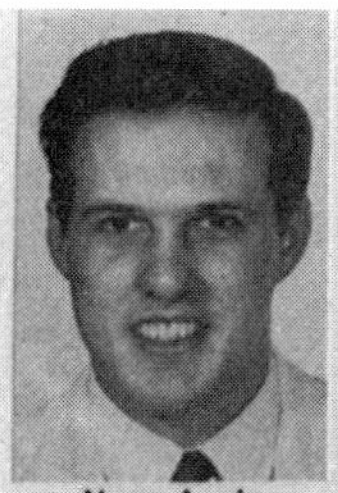

Norm Aspin
1974-75

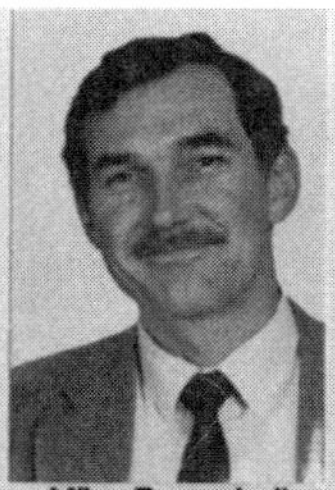

Mike Rapacholi
1977-78

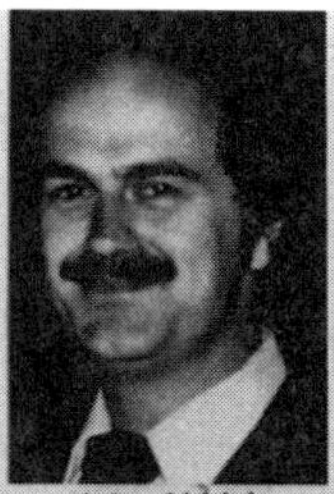

John Aldrich
1978-79

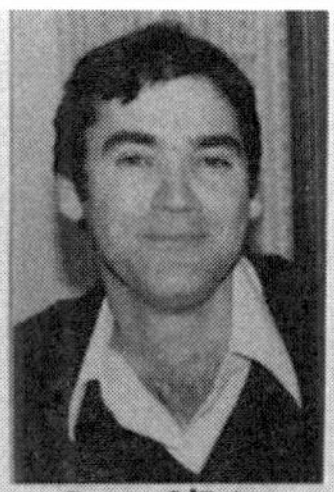

Peter O'Brien
1979-80

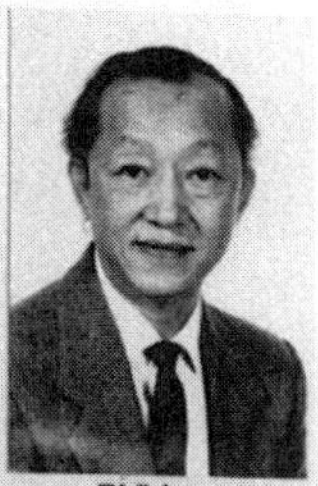

Phil Leung
1980-81

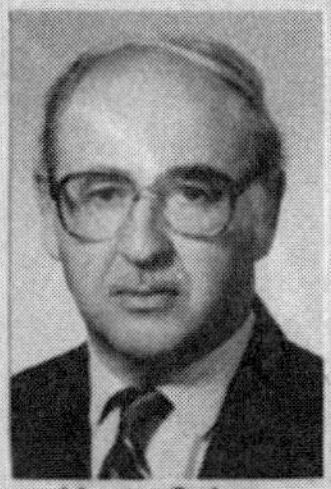

Monty Cohen
1981-82

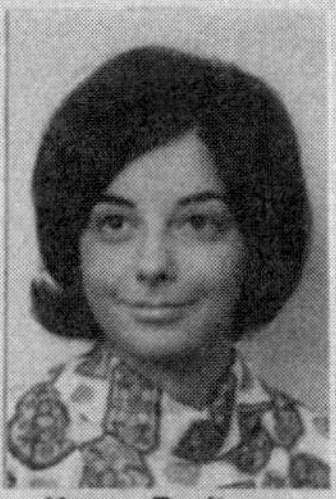

Karen Breitman
1982-83

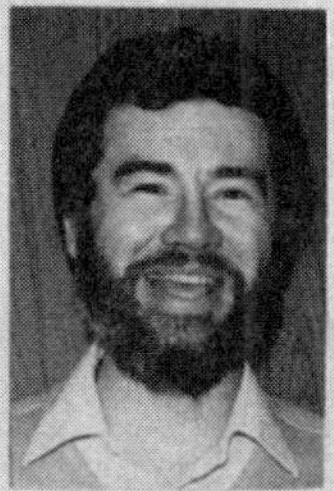

Dave Rogers
1983-84

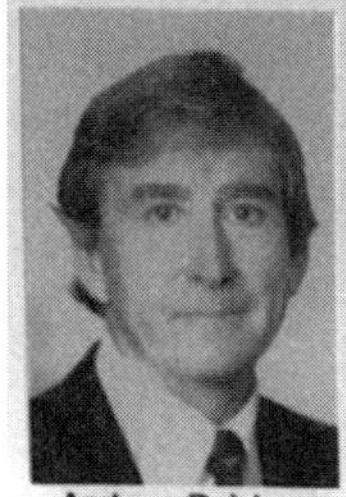

Andrew Rainbow
1984-85

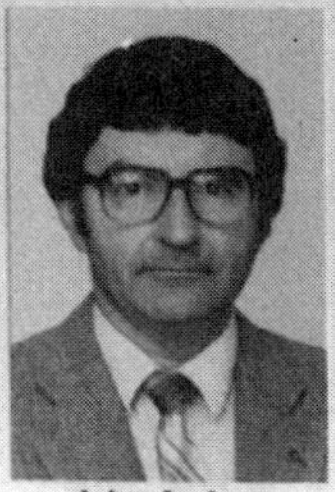

John Andrew
1985-86

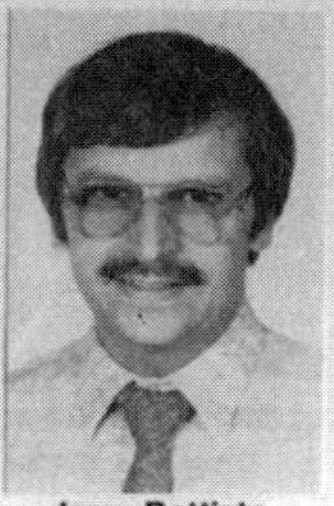

Jerry Battista
1986-87

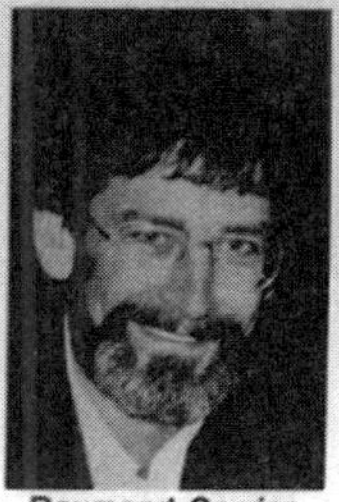

Raymond Carrier
1987-88

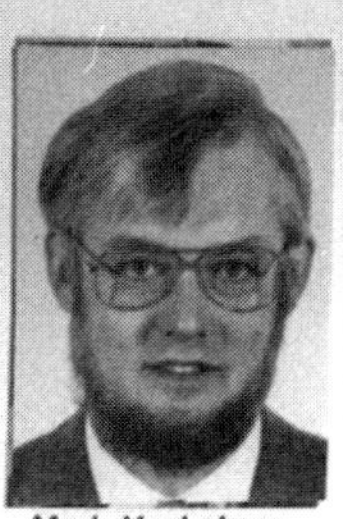

Mark Henkelman
1988-89

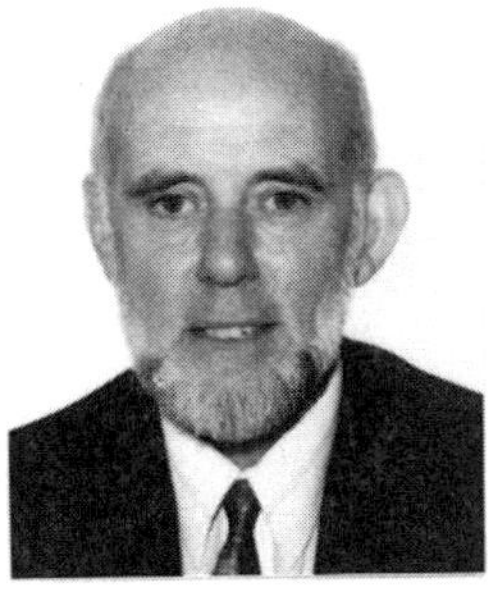

Chris Thompson
1989-90

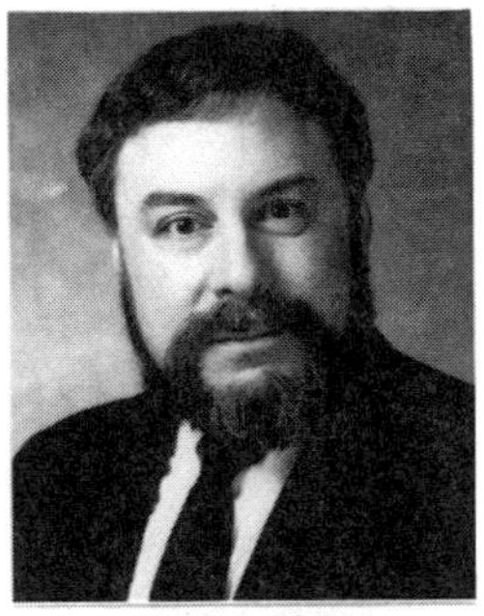

Martin Yaffe
1990-91

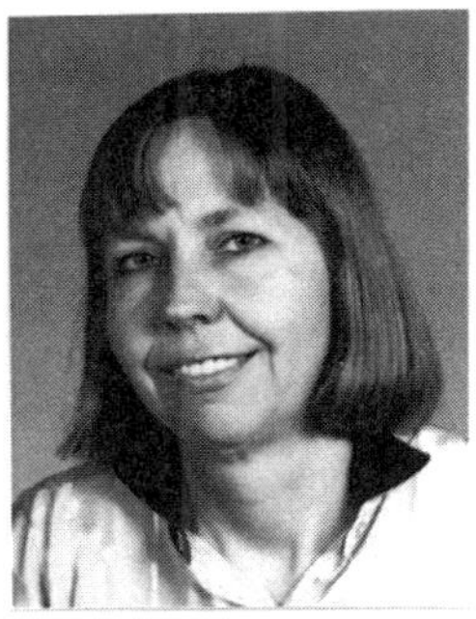

Ellen El-Khatib
1991-92

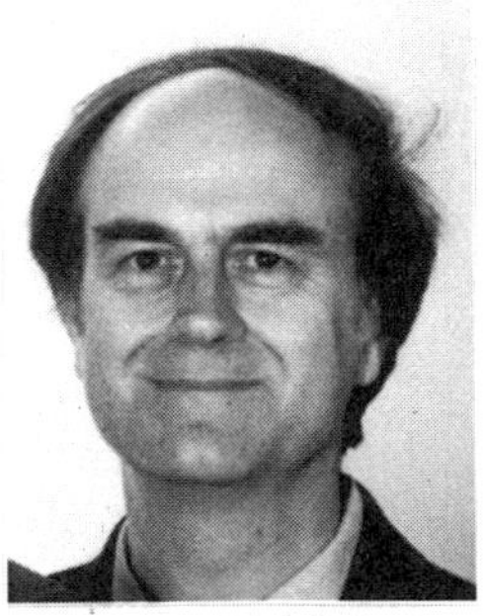

John Aldrich
1992-93

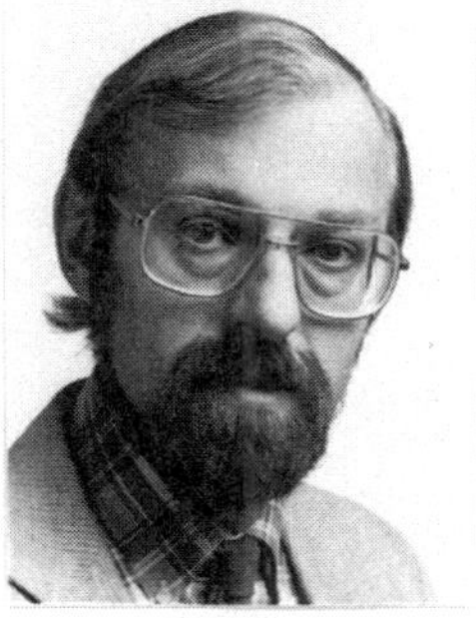

Aaron Fenster
1993-94

Chapter VII •

The Canadian Association of Nuclear Medicine *and the* Society of Nuclear Medicine in Canada

Brian Lentle

As nuclear medicine evolved into a coherent subject with its own expanding knowledge base,[1] the question of its recognition as a specialty became inevitable. The early practitioners of nuclear medicine were most often radiologists (Hector Duggan in Alberta, Leonard Rosenthall in Montréal), endocrinologists (Hamish McIntosh in Vancouver), pathologists or other specialists who grew with and into the new discipline as it developed.

The first meeting to consider the formation of a national specialty society took place in 1971. What emerged was the Canadian Association of Nuclear Medicine, whose presidents are listed in an appendix.

However, events had already moved much more quickly in Québec. In this context no less than in others, Québec led not only North America but the world. A professional association of nuclear physicians came into being in 1967; a certifying examination followed in 1969. The impetus for these developments chiefly came from Jacques Lamoureux, Étienne LeBel, Leonard Rosenthall and Joseph Sternberg.

By 1972 an examination was in place in the United States to provide for board certification in nuclear medicine. The Royal College then created a task force to examine the issue of specialty recognition. In 1976 the first certifying examinations in Canada were held in nuclear medicine, a difficult task entrusted to the chairmanship of Dr Bernard Shapiro. We who were candidates, conscious already of advancing years and declining powers, took ourselves to Toronto for a long weekend one month before the event to listen to ourselves expound upon our strengths and to remedy or hide our weakness.

The examination papers from 1976 are included in an annex. They have not become as dated as one might fear. But the instructions comprise an intelligence test in their own right, and their sheer length suggests that what was really being tested was stamina as much as knowledge.

In Canada the growth of nuclear medicine owes much to many physicians. In addition to those mentioned elsewhere can be listed Drs Bernard Shapiro, Michael Chamberlain, Brian Lentle, Albert Driedger, David Greenberg and Adel Mattar, who have served as chairs of the Royal College Examination Committee in the English language, and Alex Wilkinson and Raymonde Chartrand who have served as chairs of the Royal College Specialty Committee. Dr Jean Leveille has been particularly long serving in the chair of the Royal College Examination Committee in the French language.

The Canadian Association of Nuclear Medicine (CANM) has published a policy statement concerning the nuclear medicine physician and radiation safety. As well through the Canadian Medical Association CANM had a policy ratified to have provincial medical associations "develop standards to designate those physicians...who are appropriately qualified to direct and be responsible for nuclear medicine facilities..." A second policy had the "CMA encourage provincial authorities at the earliest possible date to require certification...in the specialty of nuclear medicine as the standard qualification for physicians who are newly designated to direct clinical nuclear medicine facilities."

The world now is pluralistic in a manner that would have astonished our distant professional forebears. And yet nuclear medicine has always depended upon the effective cooperation of technologists and physicians and often—especially in larger and academic services—radiopharmacists, physicists and computer scientists as well. In the late 1980s this interdependence has been recognized by the formation of the Society of Nuclear Medicine in Canada (SNMC), whose first two chairs were Al Driedger and John Scott. Their successors are listed in an appendix. SNMC, the birth of which is documented in Annexes B and C, arose for two reasons. One was an increasing realization that nuclear medicine faced political and regulatory problems in Canada which owed little or nothing to the boundaries between disciplines. The other was that Canadian members of the Society of Nuclear Medicine recognized that a part of their dues went to sustain a political lobby in the United States and that it was time to repatriate that money and apply it to Canadian issues.

No history is complete which looks at only one axis of time, and in a young and evolving specialty it is particularly important to use the past as a measure of the future. Paradoxically, 1990 is a period of ambiguity in that future. The opportunities are considerable. The revolution in molecular biology is providing some very specific probes to diagnose a variety of diseases, promising to change the diagnosis of cancer by the use of imaging methods. There is even renewed interest in, and success with, such approaches to treat some cancers, reviving the idea of the "magic bullet." Other new radiopharmaceuticals enable us to image blood flow to the heart and brain, while suitable receptor-binding tracers may bring the techniques of positron tomography into day-to-day clinical practice. In the midst of this growing excitement it is disappointing to note that there is a shortage of nuclear physicians in the country, particularly in academic centres.

The Canadian Association of Nuclear Medicine continues its work although, in a young specialty with persisting manpower shortages, it is necessarily small, numbering 167 Canadian members in late 1990. However, Canada has been able to host the Society of Nuclear Medicine annual meeting in Toronto in 1986 and 1993, and the association hosted the 5th Congress of the World Federation of Nuclear Medicine and Biology in Montréal in 1990. The president at the latter meeting was Dr Étienne LeBel, the secretary-general Dr Leonard Rosenthall, the treasurer Dr Raymonde Chartrand, and the scientific secretaries Drs Michael Chamberlain and Albert Driedger. Many of the scientists and physicians involved in nuclear medicine in Canada took part in the organization of this very successful meeting. It was marked both by the scientific record and by an attempt to reconcile the high technology of nuclear medicine with the human dilemmas —not only of sickness but also of poverty and other social problems. Last but not least the meeting served to cement many international friendships and collaborations.

The power of the tracer concept will likely be the measure of nuclear medicine and those who practice it. In that sense the future is secure. The quality of new Canadian graduates and the contributions to the literature of the specialty from Canadian clinicians and scientists suggest that the present problems will prove to be transient ones.[2]

Acknowledgements:
I am grateful to Raymonde Chartrand, David Greyson, Adel Mattar, Jerry Richards, Bernard Shapiro and Leonard Rosenthall, among others, for critical review of this article and for making their own recollections availableto me. I am also indebted to Jean Lentle for preparing the manuscript.

Chapter VIII •

Canadian Association of Radiopharmaceutical Scientists (CARS)

Douglas Abrams

Introduction

The beginnings of the association can be traced back to Thursday June 19, 1980 shortly after 8:00 pm in the student residence of George Washington University in St Louis at Clinton. Unofficially Brian Abeseykera, Mike Adam, Mervyn Billinghurst, Richard Flanagan, Tony Noujaim and Len Wiebe attended that first informal meeting where the formation of an official association was agreed upon in principle. This initial gathering was followed by other meetings in Banff, and Detroit that same year, where details were discussed and more structure was put into place.

The association was tentatively designated the Association of Radiopharmaceutical Scientists of Canada (ARSC) while its formation was being discussed but it was eventually incorporated under its current name in the Province of Manitoba on November 17, 1981.

Constitution, Goals and Objectives

CARS was established to both encourage communication of events of interest to people working in radiochemistry, radiopharmacy and nuclear medicine and to act as a unified body to respond to outside influences on the profession. This objective included providing a forum for monitoring and discussing political and regulatory issues impacting on radiopharmaceutical and nuclear medicine practice and research in Canada.

Merv Billinghurst, the first President of CARS, was responsible for drafting the first constitution of CARS. The original constitution remains largely intact, having undergone only minor modifications over the years.

From its very inception CARS has been an instrument for

bringing the voice of the membership to the government. The first initiative tackled was the potential imposition of a surcharge by Air Canada on the transport of radioactive goods. At this writing, CARS members are in discussion with the government regarding cost recovery for regulatory services.

CARS has also managed to facilitate communication between scientists not only within Canada but internationally through support of numerous international conferences such as the International Radioiodine Conference in Banff (organized by Tony Noujaim and Len Wiebe) and the World Congress of Nuclear Medicine and Biology in Montreal (Ray Reilly—Executive Committee and Don Lyster—Radiopharmaceutical Science Program Chair) to name a few.

MEMBERSHIP

The first executive members of CARS were Merv Billinghurst as President, Bill Welsh as Vice-President and Brian Reid as Secretary-Treasurer. The founding president, Dr Mervyn W Billinghurst, is widely recognized as the driving force behind the establishment of CARS. His influence can be seen, not only during the formative stages of the association but well after its inception, until the present. Working somewhat less visibly behind the scenes, Tony Noujaim is credited for recruiting a large proportion of the original membership of 29 people. Considering the relatively small number of people practicing in the field at that time, this was a very successful membership drive.

In order to establish a strong membership base across the country regional representatives or reporters were appointed. The first representatives were Don Lyster from British Columbia, John Scott from Alberta, Merv Billinghurst from Saskatchewan and Manitoba, Ann Warbick-Cerone from Ontario and Jacques Nadeau from Québec. At the time of publication of the first Newsletter, the initial list of reporters did not have a representative from the Maritime Provinces.

Given the excellent cooperation exhibited among CARS members today, it is probably true to say that the membership was active in getting CARS off the ground and although the list is too lengthy to publish in its entirety, all of them should be recognized for their contributions.

The membership of CARS has been very diverse in both education and working affiliation, from its inception and has remained so. Although this has been a source of difficulties in beaurocratic matters such as finding an appropriate name and defining the role of the association, this diversity has also been a source of strength for Nuclear Medicine community. CARS has continued to grow to more than 83 members, and includes men and women from all regions of Canada (and at least one from the USA) holding diverse educational qualifications including BSc's, MSc's and PhD's working in clinical, research, commercial and regulatory capacities, with most members functioning in more than one of the aforementioned areas.

ACTIVITIES

In keeping with the original mandate of CARS, many members have been actively involved with various agencies and associations in developing guidelines for the safe use of radiopharmaceuticals. CARS has representatives sitting on many committees including the Executive Council of the Society of Nuclear Medicine Canada, the Federal Advisory Committee on Radiopharmaceuticals Quality Control (John Scott and Pamela Zabel) and the Nuclear Medicine Alliance (Doug Abrams and Pamela Zabel).

The CARS executive continues to look for ways to keep the organization relevant to the membership and is currently actively working towards making a method of accrediting or certifying members available. The role of the Newsletter service is also expanding to take advantage of the global computer networking system and CARS is looking into the feasibility of setting up a bulletin to enhance communication between members.

PRESIDENTS

The original constitution used a progressive ladder format in which the President-Elect automatically progressed to President after a one year term and a new President-Elect was elected each year. This was altered in 1986 to include the Secretary-Treasurer in the ladder and have each Officer serve a two year term. In this way the executive would have more experience as their responsibilities increased and elections would only be held every second year.

The list of the people who have held the office of president of CARS is included in an appendix.

NEWSLETTER

The *Newsletter* was expected to play a crucial role in the organization and was thought pivotal in keeping interested people informed about happenings in different parts of such a large country and keeping all informed. In time it was noted that the Editor was responsible for most of the financial transactions of the association and in 1987, the duties of Treasurer were moved from Secretary-Treasurer to Editor-Treasurer which became a five year term executive position.

The first newsletter was published in the spring of 1981 with Bill Welsh as editor while also holding the office of President-Elect. This was a five page manuscript which already brought the attention to the Air Canada surcharge for restricted articles, a cause the CARS executive could rally behind to intercede on behalf of the membership. The role of the *Newsletter* has grown in importance, as envisioned by the founding members and regularly consists of more than 20 pages of information.

Given the constitutional mandate agreed upon by the founding members, it is no surprise that, in addition to the executive, the people holding the position of editor were also extremely influential in the CARS organization and are listed below:

1981–1983	William J Welsh
1984–1988	Pamela Zabel
1989–1993	Jim Ballinger
1994–1998	Neil G Hartman

Acknowledgements:

Much of this information has been obtained from the CARS *Newsletters*. I am grateful to many members for their contributions especially Merv Billinghurst for his recollections and making available correspondence assembled during the genesis of CARS. In addition, I would like to thank Barry Bowen, Richard Flanagan, Don Lyster, Ray Reilly, John Scott, Pamela Zabel and those I have forgotten to mention, for their invaluable help.

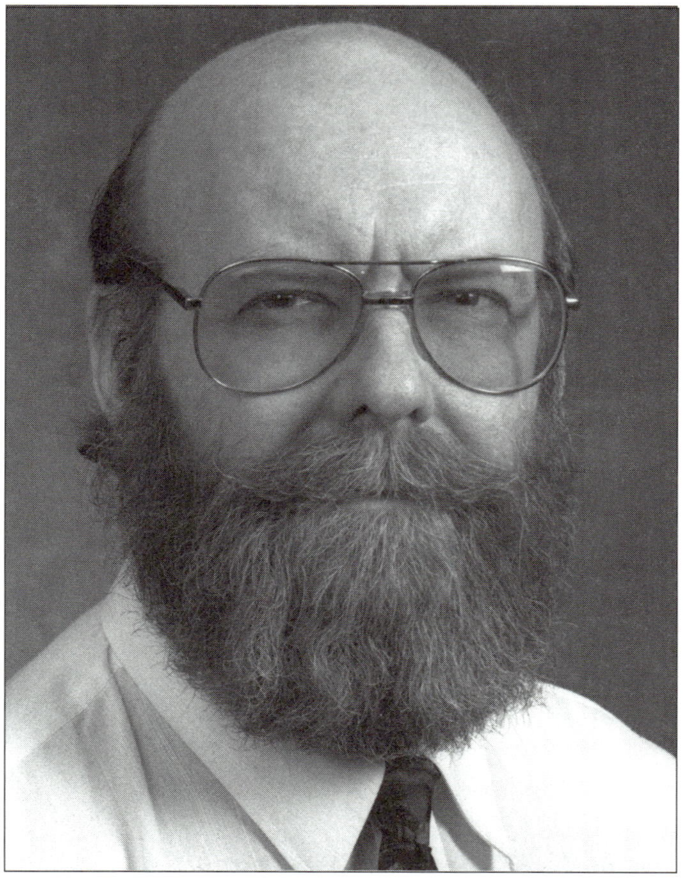

Dr Mervyn Billinghurst, first president, Canadian Association of Radiopharmaceutical Scientists

Chapter IX • *The Journal of the Canadian Association of Radiologists*

Brian Lentle

As a rule disease, as it sweeps through the land, cannot keep pace with the incurable vice of scribbling about it.
— John Mayour
De Rachitide *(1668)*

The Canadian Association of Radiologists in publishing the *Journal* in 1950 produced the first specialty journal in Canada.

However, the *Canadian Association of Radiologists Journal* (CARJ) was not the first radiological journal published in Canada. That distinction belongs to a short-lived French language journal *Les Rayons-X,* which first appeared in 1910. Dr Henri Lasnier was instrumental in its publication.[1] Dr ERN Grigg in his delightfully eclectic book *The Trail of the Invisible Light* prints a reproduction of one cover but notes that only seven issues of this journal were published before it was discontinued in 1910.[2] Copies now extant are few, and the only library copies are to be found at the Université de Laval.

As documented elsewhere in this volume, it is greatly to their credit that radiography technologists had created not only at least one regional organization before the Canadian Association of Radiologists existed but also national and regional journals and newsletters before the *Journal* came into existence.

It is also worth noting that a radiologist, Dr Léo Pariseau, was a moving force in creating *Le Journal de l'Hôtel Dieu de Montréal.* Dr HE McDermot writes:

> *One or two [Canadian Medical] journals have been concerned chiefly with historical and literary matters. In 1932, Le Journal de l'Hôtel Dieu de Montréal was founded by a group of the Hospital staff—Oscar Mercier, Léo E Pariseau, Ernest Prud'homme, and Ernest Trottier. Pariseau (1882–1944), the radiographer [sic] of the Hospital, was probably the originator; he certainly was the leading spirit. As*

Dr. Jean Saucier writes: "on peut difficilement mentionner le Journal de l'Hôtel Dieu sans parler de son animateur, le Dr. Léo Pariseau....Les Lecteurs de sa revue ouvre habituellment leur journal à sa rubrique des 'Miettes médicales de l'Histoire du Canada.'"[3] Perhaps this journal best recalls Pariseau's unusual mental powers and gift of expression, both in English and in French, his verve, his audacity, his originality. A martyr to his calling, as were others of the early radiologists (he lost an eye and developed ulcers of the hands, and died of cancer of the bowel), he never lost his eagerness, his fresh impetuous approach.[4]

Dr McDermot goes on to write as follows:

The specialties are gradually developing their own journals. The first of these to be brought out was The Journal of the Canadian Association of Radiologists *in 1950.*[5]

A scientific journal had been accepted as a purpose of the Canadian Association of Radiologists (CAR) from its early days. In the minutes of the founding meeting of CAR, a journal was identified as one of the goals of what was then the proposed organization.[6] Nevertheless, good intentions are not quite enough to launch a scientific publication. It needed a critical mass both of members of the association and of potential advertisers. No doubt the war years interrupted the affairs of CAR and further delayed production of the *Journal.*

The first issue was published in March 1950. There was an editorial board consisting of Drs EM Crawford, Origène Dufresne and Carleton B Pierce, under the chaimanship of Dr JW McKay. [7] Other documentation refers to Dr McKay as *the* editor, and there seems little doubt that that is how he functioned. It was the convention until the mid–1980s for CAR to describe the editor as the chairman of the editorial board.

The first editor of the *Journal,* Dr Joseph William McKay, had been born in Truro, Nova Scotia in 1891. He graduated from Dalhousie University in 1918. After interning at the Victoria General Hospital in Halifax he studied radiology at the Montréal General Hospital (MGH) as well as in London, England and New York City. He joined the staff of MGH in 1926 and became director of the Department of Radiology in 1948. He was later to be a president of CAR. At one time he served as chairman of the medical board and as secretary of the board of management. When he retired in 1958 it was as radiologist-in-chief and as an associate professor at McGill University. A list of subsequent editors appears in an appendix.

On the masthead of the first issue are listed the associate editors, Drs LP Belisle, Norman M Brown, G Pinsonneault and Lloyd G Stewart. In modern terms they would have chiefly served in editorial peer review.

The scientific content of the first issue was as follows:

Treatment of cancer of the skin by irradiation	RC Burr, Kingston
La contact thérapie des lesions malignes de la peau et des muqueses	O Dufresne et A Pinsonneault, Institut du Radium, Montréal
Spot film technique in Roentgen examination for duodenal ulcer	A Bernstein, Homeopathic Hospital, Montréal
Recent advances in knowledge of the biologic effect of radiation	LN Stewart and Jean Bouchard, Royal Victoria Hospital, Montréal

The subscription is listed as two ($2.00) dollars per annum.

A brief editorial in the English version (it was published in both official languages) in the first issue reads as follows:

With the rapid development of [r]adiology and allied sciences in Canada, the members of the Canadian Association of Radiologists have decided that the time has come to publish a Journal.

The purpose of the Journal *primarily is to publish articles pertaining to diagnostic and therapeutic radiology and matters of general interest to the members of the Canadian Association of Radiologists. We hope to extend the scope of the Journal by accepting contributions from other workers such as the biologists and physicists on the physical and biological phases of ionizing radiations.*

In the beginning, the size of the Journal *will be necessarily small. With this in view, the subject matter should be of satisfactory quality and suitable brevity.*

The success of the Journal *will largely depend upon the interest of and active contribution of papers by the members of the Canadian Association of Radiologists.*

THE EDITORIAL BOARD

The first two 1950 issues featured notices of the annual meeting to be held in Halifax at the Nova Scotia Hotel and lasting two days. In that year there were four issues of the *Journal* with 80 pages of scientific content in total. In subsequent years the page count was 69 in 1951, 75 in 1952 , 93 in 1953 and 57 in 1954.

As implied in the above listing it was the case from the outset that articles were published in either of the two official languages.

An anonymous editorial[8] from 1950 has as its title only the following quotation:

Come, come, and sit you down; you shall not budge;
You go not 'till I set you up a glass
Wherein you may see the inmost part of you.

[Shakespeare]
Hamlet, Act III

The quotation had no attribution and the assumption that readers might recognize its author is of interest in itself. However, the purpose of the editorial is not only to celebrate an examination of young radiologists (the "glass" is a mirror) but also to lament the developing separation between diagnostic and therapeutic radiology. The author goes on—and this in 1950—to wonder if future radiologists will ever cope with the forthcoming information explosion. However, he does so in terms much less succinct: prose styles in that era tended to the Proustian.

A striking difference between articles published in the 1950s and 1990s is that in the first decade of the *Journal* articles authored by one person were common. By the present decade multiple authorship has become the rule. In the first two issues ever published there were eight articles, four with single authors and none with more than two (and an average of 1.4 authors per article). In the first two issues of 1994 there were 28 articles and reports but only two with single authors and one article with six authors (mean, 3.6). This trend is also reflected in the publications of the founder of the Canadian Association of Radiologists, Dr Gordon Richards, which are listed in Appendix 2. Only a minority are written with a collaborator. Without a doubt science has become more complex and multidisciplinary, but it is also tempting to wonder if social pressures such as the need to publish and to include persons not directly contributing to an article in the credits do not play a role in this.

The *Journal* has without question grown. In the first year there were four issues occupying 80 pages. In 1951, its second year there were only 69 pages of editorial content in the *Journal*. In 1952, 1953 and 1954 there were 75, 93 and 57 such pages, respectively. Thereafter page numbers increased so that in 1970 the *Journal* contained 303 pages, and in 1993 all of 448 pages. In 1989 the number of issues a year had increased from four to six, with an increase in the number of pages available to the editor from 320 to 360.

In 1950 the National Research Council announced in the *Journal* the availability of funds for fundamental research "in the field of radiology."[9] The money was to be provided by the James Picker Foundation. The sum of $15 000 as income from the endowment was to be available that year, presumably in Canada alone although that is not entirely clear. "[S]tipends of the order of $3000 to $5000" for fellowships were also to be "entertained." This initiative seems not to have lasted for very long.

To anyone looking back at early issues of the *Journal* there is glimpse of a simpler era afforded by the advertising content. In the March 1952 issue Blaker, Hearns and Co offer members of CAR malpractice insurance against a single claim of up to $50 000 and a total of $100 000 in a single year. The premium is not quoted but I am reliably informed that it was less than $50. By the standards of those very modest settlements such a cost is believable.

In 1956 an article appeared entitled "The Regulation of Shoe Fitting Fluoroscopes" by Dr FD Sowby of Ottawa. The avowed purpose of the paper was to document the potential hazards of such machines and to discuss measures for their safe operation.[10] In parallel, the CAR began to pressure the regulatory agencies to have shoe-fitting fluoroscopy banned, more because of the hazard to operators than to purchasers of shoes.

To read back issues of the *Journal* is to travel once more the path of the astonishing developments in radiology that have characterized in particular the last quarter of a century. Certainly there are articles to make one wince in sympathy with our patients, like "Fabrication d'un appareil à insufflation péritonéale pour pneumopelvigraphie."[11] However, there are also reflective papers which emphasize that, for example, our present emphasis on "outcomes" is not without precedent, e.g. "The appendix: a study comparing radiological diagnosis with operative, anatomical and pathological findings and subsequent clinical results."[12]

From the outset the *Journal* carried articles concerning both diagnosis and radiation therapy. Indeed, a whole issue was dedicated to the introduction of cobalt-60 teletherapy and papers by Dr Harold Johns' group.[13] However, when most of the radiation oncologists ceased to be members of CAR in the 1980s the content of radiation oncology articles soon stopped. Contributions concerning basic science and radiation protection have always been featured and continue to appear. The *Journal* made front page headlines in an account of Taylor's analysis of variations, sometimes thirtyfold, in the radiation exposures of patients undergoing similar procedures in Ontario.[14]

The quality of medical journals can be assessed to some degree by measures such as the citation index (how often a journal is cited), the immediacy factor (how quickly it is cited) and the impact factor (to what extent its contents are quoted elsewhere). Although not perfect, and to some extent influenced by size and frequency of publication of a journal, these factors do reflect something of the merit of a journal. It will also be apparent that these measures of a journals stature are slow to appear. However, if these indices for the *Journal* are compared with those for *Radiology* and the *British Journal of Radiology* some interesting facts emerge. For example between 1978 and 1984 the citation index for *Radiology* increased by over 60 per cent, that for the *British Journal of Radiology* by 13 per cent and that for the *Journal* by 40 per cent. In that same interval the percentage changes in impact and immediacy factors were similar for the *Journal* and for *Radiology,* while both out-performed the *British Journal of Radiology*. Nevertheless in absolute terms it is a slow process to change the ranking of a journal. For example there are some 4300 journals listed in Index Medicus. *Radiology* and the *British Journal of Radiology*, between 1983 and 1988, are to be found in the first or second quartiles of the rank ordering of those journals in respect of the above measures. The *Canadian Association of Radiologists Journal* is, however, fairly consistently in the third quartile. One may conclude that, while the *Journal* has some way to go, it is slowly getting stronger. Its quality ultimately depends, of course, upon the material submitted to the editor, for no scientific journal, no matter how well presented and edited, can be better than the material submitted to it, as is implied in the editorial quoted above.

While it is usual to pay tribute to the editorial staff of a journal, any editor knows all too well that it is the people behind the editorial desk who ultimately ensure that each issue appears in the light of day. At the outset Gwendolyn A Mollison was listed as the publication manager. In June 1962 Alva I Ekstrand became editorial assistant. She became Alva Ekstrand Pentecost in 1969 and in 1976 Ms Pentecost was promoted to managing editor while also caring for the other affairs of the association as its executive secretary. In 1990 the production of the *Journal* was transferred to the capable hands of the publications section of the Canadian Medical Association.

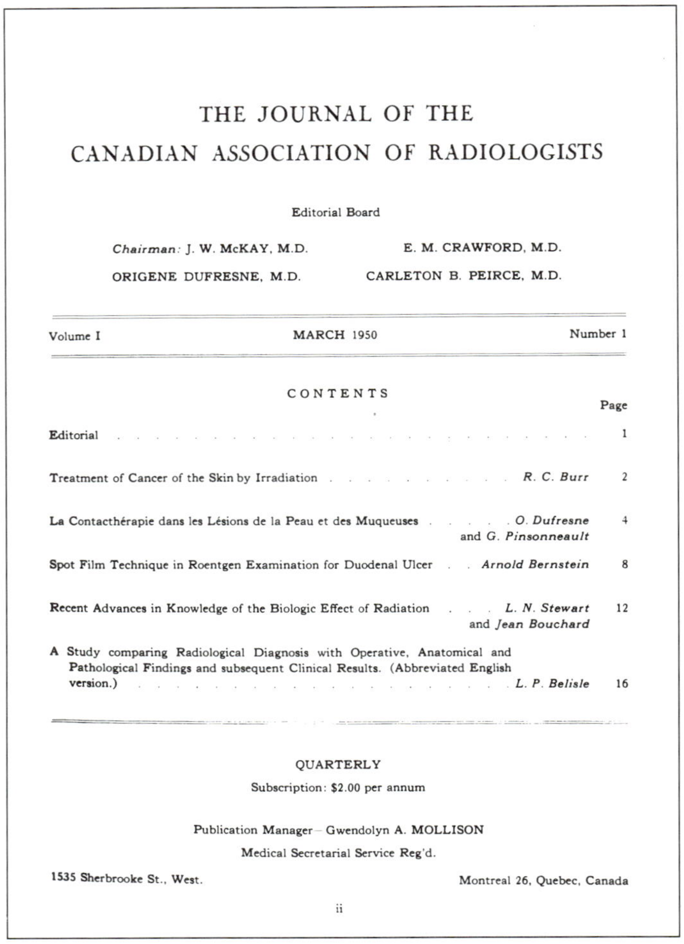

THE JOURNAL OF THE
CANADIAN ASSOCIATION OF RADIOLOGISTS

Editorial Board

Chairman: J. W. McKAY, M.D. — E. M. CRAWFORD, M.D.
ORIGENE DUFRESNE, M.D. — CARLETON B. PEIRCE, M.D.

Volume I — MARCH 1950 — Number 1

CONTENTS

QUARTERLY
Subscription: $2.00 per annum

Publication Manager – Gwendolyn A. MOLLISON
Medical Secretarial Service Reg'd.
1535 Sherbrooke St., West. — Montreal 26, Quebec, Canada

ii

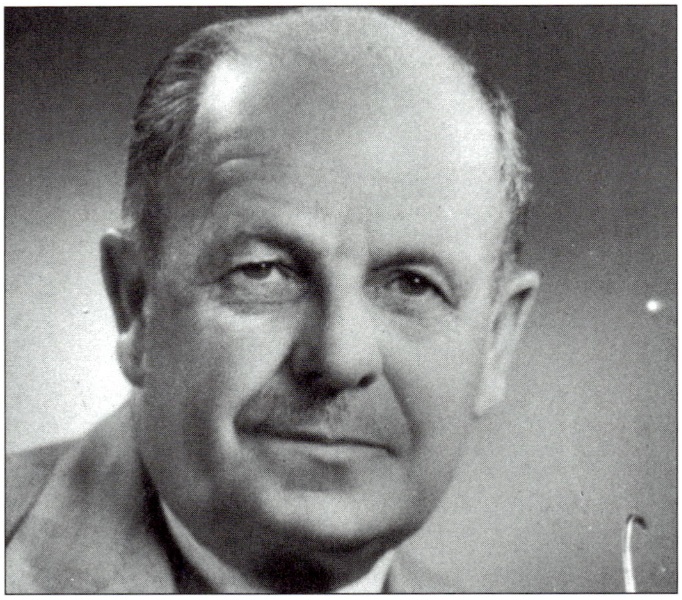

Top
Frontespiece, first issue of journal

Above
Dr JW McKay, first editor of the *Canadian Association of Radiologists' Journal*

Chapter X • History of

Radiation Oncologists

in the Royal College of Physicians and Surgeons

George B Goodman

EVOLUTION OF RADIATION ONCOLOGY IN CANADA

This discussion includes a general overview of several organizations involved in specialty practice and specific changes that took place in the 1970s concerning the evolution of radiation oncology in Canada.

CANADIAN COLLEGES AND NATIONAL SOCIETIES IN SPECIALTY PRACTICE

Because health delivery is a provincial responsibility, it is the provincial colleges of physicians and surgeons which are invested with the authority to grant licenses for the practice of medicine. The Royal College, a national body, certifies the clinical competence of a physician to practice as a specialist. However, all provinces save Québec accept the Royal College certification as the principal qualification for specialist recognition. Quebec has its own program of certification of specialists. National societies promote the general interests of individual specialties in the fields of economics, politics, technology, education etc.

HISTORICAL ASPECTS OF TRAINING AND EVALUATION— Royal College of Physicians and Surgeons of Canada

In 1938 the Royal College assumed the responsibility for recognition and certification of specialists in Canada at the request of the Canadian Medical Association. Competence as a specialist was recognized by different specialty examinations at fellowship and certification level. Pursuant to a college referendum to fellows in 1971 it was decided to eliminate this double standard. The college determined that in 1972 a single examination—a new standard—would be introduced for certification of clinical competence as a specialist and for granting of fellowship. In addition, all certificants of the college before 1972 who applied—

and would support the college objectives—could be admitted to fellowship. The effect was to bring many specialists in Canada into the college and its activities for the first time.

Mechanisms for approval of hospitals for graduate-training programs gradually evolved. Initially, some basic general requirements were introduced and site inspections of teaching hospitals began in 1960. By 1965 the minimum resources necessary for approval of hospitals for training covered 19 specialty programs.

The specialty committees of the Royal College advise on the minimum requirements for training, criteria for the acceptability of treatment institutions and programs, and the control and conduct of the examinations including appointments to the examining boards. Specialty committee chairmen are appointed by council of the college on the recommendation of the executive of the national specialty society. The remaining members are appointed, in consultation with the chairman, from nominees from the relevant national specialist societies, and with the chairmen of the examining boards in the English and French languages as ex-officio members.

DEVELOPMENT OF A SPECIALTY COMMITTEE IN RADIATION ONCOLOGY

A Specialty Committee in Radiology was created in the mid–1940s to encompass the interests of diagnostic and therapeutic radiology. The Canadian Association of Radiologists preferred that the members of its committee on training and qualifications should function simultaneously as the Royal College Committee in Radiology. This committee, a mix of diagnostic and therapeutic radiologists, with nuclear medicine and physics representation, had a nucleus group and corresponding members from all over the country. In 1972 Dr D Saunders (Toronto) was its chairman and was of great assistance in representing our interests as therapeutic radiologists to the Royal College. In 1975 the Royal College, responding to dissatisfaction among some radiotherapists at the inclusion of their affairs in the Committee in Radiology, formed a Committee in Therapeutic Radiology, which became the Committee in Radiation Oncology with the change of name of the specialty in 1976.

DEVELOPMENT OF THE NATIONAL SPECIALIST SOCIETY CARO

In the era 1960–1970 the Canadian Association of Radiologists (CAR) had a Standing Committee of Therapeutic Radiologists. The 6th meeting (Toronto 1967) was chaired by Marvin Lougheed (Montréal) and members included: Bill Rider (Toronto), Ed Smith (Calgary), I Strautmanis and Dick Walton (Manitoba) and Doug Thompson (London). The minutes record a recommendation to establish a 2nd vice-president (radiotherapy) in CAR to be on its executive and to be selected by the Committee on Therapeutic Radiology. In the same minutes, consideration of forming a Society of Radiotherapists in Canada was discussed but deferred. A separate Section of Radiation Oncology in CAR was enacted 10 years later with the support and the advice of Jean Louis-Leger, Brick Sloan, Lou Harnick, John Stevenson and Jim Sieniewicz, all past presidents of CAR. At its annual general meeting in 1980 CAR approved the establishment of a Federation of Radiological Sciences. The intent—to formalize meetings and to include under an umbrella arrangement autonomous subgroups of nuclear medicine, radiation oncology and diagnostic imaging—was not implemented, and in 1987 the Canadian Association of Radiation Oncologists (CARO) was formed.

PROBLEMS CONFRONTING RADIATION ONCOLOGY IN CANADA IN THE 1970s

In Canada, therapeutic radiology (radiation oncology) was an unattractive specialty for graduates from Canadian medical schools. Indeed, radiation oncology was identified in 1968 as having the most serious manpower shortage of all Canadian medical specialties.[1] Deterrents to recruitment included conditions of employment, negligible teaching of the specialty in universities, lack of resident-training posts and a poor image of clinical radiation therapy practice. The loss of independence associated with institutional practice (perceived as an arm of government) and much service work conjured a highly technical picture of medical practice lacking in appeal to many undergraduates. In addition, remuneration was inadequate relative to other specialties and general practice. Undergraduates were underexposed to the specialty, while the multidisciplinary approach to the teaching of cancer as a disease (oncology) did not exist. Some provincial governments also reduced the number of training posts in the specialty, compounding the problem. Another factor of importance was that most radiation oncologists were certificants and not fellows of the college and were perceived to have had little scientific and clinical training. Generally, patients were admitted to the medical or surgical services of their hospitals for medical care, with the radiotherapists providing specialty service on a consultative basis. Problems considered remediable were addressed by the specialty committee: first and foremost to establish training standards for the specialty akin to those of major clinical specialties in medicine, surgery and gynecology. New certificants had to be recognized both as competent clinicians with good medical training and as competent specialists, not only in their disciplinary expertise but also in the broad field of oncology. In addition, it was necessary to promote the clinical image of the specialty and its research and educational activities.

NEW STANDARDS FOR RADIATION ONCOLOGY IN CANADA AND A NEW NAME FOR THE SPECIALTY

The new certification examinations in therapeutic radiology were introduced in 1972. Like the old fellowship, the new examinations were of greater scope than those for the old certificate and provided broad representation of the clinical specialties of medicine, surgery and pathology on the examining boards. After the creation of the Specialty Committee in Therapeutic Radiology in 1975, it was recommended that a third paper in general oncology should be introduced and that the name of the examination be changed to radiation oncology. The College agreed promptly to the examination recommendations and later approved the change of name of the specialty.

Examinations in 1976 were expanded to include three essay type papers: 1, the principles and practice of radiation oncology; 2, basic sciences as related to radiation oncology; and 3, general oncology. Before implementing the third paper the specialty committee had explored the use of multiple choice examination (MCE) questions with the McLaughlin Examination Centre. They considered MCE too difficult to implement for our specialty because of the statistical invalidity which would result from the small number of candidates. The oral examinations consist of a clinical and a basic science component. Appended are copies of the original letter to the college concerning the "Proposal for the Change of name from Therapeutic Radiology to Radiation Oncology" and the College response (Annex 1).

The specialty committee continued to define new standards for the specialty. Revisions and rewrites of the Specialty Training Requirements and the Requisites and Guidelines for Specialty Training Programs in Radiation Oncology were undertaken with the College Training and Evaluation Committee. In addition, questionnaires with a specialty core insert were developed to provide the necessary information on which to base a judgement on the quality of programs in radiation oncology. The specialty committee was at pains to ensure the highest possible quality of training in radiation oncology and to ensure the recognition of trainees as competent clinicians with a sound background in the treatment of cancer by radiation therapy. To this end strict requirements were demanded relative to internships and residency training and in terms of training programs relative to total patient care. In addition, in response to exhortations from us (and presumably other specialties) the College accepted the principle in 1982 that where radiation therapy facilities were being accredited, that radiation oncologists be included in the cadre of experienced surveyors.

MEMBERS OF EXAMINING BOARDS AND SPECIALTY COMMITTEES IN RADIATION ONCOLOGY

I have listed such members of the examining boards and of the Specialty Committee to the Royal College as are known to me before 1971 and since that time in Annex 2.

CONCLUSION

Many radiation oncologists throughout Canada contributed to effect political changes in our national specialty society. In terms of the establishment of new standards for training in radiation oncology, the contributions of Raymond Bush and John Simpson (Toronto) are unexcelled. I believe our specialty is stronger today than ever before, and certainly our specialists are clinically competent. The 1970s represented an important time for change in our specialty, and I am proud to have played a significant part.

Acknowledgements:

I wish to acknowledge helpful comments by Drs RS Bush and WJK Simpson. In addition I would like to thank the Royal College of Physicians & Surgeons of Canada secretariat for providing lists of specialty committees and chairmen of examining boards

Chapter XI • Canadian Radiation Protection Association

Roch D DesRochers

In the period 1950–1975, many Canadian scientists worked in the field of radiation protection. A number of these were very active in international bodies and scientific associations. Scientists employed in research (in Atomic Energy of Canada Ltd (AECL) and the universities), nuclear power (AECL, Ontario Hydro, Hydro Québec and New Brunswick Power), and provincial and federal health regulatory bodies recognized their need to communicate effectively. PM Bird, after polling Canadian members of the Health Physics Society and other people working in applied radiation, organized a meeting in Ottawa in May 1967 to discuss the possible development of a Canadian organization of "applied radiation specialists." Unfortunately, he was unable to obtain an agreement on the status that a Canadian society for radiation protection should have.

Workers in the field continued to be active in international and non-Canadian bodies, especially the Health Physics Society. This is a United States-based group which publishes the journal *Health Physics* for many years *the* journal of the international radiation protection community. Canadian health physicists who were members of the Health Physics Society have been elected as directors, and named to the editorial board of the journal over the years.

In 1977–78, Richard Osborne sent a questionnaire to Canadian members of the Health Physics Society. A majority was in favour of forming a Canadian scientific society of those involved in radiation protection. A group from Ontario and Québec undertook to organize a meeting in Toronto in May 1979 for the founding of the Canadian Radiation Protection Association—Association Canadienne de

Radioprotection. This ad hoc committee included representatives of Atomic Energy of Canada Limited, the Atomic Energy Control Board, the Radiation Protection Bureau of Health and Welfare, Ontario Hydro, university and health sciences centres. The meeting was attended by approximately 125 persons, who were almost unanimous in their approval of a constitution for CRPA–ACRP. Richard Osborne, who had done a great amount of work in organizing the meeting, was elected the first president for 1979–1980.

During its first year, the Canadian association joined the International Radiation Protection Association (IRPA) and sent four delegates to the General Assembly of IRPA, held during the Fifth International Congress on Radiation Protection in Jerusalem in 1980. George Cowper, who was a member or the CRPA board of directors, was elected to the executive council of IRPA. At the next two IRPA general assemblies, IRPA6 in Berlin in 1984 and IRPA7 in Sydney, Australia in 1988, the CRPA extended an invitation to IRPA to hold its congress in Canada. The second bid was successful, and CRPA–ACRP was host to the Eighth International Congress of the International Radiation Protection Association (IRPA8) in Montréal in May 1992.

CRPA–ACRP publishes a quarterly bilingual *Bulletin* and holds an annual conference. Past presidents of CRPA–ACRP are listed in an appendix.

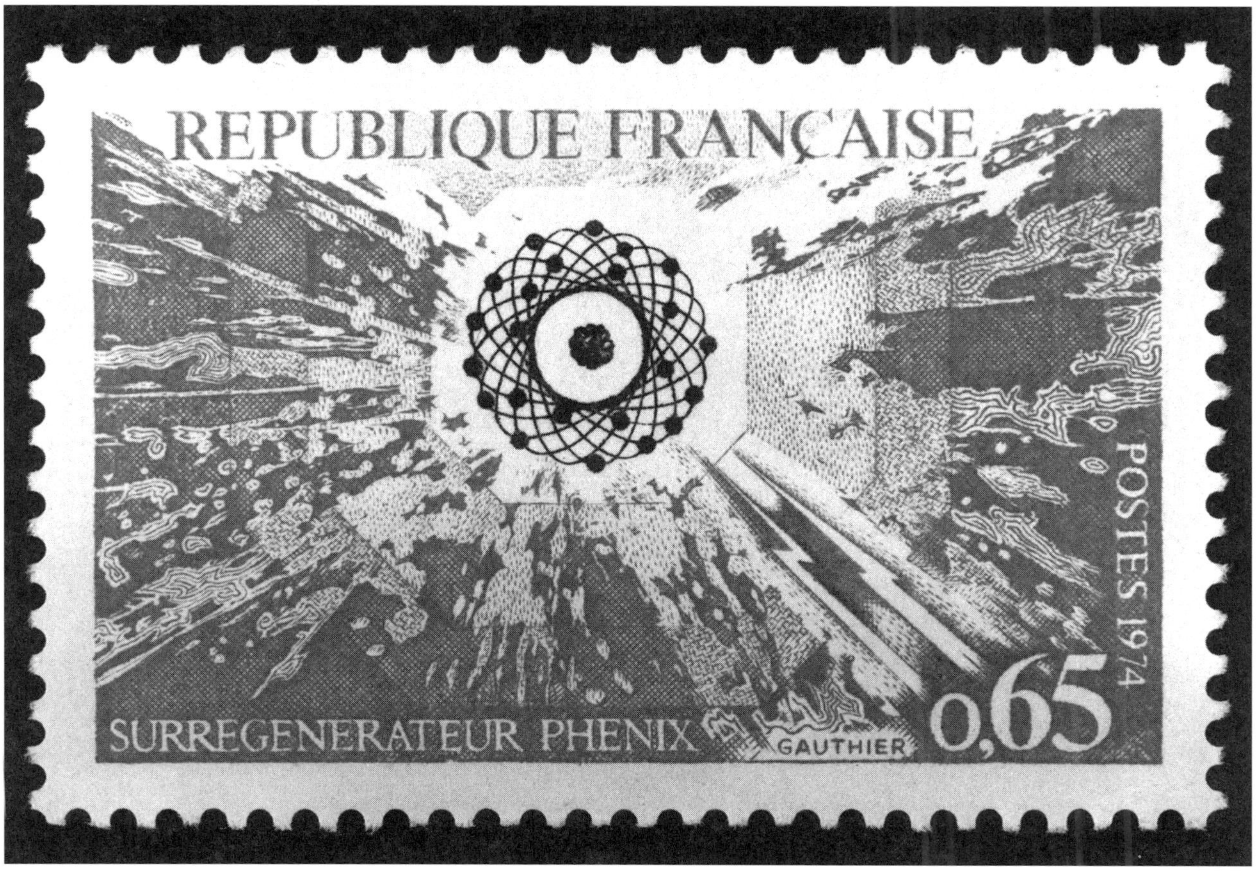

Chapter XII •

Canadian Heads of Academic Radiology

H Joachim Burhenne and Brian Lentle

Arctic char and academic radiology are not matters that seem to have much in common. But in this young country some traditions must be built very quickly.

The academic heads of radiology have come together since 1978 under the umbrella of an informal organization called the Canadian Heads of Academic Radiology (CHAR). Coming in that year from San Francisco to the University of British Columbia, one of us (JB) believed there was a need for communication and the exchange of views on academic matters such as the teaching of radiology to medical students. Also, discussion of research and fellowship programs as well as the issues of residency education might usefully be discussed by all of the chairmen of radiology in Canada for mutual benefit if such a group were created. Not least, issues related to fees and negotiations with each member's respective dean might be enhanced by the existence of a collective data base.

A call to Dr Peter Kent at the University of Saskatchewan by Dr Burhenne met with a favourable reponse, and CHAR met for the first time in Vancouver at the University Faculty Club at the annual meeting of the Canadian Association of Radiologists (CAR) in 1979. At that first meeting a tradition was established of having a dinner at which arctic char is served.

The CHAR archives, amounting to one photographic album, records that at the first meeting photography was the responsibility of Dr Hugh Morrish of Calgary, production was by Dr JDR (Jack) Miller and invitations by Dr Joachim Burhenne (University of British Columbia). Others present were Drs Lew Carey (University of Western

Ontario), Conway Don (University of Ottawa), Robert Fortin (Université de Laval), Peter Kent (University of Saskatchewan), Ted Lansdown (University of Toronto), Douglas MacEwan (University of Manitoba), Max Palayew (McGill University), James Standen (Dalhousie University) and Carl Zylak (McMaster University).

At the second meeting at the Montréal Badminton and Squash Club in May 1980 new faces were Drs Tom Challis (Queen's University), Hugh Morrish (University of Calgary), Jacques Saltiel (Université de Montréal) and BG Strom (Université de Sherbrooke). This attendance of 13 of a possible 16 chairs of radiology suggests that CHAR was already filling a need.

CHAR has always emphasized informality, no doubt because its members usually suffer a surfeit of meetings, minutes and memoranda at their desks. Indeed, Dr Don Russell (University of Alberta), then President of CHAR, wrote in the archive that in 1990 CHAR passed the first formal resolution since its inception: a vote of thanks to Dr Burhenne in 1990 for having founded CHAR, for hosting three of the meetings and for having been an active member and supporter. An agenda from the 1981 meeting in Toronto (Hart House) does survive: a workload survey, the Royal College training requirements, regional manpower constraints, relationships with nuclear medicine physicians, the teaching of physics and biological hazards, and the support of residents for attendance at conventions. Late additions to the agenda suggest that the discussion also ranged over resident representation on CAR council, a survey of the Ottawa Civic Hospital and the administrative responsibilities of a radiologist-in-chief.

Continuity within CHAR has been maintained despite the rate of change in positions which are becoming less and less attractive as fiscal constraints make the ratio of problems-to-opportunities approach infinity. Only at two annual meetings has there been no new face at the table, and on two occasions there were six. There never seem to have been fewer than 12 members present at an annual meeting. In 1990 an annual meeting was held at Chateau Lake Louise, the first annual meeting to be held independently of that of CAR, and an occasion that attracted 15 members. Indeed, on the occasion of one memorable meeting (the 16th) at Millcroft Inn in rural Ontario in March 1993, all 16 members were present, including six new ones.

A CHAR representative does sit on the CAR council to facilitate communication at a national level. Otherwise the single officer is a president—a somewhat grandiose title for general factotum. No other officers are elected although members take on fact-finding mandates. Those who have served as presidents are listed in an appendix.

The letterhead features an arctic char leaping out of the water. One recipient of the infrequent correspondence has complained that it is not serious enough, which seems to miss the point of an organization committed to mutual support and information sharing. CHAR has benefited from some generous sponsorship from Kodak Ltd on two occasions, Sanofi Winthrop, Berlex, General Electric, the 3M Company and Mallincrodt.

Times change. Having served in the past as an advisory committee to the Sterling-Winthrop Imaging Research Institute (SWIRI), CHAR has in 1994 taken over the administration of some of the residual funds from the institute. Indeed for some years the annual meeting had been combined with a meeting of the SWIRI review board. In 1995 a further innovation will see a combined meeting of CHAR with the residency program directors and the directors of research from each university academic department. The more that circumstances demand creative solutions, the better is CHAR likely to serve Canadian radiology and its faculties of medicine.

CHAR June 1st 1982: Backrow, Drs David Fraser, Carl Zylak, Max Palayew, Hugh Morrish, Jack Miller

Frontrow, Drs Tom Challis, Conway Don, Douglas MacEwan, Joachim Burhenne, and Ted Lansdown

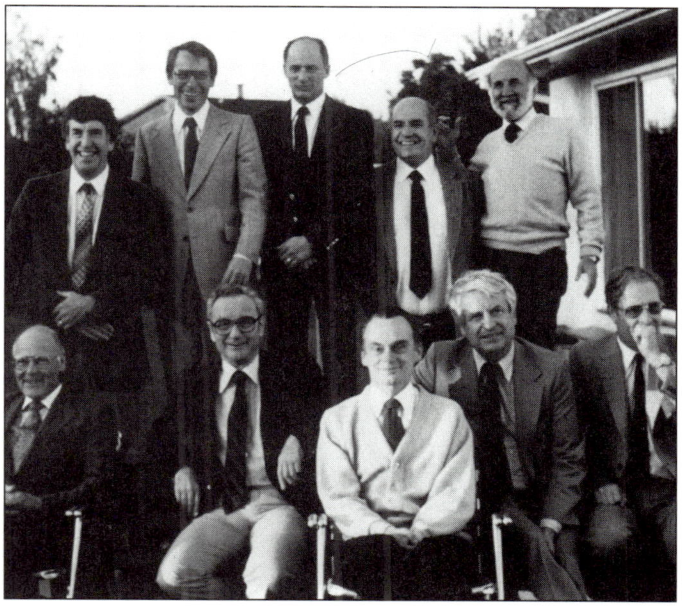

Chapter XIII •

The Sterling-Winthrop Imaging Research Institute

BRIAN LENTLE

Art is long, and grants are but yearly.
— Robertson Davies
Samuel Marchbank's Almanac

The Sterling-Winthrop Imaging Research Institute (SWIRI) was an interesting experiment which lasted all too briefly. It deserves mention because its effects may outlive its life span and because it serves as a model should anyone be brave enough to try such an experiment again.

SWIRI had its genesis in a federal government bill known as C22. This provided patent protection for pharmaceutical manufacturers in exchange for which the manufacturers committed to spend money in Canada on research and development (R&D).[1]

Sterling-Winthrop was at the time a major company in the supply of contrast media for radiological imaging. After the genesis of SWIRI, the company was to become Sanofi-Winthrop and later to merge with Nycomed.

Among several, two people in particular can claim credit for having the vision to create the brief experiment that was SWIRI. They were Jacques Boisvert of Sanofi-Winthrop and Dr Gordon Potts, then Professor and Chairman of the Department of Radiology at the University of Toronto.[2] Their vision was to identify a large sum of money to be spent on imaging research in radiology and, to a much smaller extent, cardiology. A further piece of good fortune resulted in Ms Helen Blair being appointed as managing director to administer, guide, mother and nourish the institute.

The Institute was launched with a press conference at Notre Dame Hospital on November 2, 1989. A press release at the time read in part, "The new Sterling-Winthrop Imaging Research Institute will commit $10 million during the next five years to Canadian R & D in the

the specialized field of imaging. This amount represents many times the investment being made in medical imaging in Canada today from all other funding sources." A derivative announcement appeared in the *Globe and Mail* of November 9, 1989.

An advisory board consisting of the members of CHAR formed a smaller board to advise on policy for SWIRI. It was the further great fortune of the institute that the first chair of the board was Dr Gordon Potts.

Gordon Potts' and the board's vision was of a process characterized by the highest standards of accountability and transparency. Peer review was done by experts worldwide, all names being recorded in a data bank developed by Ms Elfriede Schmidt. The reviews were collated by internal reviewers who were members of the board (chairman, Dr Gordon Potts, Ms Helen Blair, Dr H Joachim Burhenne, Dr Romeo Ethier, Dr David Fraser, Dr Gary Hebert, Dr Barry Hobbs, Dr Brian Lentle (from February 1991), Dr Khoi Nguyen (Sterling-Winthrop), Mr Ardie Nickel (Sterling-Winthrop) and Dr Giles Stevenson.

In short, the process was almost identical to that used by the scientific committees of the Medical Research Council and the National Cancer Institute. Indeed, it was more rigorous in that the taxation implications of Bill C22, an arcane world of Byzantine complexity understood only by Helen Blair—and then only sometimes—required that the board monitor spending and scientific output in annual meetings, usually held in conjunction with meetings of CAR or CHAR.

In 1990, the first year, $1045,132 was dispersed to support two career scientists (Drs John Mayo and Brian Rutt) and a variety of research projects ranging from the synthesis of acyclic and macrocyclic tetra amine bifunctional chelating agents for labeling proteins, through assessment of the effects of lung movement on pulmonary edema and the digital imaging of arteriovenous malformations, to an investigation of ultrasound-controlled, laser-induced necrosis in pig livers.[3] Conscious thought was given to trying to guide radiological investigators by a published editorial toward opportunities such as imaging function and morphology. [4]

Stirling-Winthrop Imaging Research Institute—Board. Back row, left to right: Dr Khoi Nguyen, Dr Guy Hébert, Dr Brian Lentle, Dr Giles Stevenson, Dr David Fraser, Mr Ardie Nichol, and Dr Roméo Ethier. Front row, left to right: Dr Barry Hobbs, Mrs Helen Blair, and Dr Gordon Potts

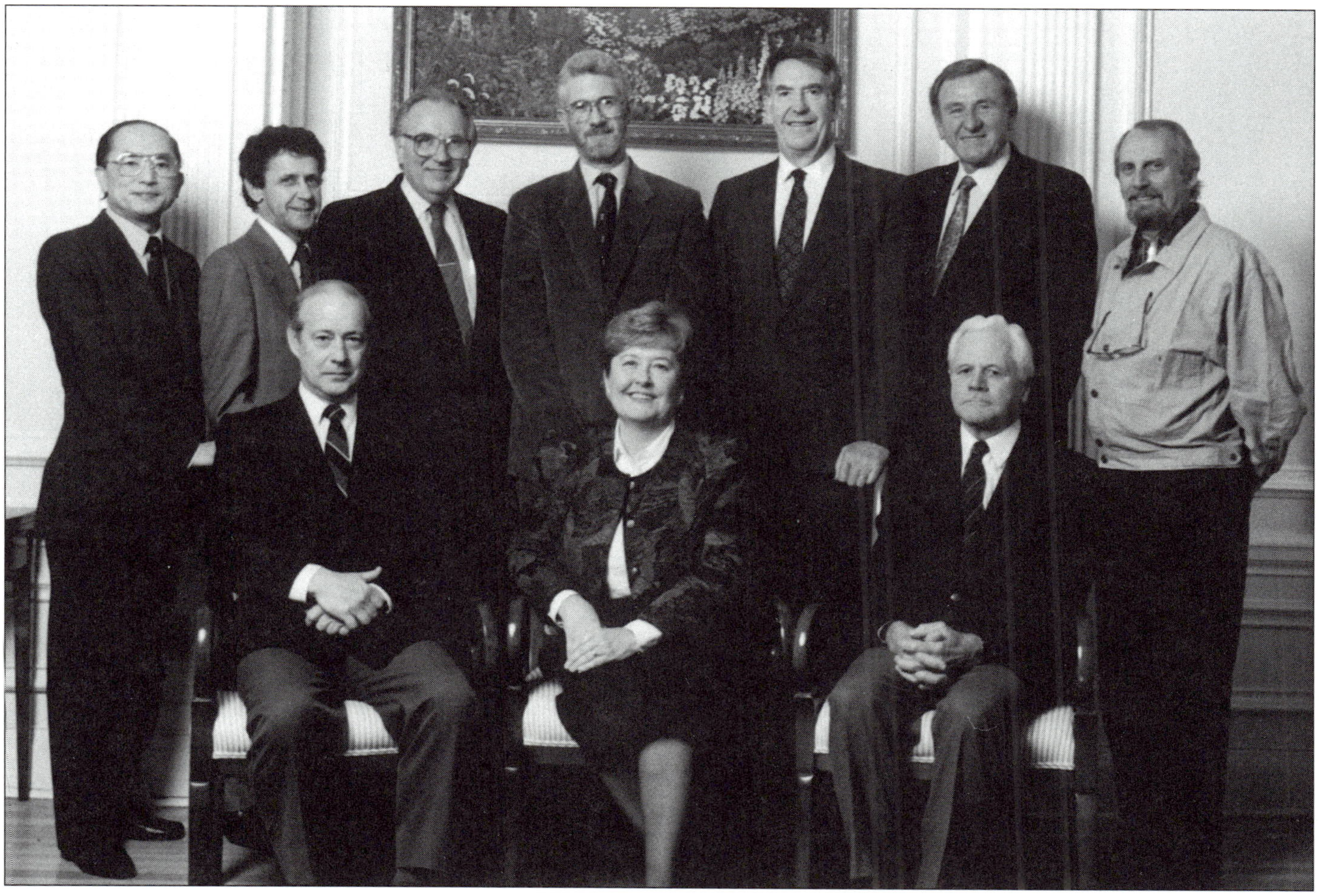

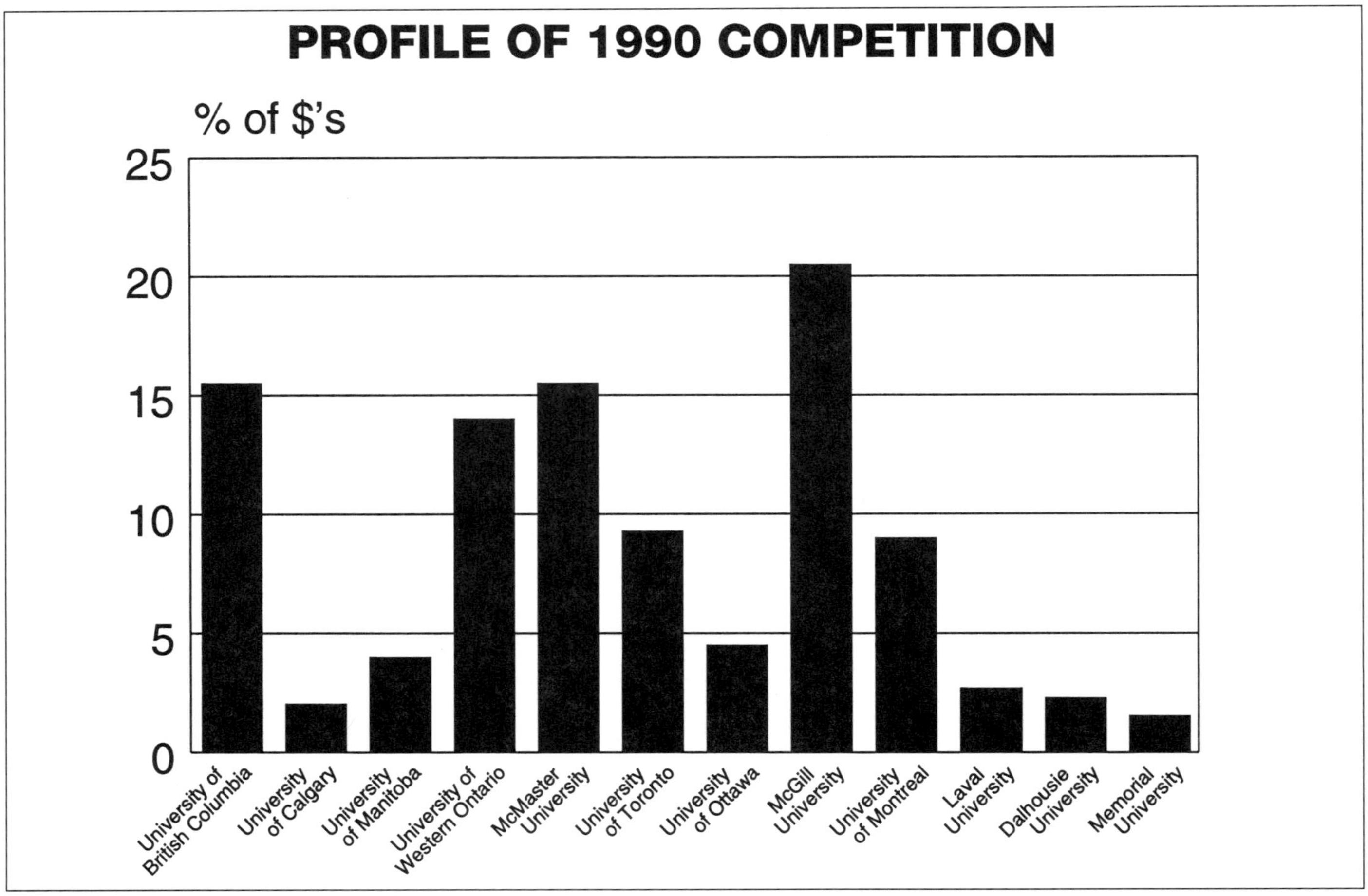
PROFILE OF 1990 COMPETITION
% of $'s
25
20
15
10
5
0
University of British Columbia
University of Calgary
University of Manitoba
University of Western Ontario
McMaster University
University of Toronto
University of Ottawa
McGill University
University of Montreal
Laval University
Dalhousie University
Memorial University

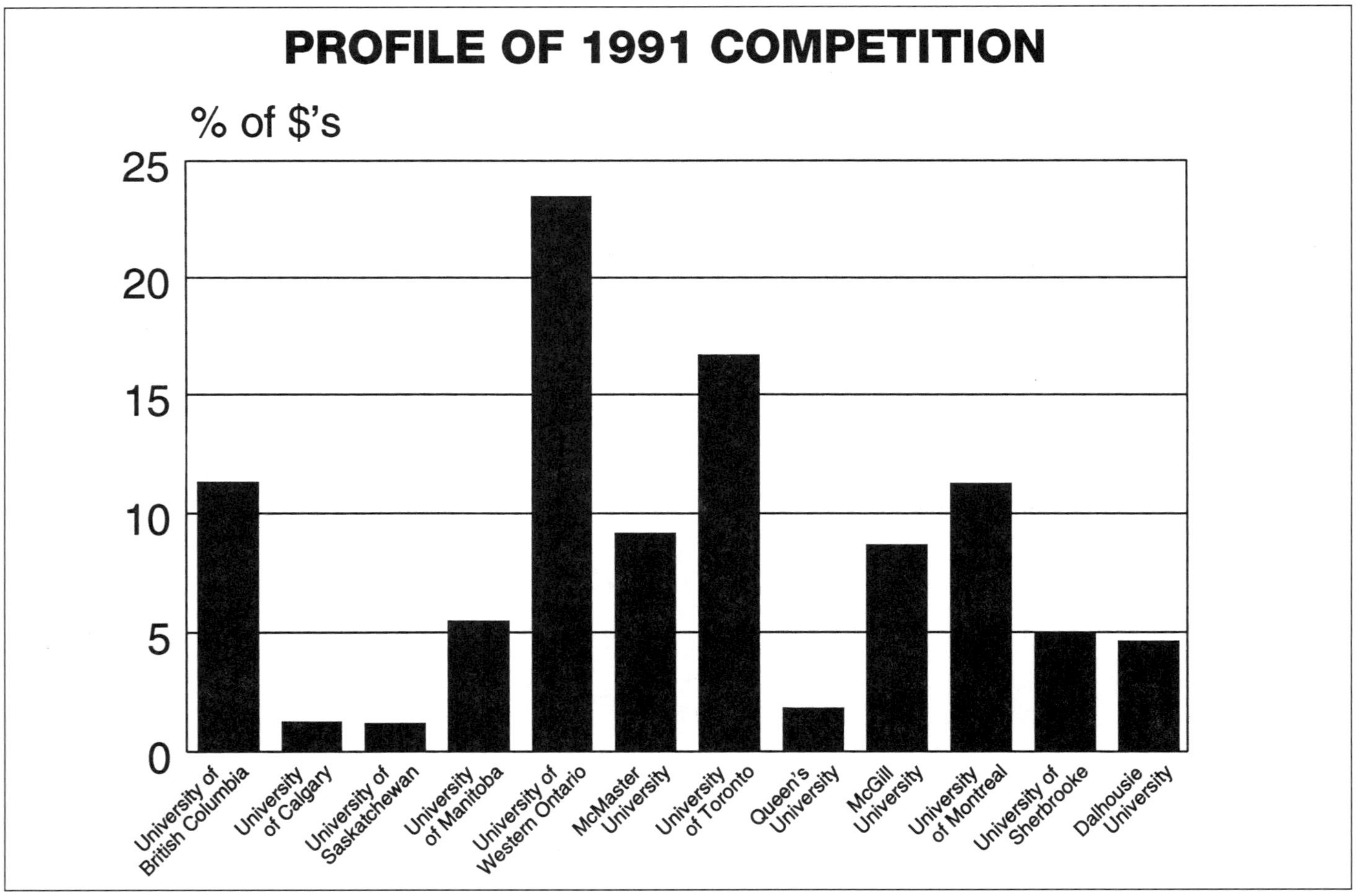
PROFILE OF 1991 COMPETITION
% of $'s
25
20
15
10
5
0
University of British Columbia
University of Calgary
University of Saskatchewan
University of Manitoba
University of Western Ontario
McMaster University
University of Toronto
Queen's University
McGill University
University of Montreal
University of Sherbrooke
Dalhousie University

In 1992 I succeeded Gordon Potts as chairman of the board and Drs Edward Lyons and Alexander McEwan were added to the board. It should also be noted that Dr Stuart Jackson was co-opted onto the review panel to provide physics input. Dr Potts' shoes were not easily filled to overflowing, but by then the process had been perfected. Ms Elfriede Schmidt, at Ms Helen Blair's right hand, was able to tell us with a touch of the keyboard how much had been spent, and how the grants were ranked.

So what went wrong? As the scientific advisors to SWIRI, my colleagues and I were not and did not expect to be privy to the corporate decisions that were involved. However, causes are not hard to find. In 1992 and 1993, the business cycle was at a low ebb. Changes in the delivery of health care in the 1990s resulted in massive reductions in health care spending throughout North America. The support of university-based research became difficult to justify when corporate viability was at risk. Consequently, the imaging component of Sanofi-Winthrop was restructured within Nycomed, itself a major manufacturing company in contrast media.

If other companies had responded in like manner to the combined challenge of SWIRI and Bill C22, the story might have had a different ending. Instead, a decision was made to complete the SWIRI story with a celebration. At the time of the spring 1994 meeting of CHAR, Mr Michael Welch and Ms Helen Blair of Sanofi-Winthrop hosted a dinner for the board. Drs John Mayo and Moni Stein were chosen to describe and present their SWIRI-supported research on behalf of the many investigators who had benefited from the institute. Other guests included Dean Martin Hollenberg of the University of British Columbia, who, while in Toronto, had given advice on the creation of the institute, Dr Gordon Potts, and Dr Brian Worthington, an old friend of Gordon's who happened to be in Vancouver as a visiting professor.

The hope must be that this brief flourishing of a notion —almost too good to last—will have instilled in a generation of Canadian radiologists the appetite and aptitude for competing for peer-reviewed research funds through the Medical Research Council and elsewhere. Time and some historical distance will tell.

Acknowledgement:
I am indebted to Ms Helen Blair for constructive criticism and factual input.

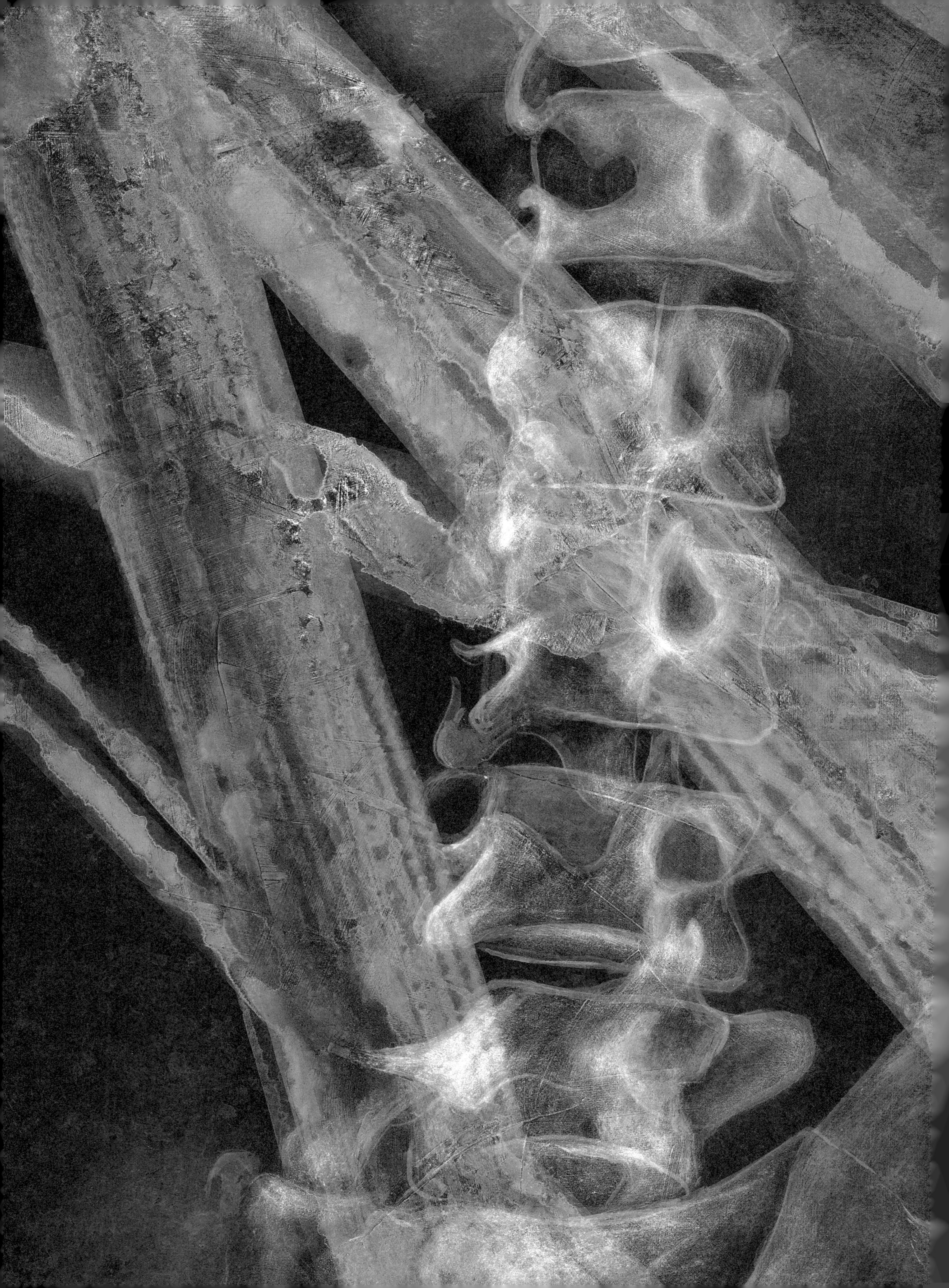

Part Seven

Groups, Programs and Activities

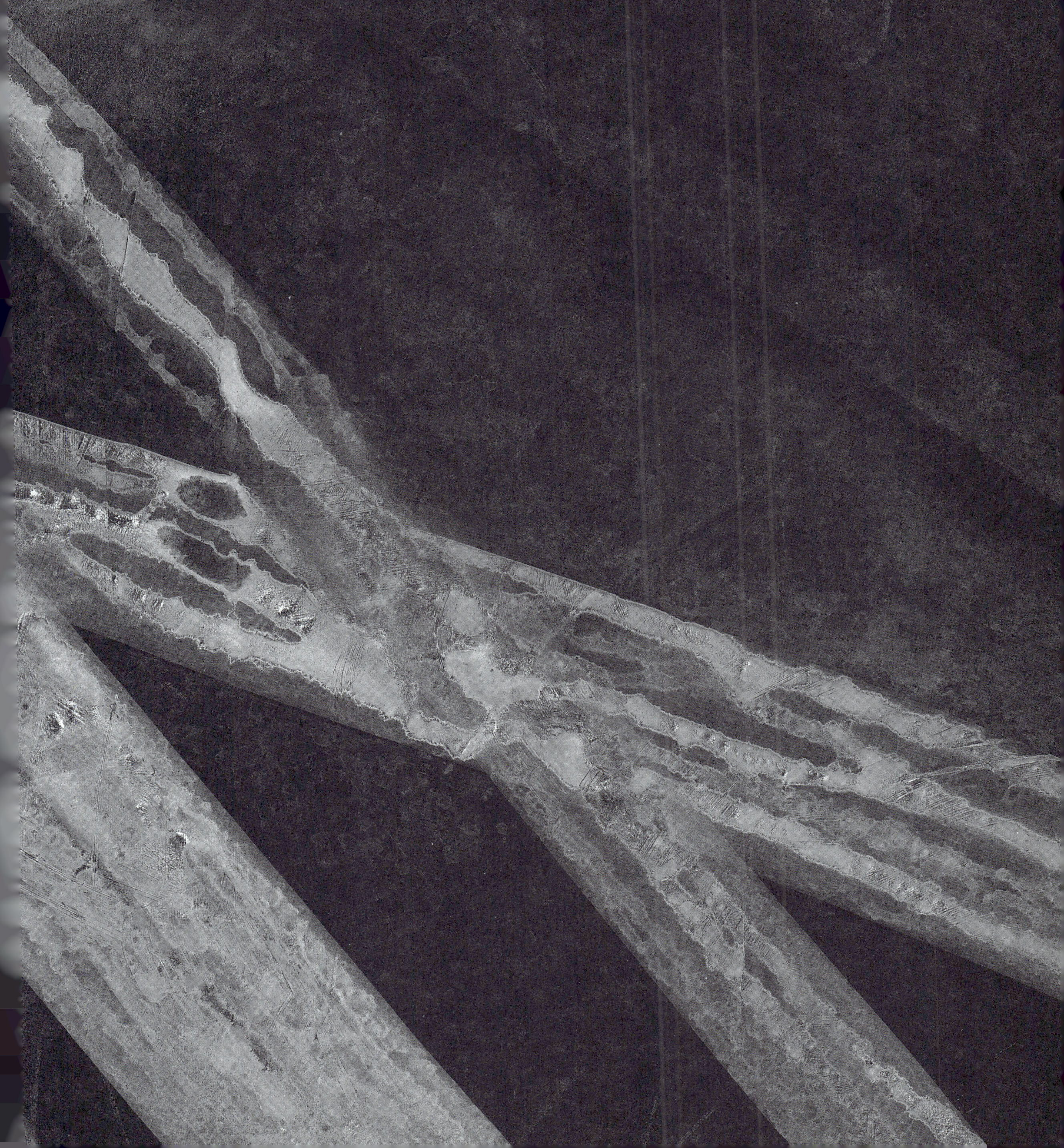

The history of the living world is that of the elaboration of ever more perfect eyes with which there is always something new to be seen.

— Teilhard de Chardin

The relationship between radiology and industry is an apparently ambiguous one. What is self-evident is that the relationship is a close one.

If there is one lesson from the alliances between radiological scientists and industry it is in the power of a collective effort. The groups described here epitomize that. Groups by their nature tend to outlive any one individual and not to be prey to simply what is fashionable in research. The individual with insight and commitment may achieve his or her research goals. However, more often a multi-disciplinary group, where the critical mass of interest, enthusiasm and critical thought is to be found, will be able to develop a self-sustaining research program. Above all this is the best environment in which to nurture the investigators and teachers of the future. It is those investigators and teachers who represent our bridge into the future: they are an investment.

— Brian Lentle

Chapter I • The Industrial Factor:

Technological Innovations which Changed Radiology

Peter Feddersen

Canadian radiologists and technologists have been extremely innovative in developing their specialties. However, these achievements have not been supported by the business climate. The Canadian diagnostic imaging market has never been an easy one from a commercial or business point of view. Companies manufacturing imaging equipment in Europe, Japan or the United States established their operations in Canada, naïvely assuming that market conditions and business opportunities would be similar to those prevailing in the United States. In the US there seemed to be no end to market growth or market opportunities, and this climate provided a comfortable business environment for most firms.

However, the sheer size of Canada, its geography, the low population density and uncertain or inconsistent government funding often made it one of the most difficult markets in the world in which imaging companies might attempt to prosper. Typically, in such circumstances, companies may be expected to limit their engagements to marginal or "niche" specialty markets. Surprisingly, this seems never to have happened, and just about all major imaging equipment suppliers are represented in Canada in full force. This begs the question: What made the difference?

The answer appears to be that the Canadian imaging market has been, in spite of its financial limitations, simply much more avant garde and quality-driven in both technical and clinical terms than other markets in the world. Everybody who has followed the diagnostic imaging market over perhaps the last 30 years is very much aware of the contributions Swedish radiologists had made in the '60s and '70s in developing angiographic equipment and procedures. Equipment or accessories were even named after radiologists such as Nordenstroem or Seldinger. What is not always realized is that Canadian physicians and hospitals were equally involved in the design and development of x-ray apparatus and that Canadian ideas and concepts led to product developments, huge commercial successes that have led to innovative machines marketed all over the world.

The keen interest by Canadian radiologists in developing new imaging technologies and their determination to be involved in research and development have made the Canadian imaging market very interesting for industry, thus sustaining the Canadian imaging industry out of all proportion to its size.

Canadian firsts or Canadian world test sites for new equipment are numerous, and only a few are mentioned here.

Some of the large commercial successes have been born on paper napkins. Not a few of the innovations have been initially viewed by industrial development engineers as purely eccentric with no hope of any commercial success or return. These engineers did not always recognize the commercial potential of some new ideas and often were resistant for a long time before committing resources to develop prototypes. Some of these innovations led to new products which have resulted in hundreds of millions of dollars' worth of sales all over the world. Also, imaging companies soon realized that Canadians felt the need to be in the forefront of testing new technologies, and many Canadian hospitals have been chosen to be the "alpha" or "beta" testing sites for new equipment designs. At the Montréal Neurological Institute, Dr Romeo Ethier installed one of the very first EMI (Electrical Musical Industries, UK) scanners ever made. The Hamilton General Hospital, on the initiative of Dr Harald Stolberg, soon followed with the second Canadian site. Hamilton General Hospital was also the first hospital in the world to install a Biplane Neuro Centrix machine engineered by CGR, and Hamilton General Hospital became the alpha testing site for the world's first universal interventional table developed by Siemens. Dr Conway Don at the Ottawa General Hospital's Department of Radiology created the first fully automated cassetteless film system in the world.[1] Such automated cassetteless systems did not become the business successes the manufacturer had hoped, simply because these systems were difficult to retrofit into existing departments. However, the operational efficiency achieved by Dr Don's cassetteless department, including the cost per examination, has not been rivalled or duplicated anywhere since.

Technology is moving forward at an ever increasing pace, and advances are continually being made with respect to image quality and radiation dose reduction. Canadian hospitals will continue to be alpha or beta testing sites for equipment produced elsewhere in the world. For example, the Royal Victoria Hospital in Barrie, Ontario, upon the initiative of Dr George Lougheed and Mr Ray Frank, has become the first hospital to use charge-coupled device (CCD)-based digital imaging technology for radiographic and fluoroscopic (R-F) applications. Modern scatter correction methods will improve image quality. This unit will be production model number five and the first one installed outside of Japan.

REMOTELY CONTROLLED R-F TABLES

(Hôtel Dieu, Montréal; l'Hôpital Jean Talon, Montréal; Radiologists: Dr Albert Jutras and Dr Guy Duckett)

Perhaps no other group of radiologists has been involved in so many technical and clinical innovations as that from the Hôtel Dieu and l'Hôpital Jean Talon in Montréal in the late '50s and early '60s. Drs Albert Jutras, Paul Roy, Guy Duckett and Marcel Longtin developed technical concepts and influenced the design of imaging equipment in a way that has remained relevant right up to the present.[2-5] The progress achieved through their work was very significant and shaped and influenced diagnostic imaging engineering in a momentous way. The innovation rate achieved in radiological engineering in the late '50s and early '60s in Montréal was tremendous, and it must have been exciting to be part of such activity. Yet surprisingly few people are aware of the milestones achieved there. Dr Albert Jutras, as Chief Radiologist at the Hôtel Dieu in Montréal, developed a strong interest in image intensifier technology as it was developing in the mid–'50s. Drs Jutras and Guy Duckett (Chief of Radiology, l'Hôpital Jean Talon) envisioned and developed the concept of the "ring stand" in 1957. This led to the development of the so-called remotely controlled R-F table later on. In 1957 they visited the Philips Co in Eindhoven and met with their engineers. A prototype was developed and built in Holland for them and installed at l'Hôpital Jean Talon in 1958. The unit was engineered with two separate 5 inch image intensifiers. One was used for video-fluoroscopy and the other one for 16-mm ciné filming and 70-mm camera operation. By 1959 a video link had been established between l'Hôpital Jean Talon and Hôtel Dieu several miles away and teleradiology was born.

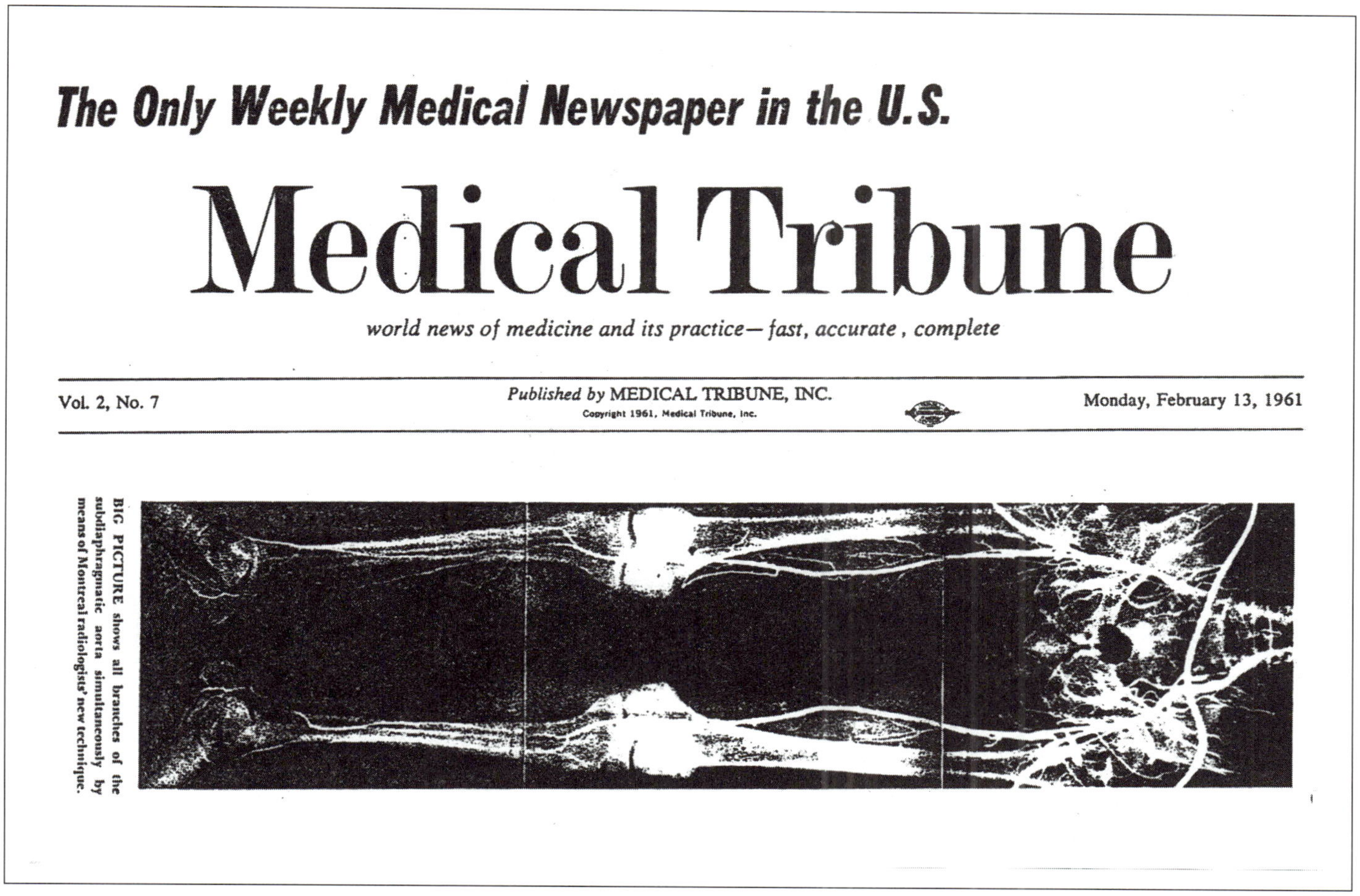

The Only Weekly Medical Newspaper in the U.S.

Medical Tribune

world news of medicine and its practice— fast, accurate, complete

Vol. 2, No. 7 | *Published by* MEDICAL TRIBUNE, INC. | Monday, February 13, 1961

Copyright 1961, Medical Tribune, Inc.

BIG PICTURE shows all branches of the subdiaphragmatic aorta simultaneously by means of Montreal radiologists' new technique.

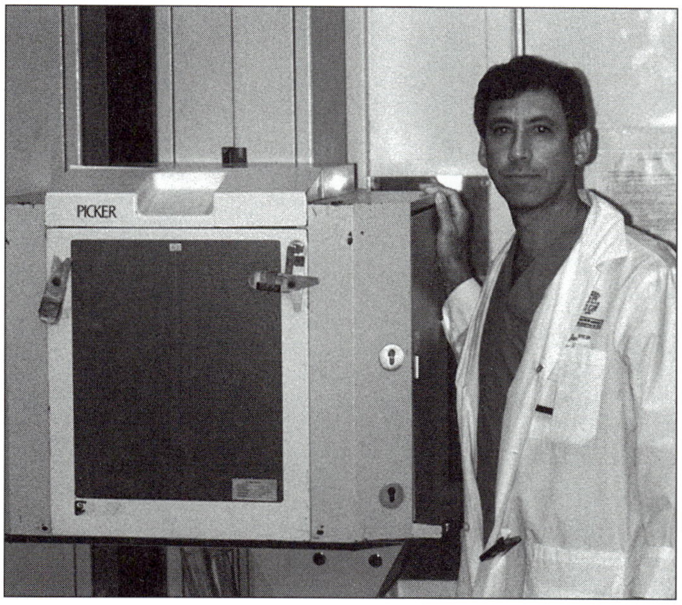

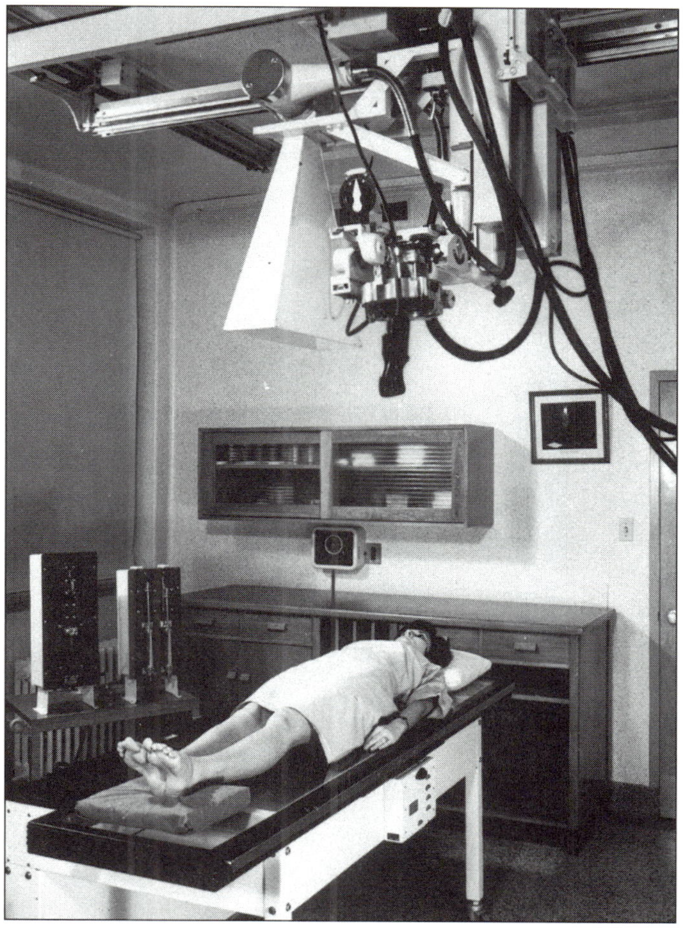

Above
Dr Larry Stein, currently Radiologist-in-Chief, Royal Victoria Hospital, Montréal, with chest unit developed by Dr R Fraser

Right
Imaging equipment with collimator for large field angiography

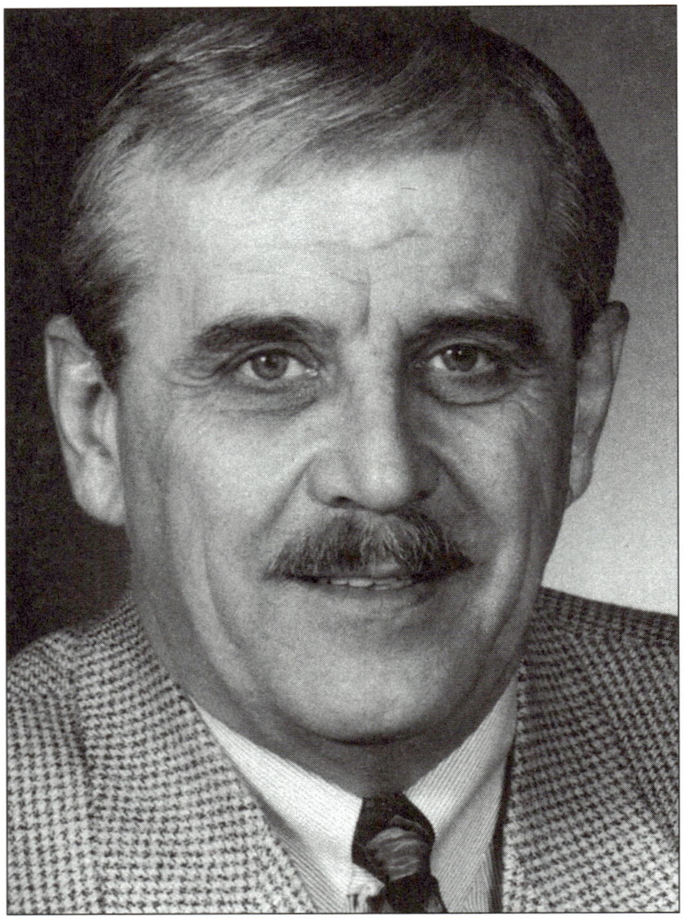

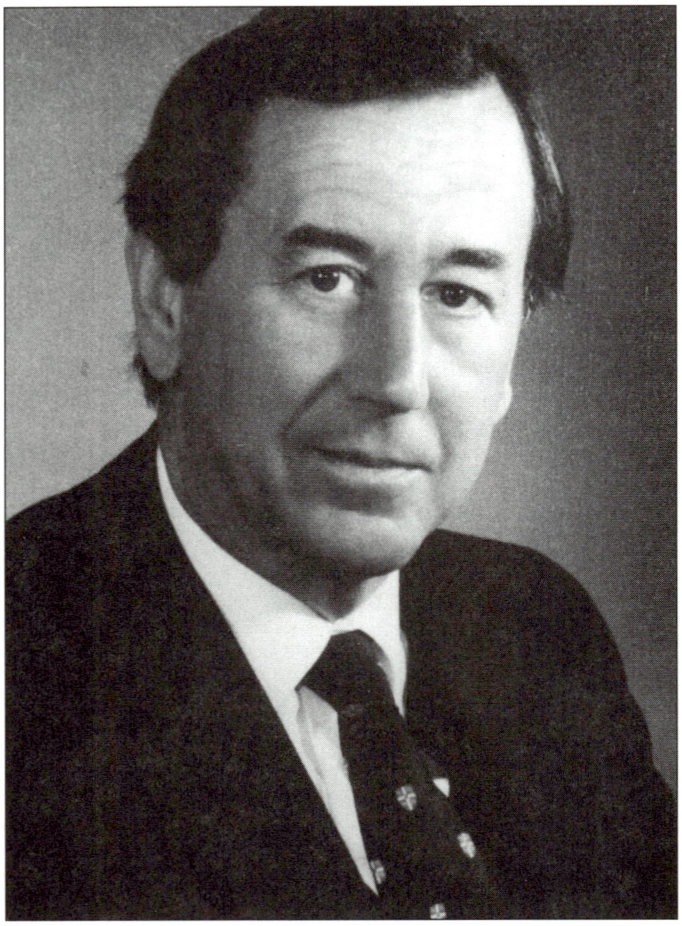

MULTI DIRECTIONAL C-ARM FOR CARDIO-ANGIOGRAPHY

(Hôtel Dieu de Montréal;
Radiologists: Drs Paul Roy and Albert Jutras)

By the late 1950s Dr Jutras was widely known as a leader in gastrointestinal radiology, and it was said that he had little interest in the radiology of other organs or systems. This suddenly changed in June 1959 when the cardiovascular surgeons from Hôtel Dieu asked him to be involved in the design of a prototype imaging unit better suited to angiographic procedures in the heart.

Dr Paul Roy had joined the Hôtel Dieu in 1959. Since he had spent many months in cardiovascular surgery during his education as a resident, he was given the task of developing a prototype angiographic unit which would better meet the needs of cardiovascular surgeons. The C-arm concept was developed and the basic design was established between Drs Roy and Mignault, assisted by Mr Art Burke of Picker Engineering in Montréal. As a result the "Saturn" prototype Floor to Wall Suspended C-Arm was built by Picker X-ray in Montréal between 1961 and 1962 and finalized just before the World Congress of Radiology held in Montréal in August 1962. Mounting the "Saturn" C-Arm on the ceiling improved it, and two units were installed in Montréal at l'Institute de Cardiologie in 1966.

It is perhaps indicative of those times with their relatively slow rate of information exchange that, when Siemens installed a new prototype of a floor-mounted cardiac C-arm with a double-pivoting patient table at the Toronto General Hospital in the mid–'70s, it was believed that this was the only cardiac system capable of certain complex projections or views. Dr Eleonore Paquet from the Institute of Cardiology in Montréal, who was discussing this matter with the vice-president of Siemens, had to tell him the disappointing news. She said: "Non, non, Monsieur Krametz. We are already doing this view for nearly 10 years."

LARGE FIELD CASSETTE CHANGER FOR LEG ARTERIOGRAPHY

(Hôtel Dieu, Montréal;
Radiologists: Drs Paul Roy and Marcel Longtin)[6,7]

At the same time as the angiographic C-arm was being created, Dr Roy also designed the first large field cassette changer for leg arteriography (1959). Again Drs Jutras and Marcel Longtin supported Dr Roy in this endeavour. The first model (RIL 400) was constructed by Research Instrumentation Limited and was ready in 1960. The first presentation about this technology was given in January 1961 at the Canadian Association of Radiologists' meeting held in Saint John, New Brunswick.

Dr Roy won the first prize *magna cum laude* for his new

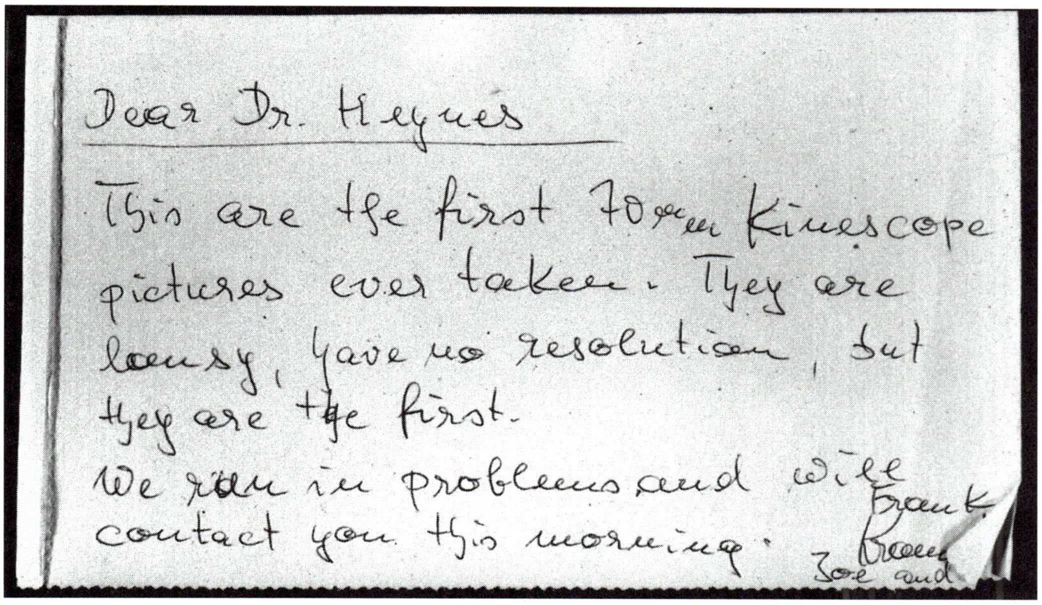
Dear Dr. Hynes

This are the first 70mm Kinescope pictures ever taken. They are lousy, have no resolution, but they are the first.

We ran in problems and will contact you this morning.

Frank

Joe and

Opposite top

Mr Ray Hanson, Technologist, University of Alberta Hospital

Opposite bottom

Dr David Hynes, Radiologist, St. Joseph's Health Centre, Toronto

Left

A note written by Dr Hynes on a paper towel by the technologist recording the first digital image

design at the scientific exhibit during the 1964 annual meeting of the Radiological Society of North America.

This large field cassette changer, which was subsequently built by various companies worldwide, achieved extremely good image quality and was extremely popular with many radiologists. Special compensation filters and tapered x-ray screens were developed, and image qualities were achieved that can, even today, easily compete with more modern complex technologies which have since become available. Large field cassette changers are still being produced and are used all over the world with many diagnosticians being very loyal to the product. Many of its users claim that large field cassette changers are very practical and can still compete in handling and in image quality with stepping table tops or stepping C-arms using Puck film changers. They can also compete in image quality with sophisticated digital stepping methods that have emerged in the early '90s.

CARDIO-ANGIOGRAPHIC EQUIPMENT

(University of Alberta Hospital; Radiologist: Dr Donald Hendin; Technologist: Mr Raymond Hanson)

With the advent of interventional procedures in radiology[1] a lot of design changes in equipment became necessary. These were implemented by all manufacturers of cardiovascular angiographic equipment in the mid–'80s.

In 1976, many years before interventional procedures employed cardiovascular imaging equipment, Dr Don Hendin invented the cardio-angiographic unit, which later became the standard incorporated by most manufacturers.

Since most movements of sophisticated C-arms are motorized, suggestions were made that these movements should be controlled remotely from behind a lead screen using predetermined standard projections. This concept of remote control suggested that all collimation be carried out by the radiographer away from the patient table. Needless to say, this method saved a lot of unnecessary radiation exposure and increased image quality dramatically.

Dr Don Hendin and Mr Ray Hanson also requested that standard projection angles should be achieved using preset protocols. At the time the presetting of standard angles was carried out in a fairly crude way by mechanical means. This subsequently led to the development of pre-programmed cardiac projections using electronic means. Today, virtually no cardiac C-arm unit is installed without this feature.

Dr Hendin and Mr Hanson also suggested that the physiological monitoring console should be moved from the examination area and placed behind the lead glass screen. With this arrangement the radiation and respiratory technologists can control the entire operation of the cardiac catheterization laboratory from behind the lead glass. From today's perspective these seem to be simple and logical steps. In the '70s it meant that a special, highly isolated pre-amplifier had to be developed which allowed physiological patient data to be monitored directly at the patient's side and sent by a special shielded cable to the physiological monitoring unit now located behind the lead glass screen.

AUTOMATIC RADIOGRAPHIC CHEST FILM CHANGERS

(The Royal Victoria Hospital, Montréal; Radiologist: Dr Robert Fraser; Technologist: Mr Archie Wilkinson)

In the 1960s, as is the case today, chest radiography comprised at least 40 per cent of all anatomic regions examined in the departments of radiography of most large general hospitals. Automated film loading and cassette handling systems have made the workload of today's radiographer somewhat easier. However, the handling and transportation of tons of film cassettes every week is still required.

During the late '60s it occured to Dr Robert Fraser (Radiologist-in-Chief) and Mr Archie Wilkinson (Chief Radiographic Technologist) that an automated unit which could feed unexposed films from a magazine into a screen-film changer and then directly into a film processor might make such time-consuming and labour-intensive work obsolete.

Based on their recommendation Picker Canada Limited, under the direction of Mr Leslie Withers, agreed to construct a prototype of an automated film-chest changer at their Bramalea plant near Toronto. The design and engineering work was completed in 1969, and the unit was installed at the Royal Victoria Hospital that same year. It incorporated such unique features as the "air-gap technique" instead of a radiographic grid and used a 10-feet focus-to-film distance with special compensatory filters mounted near the x-ray tube.

For nearly a decade the image quality achieved with this unit became the standard against which all chest radiography was judged. Other manufacturers have built automatic chest units since, and many thousands of such systems are now installed all over the world.

DIGITAL VIDEO FLUOROGRAPHY AND RADIOGRAPHY

(St. Joseph's Health Centre, Toronto;
Radiologist: Dr David Hynes)

It was mentioned above that many new concept and design ideas are sometimes born as a sketch on the back of a paper napkin. Paper napkins were very much involved in the design of the world's first practical digital radiographic systems for radiographic and fluoroscopic (RF) applications. Here, technology had constantly to catch up with the forward thinking necessary to develop a practical digital radiography system. During this time paper napkin ideas often had to bridge the gap between technical imperatives and the technical realities of the late '70s and early '80s.

In order to succeed, various technologies had to be married and a number of companies had to cooperate. Matrix Instruments, VAS Instrument Corporation, Agfa and Siemens were all involved. Making various departments within one company cooperate is difficult enough; making different companies cooperate can be a task which requires more than simply steady nerves and patience. Dr Hynes had the skills to succeed.

Thousands of digital RF units have been installed all over the world since, and virtually all such new units now

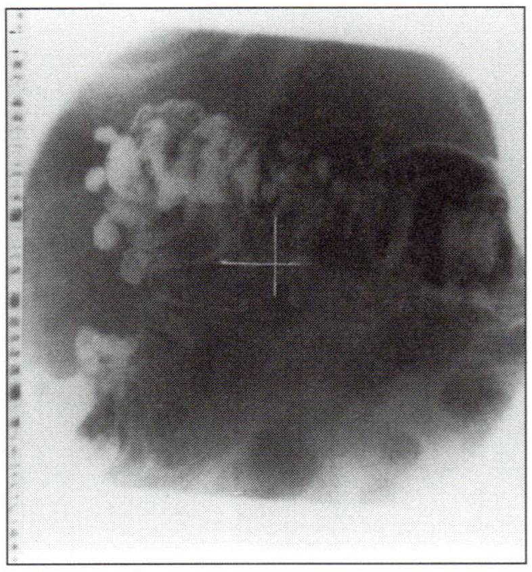

being purchased in Canada come equipped with digital imaging systems.

Dr Hynes' work began in 1976 when his department acquired an RF unit with a 512 matrix. This was soon inadequate, and in 1981 a newly developed 1024 x 1024 matrix digital storage capacity was added. In 1983 the system was futher improved by adding a digital exposure technique which allowed the image intensifier to be saturated with photons by means of high mA and milli-second exposure factors. In 1983 a practical and truly high resolution digital radiography system for RF applications with instant imaging became a reality at St Joseph's Hospital in Toronto.

In the meantime technology progressed in leaps and bounds. Image intensifiers were optimized for digital radiography through improved contrast characteristics; 10 bit storage computers became available which complemented the 1024 x 1024 matrix by providing an adequate memory capacity.

At the University of Toronto, under the leadership of Dr Martin Yaffe, a design team has developed a digital mammography device using CCD technology. Dr Aaron Fenster's group at the Robarts Institute of the University of Western Ontario is developing three dimensional display technology in ultrasonic imaging.

Not least Dr Terry Peters at the Montréal Neurological Institute produced the world's first practical work station for three dimensional stereo guided neurosurgery, and he made a major contribution to the viewing wand stereo guided work station now being successfully produced as a commercial product by ISG Technology of Mississauga.

This review of some of the Canadian initiatives in radiographic technology is one which reflects well on the past and promises much for the future. Indeed, that future is one which is already taking shape: Dr Mark Henkelman's team at Sunnybrook Hospital is pioneering, in collaboration with General Electric, the development of a low-field magnetic resonance imaging (MRI) system for real-time interventional procedures done with MRI guidance.

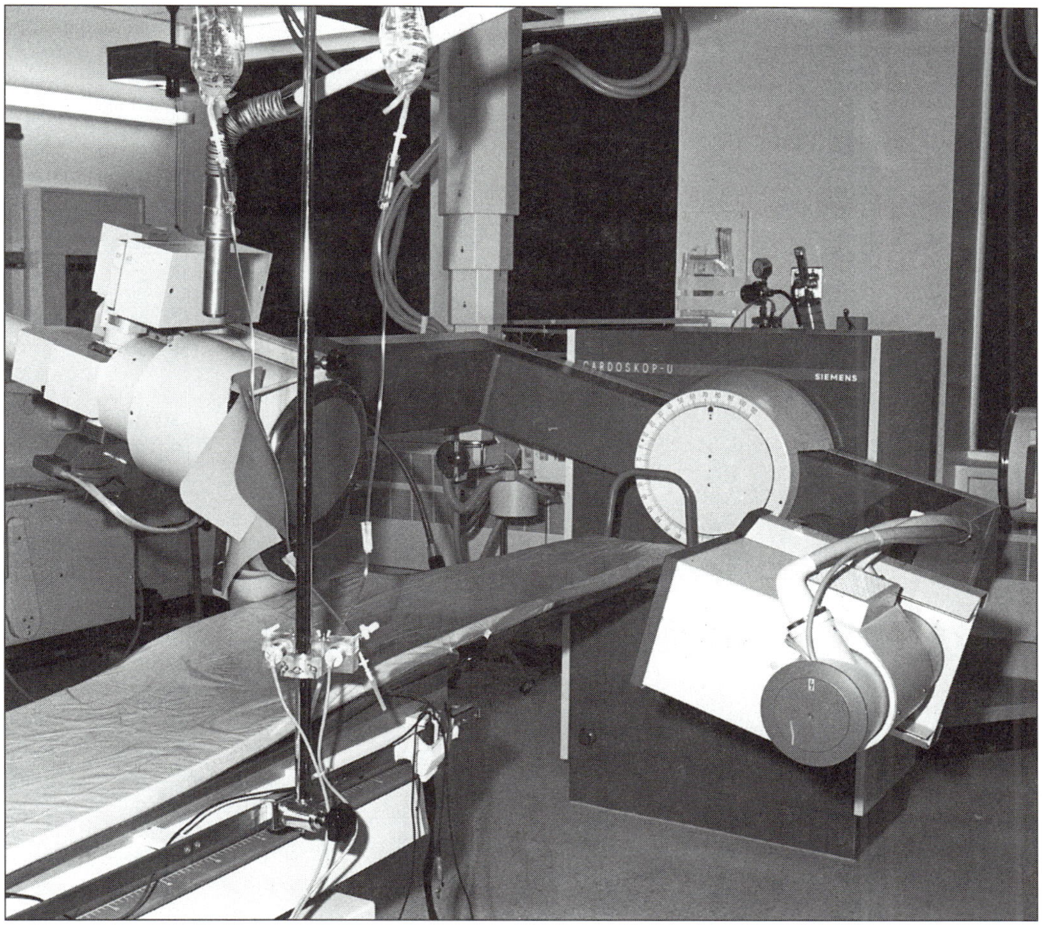

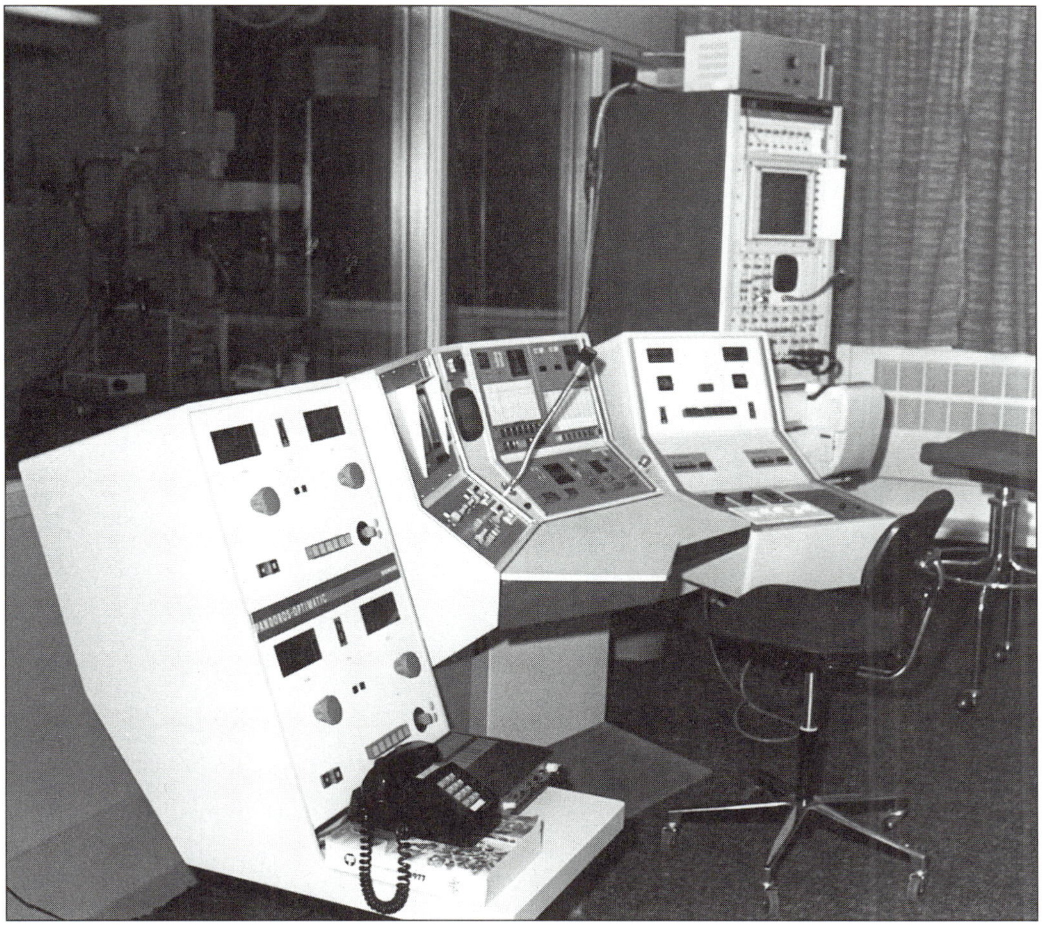

Left and below
University of Alberta cardio-angiographic unit

Opposite
First digital radiograph (courtesy Dr Hynes)

Chapter II • The History of

Interventional Radiology

of the Biliary Tract

H Joachim Burhenne

November 1979. The deposed and exiled Shah of Iran undergoes a cholecystectomy at New York Hospital-Cornell Medical Center. However, a retained common duct stone delays his return to Mexico. This further complicates the diplomatic efforts being made to obtain the release of American hostages held in Teheran by forces loyal to Ayatollah Khomeini. Physicians at Cornell want to avoid the risk of a second operation and call for a radiologist to attempt nonoperative removal of the retained stone.

This dramatic combination of political and medical events was ideally suited to bring interventional radiology of the biliary tract to the attention of physicians and the public. Radiology had been recognized as an important diagnostic specialty, but the general public was not familiar with therapeutic advances that used x-ray methods. A radiologic procedure was used in preference to surgery in this difficult clinical situation.

The retained gallstone of the Shah was removed successfully during the night of November 26, 1979. The procedure was accomplished under fluoroscopic control with the use of a wire basket manipulated through the T-tube tract into the bile duct. Worldwide press coverage of the event advanced the reputation of radiology. The front page of *The New York Times,* November 28, 1979, proclaimed "Gallstone is removed from Shah, raising chance of early departure." Years later, when the details were published in a chapter in the book, *Doctors,* by Martin O'Malley, Dr Burhenne was quoted as saying, "I was excited about being able to put radiology in the picture, to show the world what my specialty could do."[1]

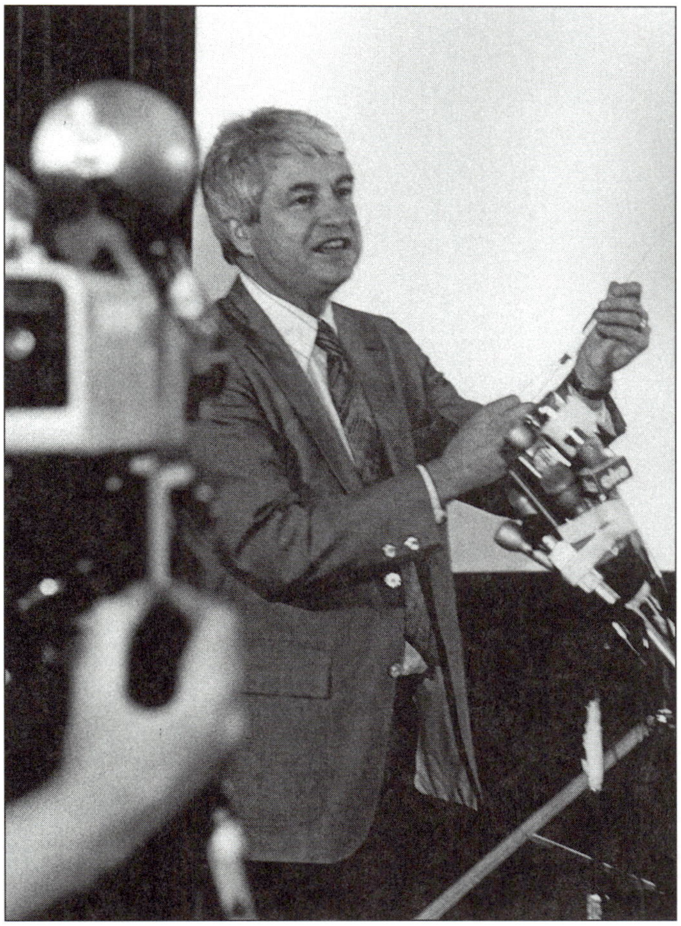

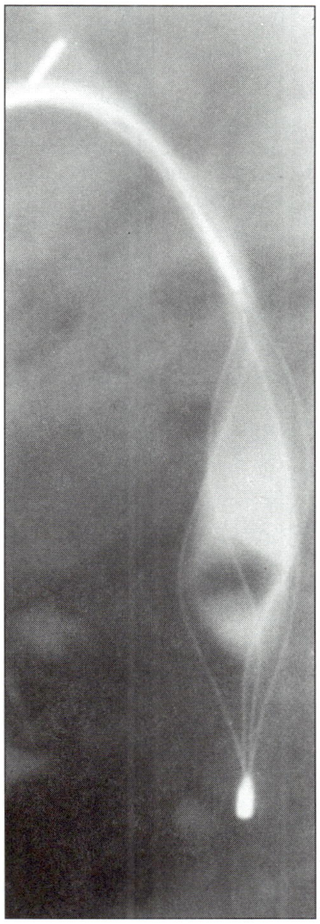

Far left
Dr J Burhenne

Left
The catheter

Below
Newspaper article from the *Vancouver Sun*

'Basket' technique avoids 2d operation

By EDWARD EDELSON
Science Editor

The procedure performed on the former Shah of Iran in New York Hospital is an ingenious technique developed eight years ago to save gallstone patients from a second operation when surgery fails to remove all their stones.

An estimated 5,000 patients a year would require further surgery for gallstones—which could be life-endangering—if the nonsurgical procedure were not available.

In essence, the procedure is simple. A thin, flexible tube called a catheter is snaked into the bile duct through an opening in the stomach wall, where the overlooked stones usually are found. At the tip of the catheter is a closed basket made of wire mesh. The basket is opened and the stone is caught and removed.

But Dr. H. Joachim Burhenne, who developed the method when he was at Children's Hospital in San Francisco, came up with some inventive ideas to make the technique a reality.

Burhenne, who now heads the department of radiology at the University of British Columbia, has become the world's acknowledged leader in the technique. His success rate has been 80%.

One of his major innovations was to change the usual medical procedure of immediately sewing up the opening in the abdomen wall that is created to allow the surgical wound to drain.

Surgeons normally remove the drainage tube after a few days. Burhenne instead began X-raying patients to determine whether any gallstones were left. If they were, he kept the tube in place for a number of weeks, to allow the body to form a fibrous channel through which the special catheter can be passed.

In the case of the shah, the official hospital statement noted that the procedure performed late Monday had to be delayed for five weeks after

(Continued on page 27)

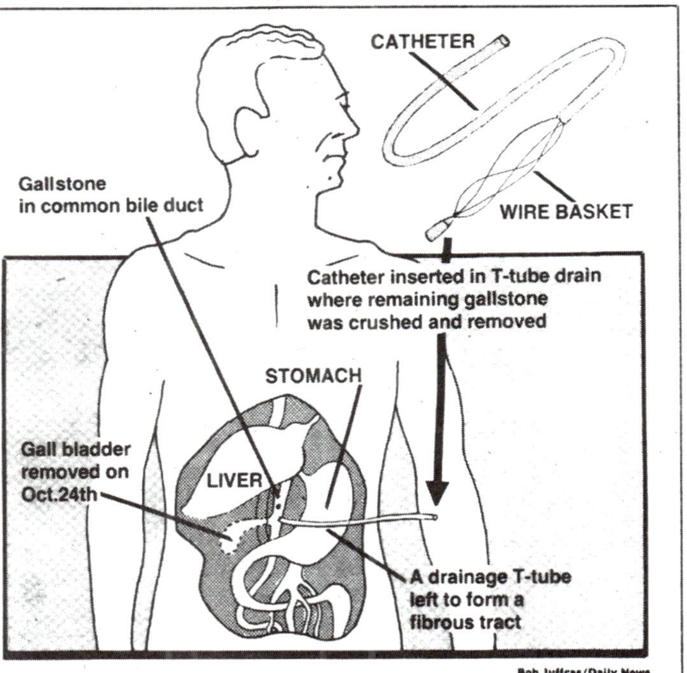

Bob Juffras/Daily News

Shah has gallstone removed without surgery by radiologist Dr. Joachim Burhenne.

The term *interventional radiology* was coined by Margulis in 1967 to describe the "growing body of manipulative procedures performed by a physician skillful in radiologic techniques and experienced in the clinical problems."[2] Successful interventional radiology had been first used in the treatment of intussusception in children in the 1920s.[3]

When was, then, the beginning of interventional radiology of the biliary tract? Credit for early work must go to Burckhardt and Mueller.[4] They reported in 1921 on percutaneous puncture of the gallbladder both in cadavers and *in vivo*. They succeeded "by injection of a shadow-producing fluid to visualize gallstones and bile ducts." The other aims of their work were to treat gallstone colic and cholecystitis percutaneously. In addition, they raised the possibility of dissolving gallstones by an injection of chemicals. We can assume that Dr Pribram in Berlin knew about the work of his surgical colleagues when he used ether in 1923 for the treatment of gallstones impacted in the common duct.[5,6] He reported success in 38 cases, but his technique of stone dissolution in the bile ducts was not used widely because of complications. Part of the success of instillation of fluids in the bile duct for stone passage probably is the result of increased fluid pressure alone. Lamis and his colleagues[7] have used catheter irrigation through the T-tube tract under fluoroscopic control with good success for the treatment of retained common duct stones.

A nonoperative surgical intervention for treatment of retained common duct stones after surgery is needed because of the increased surgical risk with re-operation.[8] Halsted, who performed one of the earliest operations on the gallbladder, was himself to die of complications after the removal of a retained common duct stone.[9]

Mondet[10] extracted retained common duct stones through the sinus tract of the T-tube as early as 1962. He developed a pliable forceps for this purpose. The same Mondet extraction forceps was used successfully by Mazzariello[11] after bougienage of the sinus tract. The first physician to use the Dormia ureteral stone basket for biliary stone extraction was Lagrave in 1969.[12] The first successful use in the United States was reported in 1971 by Mahorner.[13]

The beginnings of nonoperative intervention in the biliary tract were, therefore, contributions from our surgical colleagues. Interventional radiology came into being with US radiologists who perfected and popularized the extraction of retained common duct stones. Burhenne[14] added a steerable catheter for easier instrumentation of the T-tube tract and bile ducts. Bean[15] preferred the use of arterial catheters for basket insertion. Because the procedure was done in the ambulatory patient, there was the added advantage of the radiologist from the referring hospital performing the procedure with the interventional radiologist, and then instituting the nonoperative radiologic intervention for retained stone removal at his and the patient's own institution.

This same technique was used by Burhenne in many foreign countries where lectures were preceded by demonstrations of nonoperative stone removal with the local radiologist assisting. This method led to more ready acceptance of the procedure by surgeons and its widespread use. A success rate of 95 per cent in 661 patients treated between 1972 and 1979 also assisted in making nonoperative radiologic intervention the method of choice for retained stone removal.[16,17] This development helped inter-ventional radiology of the biliary tract become a subspecialty.

Radiologic modifications of early surgical techniques were important in the beginning of interventional radiology of the biliary tract. After its application to the management of patients with biliary stone disease proved successful, radiologists became the leaders in designing new procedures and broadened the field of intervention to include many areas of biliary tract pathologic conditions. The Seldinger[18] and other arteriographic catheter techniques were modified for use in the biliary tract. Percutaneous transhepatic techniques, already used in 1956 by Remolar[19] for external bile drainage, were expanded for interventional application. Percutaneous external biliary drainage by catheter prior to surgery[20] was followed by transhepatic catheter manipulation through benign and malignant strictures to establish internal drainage into the gastrointestinal tract.[21–23] In 1979 Ring[24] constructed a pigtail retention catheter with multiple side holes that can be positioned above and below the obstruction for drainage. The same principle of internal catheter drainage for a malignant stricture was described by a hepatojejunostomy in 1974.[25] Molnar[26] reported first, also in 1974, on relief of obstructive jaundice through percutaneous transhepatic catheter insertion. The transhepatic percutaneous route therefore evolved from cholangiography to external bile drainage[19] in 1956 and, since 1974, to internal biliary drainage in obstructive jaundice.[26] The next step was to place permanent stents or biliary prostheses in the same fashion.[27] Dotter[25] first removed bile duct stones by the transhepatic route.

Benign strictures of the bile ducts were first dilated with balloon catheters in 1974.[25] Burhenne reported on seven patients with strictures in the intrahepatic and extrahepatic bile ducts and at the hepatojejunostomy anastomosis.[29] This was before the introduction of the balloon-tipped angiographic catheter.[30] Molnar[31] first dilated choledochoenterostomy strictures by the transhepatic route in 1978. Gruntzig balloon catheters have been used for interventional dilatation since 1980.[32]

Additional palliation for bile duct cancer has been achieved with internal irradiation by iridium-192 via the decompression catheter.[33] Endoscopists have adopted successful techniques designed by interventional radiologists for the retrograde approach to the biliary tract. Nagai[34] introduced relief of bile duct obstruction through external drainage by insertion of a nasobiliary catheter in 1976. Three years later, Soehendra[35] implanted endoprostheses using the retrograde endoscopic approach for internal decompression of bile duct obstruction. Choledochoscopes have been used by the T-tube tract for removal of retained bile duct calculi,[36] and endoscopic sphincterotomy was first reported 1142 by Classen in 1974.[37] Spontaneous common duct stone passage and stone extraction thus became possible. In technically difficult cases, the transhepatic radiologic and retrograde endoscopic approaches were combined.[38]

Just as biliary interventional radiologists used the Dormia basket designed by a urologist, Fernstrom[39] adapted the radiologic technique used for missed common bile duct stones for the treatment of recurrent renal calculi through a percutaneous nephrostomy under radiologic control. Although 10 years elapsed between the first description of percutaneous nephrostomy in 1955[40] and its subsequent application for percutaneous drainage of the renal pelvis,[41] this procedure is well established. It is used for decompression, as access for a variety of endourologic manipulations and for removal of stones. More than 50 years elapsed, however, before percutaneous gallbladder puncture was extended from Burckhardt and Mueller's work in 1921.[4]

Percutaneous transhepatic cholangiography, the technical prerequisite for interventional transhepatic procedures, was described in 1937.[42] Puncture of the gallbladder then became regarded as a complication of transhepatic cholangiography. In 1967, seven cases were described in which this complication occurred.[43] Deliberate gallbladder puncture began in 1976[44] using ultrasonic guidance for direct injection into the gallbladder in dogs. Hogan *et al.*[44] used a transperitoneal approach as opposed to transhepatic puncture. The application of this technique for gallbladder decompression in patients followed in 1979.[45,46] Access to the gallbladder by the cholecystostomy tract or percutaneous puncture and subsequent sinus tract dilatation was reported for the use of stone removal in 1982.[47] Percutaneous cholecystostomy will permit access not only to the gallbladder but also the cystic duct for the removal of common bile duct stones.[48] Gallstone removal through the cystic duct was first accomplished by Mazzariello in 1974.[49] Removal of gallbladder stones via a cholecystostomy tract as a radiologic interventional technique also was described in 1974.[25] Percutaneous cholecystolithotomy was reported in 1985[50] and is now reported successful without general anesthesia.[51] Discussion continues as to whether the transhepatic or transperitoneal route for puncture is preferable to avoid bile peritonitis.[52] This complication is avoided if initial surgical mini-cholecystostomy is done under local anesthesia, then followed by radiologic stone extraction from the gallbladder, cystic duct and common bile duct. No mortality resulted in 36 high-risk patients.[53] Percutaneous cholecystolithotomy also has been described as an elective single-stage procedure but under a general anesthetic.[54]

Lithotripsy, or stone fragmentation, is an old principle in medicine. Instruments were designed for this purpose more than 200 years ago. Even electrohydrolic stone disintegration, the principle underlying the latest technique for the treatment of gallstones, was already tested in the 19th century.[55] In 1969 the Russian instrument Urat-1 was the first instrument to apply shock waves successfully to bladder stones.[56] It was followed by ultrasound lithotripsy in 1971.[57] Electrohydrolic fragmentation was first extended successfully *in vitro* and *in vivo* for the treatment of gallstones with intracorporeal probes in 1975,[58] followed by ultrasonic fragmentation of a large residual biliary tract stone by passing a flexible ultrasonic drill through the T-tube tract.[59] The most promising noninvasive technique for gallstone fragmentation is the extracorporeal shock wave application, first introduced by Sauerbruch et al in 1986.[60] Other lithotripsy centres have adopted the original method by the group of gastroenterologists from Munich to combine extracorporeal lithotripsy with adjuvant oral chemolitholysis for fragment dissolution. Comparable clinical results have, however, been reported with extracorporeal shock application alone.[61]

In all interventional alternatives to cholecystectomy the gallbladder remains *in situ*, implying that retreatment is required if symptomatic gallstones recur. This also applies to the latest technique in gallbladder stone treatment using a rotary gallstone lithotrite as a percutaneous nonoperative option[62] and gallstone dissolution with the injection of methyl tert-butyl ether.[63] Chemical ablation of the gallbladder could prevent stone recurrence. The first clinical results of gallbladder ablation are promising when combined with permanent cystic duct occlusion.[64]

Although cholecystectomy remains the gold standard

for the treatment of symptomatic gallstones, the recent developments of many nonsurgical options have stimulated surgical advancement, leading to the development of laparoscopic cholecystectomy.[65] This requires short term hospital admission and is still done under general anesthesia, but the recovery period is shortened significantly. More clinical trials with this surgical technique and with the large number of nonsurgical options are required before comparative advantages will become apparent and until the different indications for various techniques will be worked out. It is probably fair to predict that the continuing history of interventional radiology of the biliary tract will be as productive and exciting as its beginning.

Acknowledgements:
Material in this article was presented in part as the Charles T Dotter Memorial Lecture, Pacific Northwest Radiological Society, 1988, and published in *Radiological Clinics of North America* (1990; 28: 1139). It is reproduced here with the kind permission both of the author and publisher.

Dr. Joachim Burhenne on Front Page Challenge

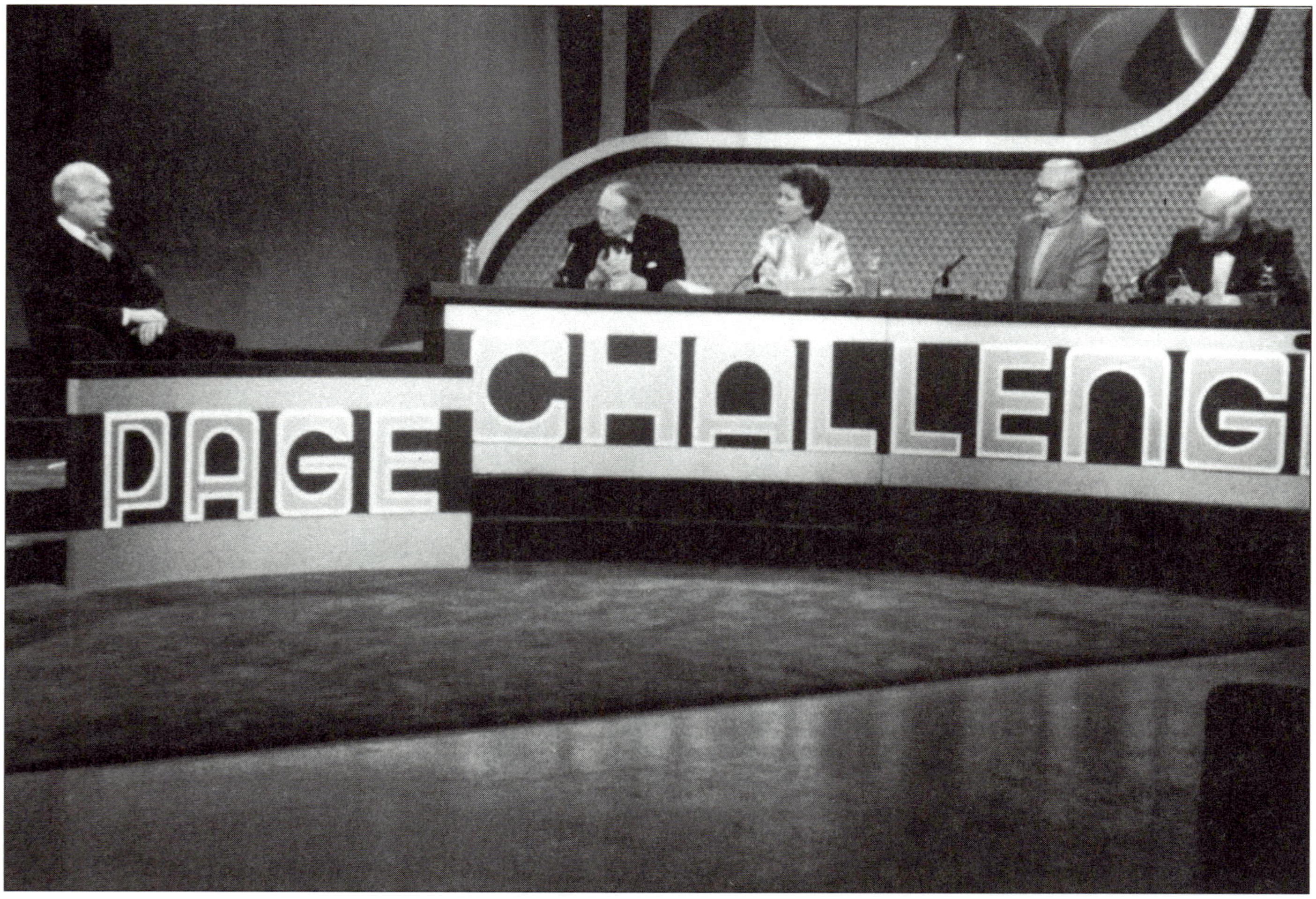

Chapter III • A History of

Ultrasound in Manitoba

1964–1980: As we saw and have remembered it

EA (Ted) Lyons, Ross E Brown and Frank A Manning

Many people were responsible for the development of diagnostic ultrasound in Manitoba, and we three played a part. Our recollections focus on the very early years: what it was like, who was there and how clinical ultrasound evolved. Our apologies to those whose contributions are not fully recognized and our thanks to those who wandered with us down memory lane and were of so much help in putting this paper together.

THE EARLY YEARS

In 1964 Dr Michael Graham Saunders, a neurologist at the General Hospital in Winnipeg, bought a Biosonar 2000–an ultrasound machine that someone had convinced him might lead to fruitful research. He was a unique individual who established the Departments of Neurology, Biomedical Engineering and Computing Sciences at what was to become the Health Sciences Centre. He was far too busy to work with the ultrasound machine so he offered it for use in a research project to any enterprising medical student. Thus it was that in the summers of 1964 and 1965 Ted Lyons investigated echopulsation of the third ventricle of the brain using the Biosonar. He earned a Bachelor of Science in Medicine for this project. Mike Saunders died in 1975 on an airplane while travelling to a meeting in Chicago.

In April 1965 Dr Ross Brown, a neurosurgery resident was the first to apply the Biosonar 2000 in clinical medicine in performing the first echoencephalogram in Manitoba. In the spring of that year Dr Saunders sponsored Ross to attend the 1965 Pittsburgh symposium on ultrasonology. At this symposium Ross found out about other clinical uses such as in obstetrics, gynaecology and cardiology.

During the next year he performed echoencephalography and some echocardiography (pericardial effusion detection) while continuing in his neurosurgery residency. In the spring of 1966 Ross and Dr Ian Morrison (an obstetrical resident) attended a clinical conference in Denver. This conference was sponsored by Dr Joseph Holmes of the University of Colorado, a nephrologist and a pioneer in the development of the new clinical scanning units made by the Wright Brothers of Boulder, Colorado. Following this conference Dr Brown enlisted the support of Dr Douglas MacEwan, then Head of the Department of Radiology at the Winnipeg General Hospital and Dr Saunders to petition the Manitoba Health Services Commission to fund the purchase of a Wright Brothers (Physionic Corporation) B-Mode static scanner for the yet to be established Department of Diagnostic Ultrasound. This bid was successful. However, in the middle of the ordering process Picker Corporation purchased the Physionics Corporation and the price of the equipment rose by approximately $3500 to the then astronomical sum of $18 000.

The department opened its doors in July 1966. Initially, Dr Brown ran the department himself (scanning patients, reporting, cleaning, doing the floors etc.) until January 1967 at which time Beverly Zack Blank was hired as a secretary. It soon became obvious that technical assistance was required as the work load increased. Beverly was trained as the first ultrasound technical specialist. She stayed for two years and then went to Vancouver. For the next three years Ross ran the department, doing echoencephalography and echocardiography with either an Ekoline 10 or 12 made by Smith Kline Instruments. In addition to abdominal scans, obstetrical and gynaecological scans were also performed with a 1966 vintage Picker B-scanner. Ross worked with Hewlett Packard to test one of their new ideas for a B-Scanner, which was great conceptually, but somehow its time had not yet come. During this time period, images were described by the uninitiated as "weather maps" or "maps of the moon." In retrospect this view might have been correct, but nonetheless they provided diagnostic information.

An on-call service was offered in emergency echoencephalography. As the department had only one physician, medical students were trained to carry out the procedure and paid a stipend to serve on a call roster. The first of these students was, quite naturally, Ted Lyons because of his previous involvement with Dr Michael Saunders. Additional students on this service were Chris Kehler, later to be an anaesthetist, and Frank Manning, later Head of Obstetrics and Gynaecology at the Faculty of Medicine and co-developer of the fetal biophysical profile.

Major clinical research was carried out in the use of Doppler ultrasound in obstetrics, with the validity of continuous-wave Doppler monitoring as a diagnostic test for fetal life established in a study of 600 patients. In addition, major research was performed in conjunction with the Head of Obstetrics, Dr Mervin Roulston, on fetal cephalometry. This data, based also on a study of more than 650 patients, was the first to clearly establish the relationship of fetal biparietal dimensions to gestational age. Other clinical investigations showed the utility of diagnostic ultrasound in differentiating solid from cystic masses and in the diagnosis of abdominal aortic aneurysms.

During the years 1967 to the end of 1969, the department grew with the addition of two more technologists, Raylene Husak and Marilyn Ball.

In the summer of 1969 Ross Brown announced he was off to Oklahoma in November to take a position as assistant professor in the Department of Radiological Sciences, and as Head of Ultrasound, under Dr Sidney Traub, himself a native of Saskatchewan. The first out of province technologist trained at the Health Sciences Centre was Mr LE Schnitzer who arrived from Oklahoma City in 1969. "LE" became the first full time American ultrasound technical specialist and was destined to work with Dr Brown in Oklahoma City.

Just prior to his departure, Ross Brown as program chairman and a board member of the American Institute of Ultrasound in Medicine (AIUM) hosted the 10th annual meeting of the AIUM in the fall of 1969. World leaders in the field of clinical ultrasound came to join with 135 other colleagues at this meeting. Notables were Joseph Holmes and John Wild from Denver, Professor Kratochwil from Vienna, Bill McKinney from Winston Salem and others. Social highlights included an evening at the Royal Winnipeg Ballet and an invitation to Government House from the Lieutenant Governor of the province.

The American Society of Ultrasound Technical Specialists (now the Society of Diagnostic Medical Sonographers) was conceived at the Winnipeg AIUM meeting in 1969 by Joan Baker (Seattle), LE Schnitzer (Oklahoma City), Marilyn Ball and Raylene Husak. Dr Brown served as the first medical advisor to this group from its inception until 1974.

With Dr Brown's impending departure in late 1969, Dr MacEwan approached Ted Lyons with an unusual offer: "Come into the Radiology residency program in July as section head of ultrasound. Run the section at noon and evenings and do a regular residency. At the end of four years you will have a dedicated ultrasound department, budget and staff."

In 1969, after completing his internship, Ted Lyons took over the Section with one secretary and two technologists—Raylene Husak and Marilyn Ball. They had one room in the radiology department and an Ekoline 20 A-mode head machine as well as a small portable Ekoline 10 head machine. The total workload was 1700 cases, mostly examination of heads. The A-mode echoencephalographic examinations were used to detect a shift of the midline echo-complex or third ventricle. We examined hundreds of patients with a history of headache or trauma. It was a useful technique but not without its flaws. In 1980 Ted ran into a former neurosurgery resident, Dr Brian Hunter in the Chicago airport. The discussion quickly led to "What are you doing now? Still ultrasound?" When Ted answered in the affirmative he pulled out of his wallet a faded polaroid picture of an echoencephalogram we had done on a patient of his several years previously. We had missed the diagnosis, and he had kept the picture ever since! The original technique was also used to detect third and lateral ventricular dilatation in adults and children, but in 1976 a computed tomographic scanner was installed and this superior tool marked the end of A-mode ultrasound encephalography.

In the early years, with Ted as the only physician in ultrasound, there was a problem with coverage when he was away lecturing. For two years he carried a portable Xerox transceiver to meetings and every evening Kathy McDiarmid would spend hours on the phone transmitting the polaroid A-mode echoencephalographic images for official interpretation. The phone bills were impressive. When Ted was visiting Oklahoma in 1976 Ross Brown, not to be outdone, demonstrated the use of *his* xerox transceiver which was hooked up to the mobile telephone of his red Shelby AC Cobra car. A prerequisite for practice in clinical ultrasound was and is a love of toys and gadgets!

Shael "Chuck" Harris and Kathy McDiarmid were trained as technologists and replaced Raylene and Marilyn upon their departure in 1971. Diane Atkins was hired by St Boniface General Hospital, and trained at HSC going to do "midline heads" and M-mode echocardiography. Diane taught Kathy the art of echocardiography. In the early days the department was held together by a series of secretaries, namely Linda Howatt, Anne Oleksiuk and Marg Potts.

1971 was also a year in which it was decided to investigate the possible bioeffects of ultrasound waves. In cooperation with researchers at the university's Animal Sciences department, a group of chick embryos were exposed to ultrasound energy and the offspring examined. Nothing untoward was found so they gave us two of the unhatched eggs. We hatched them in a "hot" box in the one-room department and at delivery named them Chuck and Doug. They remained in the lab until six weeks of age when they began to make a lot of noise with their clucking and banging against the side of the box. It was time to find them a new home. Harriet Lyons, Ted's wife, taught Grade 5 at Pinkham School on Lulu Street close to the hospital. A cage was built, and Chuck and Doug went to school. They were class pets until June when the class donated them to Aunt Sally's farm at the zoo.

Ted was awarded the first SERF (Scientific Educational and Research Fund) travelling fellowship from the HSC. In July 1971 he went to Glasgow Scotland to spend a year doing research with Professor Ian Donald, a leading obstetrician in Great Britain and head of the Queen Mother's obstetrical hospital. Ian Donald was an innovator in clinical ultrasound using the first B-scan machine, a Diasonograph manufactured in Edinburgh. He started the genetics department and was an accomplished painter, pianist and yachtsman.

In 1970 Ted was asked by St Boniface Hospital to set up an ultrasound laboratory. Diane Atkins, a laboratory technician who had been trained at HSC, became the first technologist there. Gene Charney was later hired. Dr Andrew Morris was the cardiologist responsible for the interpretation of the echocardiograms at St Boniface General Hospital. In addition Denis Gratton was hired to work at St Boniface after his training but since they had no B-scan equipment he stayed at HSC working with Bruce Goalen and Kathy McDiarmid. Later Denis worked at St Boniface one or two days a week using a Unirad B-scanner for obstetrical and abdominal ultrasound examinations. Shortly thereafter, Gene Charney was trained in B-scanning.

Gerry Ballard, who had trained in 1975, became the chief technologist in 1980 and continued to run the department until 1993. Patrick Lawrence returned from Victoria to fill the new position of Educational Coordinator.

One of the more memorable departmental accomplishments was the publication of a *Color Atlas of Sectional Anatomy*. The material was collected by a combined effort of many of the technical staff and key members of the departments of Anatomy and Medical Photography. Saturdays were devoted to visits to the provincial veterinary laboratory at the Fort Garry campus where frozen specimens were sectioned with a bandsaw, placed on plexiglass sheets, cleaned, photographed and frozen. Many of the sections were embedded in plastic and are on display in the Department of Anatomy.

In 1975 at the HSC we set up a long term follow-up study of fetuses exposed to diagnostic ultrasound *in utero*. Margaret Cograves led the study for eight years supported by a group of part-time helpers, namely Evelyn Osborne, Florence Minty and Val Theissen. The work was published ten years later showing no untoward effects on the children.

Also in 1980, Ross Brown returned to Winnipeg from Oklahoma to work in ultrasound at both HSC and St Boniface Hospital. In 1987 he was appointed Vice President —Medicine at St Boniface's Hospital and was succeeded by Dr Gordon Askew. Dr Julie Schollenberg and, more recently, Dr Fern Karlicki comprise the current ultrasound physician staff at St Boniface.

Dr Clifford Levi joined the staff of HSC in October 1981 and was joined by Drs Dan Lindsay, Suzie Holt, Sid Dashefsky, and for a short time, Dr Chris Caco. Cliff is now the Section Head of Ultrasound after eight years of untiring contributions to service and research.

The staff has published three books, 40 scientific papers and at least 17 chapters in most of the leading texts concerning ultrasound. In 1979 Frank Manning returned to Winnipeg having spent time at the University of California at Los Angeles, where he had worked with Larry Platt developing the planning score, and at Oxford where he had worked with Geoffrey Dawes on fetal breathing.

In the 1980s subspecialization struck at the HSC, and individual ultrasound units were established for fetal assessment (Drs Frank Manning, then Chris Harman and Savas Menticoglou); pediatric cardiology (Drs George Collins, then Andy Pellich and Nils Giddens); pediatric ultrasound (Drs Dan Wilmot, then Bruce Shuckett and Alice Patton) and adult echocardiography (Drs Ted Cuddy then Norman Patton).

Chapter IV • *Imaging Research at the*

Montréal Neurological Institute

TERRY PETERS AND WILLIAM FEINDEL

THE EVOLUTION OF NUCLEAR MEDICINE IMAGING EQUIPMENT

The first clinical radionuclide localizing scanner based on the principle of a scintillation detector was developed by Herbert Cassen in the early 1950s. This rectilinear type of scanner had low sensitivity, and further development was necessary to make the device suitable for brain scanning. The first work in Canada was carried out by Drs Harold Johns and Bill Reid in Saskatoon[1] and was continued at the Montréal Neurological Institute (MNI). The first scanner produced in 1956 had a novel scanning mechanism. The device was designed so that both halves of the head would be scanned simultaneously, that the parasagittal regions would be included, and that the ends of the detectors would follow fairly closely the contour of the average adult skull maintaining a fairly constant distance and geometry. The two detectors consisted of one-inch thick and one-inch diameter thallium-activated sodium iodide crystals coupled to photomultipliers and mounted in one-inch thick lead shields. The collimator consisted of a single hole 3/4 inch in diameter and 3 1/4 inches long. The detectors scanned the head in a series of eight parasagittal arcs, starting at the nose, each describing 180°, and separated in coronal section by approximately 7.5°. The scan took about 30 minutes.

In clinical use the patient wore a rubber bathing cap in order to present a smooth surface to the detectors and allow fixation of the head in a cushioned clamp. The data were visualized by printing dots in proportion to the measured count rate and obliques in proportion to the difference in count rate between the two detectors.

Using I-131 labeled human serum albumin the device showed considerable promise, showing excellent correlation with other

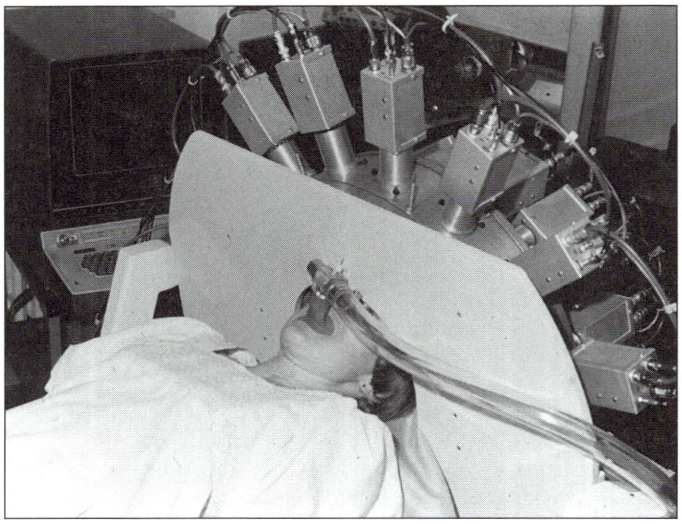

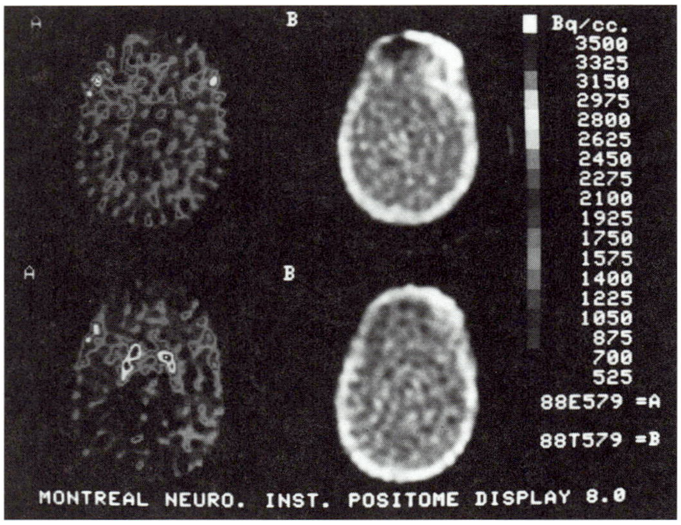

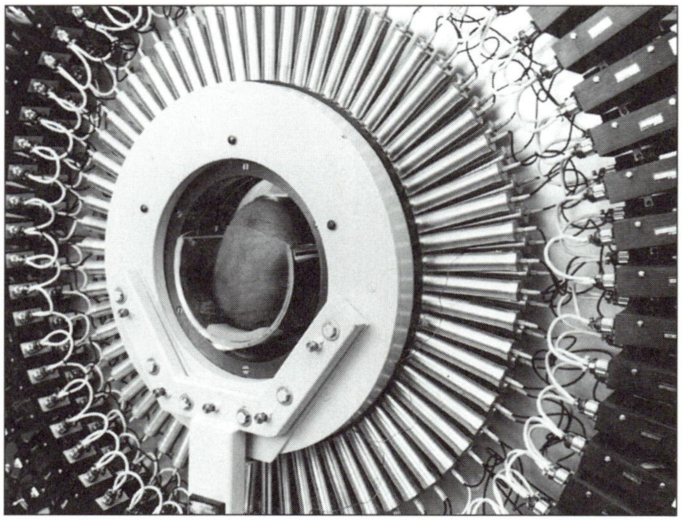

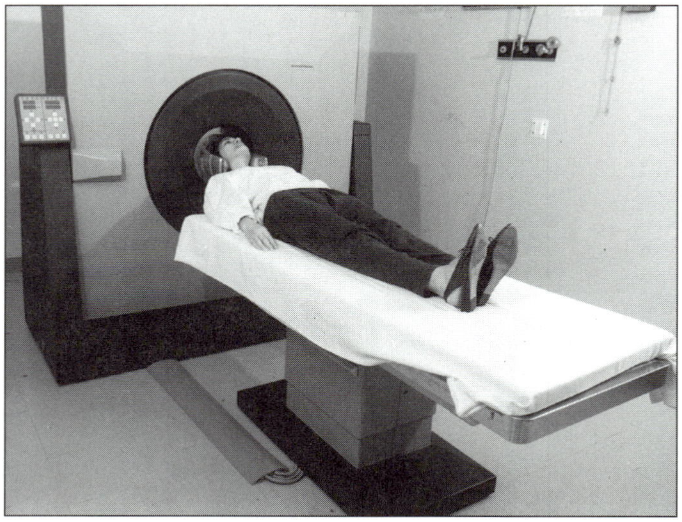

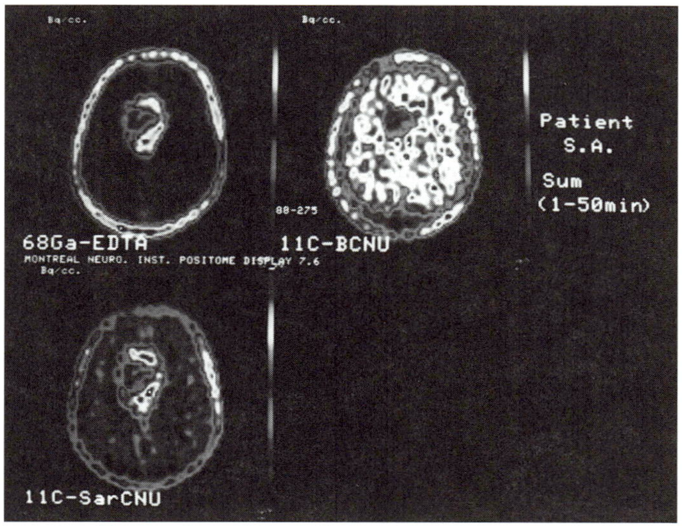

Top left
The first positron emission tomography scanner in Canada. It had originally been built in Brookhaven in the late 1960s and came to Canada in 1975. It consisted of a ring of 32 sodium iodide crystals as detectors interfaced with a PDP 12 computer

Centre and bottom left
A 'wobble motion' was added to the Positome (built in 1978 and the first such system to use bismuth germanate [BGO] crystals) in 1985 to allow the centre of the detectors to move on the circumference of a 1cm radius circle. This system had 64 detectors interfaced to a PDP 11/34 computer. The result was an ability to do high resolution studies in short times

radiological procedures in 90 per cent of 115 cases studied with no false positives.[2]

The scanner was improved over the years[2] but still maintained the original scanning geometry. It was used for nearly 20 years.

POSITRON EMISSION TOMOGRAPHY AT MNI

The use of positron emitting radioisotopes in medicine was first proposed by Wrenn[3] in 1951, but it was not until the 1970s that positron emission tomography (PET) scanners were designed and produced. The MNI developed and installed the country's first PET scanner in 1975 and has been heavily involved in the development of PET in this country ever since. The design was an updated version of that designed at the Brookhaven Laboratory, and the device was further updated by Thompson[4] with the use of bismuth germanate (BGO) detectors. This scanner utilized 64 BGO crystal detectors in a circular array, and a modified version was commercialized by Atomic Energy of Canada.

OTHER IMAGING MODALITIES

In 1973 the Montréal Neurological Institute (MNI) was the first institution in Canada to install a computed tomographic (CT) scanner (EMI Mk 1). A second EMI scanner was installed in 1976, and during the period 1976–80 we worked closely with EMI to develop various enhancements of this machine, particularly high-resolution imaging of the spine. In 1985 the MNI was the first site in Canada to install a high-field (1.5T) magnetic resonance imager/spectrometer.

In 1982 we were the first group in Canada to begin using CT and digital subtraction angiographic (DSA) images to plan neurosurgical procedures using computer analysis, and this subsequently developed into the stereotactic surgery and ultimately the image-guided surgery programs that are now in place, incorporating images from CT, DSA, MRI, MRA, PET and EEG. An outgrowth of the early work in this area was the establishment in 1987 of a company—CMI Services—by Peters, along with John Clark and Bruce Pike (his graduate students at the time) to develop and market PC-based stereotactic planning software. At the same time, our interaction with Dr Ervin Podgorsak of the medical physics and radiation oncology departments at the Montréal General Hospital resulted in one of the first uses of linear accelerators to perform radiosurgery as well as the development of the McGill Dynamic Radiosurgery technique.

Over the years since the founding of MNI, stereoscopic radiological imaging has been the rule rather than the exception. Even today, most radiographic procedures are performed here in stereo, and with the advent of DSA, quantitative analysis of stereoscopic images has been routine in the planning and guidance of neurosurgical procedures. We installed a prototype stereoscopic DSA unit in 1986, which in 1989 was upgraded to enable stereoscopic fluoroscopy also. Stereo displays have now moved into the operating room, allowing the surgeons an even more realistic appreciation of the brain depicted by 3D models based on multi-modality images.

With this focus of neurological imaging MNI established the McConnell Brain Imaging Centre in 1983 as a vehicle for research in brain function and mapping using PET (and more recently functional MRI), the use of multiple imaging modalities in surgical planning, and the use of MR spectroscopy to understand brain and neuromuscular function. Significant in the history of the Brain Imaging Centre was the awarding in 1992 of a $5 million grant by MRC to fund much of the functional imaging research at MNI.

Opposite top right
The ability to correct transmission scans for attenuation correction was added in 1987, and the first simultaneous emission/transmission scans were performed in 1987

Opposite centre right
A Scanditronix PC 2048B scanner was installed in 1989. It has 2048 BGO crystals coupled in blocks of 16 to 128 photo-muliplier tubes and is coupled to a VAX station 4000/90 computer which constructs 128x128 images in 1.5 seconds

Chapter V • Imaging Research at

Sunnybrook Health Science Centre

Michael J Bronskill

The Imaging Research Group at Sunnybrook Health Science Centre includes scientists working in all the modern diagnostic techniques, using ultrasound, x-rays, nuclear medicine methods, and magnetic resonance (MR) imaging. The group has its origins at the Ontario Cancer Institute (OCI), where in the early 1970s Dr Harold Johns, as head of the Physics Division. initiated a new research direction in the medical physics of imaging. Many of the current imaging group at Sunnybrook received their graduate training at the OCI under Harold Johns.

In the late 1980s Sunnybrook Health Science Centre decided to make research a strategic priority, and initially the Reichmann Research Building was designed and built. As construction progressed in 1989 the imaging research program was recruited from OCI, providing Sunnybrook with a major, intact research group with an established graduate training program within the Department of Medical Biophysics at the University of Toronto. An initial group of about 40, including seven scientists, moved from the OCI in late 1990. In late 1994 the complement was a total of 70, including 10 scientists and 30 graduate students.

A wide spectrum of imaging research is now supported by an annual budget of about $4 million with core funding from the Sunnybrook Research Foundation and multiple grants from national agencies and medical imaging industries. A common thrust in all the research is the development of techniques which incorporate functional as well as structural information. Ultrasound research has made major contributions to ultrasonic biomicroscopy and

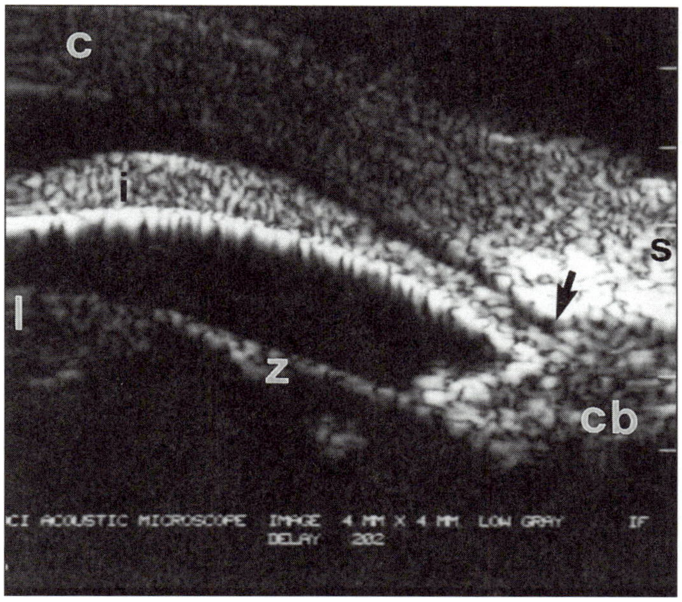

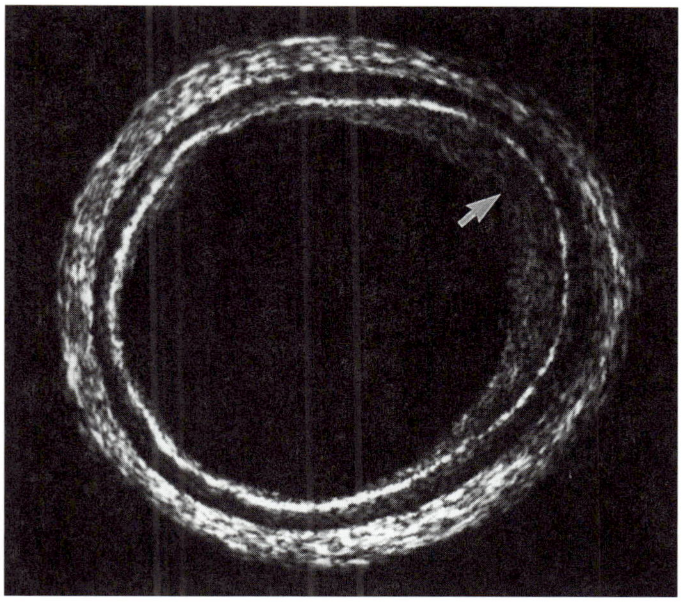

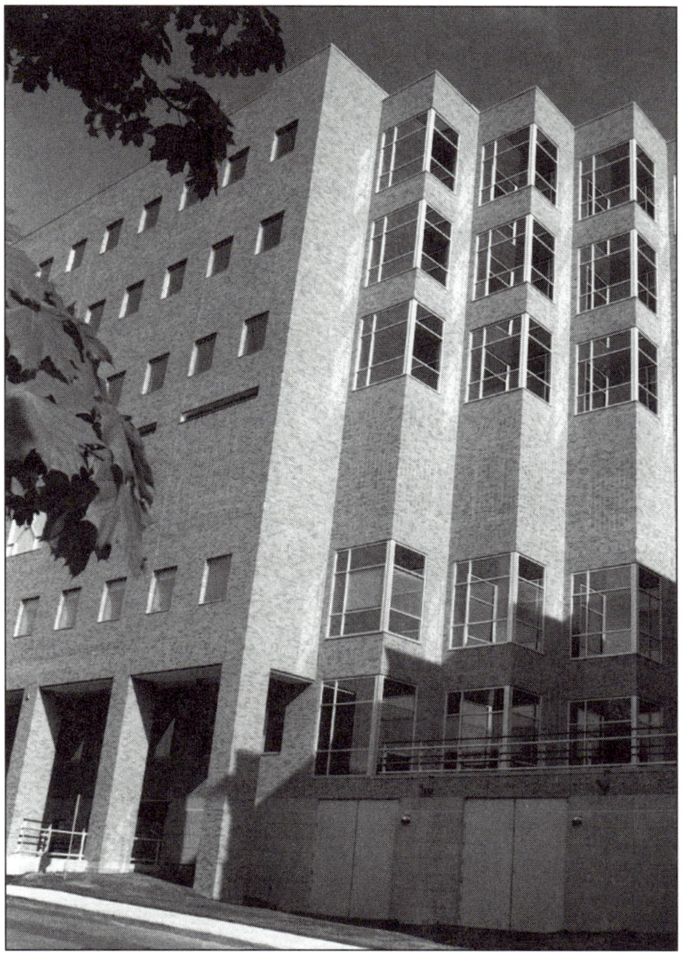

quantitative methods are being developed to assess perfusion and blood flow in small vessels. X-ray research covers a broad range of topics. One highlight is research and development in respect of mammography. Sunnybrook is the coordinating centre for the National Institute of Health-funded US National Digital Mammography Development Group, a consortium of research, clinical and industrial partners. Research in MRI also covers a wide range of topics. The current focus is on MR techniques to provide real-time image guidance during minimally invasive therapy; this involves a partnership with ISG Technologies, General Electric Medical Systems and the Toronto Hospital. The multimillion dollar project has stimulated the installation at Sunnybrook of a second 1.5T imager devoted to research, which incorporates a unique open-concept magnet, allowing access to the patient during imaging.

Top left
Ultrasound biomicroscope image of the corneal-scleral junction in a patient with glaucoma. Note that the channel to the iris root (arrow) is almost blocked by the iris, i, which is displaced toward the top of the image. In this image, the field of view is 4mm by 4mm with resolution of approximately 50 μm. Other structures shown include the cornea (c), sclera (s), ciliary body (cb), zonules (z), and lense (l)

Top right
High frequency ultrasound (45 MHz) intravascular ultrasound showing sharp definition of the wall of a femoral artery *in vitro*. Early plaque developement is evident (arrow)

Left
The Reichmann Research Building completed in 1990 on the Sunnybrook Health Science Centre campus, houses the Imaging Research Program which occupies nearly two floors of the building

Chapter VI • *Radiation Protection*

Roch D DesRochers

The history of radiation protection dates from the late 1890s. The first report in a Canadian publication of adverse effects from radiation exposure appeared in 1896.[1]

Although Canadian specialists were aware of earlier international developments, specific Canadian recommendations on radiation protection date from about 1945. The Canadian Atomic Energy Project was established in 1942 and operated at the Montréal laboratories and later at Chalk River, Ontario[2] under the auspices of the National Research Council. Radiation protection was from the beginning a major concern. The risks of cancer induction and genetic mutation from repeated small doses of radiation had been recognized early.

Within the Canadian Atomic Energy Project recommended maximum radiation doses were reduced to about 15 röntgen per year* (down from 50) before the International Commission on Radiological Protection (ICRP) recommendations to this effect. Early recognition of a linear, non-threshold dose-response relationship for induced genetic changes and the possibility of a similar relationship for radiation-induced leukemias was not completely incorporated into ICRP recommendations until 1959. The possibility of fetal harm, notably defective development of the central nervous system, was also considered.[3] It was recommended in 1945 that women should not be employed in the Canadian Atomic Energy Project in areas where there was "any serious possibility of irradiation hazard."[3]

In 1946 the Atomic Energy Control Act was made law and led to the creation of the the Atomic Energy Control Board (AECB) under its first president, General AGL McNaughton who was succeeded by Dr CJ Mackenzie.[4,5] The Act made provision for legislation in the field of atomic energy. The first Canadian regulations appeared in 1947, but these were preoccupied with security of information and materials. Since health and safety matters were traditionally the concern and responsibility of provinces, there was little detailed reference to radiation protection. "Reasonable and proper precautions" were prescribed. The AECB urged provincial authorities through the Dominion Council of Health to issue radiological safety regulations. The revised regulations in 1954 at the end of this period were unchanged with respect to health and safety matters.

An event which was to have a significant influence on the development of the regulation of radiation exposure took place in Canada. In 1949 a tripartite conference was held at Chalk River with 23 participants from the United States, Great Britain and Canada. The notes and the minutes document an explosion of concepts, ideas, questions and decisions that set the scene for decades to come in international and national regulation of radiation exposure. There were eight Canadian participants, including GC Laurence, who was to become a member of ICRU in 1950 and later president of AECB. Other presidents of AECB are listed in an appendix.

Some of the topics discussed and conclusions drawn are of note. Parameters for the average or "standard" man were defined for the first time, largely based on data assembled by AJ Cipriani from Chalk River. "Standard man" had a mass of 70 kg and was given the basic chemical composition, organ masses and metabolic parameters in use today. The first lung model, the concept of relative biological effectiveness (RBE) and values for differing kinds of radiation were agreed upon. Arguments developed as to whether one should use 200-kV x-rays or radium gamma-rays as the reference radiation. The conference participants agreed that radium gamma-rays would be more appropriate: although x-rays were more often used for comparison in experiments, radium gamma-radiation would provide a better defined reference. This recommendation was rejected, and ICRP later selected 200-kVp x-rays as the reference radiation.

ICRP recommendations of 1950 did indicate that "while the values proposed for maximum permissible exposures are such as to involve a risk that is small compared to the other hazards of life, nevertheless in view of the unsatisfactory nature of much of the evidence on which our judgements must be based, coupled with the knowledge that certain radiation effects are irreversible and cumulative, it is strongly recommended that every effort be made to reduce exposures to all types of ionizing radiations to the lowest possible level." ICRP recommendations of 1954[6] include the statement that no increment in radiation dose 0 can be regarded as absolutely safe. Such basic principles have been adhered to in ICRP recommendations since then.

In 1950 a radiation protection service was inaugurated within the Industrial Health Division of the Department of National Health and Welfare. At this time, AECB staff consisted of a very few persons. The problems arising from developments in the fields of nuclear energy and nuclear medicine, the growing recognition of the need for increased safety precautions in the use of x-rays, and concern about the possible effects of radiation exposure of members of the public from all sources, led to a rapid expansion of radiation protection activities. These activities resulted in establishment of the Radiation Protection Division (later designated Radiation Protection Bureau) as a separate division within the federal department of Health and Welfare; one of its principal functions was to act as health advisor to AECB and to the provinces. A film monitoring dosimetry service for radiation workers in Canada was established in 1951[7] at the request of the Dominion Council of Health. Shortly after the first US hydrogen-bomb tests in the Pacific Ocean in 1954, increased efforts were devoted to measurements of radioactive fallout and assessment of its potential health effects on members of the general population.

After 1956 ICRP developed its Publication No 1, which appeared in 1959;[8] some key changes in ICRP's approach are reflected in this document. The previous permissible levels of exposure had been expressed in terms of the dose in a rather short interval of time—one day or one week—and it had been assumed that if this average dose rate was low enough, no appreciable bodily injury would become apparent in the lifetime of an individual. But increasingly scientists believed that the accumulation of small doses might result in some long-term biological damage being expressed, notably genetic effects in the descendants of exposed individuals. The concept of a linear, non-threshold dose-response relationship for induction of late effects was apparently accepted by the commission, although some doubt was expressed as to whether there might be a threshold for induction of leukemia by x-rays and of bone cancer by radium.[7]

Accumulation of both somatic and genetic damage in the individual was, therefore, theoretically limited by a formula which ensured that the average annual dose to the whole body or to critical organs would not exceed 5 rem* per year from age 18 onward whereas *the recommended* *maximum for any given year was 12 rem.*[7] A quarterly limit of 3 rem in any period of 13 consecutive weeks was also recommended. Single doses of the order of 3 rem were to be avoided as far as practicable, especially in the case of women of reproductive age. Concurrently with the production of this publication, the draft for a new set of regulations to the Atomic Energy Control Act in Canada was being prepared by AECB, which was advised by staff from the Radiation Protection Division of National Health and Welfare, from Atomic Energy of Canada Limited (AECL) and from the Departments of Health and Labour in Ontario. Following a 1959 recommendation of the Dominion Council of Health, health and safety matters were specifically addressed in the new Atomic Energy Control Regulations which appeared in 1960. These regulations were, by and large, consistent with ICRP Publication 1.[8] They were slightly more conservative, for in addition to *a quarterly limit of 3 rem to radiation workers there was also a limit of 5 rem in any 52 consecutive weeks.* Special dispensation by the board was needed in order to invoke the age formula.

Employment of pregnant women as atomic-radiation workers was prohibited. These regulations applied specifically to persons using radioactive materials; the use of medical x-rays was not and is not regulated by AECB. However, several of the provinces had passed legislation governing the use of x-rays by then;[7] in general, this legislation also conformed to ICRP recommendations.[9]

The Canadian Atomic Energy Project had meanwhile been reorganized as Atomic Energy of Canada Limited (AECL). It is interesting to note that AECL never used the age formula and, because of its contacts with the ICRP, adopted the 5-rem, whole-body annual limit toward the end of 1956. There were, however, some problems with the film badges used to record whole body exposures of radiation workers. These films overestimated the radiation doses from low-energy x-rays[8] so that the whole body doses recorded were somewhat higher than those actually received. Although various improvements in the film badges were made during this period, this problem was not really solved until thermoluminescence dosimeters were introduced in 1973.

The annual maximum permissible exposures did not change appreciably in the next formal recommendations of ICRP in its Publication 9: five rem per year for gonads, red bone marrow and the whole body, with special restrictions for women of reproductive age and for pregnant women. For individual members of the general public, this value was to be divided by 10. These recommendations of ICRP were incorporated in the revised Canadian regulations which were issued in 1974 and which remained in effect through 1986 with only two additions, which are noted later. The protection of uranium miners continued to be regulated mainly by the provinces, as it had traditionally been, until 1978.

Ontario Hydro began to play a major role in practical radiation protection in Canada[10–12] with the establishment of large nuclear power generating stations at Douglas Point (1967), Pickering (1971) and Bruce (1975). The tradition was continued with the entry of the provinces of Québec and New Brunswick into the area of nuclear power generation. Courses in radiation protection were established for workers in the nuclear generating division of Ontario Hydro and the ICRP principle of keeping radiation exposures of workers as low as reasonably achievable was emphasized from the beginning of this program. Equally important has been improvement in the design criteria for these reactors. The design target for the Pickering reactors, a target which has in fact usually been achieved, was a maximum of 5 millirem per year, or 1/100th of the ICRP recommended limit, for those maximally-exposed members of the general public who might live continuously and grow their own food near the generating site. Ontario Hydro was the first Canadian organization to establish during this decade a continuing annual follow-up of the mortality of its current and pensioned employees in order to ascertain the potential impact of occupational exposure to radiation on the health of its employees.[13]

Although ICRP has long recommended that exposures of patients resulting from the application of x-rays and other sources of ionizing radiation in the healing arts should be exempt from legislative limits, it continues to follow the established tradition[6] of recommending practical methods for protection of the patient in diagnostic radiology.[14] A new set of Canadian regulations was drafted by AECB,[15] based on ICRP Publication 26. AECB established a system of issuing consultative documents for public and scientific comment before new regulatory measures are established. The new regulations will be issued only after due consideration of all comments received. Again in 1992, after the important changes in ICRP Publication 60,[16] further changes to the regulations were developed and public consultations were held.

SUMMARY:

Soon after the initial period of discovery of ionizing radiations in the 1890s came the realization that protection was needed. A growing concern led to collective appraisals and to the development of the relevant basic sciences. The advent of atomic energy in 1945 brought increased emphasis on and capability for protection. The Atomic Energy Control Act was part of the worldwide expansion of atomic energy and public awareness that led eventually to quantitative federal and provincial regulations in Canada. As ICRP has developed its ideas, with considerable input from Canadian scientists, so the Canadian and provincial regulations in the field of radiation protection have been developed. Currently, we are anticipating a new set of Canadian regulations based on ICRP Publication 60.[16]

Acknowledgements:

This chapter reproduces extensive excerpts from a summary by DK Myers of a paper by Drs AM Marko and RV Osborne presented at the annual meeting of the Canadian Radiation Protection Association in Saint John, New Brunswick, June 11–13, 1985, on the 90th anniversary of the discovery of x-rays.

* These are the older units for expressing quantities of radiation, since replaced by SI units.

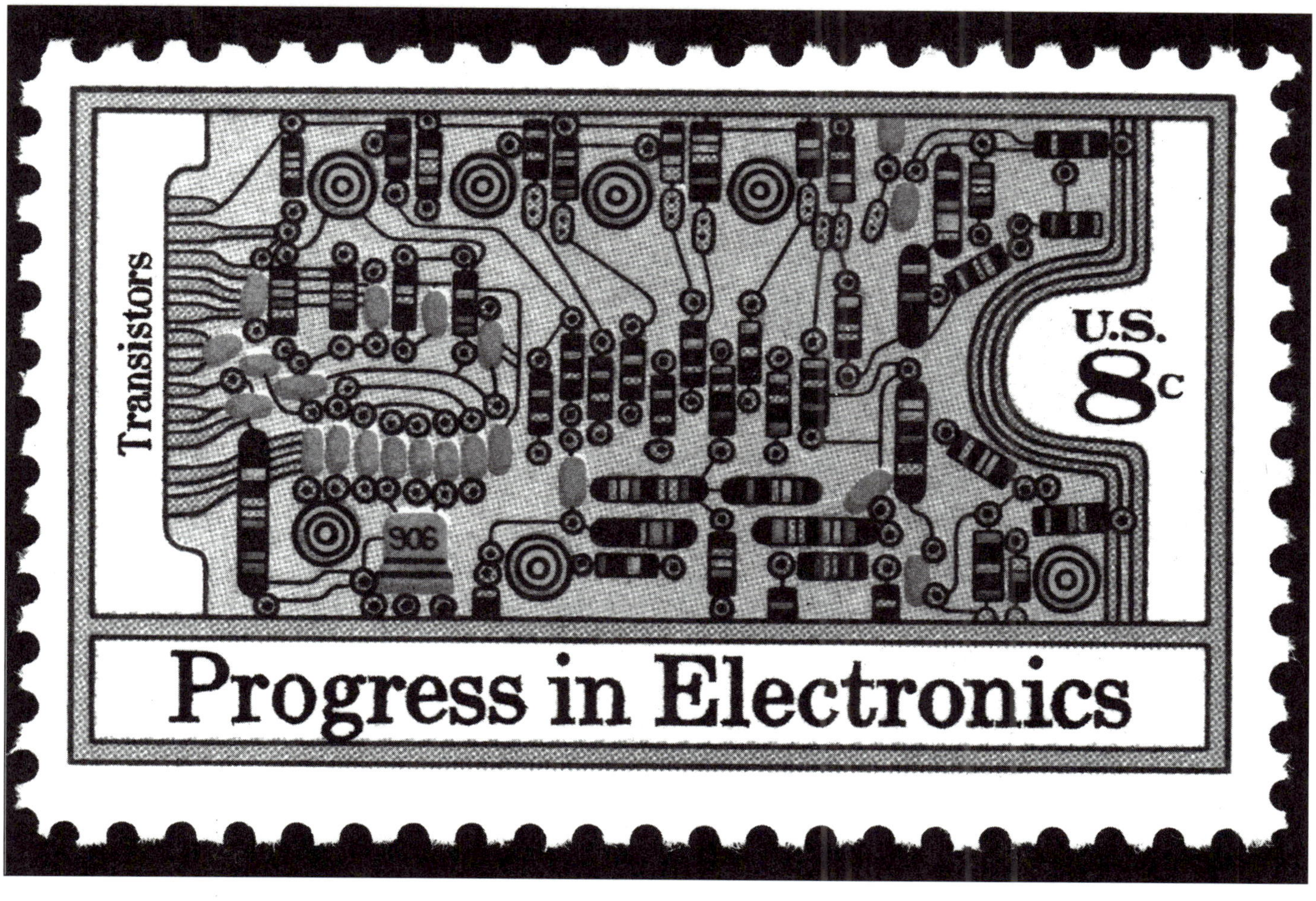

Canadian Association of Radiologists

1937–1938

J Kenneth Lipinski

SUMMARY

The original applications of 94 physicians who joined the Canadian Association of Radiologists in 1937 and 1938 were reviewed. The sex, birthplace, age, medical schooling, training in radiology and practice location were analyzed to obtain a profile of these founding members.

SOMMAIRE

L'auteur revoit les 94 demandes originales du statut de membre auprès de l'Association canadienne des radiologistes en 1937 et 1938. Il fait aussi une analyse du sexe, de l'âge, de la formation médicale, de la formation radiologique et des lieux d'exercice de ces 94 médecins et en trace le profil.

INTRODUCTION

The Canadian Association of Radiologists (CAR) was formed in 1937. A review was undertaken at its 50th anniversary to examine the profiles of the founding members.

METHODS AND RESULTS

The original applications of the 94 members of the CAR who joined in 1937 and 1938 were reviewed. The detailed application form included many important biographical details.

The material summarized from the application forms is presented in Tables 1 to 9.

Table 1

PLACE OF BIRTH

Ontario	47
Québec	28
Manitoba	5
British Columbia	2
New Brunswick	2
Prince Edward Island	1
U.S.A.	4
Australia	1
Scotland	3
England	1
Canadian	85
Non-Canadian	9
Total	94

DISCUSSION

The worldwide rise of specialization in medicine led to the formation of specialty organizations to meet new needs. Although the histories of many such organizations are available from the minutes of the annual meetings and the published memoirs of members, there is not available a profile of the individual members.

The 50th anniversary of the founding of the CAR provided a unique opportunity to review such material. The original applications of the members who joined in the first year of the organization (1937–1938) were available for analysis. The striking finding from the analysis has been the homogeneity of the founding members.

The group of 94 was male-dominated, with only two women members. Most were born in Canada (Table 1), and attended Canadian medical schools (Table 2). What led these individuals to choose diagnostic radiology is not apparent from the applications. Most had at least three years of clinical experience, and almost half had at least five years before entering radiology (Table 4). This practical clinical experience was obtained almost without exception in Canada, yet only 17 members completed their entire radiology training in Canada. The others either obtained all their training in the United States, England or on the continent, or had taken part of their training in Canada with supplements from these foreign centres (Table 5). Most individuals spent their time in formal observation of the practice of radiology and informal study courses in physics rather than in direct apprenticeships. Six of the members had no specialty training experience before limiting their practice (Table 6).

Table 2

MEDICAL SCHOOL ATTENDED

Toronto	24
McGill	18
Laval	12
Western	10
Manitoba	9
Queen's	6
Montréal	5
Dalhousie	2
Alberta, Toronto	2
Syracuse	1
Sydney, Australia	1
Edinburgh	1
Heidelberg, Toronto	1
Paris, Montréal	1
Paris, Laval	1
Total	94

Table 3

NUMBER OF YEARS OF MEDICAL EXPERIENCE BEFORE STUDY AND PRACTICE OF RADIOLOGY

None	28
Less than 2	9
3 to 5	14
6 to 10	28
10 to 15	7
16 to 20	4
21 to 25	4
Total	94

Table 4

TYPE OF PRACTICE BEFORE STARTING PRACTICE OF RADIOLOGY

General practice	62
Internal medicine	3
General surgery	1
None	28
Total	94

Only 20 formal certificates were obtained among all the members, of which three members held multiple diploma (Table 7). This reflects the infancy of the specialty and the lack of a formal examination process, not only in Canada, but worldwide.

Canadians obtained their training in the United States and overseas in the major centres of activity of the new specialty, but most often in London, Paris, New York and Chicago. World War I also provided a venue for experience with the Canadian Army Medical Corps in Europe. Many army doctors used x-rays in their daily clinical practice, mainly in the extraction of bullet fragments and bone setting.

Most practiced in Québec and Ontario and 32 (one-third) of them in either Montréal or Toronto (Table 8). Of the total 71 limited their practice to radiology only (Table 7). Many of the individuals maintained contact with university centres, and were involved in the teaching of radiology. Sixty papers had already been published by 20 members, an average of three papers each.

Table 5
PLACES OF TRAINING

No specialized training		6
Canada	entirely in Canada	36
	Canada and partly overseas	21
U.S.A.	entire training	16
Overseas	entire training	15
Total		94

Table 6
TYPE OF TRAINING IN RADIOLOGY

No training	6
Formal university or hospital	
Study course	10
Observers	55
Apprenticeship	48

Note: 25 followed two types of training.

Table 7
QUALIFICATIONS

American College of Radiology	3
American Board of Radiology	4
Fellow of the Board of American Radiology	3
Diploma of Medical Radiology and Electrotherapy	2
Paris University Certificate	6
Cambridge Diploma	1
State of Michigan Diplomate	1
Total	20

Table 8
PRACTICE LOCATION IN 1937–1938

Québec	(Montréal 18)	25
Ontario	(Toronto 14)	38
British Columbia	(Vancouver 3)	12
Alberta		5
Saskatchewan		5
Manitoba		5
Maritimes		3
New York State		1
Total		94

Table 9
PRACTICE PATTERN

Limited to radiology	71
Limited to radiology, physical medicine and electrotherapy	15
Radiology and general practice	5
Radiology and internal medicine	1
Radiology and chest disease	1
General surgery	1
Total	94

Acknowledgement:
This article originally appeared in the *Annals of the Royal College of Physicians and Surgeons of Canada*[1] and is reprinted with the permission of the author and that journal.

Chapter VIII • *Profile of the Founding Members of the*

Canadian Association of Radiation Oncologists

Stewart M Jackson

SUMMARY

The profiles of the 149 founding members of the Canadian Association of Radiation Oncologists are reviewed. Data focus on medical school, radiation oncology training and specialty qualifications. A comparison is made of all members with those qualifying from medical school in the last 10 years.

SOMMAIRE

L'article trace le profil des 149 membres fondateurs de l'Association canadienne des radio-oncologues en s'inspirant de l'école de médecine concernée, de la formation en oncologie radiologique et des qualifications de spécialisation. Une comparaison est faite de tous les membres avec le groupe issu des Facultés de Médecine au cours des dix dernières années.

INTRODUCTION

The Canadian Association of Radiation Oncologists (CARO) was formed in 1988. Despite its long history in Canada, radiation oncology remains misunderstood. Therapeutic radiology has been recognized by The Royal College of Physicians and Surgeons of Canada (RCPSC) since the 1940s. On its 50th anniversary, the Canadian Association of Radiologists (CAR) reviewed the profiles of its founding members.[1] The recent establishment of an independent CARO and a report about the founding members of CAR stimulated an examination of the founding members of CARO. Specialist qualifications and the changing profile of more recently qualified members were examined.

METHODS AND RESULTS

The by-laws of CARO allow two-year terms for the principal officers. During 1988 and 1989, its first two years, 203 individuals joined CARO. Of these, 149 were full or regular members. Residents, fellows, associates and honorary members were excluded in this analysis. The demographic details listed in the first two CARO directories of 1989 and 1990 exclude the place of birth of members, but their medical schools were recorded. Universities and training positions for radiation oncology were known for all but two members. Fellowship (FRCPC) or Certificat de Specialiste de la Province de Québec (CSPQ) was known, as were other similar qualifications. The profile of all regular members was compared with that of those graduating from medical school since 1978 (Tables 1–6).

DISCUSSION

In contrast to the findings about the founding members of CAR in 1937–1938, CARO members had attended many different medical schools (Tables 1, 2). Of the members, 64 were graduates of Canadian medical schools, and 85 were graduates of schools in 26 other countries. Of the 64 Canadian graduates, 21 were from the University of Toronto, and 16 from Quebec universities. Of the members, 102 received their principal training in radiation oncology in Canada (Table 3); 24 of these members took additional training outside Canada, mainly in the United States or France. Of those trained in Canada, most received their training in Toronto at the Princess Margaret Hospital (PMH). Of those trained exclusively outside Canada, most received it in the United Kingdom or Ireland (Table 4). The importance of formal qualifications, either through the RCPSC or similar authorities, is in contrast to the case of the founders of CAR. Of the CARO members, 130 were fellows in radiation oncology, and 12 had CSPQs. Nine of the 15 who held neither the FRCPC nor the CSPQ had fellowship in the Royal College of Radiologists. Of the members, 12 had additional fellowships in other specialties such as internal medicine or surgery, whereas 64 members held FRCR, FRCS, FRACR or MRCP degrees.

Also in contrast to the situation 50 years ago, 28 members were female, and 12 of the 32 members who graduated from medical school since 1978 were female. More than half of the members practice in Ontario and Québec, and all but one in Canada (Table 5). Those members who had qualified in medicine in the last 10 years were significantly different from their more senior colleagues. Of the 32, 25 were graduates of Canadian medical schools; 30 hold an FRCPC degree, and the other two hold FRCR qualifications. Their training has been mainly confined to Canada (Table 6), but it has been dispersed across the country. The 12 females were, with one exception, Canadian graduates, and eight were trained at the PMH.

Table 1

MEDICAL SCHOOL

Toronto	21	McMaster	4
Dalhousie	5	Queen's	3
McGill	1	Western	3
Montréal	6	Saskatchewan	2
Laval	9	Calgary	1
Sherbrooke	1	Alberta	2
Ottawa	2	British Columbia	4

Table 2

MEDICAL SCHOOL OUTSIDE CANADA

UK and Ireland	48	North Africa	7
India, Sri Lanka	9	South Africa	3
USSR	1	Middle East	2
SE Asia	4	South America	2
Europe	7	West Indies	1

Table 3

RADIATION ONCOLOGY

	Training in Canada	Additional training outside Canada
PMH	*49	8
Ontario	8	1
Québec	5	11
BC	8	1
Alberta	6	–
Saskatchewan	1	1
Manitoba	–	1
Various	1	2

*Nine of these received part of their training in other Canadian centres.

Table 4

RADIATION ONCOLOGY

Training Exclusively Outside Canada

UK and Ireland	40	South Africa	1
France	1	Egypt	1
Sweden	2	Unknown	2

Table 5

PRACTICE LOCATION

Ontario	66	Saskatchewan	5
Québec	24	New Brunswick	5
British Columbia	20	Nova Scotia	5
Alberta	13	Newfoundland	2
Manitoba	7	Prince Edward Island	1

Table 6

RADIATION ONCOLOGY

Training of Those who Graduated in the Last 10 Years

PMH	11	Alberta	2
PMH and elsewhere in Canada	3	Ontario	3
PMH and outside Canada	1	Québec	3
British Columbia	5	France	1
		UK 3	

Acknowledgements:

The author acknowledges the contribution of Susan Broadbar, office manager, Radiation Oncology, British Columbia Cancer Agency, for the production of the first two CARO directories, which made this analysis possible.

Chapter IX • *Flashback—Saskatoon, 1962*

Trevor Cradduck

In the early 1960s two new radionuclide imaging systems were developed in Saskatoon. The first, a whole body rectilinear scanner, was part of work carried out by the writer Trevor Cradduck for completion of his MSc thesis in 1962. The scanner was soon joined by one of the first gamma cameras, designed by Sylvia Fedoruk and Trevor Cradduck in collaboration with Nuclear Enterprises of Winnipeg. It was installed at the Cancer Clinic in Saskatoon in 1964.

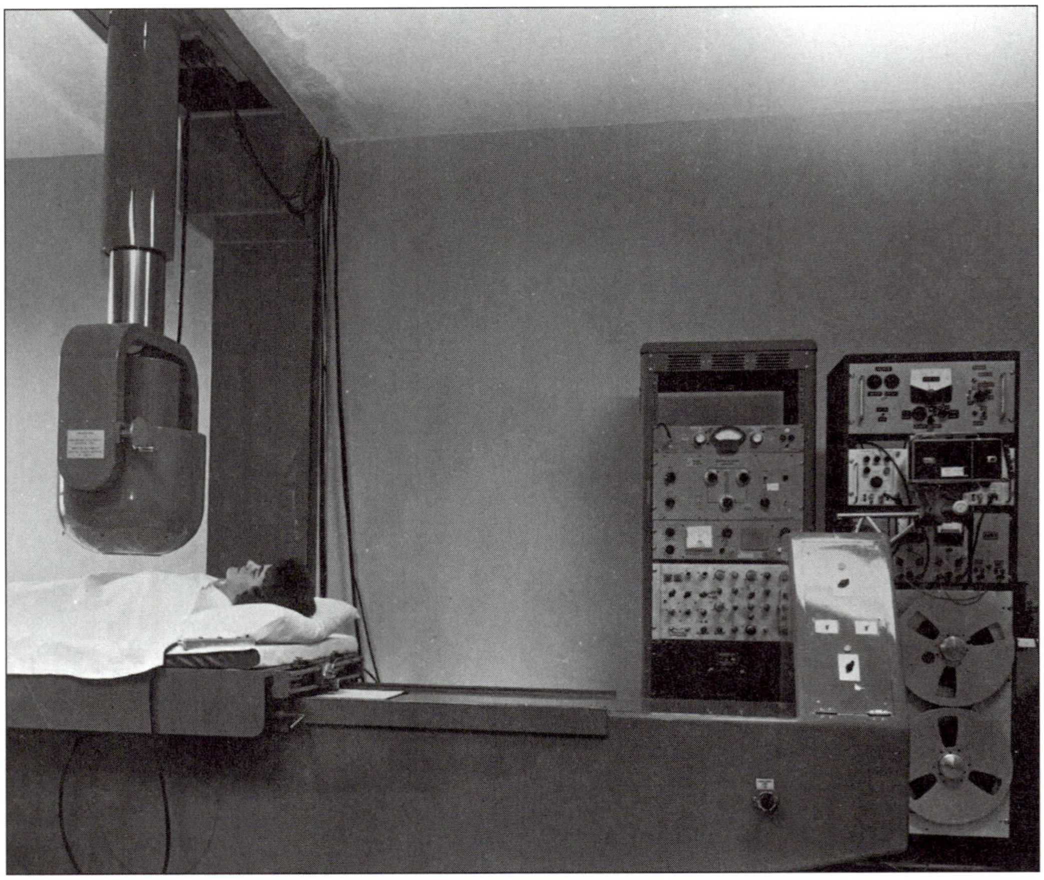

Left and below
The gamma camera

Right
Trevor Cradduck

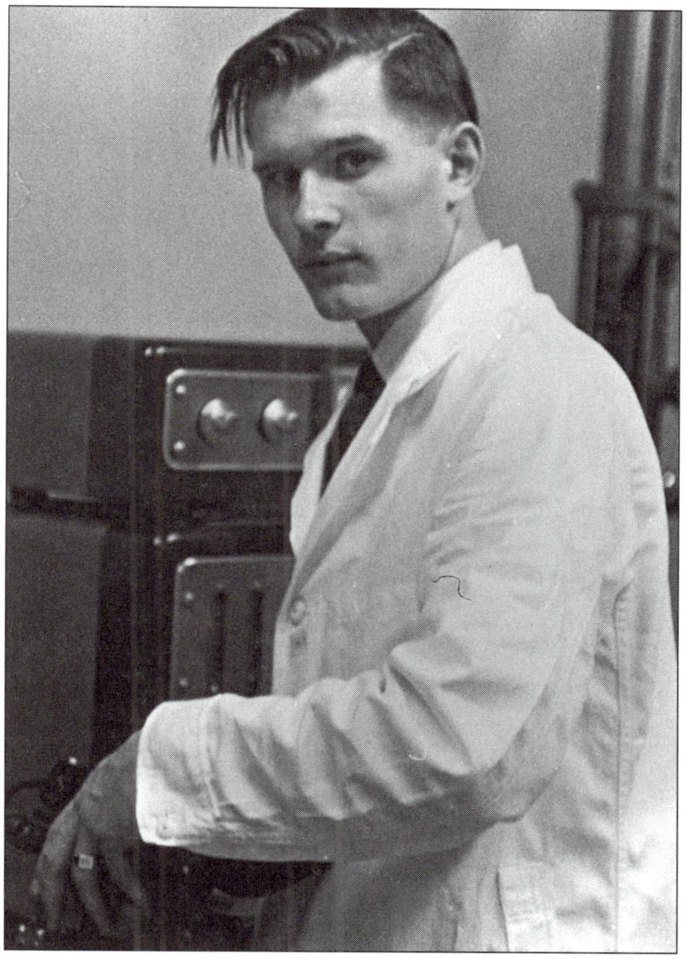

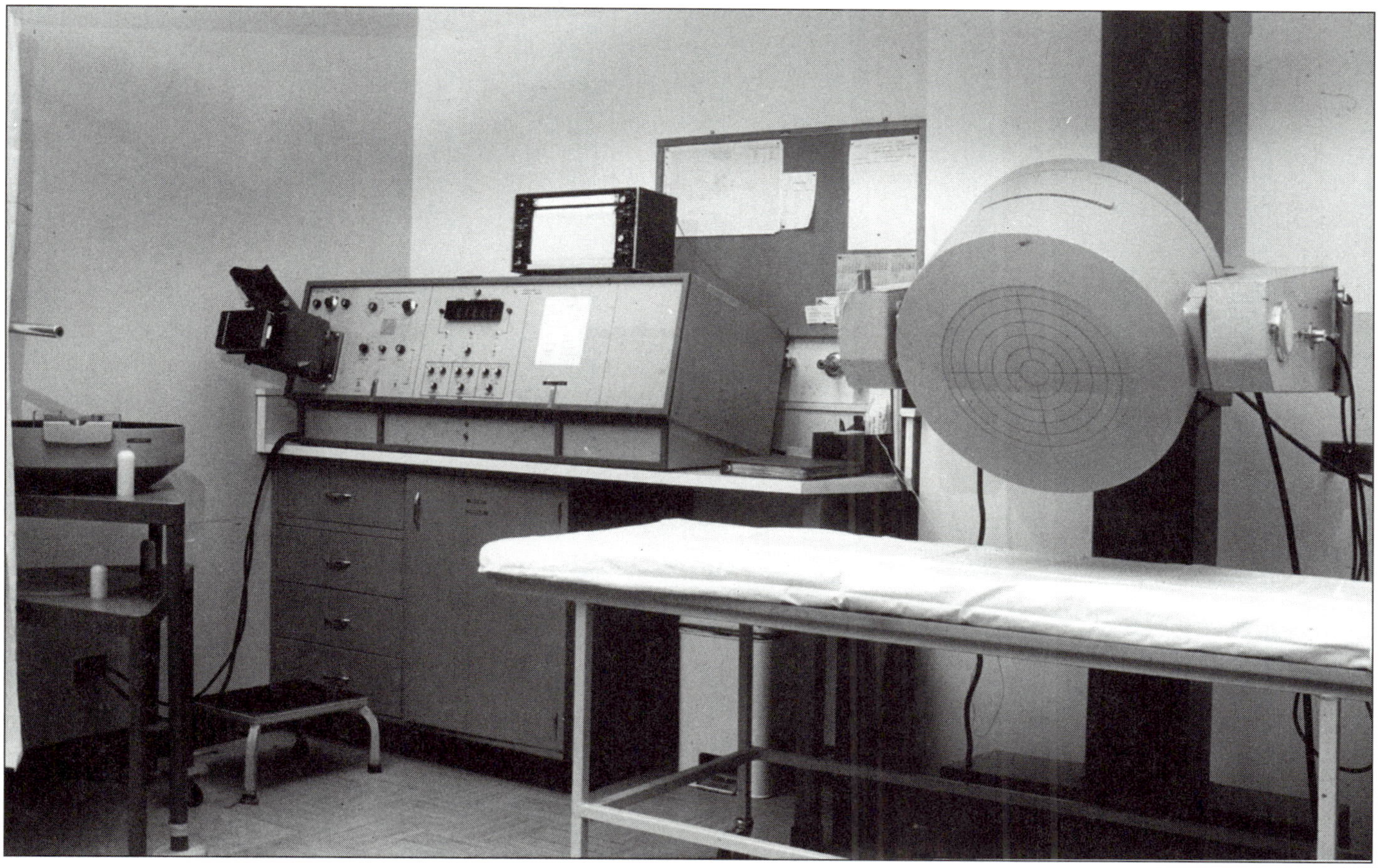

Chapter X •

Cancer Radiotherapy

Using Negative Pi-Mesons

GKY Lam, GB Goodman, RW Harrison, LD Skarsgard and RO Kornelsen

INTRODUCTION

During the 1950s, significant improvements were made in cancer cure by the introduction of cobalt-60 gamma rays compared to the conventional x-rays. Charged particle beams are expected to further enhance this physical dose localization because of their finite ranges in tissue and the high-dose Bragg peak at the end of their ranges. Among the charged particle beams, negative pi-meson (pion) has a particular advantage for deep-seated radiotherapy because, unlike most other charged particles, it can be captured by the nucleus of an atom at the end of its range and subsequently cause disintegration of the nucleus. This results in the release of a large amount of energy (from the 139-MeV rest mass of a pion), part of which appears in the form of short range, highly ionizing, heavy secondary charged particles, which tend to deposit energy in the close vicinity of the point of interaction (star formation). It is commonly observed that intense ionizations such as those produced by pion stars is much more efficient in killing cells than conventional radiation. Clinical use of pions required an intensity of the order of 108 pions per second and thus had to wait for the arrival of the high intensity medium energy accelerators called meson factories in the early '70s. Dedicated biomedical pion channels and clinical research programs were established in all three meson facilities: the Clinton Anderson Meson Facility (LAMPF),[1] the Swiss Institute of Nuclear Research (SIN),[2] and the Tri-University Meson Facility (TRIUMF).[3]

The TRIUMF biomedical channel received its first beam in June 1975, but deep-seated-tumor radiotherapy was not initiated until May 1982.

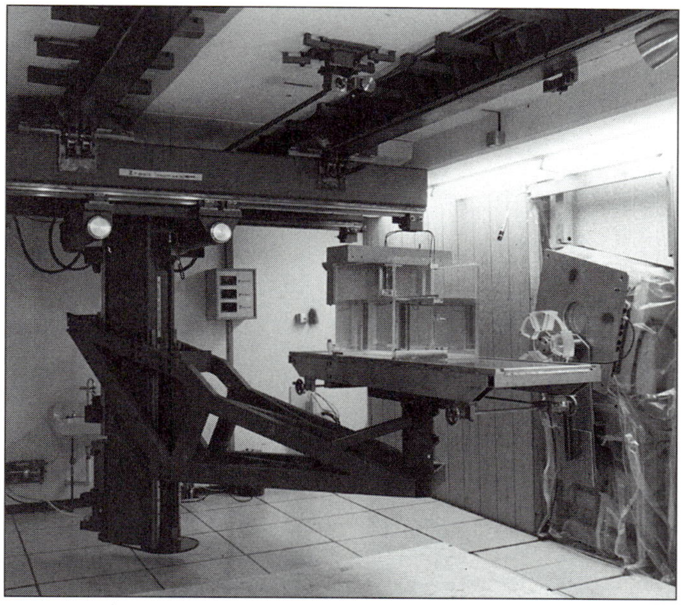

Left and below
Tri-University Meson Facility
(TRIUMF)

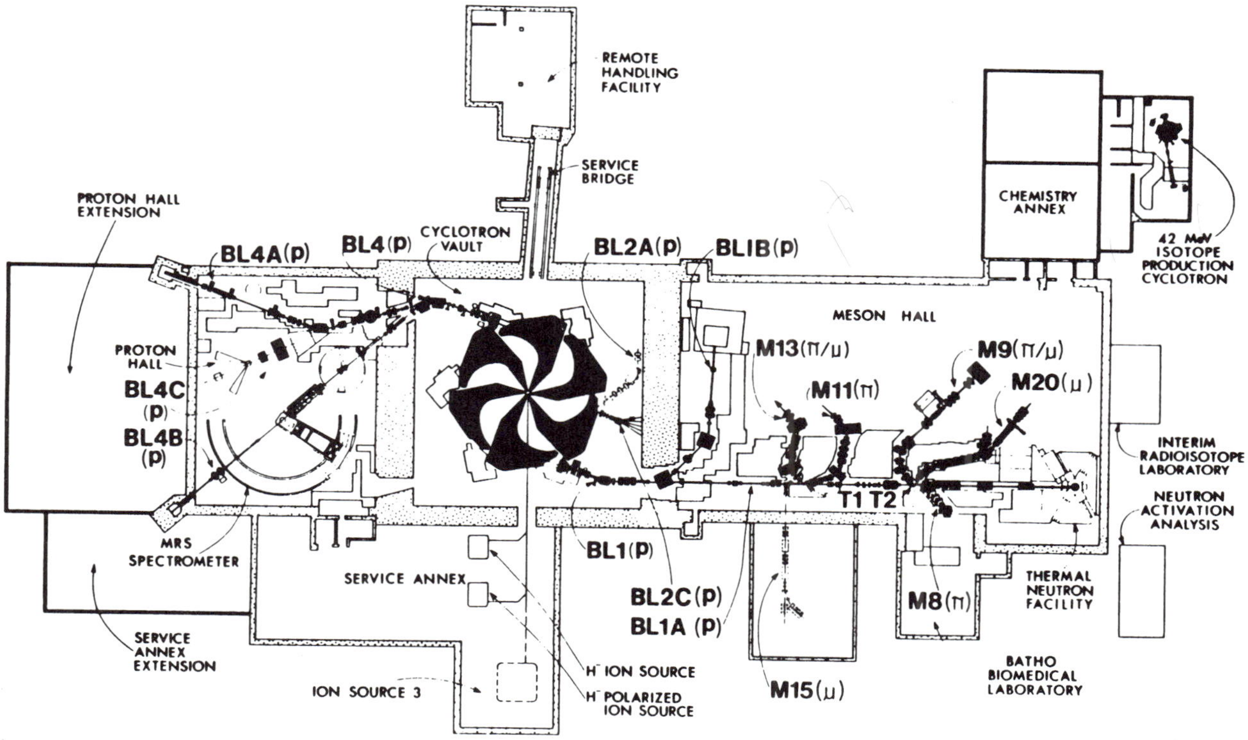

BEAM CONTROL AND MONITORING

Pion beams are inevitably contaminated with other charged particles, such as muons and electrons, depending on the pion production target material and the momentum selection of the channel.[4] These contaminant particles have the same particle momentum and longer ranges than the pions, somewhat diluting the dose localization advantage of a pure pion beam. The contamination of the TRIUMF pion beam is routinely monitored by a modified time-of-flight method, using signals from the scintillator telescope and the RF pulses of the cyclotron. The TRIUMF beam time structure of 44-ns periods is ideal for these studies. The pion production from targets has turned out to be only about 60 per cent of what was expected from cross section data available over 10 years ago and, furthermore, the channel only collects about 70 per cent of its design particle acceptance, resulting in a factor of two lower flux than originally expected.[4]

DOSIMETRY

The dosimetry of a pion beam is, in general, more complicated than other charged particle beams because (1) the composition of a contaminated beam varies from point to point due to pion in-flight interactions and differential scattering;[4] and (2) the secondary charged particle spectrum on pion capture depends on the atomic composition as well as the chemical structure of the medium.[5] The dosimetry of the TRIUMF pion beam is being studied as a joint effort with the other charged particle facilities through a task group (Charged Particle Radiation Therapy Committee) of the American Association of Physicists in Medicine.[6]

DEVELOPMENT OF LARGE UNIFORM FIELDS FOR CLINICAL USE

The raw beam that is extracted by tuning for maximum flux and minimum momentum chromaticity has a uniform dose only over about a 10 cc volume, which is far too small for direct clinical use. Large uniform dose fields are generated by spot scanning in three dimensions. The lateral scanning is done by moving the patient on a couch through a raster of spot patterns which conform closely to the tumor cross-section. The depth-wise scanning is handled by a multi-step plastic rotary range shifter[7] which can produce extended uniform dose profiles using the simple technique of linear programming to handle addition of dose profiles.[8]

It is expected that the biological effect of a pion beam depends not only on the physical dose but also on the spatial density of ionization. Biological studies using cultured cells[9] and small animals[10] were therefore conducted on some of the standard beam tunes, and the results were used to generate large volume fields with uniform biological effect. Some large-animal studies[11] were also conducted prior to clinical trials in order to monitor for possible unexpected long term effects of pion irradiation.

CLINICAL TRIALS

Before actual trial on the deep-seated tumors for which pions are really designed, it was considered essential to have some preliminary studies directly on patient tissue as a precaution to confirm the positive findings of previous biophysical studies. Skin nodule irradiations[12] were therefore conducted from November 1979 to February 1982 on patients with subcutaneous metastases from a wide variety of malignancies. The relative biological effectiveness compared to conventional radiation from these human skin studies agreed very closely with those obtained from biological experiments and no untoward intermediate to long term effects were observed.

In May 1982, when the three-dimensional scanning treatment couch was installed and the TRIUMF cyclotron could deliver large blocks of high intensity beam time suitable for patient treatment, deep-seated phase I radiotherapy was initiated using two approved protocols: advanced pelvic tumor (including rectum, prostate and bladder) and brain tumors (glioblastoma).[13] By 1988 the phase II dose escalation studies were completed and a phase III glioblastoma trial was initiated. Two years later, a similar trial for prostate cancer was also started. Both of these trials were completed by the end of 1994. The patients are being followed up for several more years for a final analysis.

Chapter XI •

The Saskatchewan Radon Plant

1931–1962

DV Cormack

A device to collect the radon emitted from a radium solution and subsequently use it for the treatment of cancer patients was designed and constructed in the 1930s by EL Harrington, head of the Department of Physics at the University of Saskatchewan. Harrington, a native of Missouri, obtained a Bachelor of Arts degree from the University of Missouri, a master's degree from Harvard and a PhD from the University of Chicago. As a post-doctoral fellow at the University of Chicago under Millikan, he undertook a precise redetermination of the viscosity of air,[1] the value of which is an essential ingredient in deducing the charge of the electron from the oil-drop experiment. Harrington's value of *e* was used by Millikan in obtaining the value of 4.774×10^{-10} esu (1.593×10^{-19}C) included in a compilation of values of physical constants.[2] This value of *e* remained the standard until 1935 when it was superseded by the current value of 1.602×10^{-19}C, based on more precise and reliable methods which had been developed in the intervening years.

Harrington joined the faculty of the Department of Physics of the University of Saskatchewan in 1920 and was appointed head of the department in 1924. In 1929 he was appointed the only nonmedical member of the Cancer Committee established by the Saskatchewan Medical Association to set up a comprehensive cancer program to provide the "most modern scientific treatment," including the availability of a supply of radium to be used in "centres where the treatment could be administered to patients under thoroughly trained and competent physicians." In view of Harrington's work with, and on behalf of the committee, he can probably be considered

Canada's first medical physicist. His advice was sought and heeded by the Minister of Public Health FD Munroe in drafting the act which established the Saskatchewan Cancer Commission in 1930.

A major concern of the Cancer Committee in 1930 and 1931 was the form in which the radium should be obtained. In one form the radium salt was sealed in needle-like metallic tubes which were inserted into cancerous tissue for a period of some tens of hours and then removed. In the other form, the radon (or radium emanation) was collected in small gold tubes or "seeds," which were inserted in the tumor and could be left indefinitely to deliver the radiation dose as the activity of the radon decayed (3.8-day half-life). Harrington is said to have used the analogy of a cow supplying milk to illustrate the way a quantity of radium in a central location could be used to provide a continuing source of radon for use in various hospitals in Saskatchewan and even beyond. The final decision was to purchase 500 mg of radium in the form of radium bromide to be put into solution in the radon collecting apparatus and 1000 mg sealed in a number of needles. The radium for the radon plant was delivered in February 1931, and the remainder in July of that year.

The commission had accepted the recommendation of the Cancer Committee that the "emanation plant be situated in the University of Saskatchewan in charge of the Professor of Physics" but the question remained, who should build it? Several types of apparatus were already in use at the time including one patented by Failla of Memorial Hospital, New York. Failla was then in the business of constructing radon plants and quoted a price of $6800, including placing the radium in solution. This, however, was judged to be "entirely too expensive" for Saskatchewan at the beginning of the Depression. During his Christmas holidays in 1930, Harrington inspected radon plants in the Mayo Clinic, Edward Hines Hospital in Maywood, Illinois, Simpson Laboratories in Chicago, and the University of Wisconsin. With the prospect of a substantial saving in cost and the potential of making a number of improvements in the design, Harrington was authorized by the commission in April 1931 to proceed with the purchase of supplies and the construction of the plant.

EL Harrington was a proficient and enthusiastic glassblower and constructed much of the apparatus for the undergraduate "modern physics" labs. To insert a personal note, I recall vividly an experience shortly after I arrived in Saskatoon as a graduate student in the fall of 1950. I had been assigned a desk in a room adjoining Harrington's office which also contained a bench where Harrington did some of his glass-blowing. One day he asked me to give him a hand constructing a glass coach horn with which he was going to demonstrate some acoustic principles to his first-year class of premeds. My job was to support the bell end of a ten-foot section of the horn while he attached the mouthpiece. Although his hands were rather shaky, the right and left were perfectly synchronized, and he produced a beautiful joint. Later that morning, I heard a melodious blast from the direction of the physics theatre.

Harrington was somewhat hesitant to undertake the construction of the entire radon plant and attempted to recruit Fred Gleave, the technician in the Department of Physics at the University of Alberta. Gleave was unable to undertake the job and with the encouragement of GH Henderson of the Department of Physics at Dalhousie—who had a radon plant of his own—Harrington began construction of the plant in April 1931 with the assistance of EO Braaten, the first radon plant technician. By August 5, Harrington was able to report that the plant was assembled and holding vacuum.

A major problem was how to get the radium bromide safely and efficiently into solution. In Winnipeg, Manitoba a Failla plant had been acquired to be operated under the direction of Professor Frank Allen, head of the Department of Physics at the University of Manitoba and Dr Pat MacDonald, physicist for the Manitoba Cancer Institute. Failla came to Winnipeg and placed the radium in solution in April 1931. After some correspondence with MacDonald, Harrington secured the assistance of JWT Spinks of the Department of Chemistry, University of Saskatchewan, who installed the radium solution in the plant without a hitch. (Two years later Spinks spent a 10-month sabbatical in Darmstadt where he collaborated on a project with Gerhard Herzberg. This association played a major part in Herzberg's move to Saskatoon in 1935.) Spinks himself was later to become president of the University of Saskatchewan.

A schematic of the proposed plant was drafted by Harrington[3] in early 1931. A simplified drawing of the plant as constructed later that year is provided in an accompanying illustration. The radium solution was contained in a flask (1 in the illustration) which was surrounded by a lead-lined safe (2). A Toepler pump (4,5,6,7) served to collect the radon and crowd it past the mercury in the pig-tail trap (8) into the purification chamber (9,10,11), which included a KOH tube to absorb CO_2, a $P_2 0_5$ tube to absorb water vapor and a CuO tube. The CuO was heated electrically to catalyze the recombination of the hydrogen and oxygen formed by radiolysis in the radium solution. The purified radon was removed from the purification chamber by a second-stage Toepler pump. It was important that as nearly perfect a vacuum as possible be achieved in this part of the

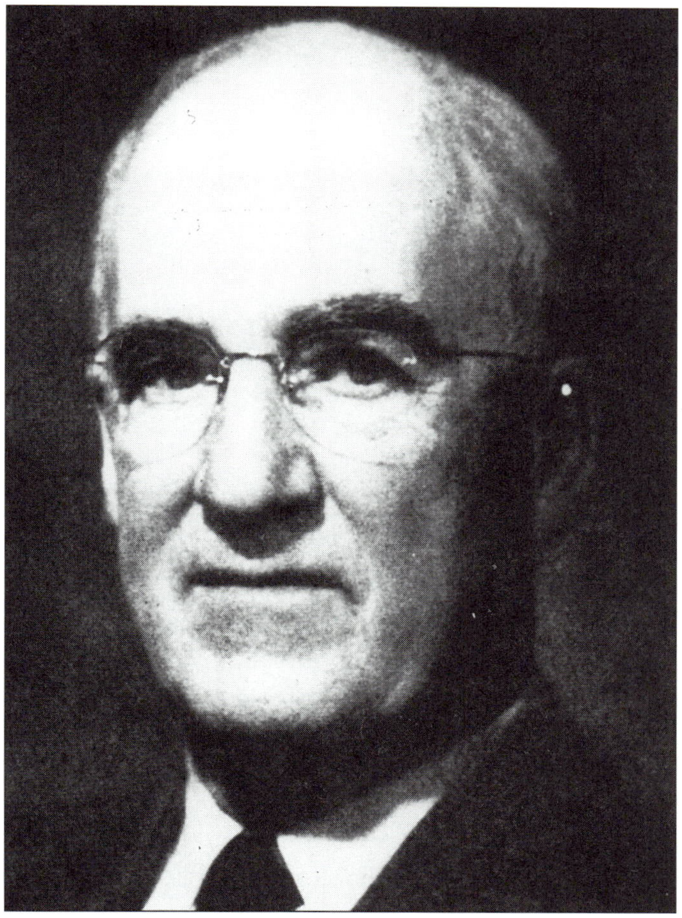

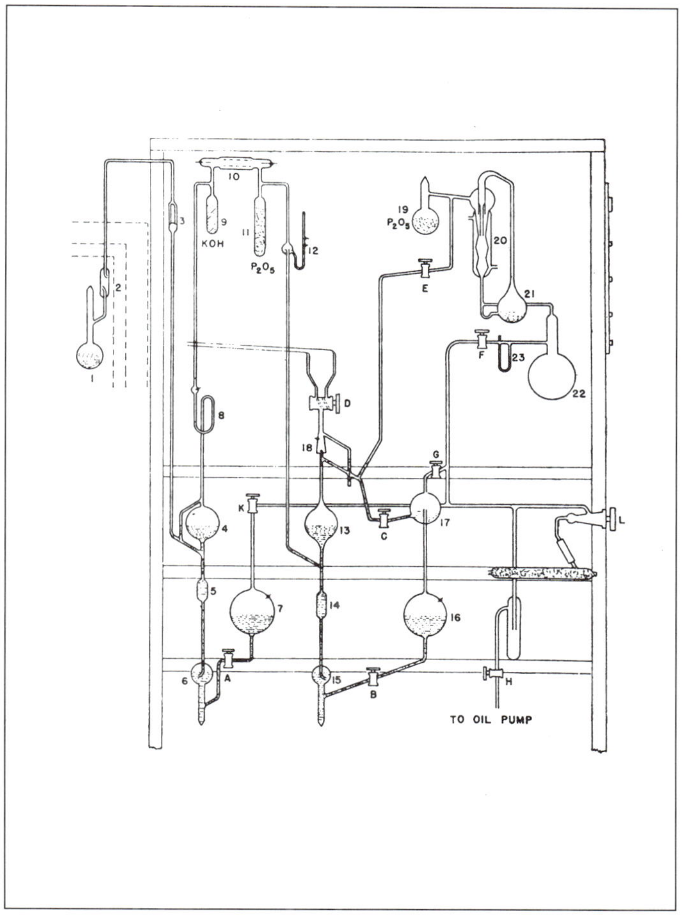

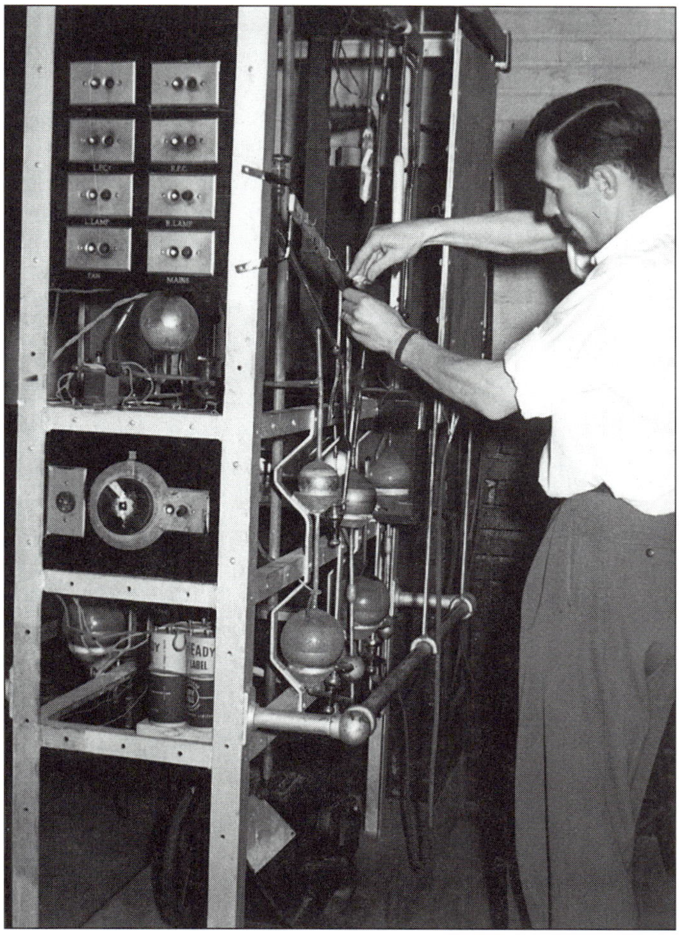

Top left
EL Harrington

Left
Gerd Froese, 1953

Above
Schematic of the radon plant 1931

system and Harrington added a mercury vapor diffusion pump of his own construction (19–23) to Failla's basic design. When gold seeds were required, fine gold tubing was attached to the end of the glass capillary with sealing wax. Radon was compressed into the tubing by raising the level of mercury in the tubing leading to stop-cock D.

The day-to-day operation of the plant was carried out by a technician, usually a senior undergraduate student in honors physics or engineering physics. The duties of the technician included "pumping," that is, removing the accumulated radon from the space above the radium solution, extracting the bulk of the contaminating gases and compressing it into the gold tubing. He would then measure activity of the sample by comparison with a known radium source and cut the tubing according to the number and strengths of sources requested by the radiotherapists, who would now be called radiation oncologists. Another important function was to accumulate the unused seeds, and after a year or so, send the gold to the Royal Canadian Mint in Ottawa to return a little revenue to the Cancer Commission.

The employment of students to operate the radon plant provided a much-appreciated source of financial support for the students and also introduced them to medical physics as a career. Table I gives a partial list of individuals who served as radon plant technicians over the years. Many of them have gone on to acquire senior positions in universities and cancer centres.

Radon seeds from the Saskatoon plant were used not only in the clinics in Saskatoon and Regina but also in Edmonton, Calgary, Brandon, Winnipeg, Montréal and Vancouver. There were also a few non-medical applications. In 1943, Harold Johns, then on the faculty of the University of Alberta in Edmonton, acquired radon seeds from Saskatoon for use in radiographing aircraft castings. Two years later, Johns was given a joint appointment with the University of Saskatchewan and the Saskatchewan Cancer Commission. Upon Harrington's retirement in 1952, Johns assumed supervision of the radon plant.

By 1961 the plant had been in operation for more than 30 years and was showing signs of old age. In particular the Pyrex and soft glass components, including the bulb which held the radium solution, were grossly discoloured and brittle from massive doses of radiation. Moreover, radioactive gold seeds were commercially available with which to carry out equivalent radiotherapy. The final closure of the plant in 1962 was precipitated by the discovery of a leak of some of the radium solution which, however, was safely contained, thanks to the efforts and cooperation of many people and groups, including the Occupational Health Branch of Saskatchewan, the Department of National Health and Welfare and the Commercial Products Division of Atomic Energy of Canada Limited.

Like the 4.774 x 10^{-10} esu value for *e*, the Saskatoon radon plant has been superseded. However, it served us well in its time not only for the treatments which it made possible but in stimulating the development of medical physics in Canada.

Radon Plant Technicians

EO Braaten	1931–32	RV Theobald	1944–46
Mr Clark	1932–33	JB Harrington	1948–49
HH Penley	1934–35	JR Cunningham	1949–51
GA Wrenshall	1935–36	RG Baker	1951–52
GJ Thiessen	1936–37	W Harms	1952–53
WA Morrison	1937–38	G Froese	1953–54
JL Stewart	1938–40	ECB Pederson	1954–55
FK Wilson	1940–41	DO Schneider	1955–56
AS McKay	1941–42	EG Rawson	1957–59
L Kovach	1942–43	C Vandenberg	1958–60
JJS Hamilton	1943–44	RF Cripps	1960–62

Acknowledgement:

I take pleasure in acknowledging the assistance and encouragement of Jack Cunningham, Sylvia Fedoruk, Gerd Froese and Harold Johns.

Editorial Acknowledgement:

This article has been reprinted from *Physics in Canada*[4] with the kind permission of the author and publisher.

Chapter XII •

A Radioactive Gold Ring

John E Aldrich

As can be appreciated from the preceding article, radon had been important in radiation therapy for many years. However, as the technique was gradually abandoned, a considerable amount of radioactive apparatus was left behind. In some cases the "valuable components" were sold as scrap. In particular the gold could easily be recycled and turn up again in quite a different form. There had been several reports in the United States of radioactive jewelery, but this was the first reported case in Canada.

In 1988 a 56-year-old woman presented with a ten-year history of chronic irritation under the ring on the ring finger of her left hand. Neither topical steroids or removal of the ring resulted in improvement. Physical examination revealed erythema and scaling localized to a well-demarcated circumferential area on the finger. There were also similar changes on the medial aspects of the adjacent fingers. A 4-mm punch biopsy showed a well-differentiated squamous cell carcinoma that was superficially invasive.

On simple examination with a Geiger–Muller counter the ring was clearly radioactive. The ring was placed on an x-ray film and left in a darkroom for two days. The result was an autoradiograph. Only the band of the ring was radioactive.

At the time the ring was purchased in 1951 settings were often chosen and the band attached by the jeweller in the shop. Clearly, the spool of gold for the band had come from radioactive stock. To try to estimate the dose, a lithium fluoride PTFE thermoluminescent dosimeter was taped to the inside of the ring. The dose was estimated to be 2.4 Gy per week.

Although there had been reports in the United States of such radioactive gold rings, this was the first documented case in Canada.[1] At about the time that radon plants were being dismantled in the 1940s the valuable gold, which had been used to hold the radon gas, was sometimes inadvertently sold off. It would have been sent with all other scrap gold to be refined in New York and in this case, made into gold wire. After 30 years the main radionuclide remaining would be lead-210 from which the beta and gamma rays would contribute the main dose to the basal cell layer.

The ring was worn by the patient virtually continuously for 30 years before she noticed any irritation. The dose to the basal layer would have been in excess of 4000 Gy.

Ackowledgement

This article was published in part in the *Journal of the American Academy of Dermatology* and is reproduced with permission.

Below left and right
The gold ring

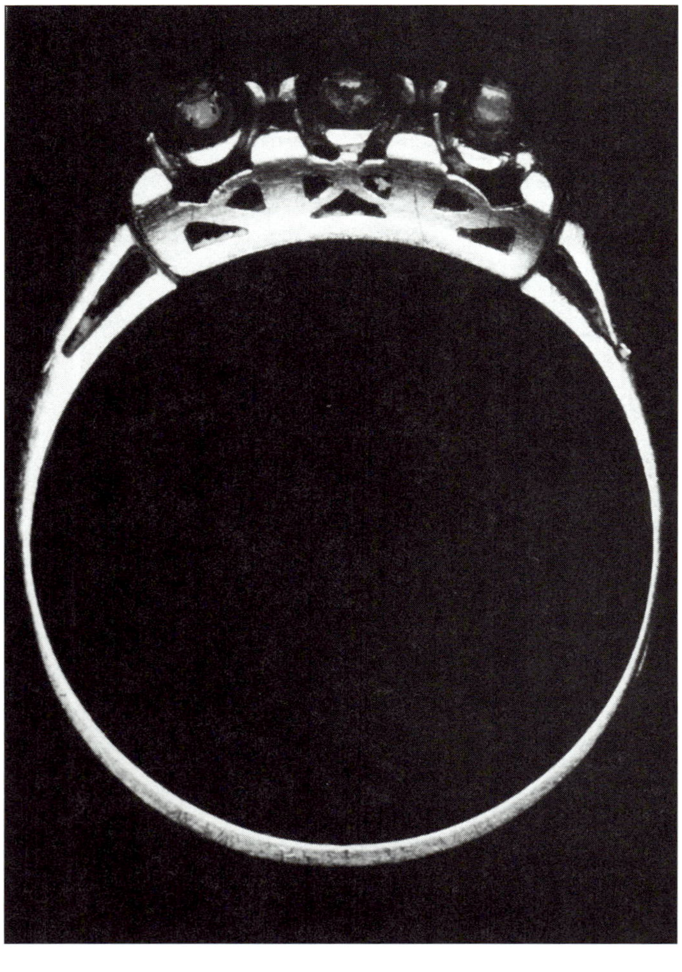

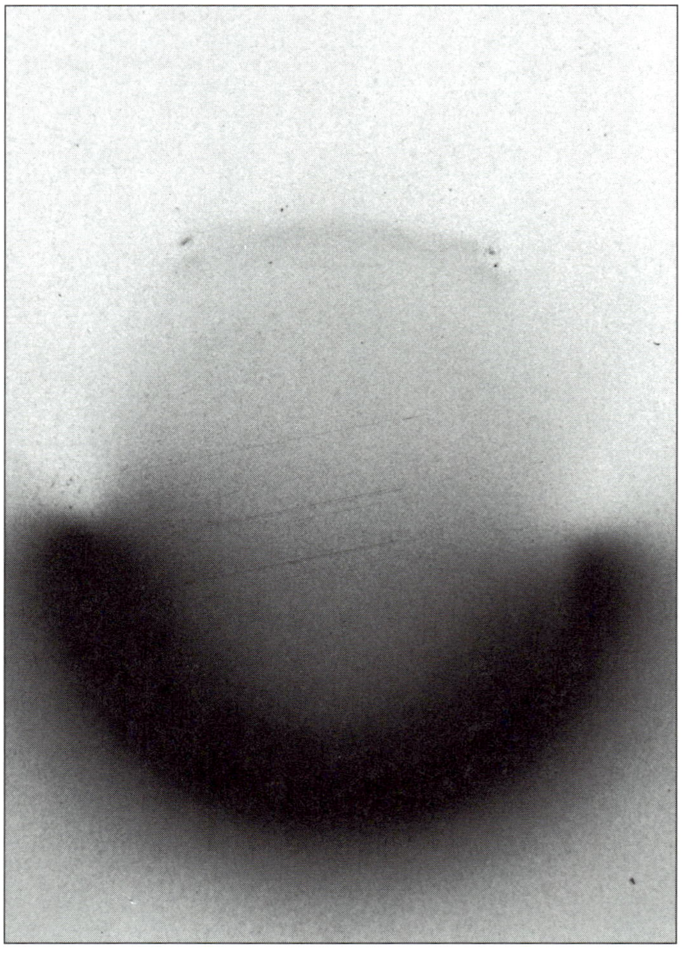

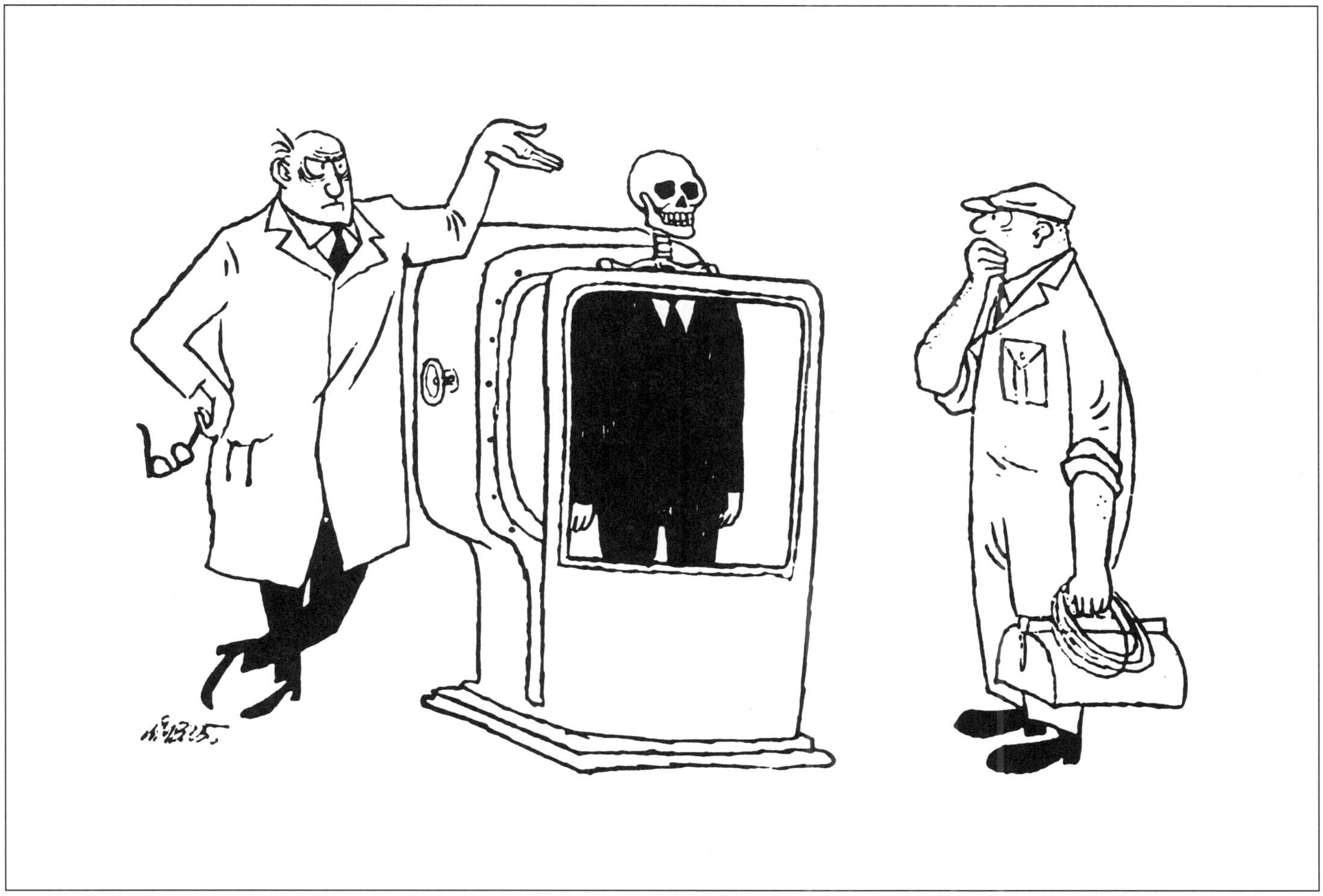

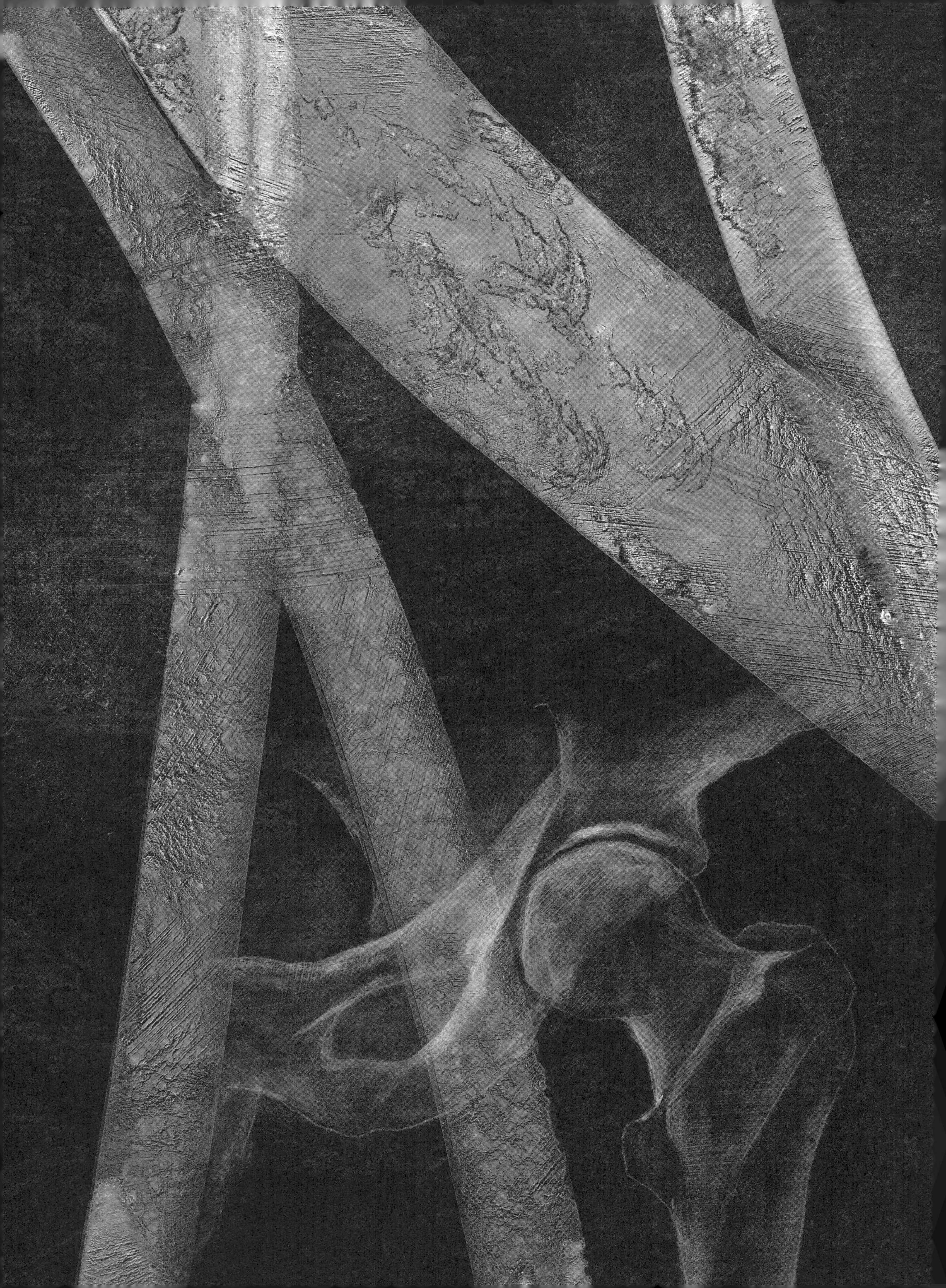

Part Eight

Radiological Sciences and the Graphic Arts

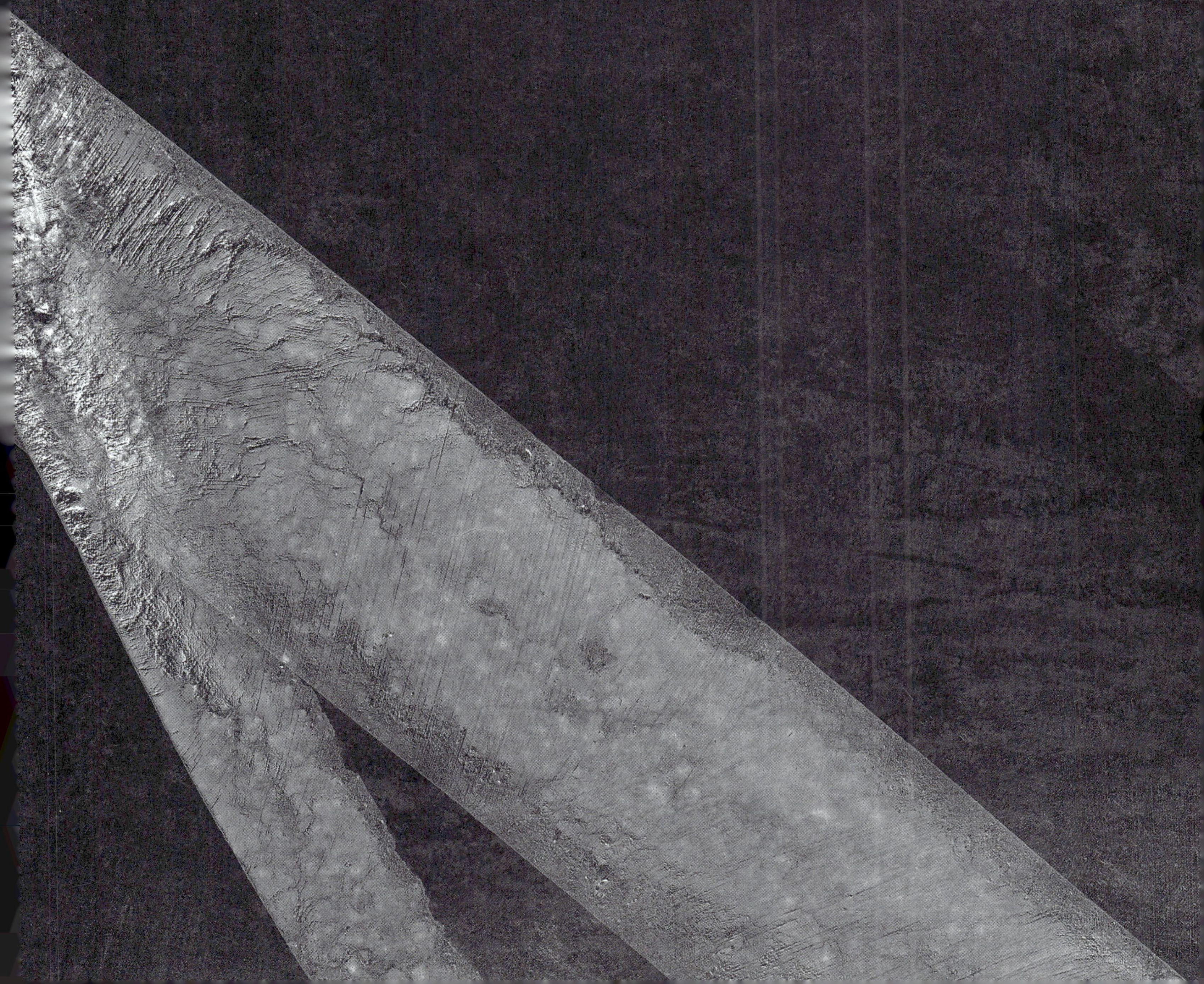

One school of anthropology has suggested that art is derived from shamanism and that art and medicine have, to that extent, roots in common.[1,2] Images and image processing are fundamental parts of the radiological sciences. In that context images come the full circle from religious utility to imaginative content to practical application.

As Professor Tom Hudson of the Emily Carr Institute points out in his television series *Mark and Image,* images may have both esthetic and information content. He used medical diagnostic images in that series to illustrate images being used for their information content. However, we usually choose to keep these domains distinct, separated by that chasm which some wish to believe separates artistic from scientific sensibilities.

Radiographs are certainly not made with a view to satisfying esthetic criteria, but the compelling nature of the images that result has been recognized by creative artists. Film director Donald McWilliams made a film for the National Film Board of Canada called *Creative Process: Norman McLaren,* a 116-minute montage of McLaren's experimental cinematic images, including some radiographs on which he had drawn fanciful abstract patterns. McLaren had a remarkably creative career at the National Film Board and pioneered the technique of drawing directly onto film. After viewing his film *Hen Hop,* Picasso remarked, "At last, something new in the art of drawing."[3]

Other artists have used radiographic images in their creations. Barbara Bloom, for example, has used bite-wing radiographs in her mixed media montage *The Reign of Narcissism: Tooth X-ray Chair 1989,* and Canadian Verlé Harrop, artist-in-residence at the Faculty of Medicine, Dalhousie University, has systematically explored the use of radiographic images combined with other graphic material and has achieved results with great emotional content. One of her images is used on the cover of this volume.

It is one thing to use radiographic imagery in works of art. However, Bronowski seems to have gone so far as to suggest that the insights provided by x-rays and radiographs have catalyzed some of the Western art of the 20th century:

> *Since the time of Newton's* Opticks, *painters had been entranced by the coloured surface of things. The twentieth century changed that. Like the [x]-ray pictures of Röntgen, it looked for the bone beneath the skin, and for the deeper, solid structure that builds up from the inside the total form of an object or a body.*[4]

Radiographic images have often been used in the graphic designs of postage stamps. In such a context it becomes possible to recognize that images such as a chest or hand radiograph or a radionuclide bone scan have an iconic quality that transcends their diagnostic utility.

Dr Douglas McEwan, a Canadian radiologist who has served not only as professor and chairman of the Department of Radiology at the University of Manitoba but also as president of the Canadian Association of Radiologists and of the Radiological Society of North America, has approached the esthetic content of images from another perspective. He has recognized that primitive images often achieve a radiographic vision in seeing beneath the surface of either animals or people. This is strikingly different from the traditional concern of Western art with the surface qualities of texture and colour, shade and colour saturation. In that sense the art is not so primitive. In reality it anticipates, as noted above, what is described in the Western/Eurocentric world view as modern art.[2] Such penetrating primitive images often transcend conventional representative art by adding an esthetic dimension that makes one look at objects in a new way.

Finally, in this brief review, it is evident from many of the images which appear on the cover of the *Canadian Association of Radiologists Journal* that a number of Canadian radiologists use their insights into the photographic process to create something more than ephemeral records. Dr Orest Semchishen, a radiologist in Edmonton, has achieved considerable fame for his spare, silver prints of scenes from the Ukrainian communities of the western prairies.[6] These are to be found in many galleries, including the National Gallery of Canada Museum of Contemporary Photography. Few of us will be able to look at such images without experiencing a reaction that defines such images in unquestionably esthetic terms.

— Brian Lentle

Chapter I • Norman McLaren

NATIONAL FILM BOARD ARCHIVES

Norman McLaren's career has been characterized by creative and technical brilliance, and by humor and sympathy for the human condition. His sense of movement has brought life to everything from a straight-back chair to scratches on raw filmstock. He was one of the first to experiment not only with picture but also with sound drawn or engraved directly on movie film, and was a pioneer in 3-D animation.

In *Narcissus*, his 59th film and in his words his last film, he continues to experiment with intricate optical printing processes. McLaren's *Narcissus* treats an age-old theme with stunning impact. Longer and more dramatic than his other films, it illustrates the tragedy of the Greek youth who condemns himself to a trapped existence, the victim of excessive self-love. As in his films *Pas de deux* and *Ballet Adagio*, McLaren has again chosen dance over animation as the more subtle vehicle for portraying human emotion.

Norman McLaren was born in Stirling, Scotland in 1914. The son of a house-painter and decorator, he had his first contact with film when he was around seven years old. As he describes it, "Before moving away, a neighbor, wishing to get rid of some unwanted possessions, presented my parents with a box containing a small projector and some strips of film. These mysterious strips immediately attracted me—by their smell."

At 18, McLaren began a five-year course at the Glasgow School of Art, specializing in his last three years in Interior Design. At Glasgow in 1934 he made his first film using a worn-out 35mm print he begged from a local movie house. Tying up the family bathtub for several

Norman McLaren's Noodle Doodles

In 1955 (the year he made Blinkity Blank*), McLaren went into the hospital to get his head examined. He had been suffering from headaches. After X-raying his skull, the hospital gave him the plates.*

Random Interpretations of the Things I Doodled

"I was going to fling them out and then thought, well it is a sort of portrait of me, so I'll just fill the head with doodles, improvising with anything that comes into my head when it is swirling with thoughts."

X's & O's
represents my interest in things that are kind of puzzling.

1,2,3,4
I was working on a film called 1,2,3, which I got stuck on. I finally picked it up again, and that became Rhythmetic.

Hearts
I hope that my films would move people, not intellectually but emotionally. I had a tendency to be too abstract, and I wanted to put more human emotion into my films.

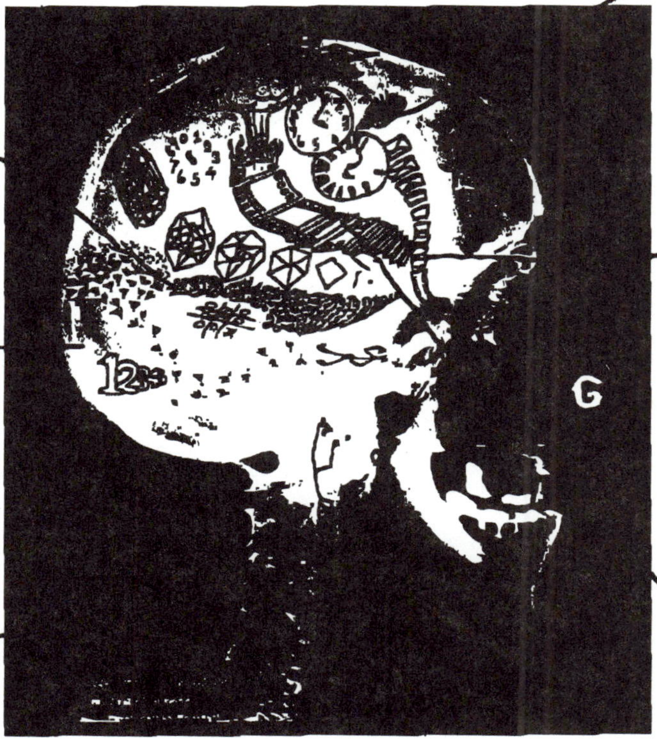

Clocks
indicate my obsession with time in film-making ... number of seconds, number of frames, 24 frames per second.

Film Transforms to Letters
At that period I was receiving a lot of mail from all over the world wanting to know about my techniques. It was disturbing my filmmaking & thinking. It led me to produce technical notes on all my work that I could send out.

Stairway with Film
I was trying to get better & better with every film... atomic bomb at that time and its potential for destroying all. Right at the top is a little flower with wings. That represents hope, I think.

The McLaren Package
2 videos:
Creative Process: Norman McLaren
exploring McLaren's genius 117 min.
Selected Films: Norman McLaren
14 films 114 min.
plus the 104-page book,
Norman McLaren on the Creative Process
featuring McLaren's own technical notes on his films
C 0191 132 $49.95 plus taxes

Above
Still frame from "The Creative Process: Norman McLaren"

days, Norman soaked off the film's emulsion and then applied colored dyes to the clear celluloid, resulting in a three-minute abstract film. His third film, *Colour Cocktail*, was entered in the Scottish Amateur Film Festival in 1935 where John Grierson, acting as a one-man jury, judged the film bad, but, recognizing McLaren's potential, gave him a prize, and on the strength of the film, offered McLaren a job at the General Post Office Film Unit in London. Before starting work with Grierson, however, McLaren first traveled to Spain to shoot footage of the civil war for Ivor Montagu's documentary *Defense of Madrid*.

McLaren's trip to Spain had a profound effect on him, and when war in Europe was imminent, he decided to go to America. Arriving by boat in New York as a landed immigrant in October 1939, McLaren spent several months looking for work before joining a company that produced industrial and public relations films.

Meanwhile, John Grierson was in Canada where he had founded the National Film Board in 1939. Grierson contacted McLaren in New York and asked him to come to Canada to work at the NFB. In 1941 McLaren joined the NFB, spending much of his early time there setting up an animation unit and training young filmmakers. Because most of the Board's duties became involved with war propaganda, civilian morale and promoting war bonds, McLaren's works during this period were theatrical trailers which addressed such topics as war gossip, inflation, and the need to buy Victory Bonds.

In 1944, McLaren was given the job of supervising the *Chants Populaires* series, which attempted to illustrate French-Canadian folk songs for audience sing alongs. *Le Poulette grise* (1947) was one of two films McLaren produced for this series.

In 1952, following a trip to China, where he taught fundamental animation techniques to Chinese artists under the auspices of UNESCO, and where he witnessed the civil war, McLaren made his Oscar-winning film, *Neighbors*. McLaren made the film as a reaction to the climate of fear and suspicion that had been building in North America since the end of World War Two.

During his work in Asia, McLaren's health had suffered, and upon his return to Canada it deteriorated further and he was hospitalized with severe rheumatic fever that permanently damaged his heart. He was, nevertheless, strong enough to produce the film *Blinkity Blank* in 1955. In *Blinkity Blank* McLaren experiments with the use of "intermittent" animation and spasmodic imagery, making play with "persistence of vision" and "after-image" in the retina of the eye. The visuals were engraved and colored on opaque black film stock.

In the latter half of the 1960s and in the 1970s, McLaren returned to what he had already been drawn to in *Neighbors* and *Chairy Tale* (1957)—the use of the human image to reflect upon mankind's condition. His elaboration of "live-action" through control of camera speeds and through intricate optical printing processes was pushed far in *Pas de deux* (1967) and even farther in *Narcissus*.

It would be criminal not to recognize the work of McLaren's close collaborators who have contributed to his films. As McLaren once stated, "Sometimes I get the impression from articles people write about me that I make my films almost single-handed. Now, this is a quite erroneous impression. Usually it's with one or two people. We form a small team. Most often it's been with Evelyn Lambert, but almost as frequently with Grant Munro. On the music side it's with Maurice Blackburn. So there's usually three people on the team."

Donald McWilliams has been working with McLaren on *Narcissus* since 1981, allowing McWilliams to explore further his special interest in optical effects. Their skills were most tested in the third sequence of *Narcissus*, when *Narcissus* and his self-image dance a series of pas de deux in which they act out a ghostly hide-and-seek.

While in China in 1953 McLaren received a telegram that read, "Congratulations. *Neighbors* wins Oscar." Puzzled, McLaren sat down to compose a reply. "I am pleased with your news," he began his letter, unable to see that any of this called for costly telegrams, "but who is Oscar?"

Throughout his career Norman McLaren has shied away from the trappings of success and his fame. Even with this tribute we have take liberties counter to his lifelong desire to let his films speak for themselves. We hope he will understand our intentions, which are to introduce his latest film to New England and to provide his audiences with an all-too-rare opportunity to review his films in the format in which they were made, and ideally in which they should be viewed.

Chapter II •

Dr Orest Semchishen

Brian Lentle

Orest Semchishen might well have been content to rest on the laurels he earned as a radiologist at the Edmonton General Hospital. Instead, he has fashioned a second and parallel career which lesser mortals might be content to regard as enough of a contribution to our national life. Orest is an extraordinary photographer. He has recorded the presence on the prairies of those who share his East European background. His spare, silver prints—typically of villages, Eastern Orthodox churches and their peoples—have come to be seen as deeply reflective of the Ukrainian and other cultures of western Canada. Technically superb as photographs, his work also displays the humanity of his other vocation.

It is no surprise, therefore, that Orest's work has been sought by some of the major collections of art photography in the country. These include the Canadian Museum of Contemporary Photography, the Alberta Art Foundation, the Ukrainian Museum and Archives, the Edmonton Art Gallery, the Winnipeg Art Gallery, the Canadian Centre for Architecture, Athabasca University and the Chinese Multicultural Centre. His work has been included in group shows arranged by the National Film Board, the Department of External Affairs, the Edmonton Art Gallery, the Muttart Gallery and the Walter Philips Gallery in Banff, among others. Photographs by Orest were included in the opening exhibit of the Canadian Museum of Contemporary Photography (CMCP), an affiliate of the National Art Gallery.

Ten exhibits, four slide collections and nine publications have brought his work to the public. His latest book, *Orest Semchishen—In Plain View,*[1] brings together some 140 photographs shown at an exhibit in Ottawa in 1994. The photograph he elected to have published in this volume is called "Hutterite Boys." It is to be found in several collections in Canada, including that of CMCP.

Orest is reflective about his art and craft. When questioned some years ago about the status of photography as an art form, he replied about his own work "I call it documentary photography because that avoids the question." I suspect that an answer is to be found in looking at his photographs.

Below
The Hutterite Boys

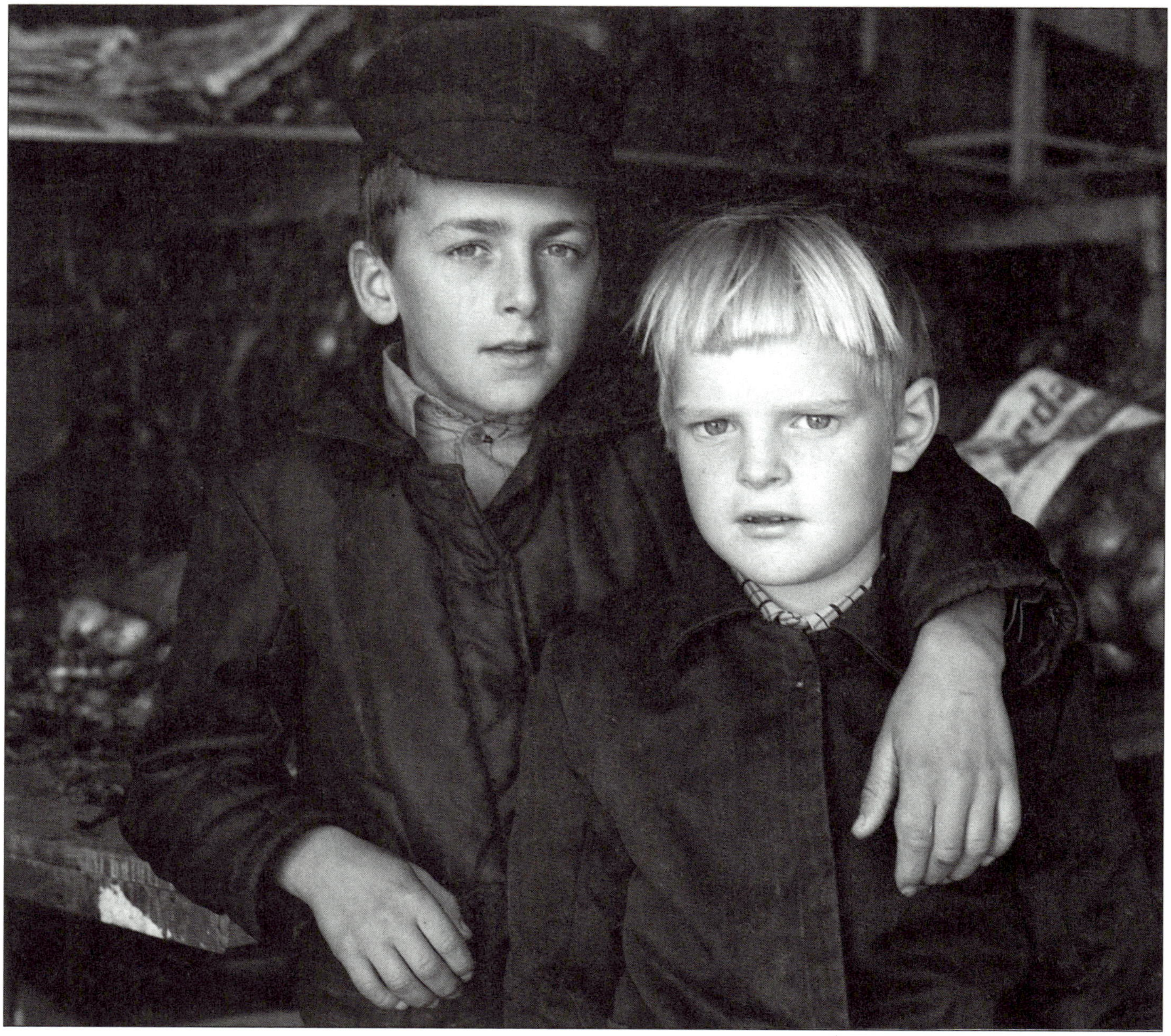

Chapter III •

Canadian Stamps and the Radiological Sciences

Brian Lentle and Peter Munk

Stamps are often used to recognize contributions to or the characteristics of a nation's life. Winners of Nobel Prizes can certainly expect to find their likenesses on the stamps of Sweden; such is the case with Röntgen, the Curies, Bequerel and Rutherford.[1] Indeed, the Nobel Prize seems to be a guarantee of philatelic fame not only in one's native country but elsewhere. A likeness of Röntgen has appeared on the stamps of at least ten countries or city states (Afars and Issas, Central Africa, Danzig, Germany, German Democratic Republic, St Vincent, Surinam, Sweden, Spain and Togo), while Madame Marie Curie has had her likeness used by over 20 countries, particularly since a French issue was also produced in many colonies of the French empire (see, for example, Cameroun, Scott B1: 1938).

Several Canadian physicians have been the subjects of commemorative stamp issues. Tupper, in his role as politician rather than physician, appears in some group scenes commemorating the 1867 Charlottetown Conference (Scott 142: 1927) and he has also been the subject of a commemorative issue (Scott 358: 1955). Dr Norman McRae, the physician-poet of "In Flander's Fields" has been portrayed on a stamp (Scott 487: 1968), as has been the work of Dr Tait MacKenzie, the physician-sculptor (Scott 656–657: 1975).

Physicians commemorated upon Canadian stamps primarily for their medical contributions have been Drs Banting and Best (Scott 533: 1971), Dr Norman Bethune (Scott 1264–1265: 1990), Sir Wilfred Grenfell (Scott 438: 1965), Dr Emmanuel-Persillier Lachapelle (Scott 877: 1980) and Sir William Osler (Scott 495: 1969). Bethune was celebrated most unusually by stamps of the same design issued

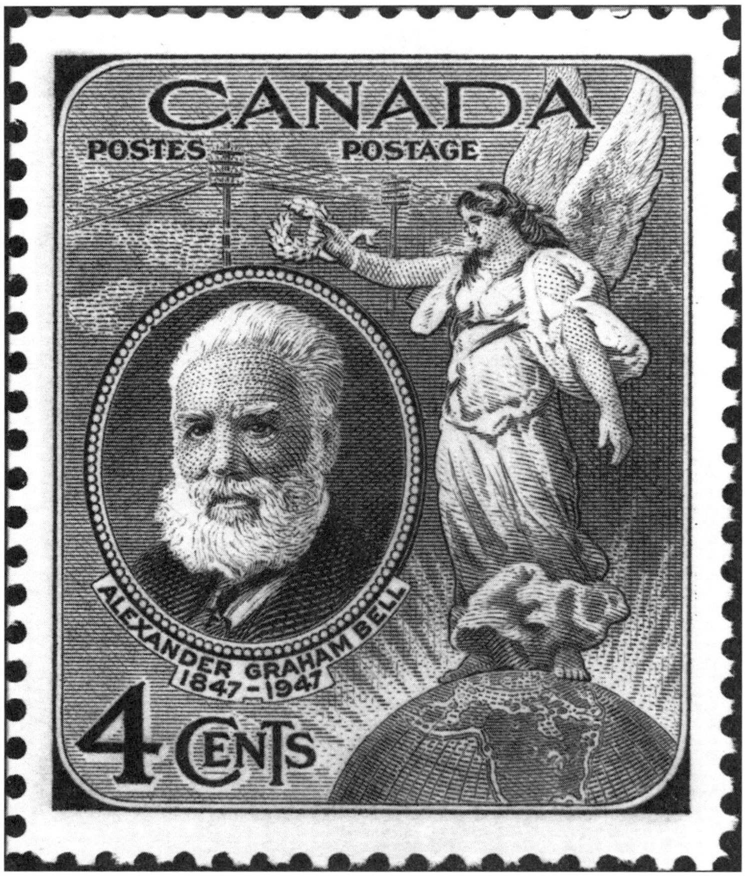
CANADA
POSTES POSTAGE
ALEXANDER GRAHAM BELL
1847–1947
4 CENTS
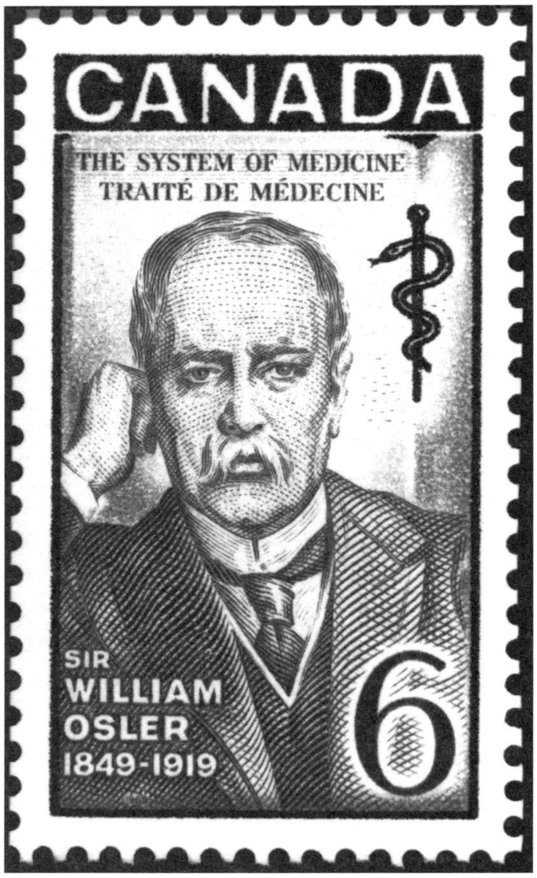
CANADA
THE SYSTEM OF MEDICINE
TRAITÉ DE MÉDECINE
SIR
WILLIAM
OSLER
1849-1919
6
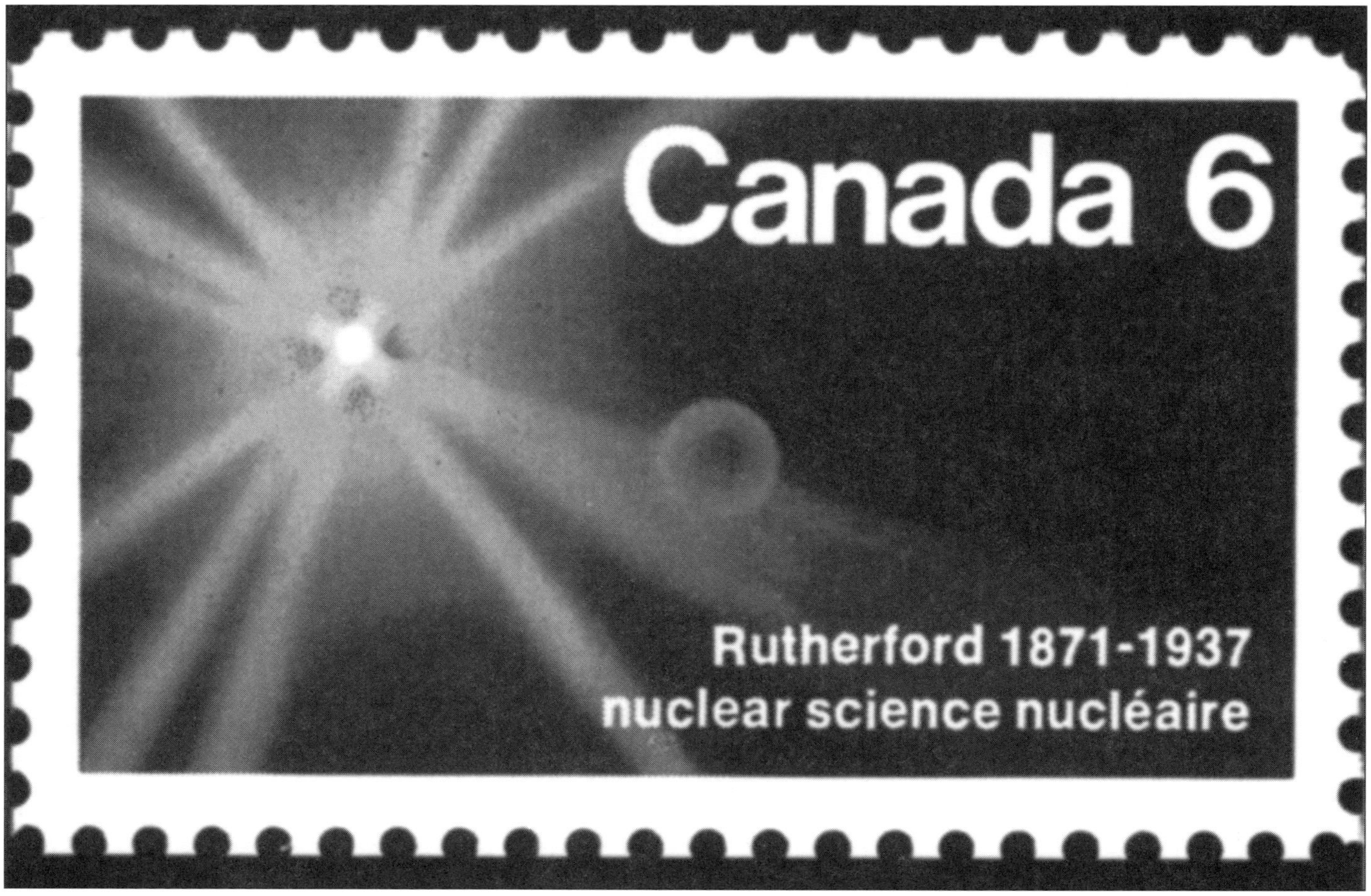
Canada 6
Rutherford 1871-1937
nuclear science nucléaire

simultaneously in Canada and in China, where he did most of his work.

Osler's life bridged the introduction of x-rays into medicine. While he appears to have had no particular interest in radiology it is reflective of his alert and enquiring mind that within months of the discovery of x-rays he unsuccessfully radiographed some gallstones both held in his hand and folded into a beefsteak. He was unlucky in choosing non-radio-opaque stones, for we now know that a minority of such stones would have been detectable.[2]

Dunlop has written an account of Nobel Prize winners whose work has influenced the course of medicine, entitled "Medical Nobels—stamp of genius."[1] There are other published accounts of the philatelic documentation of the history of the radiological sciences.[3,4] These articles manage to avoid any reference to Canadian stamp issues.

It is perhaps appropriate in a country with such a strong tradition in medical physics that such pioneers have been recognized on stamps for their contributions to medicine. Foremost is the work of Dr Harold Johns and his group at the University of Saskatchewan,[3] which was celebrated in a science and technology issue (Scott 1209: 1988). Dr Johns' team developed, among other things, the cobalt-60 radiation treatment unit, and his textbook of radiological physics has been required reading for generations of radiology residents. Inexplicably, not only is this stamp ignored in the articles published on this subject,[4,5] but it is not reproduced in the otherwise excellent slide set "A philatelic history of radiology" produced by Radiology Centennial Inc of the United States.[6]

A stamp was also issued to celebrate the work of Rutherford (Scott 534: 1971). Unlike the stamp issued by his native country of New Zealand, the Canadian issue does not bear his likeness. Rutherford has also been the subject of a stamp issued by Romania. Rutherford did his major scientific research at McGill University in Montréal.[7] Donizetti describes the work of Rutherford in revealing the structure of the atom as fundamental to the development of nuclear medicine, although the development of the tracer principle by Georg de Hevesy is usually seen as the defining moment in that history (Sweden: 1983).[8]

Alexander Graham Bell, best known as the inventor of the telephone, has been much celebrated on stamps, both in Canada (Scott 274: 1947) and elsewhere (Gabon, Scott 363: 1976; Luxemborg, Scott 590: 1976; Madagascar, Scott 553–557: 1976). Bell's interests were numerous and eclectic. However at home and while on vacation in Baddeck, Nova Scotia he was among the first to make radiographs. He also may have been the first to suggest the use of radium to treat cancer; his diaries indicate that he proposed what we now call telemedicine in the earliest years of this century.[9] A Canadian stamp has also honoured Marconi for his invention of radiotelegraphy. He is otherwise reputed to have been the inventor of radiographic fluoroscopy.

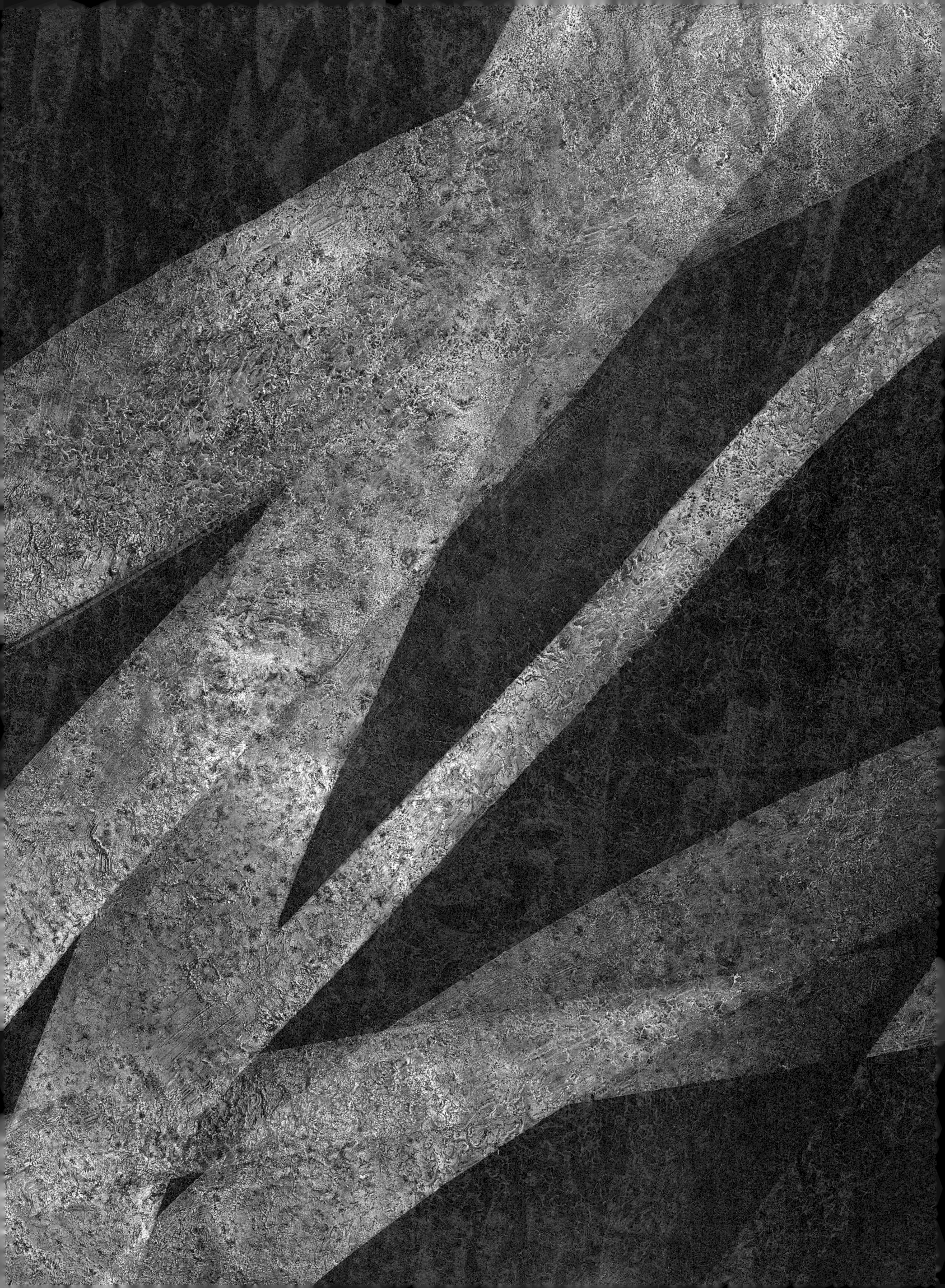

Part Nine

Postscript

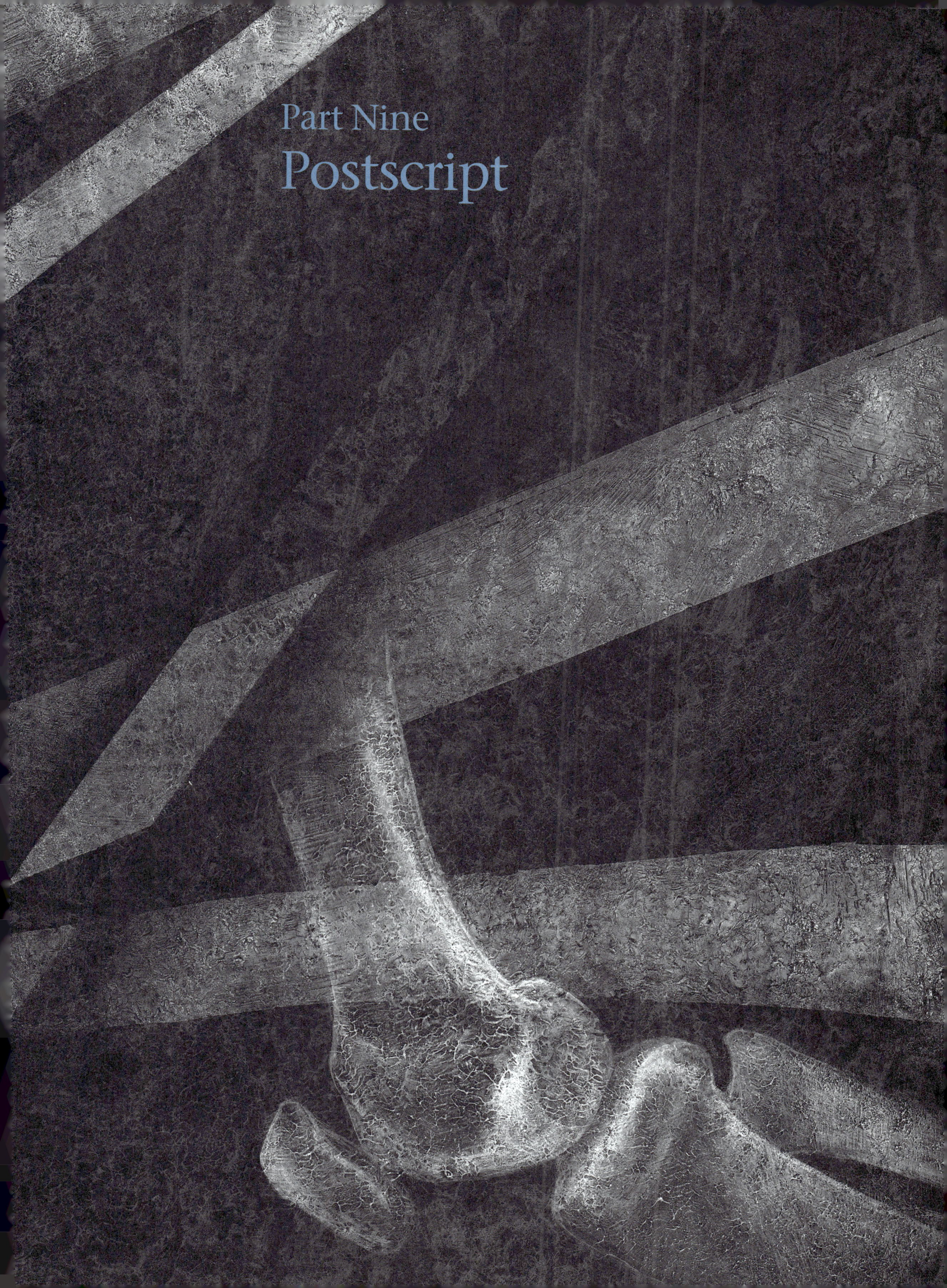

Chapter I • Postscript

Brian Lentle

Nothing endures but change.
— Heraclitus
(c540–c480 BC)

While preparing this volume for publication it has been impossible to ignore a wider issue: that Canada may not even be a relevant concept when the bicentennial of Röntgen's discovery is reached. And yet this account teaches us that in a number of successful enterprises and organizations, colleagues from the anglophone and francophone cultures have found a common purpose and a source of mutual support in their professional undertakings. Canadians in the radiological sciences—whether physicians, physicists or technologists—appear to have found it beneficial to preserve the best of regional and subspecialty affiliations while seeking a larger national identity. Only time will tell if that is a source of strength or a serious weakness in the structures described. Certainly, the leaders in the early years of the radiological sciences in Canada were people of vision but also of humility, wisdom, tolerance and forbearance. Those are attributes to emulate at any time and never more so than now. It has always seemed to me that we must make Canada work as an emblem for the future of the human race, if it is to have one.

My interest is in the future because I am going to spend the rest of my life there.
— Charles F Kettering

Someone has suggested that the search for the Canadian identity is in fact the Canadian identity. And yet these pages tell a somewhat different story: that the nation has had a strong radiological identity. But just as it has taken a pair of grateful immigrants to collect that story together here, one of the more refreshing aspects of the collective Canadian psyche is that we find little compulsion, as a group, to parade our strengths.

Health care and medicine are going through a time of massive change at the end of the 20th century. If there is a lesson in these pages it is, as Heraclitus observed 2500 years ago, that change is in fact a constant. Indeed, given the gulf between that blurred and now nearly uninterpretable radiograph made by Professor Cox in early 1896 and a cerebral activation scan done with an echo-planar magnetic resonance sequence or a neuroreceptor image of the basal ganglia made with positron emission tomography in 1995, the radiological sciences have compressed an incredible series of changes into just 100 years. For us, therefore, more than for most, change is an elixir of opportunity.

Change there will be. Hospitals are now viewed with scepticism as anachronisms. Society no longer concedes autocratic authority to physicians. Their role and status are changing just at a time when their real power to intervene in illness has reached a point unimaginable as little as 50 years ago. Again, a more pluralistic world is one that fits the radiological model well. A diagnostic service, if it was to achieve anything more than survival, has always brought together a host of different skills. In that context, to be a leader in a radiological service is to be the conductor of an orchestra and not necessarily the soloist. And yet time and again these pages point to the critical need for and the value of leadership in all professions, in coaching for and pointing the way to the future.

The emphasis in health care is changing to primary care in the community; it is ceasing to be technology-driven and will instead become cost accountable and concerned with human values; and the emphasis is shifting from treatment to prevention and chronic care. The team and the managerial approach is supplanting the professional as an individual provider. Competition is giving way to cooperation; high technology to more personal care; large hospitals to community care; treatment to prevention and acute to chronic care. But these changes are certainly consistent with strong services in the radiological sciences, if with some change of emphasis.

Among other changes in the present world-view, scepticism concerning the "technological fix" is a real one. Too often we have been led falsely down that path. The words of Feynman bear repeating: "For a successful technology, reality must take precedence over public relations, for Nature cannot be fooled."[1] And yet what we do in the radiological sciences is incurably rooted in high technology. It is not difficult to reconcile these facts. Much of what technology has given us in contexts outside our own has done a great deal for the public health. The refrigerator and microwave oven are not trivial examples. Our task, in whatever branch of the radiological sciences we work, will be not only to exploit but also to make human our technology.

That is not to deny some of the issues which confront medicine as a whole and radiology in particular: the need to ensure that only appropriate testing of patients is done; the need to expand the evidentiary basis for the practice of medicine and to be sure that our tools are not only effective but cost-effective; the need for sustained quality, for improved safety, and for improved communications. Our waiting rooms should be resting places, not residences. And will the digital archiving of images finally mean that x-ray films will not be lost, or secretly stored in someone's files, or simply left to self-destruct? For too long we have allowed physicians using radiological services in a hospital to believe that film loan libraries are irrefutable evidence of the existence of black holes!

It is possible to imagine a future in which technology, as a servant not a master, will radically change the nature of all the healing professions. One of the new paradigms is the "patient-focussed hospital." (It would be nice but not true to think that they always had been.) What better way to have the patient involved in his or her own care than to let that patient view the images made of his or her own body? At the same time the focus of anatomical, physiological and pathological teaching in the 21st century cannot remain in dissecting the dead in the laboratory and in the morgue. We as radiological scientists have an important part to play in teaching these subjects.

One of a surgeon's fears in the operating room is what lies behind the tissue he is about to cut into. His or her work, therefore, will increasingly be done under image guidance, with the images revealing what the knife is about to sever or the catheter is about to enter. That future is already here to some extent in interventional radiological methods, which have already replaced some surgical ones.

As the targeting of radiotracers becomes more specific, more and more they will be used in treatment as well as diagnosis. This will complement the therapeutic uses of high-energy radiations for treatment in radiation oncology.

Radiology was born into the second industrial revolution. This saw the introduction of electricity and the telephone. It is now poised to enter the third industrial revolution in which knowledge, information, and their transfer will continue to transform the world. The computer and the information network may well be a major part of the infrastructure for the future. Images will be moved and blended, analyzed and distributed, compared and archived, while information on appropriate and optimal pathways of care may be found only a keyboard away. We shall model treatment regimes, plan interventions and teach in such an environment. Information will be the substance of education[2] and indeed of survival, the computer and knowledge—coupling the tools.

This is not idle speculation but imminent reality. It does not deny the role of care-givers. There is no prospect of touch, of compassion or of intuition being automated.

This will change our medical schools, universities and colleges. Hospitals will ignore this future at their peril, because the patient who understands his or her care and has been treated by means inherently less damaging will be home sooner, to say nothing of being much happier and less disabled. In this way we will help to deal with the need to achieve more while spending less of the diminishing resources available for sickness care.

To manage change has been raised into a profession by the ubiquitous consultants who are conducting the last rites on so many hospitals and programs in this decade. We have been managing change very well in radiology for 100 years (by ourselves). We must now ask ourselves how best to do so in the future. We must also determine what shape our national organizations will take. As groups with strong national identities? As organizations not rooted in the past but alive to the future and with the ability to properly represent what is best about what we do best, without being self-serving? Will they, above all, act in concert, not in mutually antagonistic factions?

The issue of the size of the stage on which the future is to be played out is not within our control. It is only possible to reflect on the advantages we have enjoyed to date from our national affiliations. And to trust that wisdom and tolerance shall prevail.

It has been fascinating to look back into the past. But how much more promise we may anticipate in the future, our future, as the second and subsequent centuries after Röntgen's discovery unfold. To that extent there will always be "a new kind of ray."

Destiny is not a matter of chance,
it is a matter of choice;
it is not a thing to be waited for,
it is a thing to be achieved.
— William Jennings Bryan

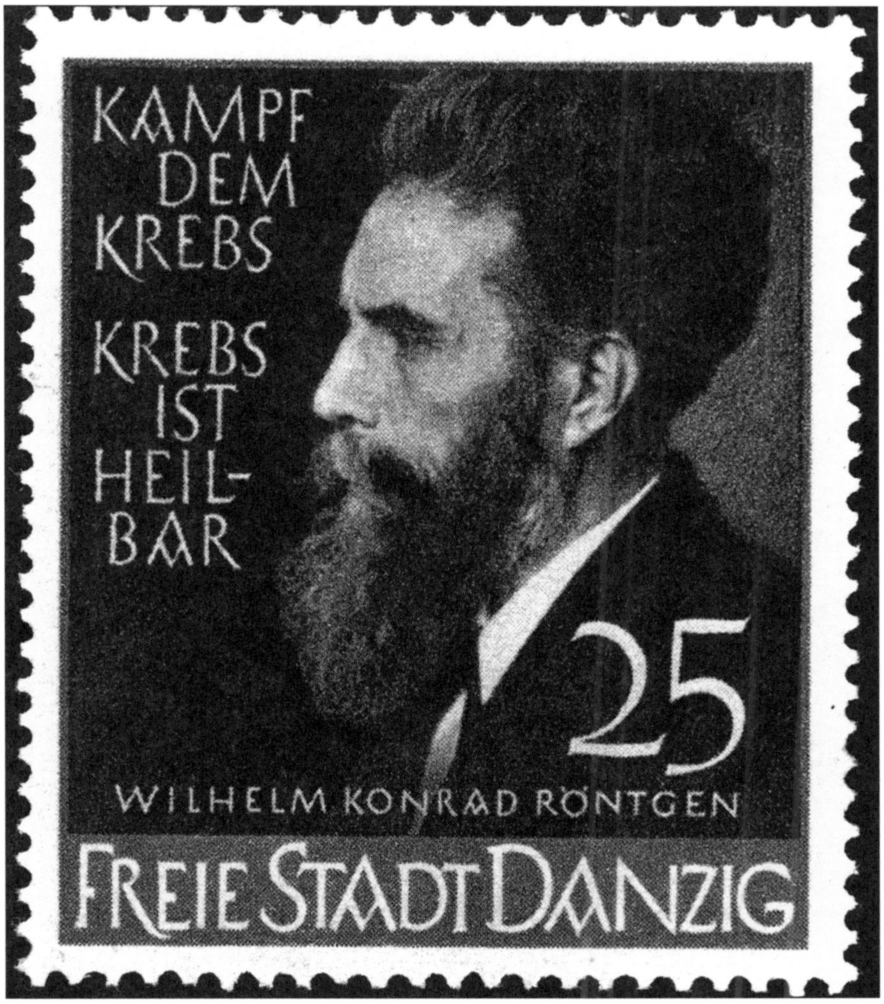
KAMPF
DEM
KREBS
KREBS
IST
HEIL-
BAR
25
WILHELM KONRAD RÖNTGEN
FREIE STADT DANZIG

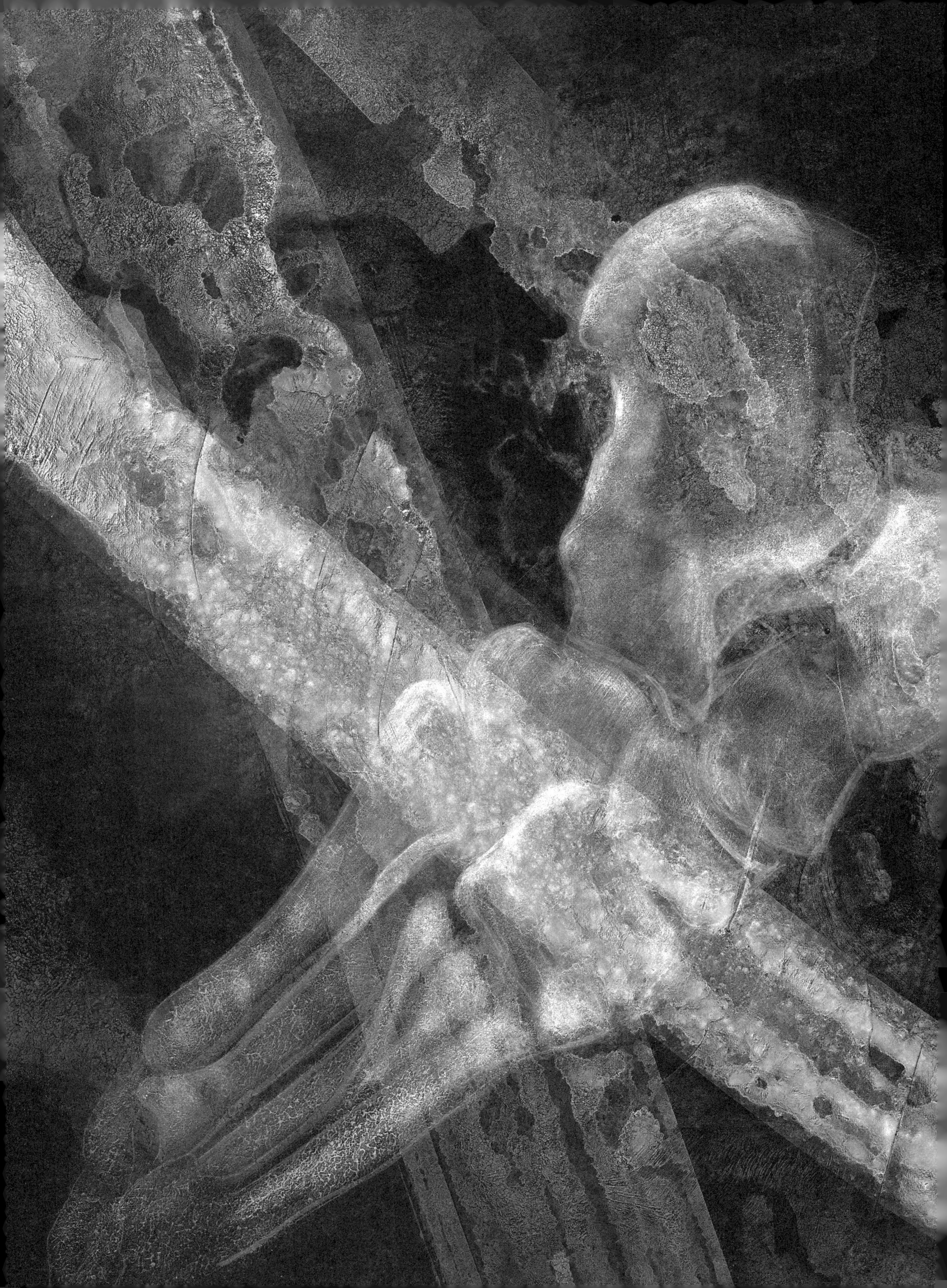

Part Ten

Annexes, References and Notes

A New Kind of Ray: References

Introduction **xxiv**

1. Roberts RM. Serendipity: accidental discoveries in science. New York: Wiley, 1989.
2. Judson HF. The search for solutions. New York: Holt, Rinehart and Winston. 1980.
3. Feddersen P. The industrial factor: technological innovations which changed radiology. In: Aldrich JE, Lentle BC, editors. A new kind of ray: The radiological sciences in Canada 1895–1995, Montréal: The Canadian Association of Radiologists, 1995.
4. Young IR. The interaction of industry and academia in diagnostic imaging. Invest Radiol 1993;28:S61.
5. Blume SS. Insight and industry. Cambridge MA:MIT Press, 1992.
6. Peabody FW. The care of the patient. J Am Med Ass 1927; 88:879.
7. Jolesz FA, Shtern F. The operating room of the future: report of the National Cancer Institute workshop—Imaging-Guided Stereotactic Tumor Diagnosis and Treatment. Invest Radiol 1992; 27:326.

Part One: Origins

I *Röntgen and the Discovery of X-rays* **5**

1. Bruwer AJ. Classic descriptions in diagnostic radiology. Volume 1. Illinois: Thomas, 1964.
2. Dibner B. The new rays of Professor Röntgen. Norwalk, Conn.: Burndy Library, 19.
3. Glasser O. Dr WC Röntgen. Springfield, Illinois: Thomas, 1945.
4. Glasser O. Wilhelm Conrad Röntgen and the discovery of the Röntgen rays. Springfield, Illinois: Thomas, 1934.
5. DelRegato J. Wilhelm Conrad Röntgen. Int J Radiat Oncol Biol 1976; 1:1.

Part Two: The Pioneers

I *Gas Tubes* **14**

1. Brecher R and Brecher E. The x-rays. Baltimore: Williams and Wilkins, 1969.
2. Grigg ERW. The trail of the invisible light. Illinois: Thomas, 1965.
3. Mould RF. A history of x-rays and radium. London: James Cond, 1980.

II *Canada's First Clinical X-Ray* **17**

1. Wright A. Experiments upon the cathode rays and their effects. Am J Sci 1896 March; 1(Ser 4): 235.
2. Frost EB. Experiments on the x-rays. Science 1896; Feb 3: 235.
3. Cox J, Kirkpatrick RC. The new photography with report of a case in which a bullet was photographed in the leg. Montreal Medical J 1896 March; 24: 661.
4. Cox J, Callendar HL. Some experiments on the x-rays. Trans Roy Soc Can 1896 May; 2 (Ser. 2 Sec. III): 171.
5. Rowland S. Report on the application of the new photography to medicine and surgery VII. Brit Med J 1896 March; 1:748. (This report includes a diagram and short description of the "focus tube" but does not identify the inventor of the tube.)

Secondary sources:

Rowland CG. Priority of clinical x-ray reports: a classic dethroned. Can J Surg 1962; 5: 247.

MacDermot HE. The earliest clinical applications of the x-rays. Can Med Ass J 1933 March; 321.

Brecher R, Brecher E. The x-rays. Baltimore: Williams and Wilkins, 1969.

III *Alexander Graham Bell* **21**

1. Bruce RV. Alexander Graham Bell and the Conquest of Solitude. Boston: Little, Brown and Company, 1973.
2. Bell AG. Home Notes. 1896 May 24.
3. Bell AG. Home Notes. 1896 June 18.
4. Bell AG. Home Notes. 1898 June 25.
5. Bell AG. Radium and Cancer. Science 1903; 18: 155.

IV *Some Observations on Early Diagnostic Radiology in Canada* **25**

1. Cox J, Kirkpatrick RC. The new photography with report of a case in which a bullet was photographed in the leg. Montréal Medical Journal 1896; 24: 661.

V *Ernest Rutherford at McGill University* **29**

A. Papers by Rutherford

1. Rutherford E. Uranium radiation and the electrical conduction produced by it. Phil Mag 1899; 47(Ser 5): 109.
2. Rutherford E, Owens R.Thorium and uranium radiation (preliminary note). Trans Roy Soc Canada 1899; 2 (Sec III): 9.
3. Rutherford E. A radioactive substance emitted from thorium compounds. Phil Mag 1900; 49(Ser 5): 1.
4. Rutherford E. Radioactivity produced in substances by the action of thorium compounds. Phil Mag 1900; 49(Ser 5): 161.
5. Rutherford E. Einfluss der Temperature auf die 'Emanationen' radioaktiven Substanzen. Physikalische Zeitschrift 1901; 2: 429.
6. Rutherford E, Brooks HT. The new gas from radium. Trans Roy Soc Canada 1901; 7(Sect iii, Ser ii): 21.
7. Rutherford E, Soddy F. The Radioactivity of thorium compounds, Part I: an investigation of the radioactive emanation. Trans Chemical Soc 1902; 81: 321; Part II: The cause and nature of radioactivity. ibid:837.
8. Rutherford E, Soddy F. The cause and nature of radioactivity, Part I. Phil Mag 1902; 4(Ser 6): 370; Part II. ibid:569.
9. Rutherford E, Soddy F. Condensation of the radioactive emanations. Phil Mag 1903; 5(Ser 6): 561.
10. Rutherford E. Excited radioactivity and the method of its transmission. Phil Mag 1903; 5(Ser 6): 95.
11. Rutherford E. The magnetic and electric deviation of the easily absorbed rays from radium. Phil Mag 1903; 5(Ser 6): 177.
12. Rutherford E, Soddy F. Radioactive change. Phil Mag 1903; 5(Ser 6): 576.
13. Rutherford E, Soddy F. The cause and nature of radioactivity, Part II. (See ref. 8: p 582).
14. Rutherford E, Soddy F. A comparative study of the radioactivity of radium and thorium. Phil Mag 1903; 5(Ser 6): 445 (specifically, p 453).
15. Rutherford E. The amount of emanation and helium from radium. Nature 1903; 68: 366.

16. Rutherford E, Royds T. The nature of the α-particle from radioactive substances. Phil Mag 1909; 17(Ser 6): 281. (A preliminary version of this paper was published in the Memoirs of the Manchester Literary and Philosophical Soc 1908; 53(No: 1): 1.
17. Rutherford E. The radiation and emanation of radium. Part I, Technics. 1904 July; 11; Part II, ibid. 1904 Aug; 171.
18. Rutherford E. The succession of changes in radioactive bodies (Bakerian Lecture). Phil Trans Roy Soc 1904; 204(A): 169.
19. Rutherford E. Slow transformation products of radium. Phil Mag 1905; 10(ser 6): 290.
20. Rutherford E. Bakerian Lecture (ref. 18): 213.
21. Rutherford E. Charge carried by the α- and β-rays of radium. Phil Mag 1905; 10(Ser 6): 193.
22. Rutherford E. The mass and velocity of the α-particles expelled from radium and actinium. Phil Mag 1906; 12(Ser 6): 348.
23. Rutherford E, Hahn O. Mass of the α-particles from thorium. Phil Mag 1906; 12(Ser 6): 371.
24. Rutherford E. Retardation of the α-particle from radium in passing through matter. Phil Mag 1906; 12(Ser 6): 134.
25. Rutherford E. The scattering of alpha and beta particles by matter and the structure of the atom. Phil Mag 1911; 21(Ser 6): 669.
26. Rutherford E, McClung RK. Energy of Röntgen and Becquerel Rays, and the energy required to produce an ion in gases. Trans Roy Soc 1901; 196 (A): 25.
27. Rutherford E, Barnes HT. Heating effect of radium emanation. Phil Mag 1904; 7(Ser 6): 202.
28. Rutherford E, Barnes HT. Heating effect of the α-rays from radium. Phil Mag 1905; 9 (Ser 6): 621.
29. Rutherford E. Radium—the cause of the earth's heat. Harper's Magazine 1905:390.
30. The number of papers given here is derived from the contents of Vol I of the Collected Papers (Ref. 31) and differs slightly but not significantly from Heilbron's analysis in "Physics at McGill in Rutherford's time" (Ref. 54). The bibliography in Rutherford in Manchester (ed. Birks JB. London: Heywood, 1962) includes several items not reprinted in the Collected Papers, but the additional items are abstracts and letters of a popular nature.
31. The collected papers of Lord Rutherford of Nelson. (3 Vols.) Vol. I: New Zealand–Cambridge–Montreal. London: George Allen and Unwin, 1962.
32. Rutherford E. Radio-activity. Cambridge: Univ Press, 1904 and 1905.
33. Rutherford E. Radioactive transformations (Silliman Lectures), New York: Charles Scribner's Sons, 1906.

B. Other Authors

34. Villard P. Sur la réflexion et la réfraction des rayons cathodiques et des rayons déviable du radium and Sur le rayonnement du radium. Comptes Rendus Acad Sci 1900; 130: 1010– and 130: 1178.
35. Wilson D. Rutherford. Simple Genius. (ref. 52) p 127.
36. Schmidt CG. Ueber die von den Thorverbindungen und einigen anderen Substanzen ausgehende Strahlung. Annalen der Physik u Chemie 1898; 65:141–151. See also: Badash L. The Discovery of Thorium's Radioactivity. J Chem Education 1966; 43: 219.
37. Wilson D. ibid., (ref. 52): 168.
38. Curie P, Curie Mme M-P. Sur la radioactivité provoqué par les rayons de Becquerel. Comptes Rendus Acad Sci 1899; 129: 714.
39. A recent full-length biography of Brooks is: Rayner-Canham MF and Rayner-Canham GW. Harriet Brooks, Pioneer nuclear scientist. McGill-Queen's University Press, 1992. However, the description "Canada's Marie Curie" is attributable to the present writer, not to the biography.
40. Curie, Mme Sklodowska. "Sur les poids atomique du métal dans le chlorure de baryum radifère." Comptes Rendus Acad Sci 1899; 129: 7.
42. Baskerville C. On the existence of a new element associated with thorium. Chem News 1901; 84: 179 and 84: 187.
43. Becquerel H. Sur la radioactivité de l'uranium. Comptes Rendus Acad Sci 1901; 133: 977.
44. Trenn TJ. The self-splitting atom, (Ref. 51) Appendix 3 (pp. 156–159) includes a reprint of E von Schweidler, "Uber Schwankungen der radioaktiven Umwandlung" (1905).
45. Ramsey W, Soddy F. Gases occluded by radium bromide. Nature 1903; 68:246 and Experiments in radioactivity, and the production of helium from radium. ibid 68: 354.
46. Geiger H, Marsden E. On a diffuse reflection of the alpha particles. Proc Roy Soc 1909; 82(A): 495.
47. Curie P, Laborde A. Sur la chaleur dégagée spontanément par les sels de radium. Comptes Rendus Acad Sci 1903; 136: 673.
48. Pyenson L. The incomplete transmision of a European image: physics at Greater Buenos Aires and Montreal, 1890–1920. Proc Amer Phil Soc 1978; 122(No. 2): 92.
49. Wilson D. ibid. (ref. 52) p189.
50. Terroux FR. The Rutherford collection of apparatus at McGill University. Trans Roy Soc Can (Sec. III) 1938, 32: 9.

C. Bibliography:

There are over 30 biographies of Rutherford and books or articles discussing particular phases of his career. Only those of particular relevance to Rutherford's work at McGill are listed here:

51. Eve AS. Rutherford. Being the life and letters of the Rt Hon Lord Rutherford OM. (The "official" biography.) Cambridge: Univ Press, 1939.
52. Wilson D. Rutherford—Simple genius. Cambridge, Mass: MIT Press, 1983.
53. Feather N. Lord Rutherford. London: Privy Press, 2nd ed, 1973.
54. Bunge M, Shea WR (eds.) Rutherford and physics at the turn of the century. New York: Dawson and Science History Publications, 1979. In particular, the following chapters: Badash L. "The origins of big science: Rutherford at McGill." pp 23–41; Heilbron JL. "Physics at McGill in Rutherford's time." pp 42–73; Feather N. "Some episodes in the α-particle story, 1903–1977." pp 74–88.
55. Trenn TJ. The self-splitting atom. The history of the Rutherford–Soddy collaboration. London: Taylor and Francis, 1977.
56. Howorth M. Pioneer research on the atom. The life story of Frederick Soddy. London: New World Publications, 1958.
57. An excellent short biography of Rutherford is that of del Regato JA in Radiological Physicists. New York: Amer Inst of Physics, 1985. (The original version of this chapter was published in Int J Radiation Oncology Biol Phys 1979; 5:539).

VI *Rays of Hope: The Establishment of Radiation Oncology in Canada 1895–1976* **45**

1. Groves Abraham. Roentgen rays in relation to cancer. Canadian Practitioner 1902; 27:313.
2. Third, James. Some of the diagnostic and therapeutic uses of the x-rays. Canada Lancet 1902; 35:526.
3. Hett FW. The use of x-rays in cancer, lupus and Hodgkin's disease. Dominion Medical Monthly 1902; 9:76.
4. Hayter Charles. History of radiotherapy in Saint John, NB. CARO Newsletter 1991; 2:4, and 1992;1:4.
5. Gray TL. Uses and abuses of x-rays. Canad Med Ass J 1928; 18:686.
6. Cosbie WG. Gordon Richards and the Ontario Cancer Foundation. Can Assoc Radiol J 1958; 1:1.
7. Jones WA. Gordon Earle Richards—a little about his life and times. Can Assoc Radiol J 1955; 6:1 (and reprinted in this volume).
8. Richards GE. The radiological treatment of cancer: methods and results 1928–1935. Canad Med Ass J 1936; 35:299.
9. Blair, Allan. Cancer in Canada: Summary of report of national survey 1947. Toronto: National Cancer Institute of Canada, 1947.
10. Jackson SM. History of radiotherapy in Canada. CARO Newsletter 1990; 1:2.
11. Houston CS, Fedoruk SO. Saskatchewan's role in radiotherapy research. Canad Med Ass J 1985; 132:854. See also Houston CS, Fedoruk SO. The history of radiation therapy in Saskatchewan. In: Aldrich JE, Lentle BC, editors. A new kind of ray: the radiological sciences in Canada 1895–1995. Montréal: The Canadian Association of Radiologists, 1995.
12. Johns HE. Impact of physics on therapeutic and diagnostic radiology. Canad Assoc Radiol J1979; 4:192.
13. Peters MV. A study of the survival in Hodgkin's Disease treated radiologically. American J Roentgenology 1950; 63:299.
14. Fitzpatrick PJ. Dr Vera Peters: Obituary. Int J Rad Oncol Biol Phys 1994; 29:195.
15. Bush RS. The compleat oncologist. Int J Rad Oncol Biol Phys 1982; 9:1019.
16. Goodman GB. History of radiation oncologists in the Royal College of Physicians and Surgeons. In: Aldrich JE, Lentle BC, editors. A new kind of ray: The radiological sciences in Canada 1895–1995. Montréal: The Canadian Association of Radiologists, 1995.
17. Jackson SM. Profile of the founding members of the Canadian Association of Radiation Oncologists. Ibid.

VII *The Rutherford Legacy: Nuclear Medicine in Canada* **57**

1. Brucer, MA. Chronology of nuclear medicine. St. Louis, Miss: Heritage Publications; 1990.
2. Kaplan E, editor. Selected historical aspects of nuclear medicine. Semin Nucl Med 1979; 9: 147.
3. Donizetti P. Lord Rutherford and nuclear medicine. In: Shadow and substance. The story of medical radiography. Oxford: Pergamon Press, 1967, p 151.
4. Ibid, p 50.
5. Levi H. George Hevesy and his concept of radioactive indicators—in retrospect. Eur J Nucl Med 1976; 1: 3.
6. Hevesy G. The absorption and translocation of lead by plants. Bioch 1923; 17: 439.
7. Anger HO. Scintillation camera. The Review of Scientific Instruments 1958; 29: 27.
8. Judson HF. The search for solutions. New York: Holt, Rinehart and Winston. 1980.
9. Fedoruk S. Remarks by Her Honour the Lieutenant Governor of Saskatchewan. Conference of the Canadian Nuclear Association and the Canadian Nuclear Society, Ottawa, June 6. 1989. Archives of Canadian Association of Radiologists—courtesy of Dr A Wilkinson.
10. Lentle B. The Canadian Association of Nuclear Medicine. In: Morley TP, editor. Medical specialty societies of Canada. Toronto: Associated Medical Services Inc, 1991.

Part Three: Progress by Province

Preamble **64**

1. Posner E. Reception of Röntgen's discovery in Britain and USA. Brit Med J 1970; 4: 357.
2. Roberts RM. Serendipity: accidental discoveries in science. New York: Wiley, 1989.
3. Judson HF. The search for solutions. New York: Holt, Rinehart and Winston. 1980.
4. Blume S. Insight and industry. Cambridge: MIT Press, 1992.

I *Public Perception: X-rays as Metaphor* **67**

1. Conrad J. Youth. New York: Doubleday, 1903.
2. Woodcock G. Canada and the Canadians. Toronto: Oxford University Press, 1970, p 163.
3. Tannahill R. Sex in history. New York: Stein and Day, 1980, p 348.
4. Connor JTH. The adoption and effects of x-rays in Ontario. In Aldrich JE, Lentle BC, editors. A new kind of ray: The radiological sciences in Canada 1895–1995. Montréal: The Canadian Association of Radiologists, 1995.
5. Gingras Y. La Réception des Rayons X au Québec: Radiographie des Pratiques Scientifiques. In: Aldrich JE, Lentle BC, editors. A new kind of ray: The radiological sciences in Canada 1895–1995. Montréal: The Canadian Association of Radiologists, 1995.
6. Jack D. Rogues, rebels, and geniuses. The story of Canadian medicine. Toronto: Doubleday, 1981, p 310.
7. Tannahill R. Sex in history. New York: Stein and Day, 1980, p 352.
8. Anon. Quoted by Graves R, Hodge A. The long weekend: A social history of Great Britain 1918–1939. London: Readers Union Ltd (Faber and Faber), 1941, p 200.
9. Feynman RP. What do you care what other people think? Further adventures of a curious character. New York: WW Norton, 1988.
10. Eddington AS. The nature of the physical world. New York: Macmillan, 1928, p 1.
11. Baumer FL. Modern European thought. Continuity and change in ideas 1600–1950. New York: Macmillan, 1977, p 462.
12. The Globe and Mail, Thursday, October 20th, 1994
13. Woodcock G. Canada and the Canadians. Toronto: Oxford University Press, 1970, p 221.
14. Feddersen P. The industrial factor: Technological innovations

which changed radiology. In: Aldrich JE, Lentle BC, editors. A new kind of ray: The radiological sciences in Canada 1895–1995. Montréal: The Canadian Association of Radiologists, 1995.
15. Metcalf F, editor. The Penguin dictionary of modern humorous quotations. London, England: Penguin Books, 1987.

II *Radiology in Newfoundland* **73**

1. Grenfell WT. A Labrador doctor: autobiography of Wilfred Thomason Grenfell. Boston: Houghton Mifflin Co, first edition, 1919.
2. Hodson CJ, Edwards D. The urinary tract. In: Shanks SC, Kerley P (eds). A textbook of x-ray diagnosis by British authors. London, HK Lewis, fourth edition, 1970: p 297.

III *History of the Use of X-rays in Nova Scotia* **77**

1. The new photography. Maritime Medical News 1896; 8: 90.
2. Bruwer AJ. Classic descriptions in diagnostic radiology. Volume 1. Illinois: Thomas, 1964.
3. Archibald BO. X-ray vignette, Nova Scotia Medical Bulletin 1951; 30: 237.
4. Maritime Medical News 1897; 9: 419.
5. Maritime Medical News 1900; 12: 173.
6. Farrell ED. Fracture-dislocation of spine—lympho-sarcoma of lung. Maritime Medical News 1901; 13: 290.
7. Obituary. Nova Scotia Medical Bulletin 1942; 21: 284.
8. Matters personal and impersonal. Maritime Medical News 1898; 10: 391.
9. Matters personal and impersonal. Maritime Medical News 1901; 13: 329.
10. Maritime Medicine News 1901; 13: 442.
11. Maritime Medical News 1904; 16: 269.
12. Codman EA. A study of the accidental x-ray burns hitherto recorded. Philadelphia Medical Journal 1901; 9: 438.
13. Becker A. Radiological pioneers in Saskatoon. Saskatchewan History 1983; 36: 31.
14. Scammell HL. History of the Victoria General Hospital, unpublished, 1937.
15. Honor where honor is due. Editorial. Maritime Medical News 1905; 17: 178A.
16. Kinley K. One hundred years of pharmacy service in the Victoria General Hospital. Unpublished, 1976.
17. Victoria General Hospital Annual Report, 1903.
18. Ernest Amos Codman 1869–1940. New Engl J Med 1941; 224: 296.
19. Codman EA. A study in hospital efficiency. Boston: Todd, 1917.
20. Codman EA. The shoulder. Boston: Todd, 1934.
21. Victoria General Hospital Annual Report, 1917.
22. Bird MJ. The town that died. Toronto: McGraw-Hill Ryerson, 1962.
23. Metson G. The Halifax explosion. Toronto: McGraw-Hill Ryerson, 1978.
24. Archibald BO. December 6th 1917, Nova Scotia Medical Bulletin, 1950; 29: 303.
25. Raddall TM. Halifax—warden of the north. Toronto: McClelland and Stewart, 1971.

V *Histoire de la Radiologie au Canada Français* **93**

1. Le Naturaliste Canadien, février 1896, contient également une mention brève de la découverte sous la signature de l'abbé Poirier.
2. Cf Star et Witness, 6 février 1896.
3. Voir à ce sujet l'excellente biographie par René Bureau: Le Naturaliste Canadien 1950; 77: 185
4. Weston TC. Reminescences among the rocks, 1890
5. Mgr J-C-K Laflamme: Le Naturaliste Canadien 1950; 77: 197.
6. Arthur Maheux. Propos sur l'éducation, Québec 1941: 107.
7. Archives du Séminaire de Chicoutimi, lettre Laflamme-Huard, 10 mars 1892.
8. Archives du Séminaire de Chicoutimi, lettre Laflamme-Huard, 12 mai 1896.
9. Archives du Séminaire de Chicoutimi, lettre Laflamme-Huard, 8 février 1899.
10. Docteur J-Edmour Perron: discours présidentiel 7ème Congrès de l'ACFAS, oct 1939.
11 Journal du Séminaire; IV: 605.
12. On sait que l'appareillage français était depuis toujours populaire chez nous. L'Hôtel-Dieu de Montréal recevait en 1896 ses premiers appareils Apostoli. En 1897, Radiguet et Massiot, de Paris faisaient ici avec Ducetret et d'autres maisons françaises, une concurrence sérieuse à la maison Max Kohl de Chemnitz.
13. Journal du Séminaire; IV: 625.
14. ...dont le perfectionnement fut attribué à tort à Thomas Edison, cf. J. Edmour Perron, ibidem.
15. La Presse 16 février 1896.
16. Reardon V. Ville de Montréal. La Presse, 6 juin 1896.
17. La Presse. 24 mars 1896.
18. Journal du Séminaire; IV: 642.
19. Archives du Séminaire de Chicoutimi, lettre Laflamme-Huard, 12 mai 1896.
20. Archives du Séminaire de Québec, Papiers Laflamme, carton 60.
21. Archives du Séminaire de Québec, Papiers Laflamme, carton 60.
22. L'Union médicale, juin 1897
23. Papiers personnels.
24. Le regretté docteur Edmour Perron possédait six de ces sept numéros; Mme Perron en a fait don à la Société canadienne-française d'Electroradiologie en même temps qu'un grand nombre de documents inestimables pouvant servir à une histoire élaborée de la radiologie. Je suis redevable à sa gentillesse d'avoir pu les consulter pour la rédaction de ces quelques notes et je lui en exprime toute ma reconnaissance. Mes remerciements vont également au docteur René Bureau, du Département de physique de l'Université Laval, pour ses sages conseils, et à M l'abbé Prévost, archiviste de l'Université Laval, pour m'avoir donne avec tant de gentillesse accès à tous les documents d'intérêt.
25. Les anciens présidents de la Société Médicale de Montréal, in Annuaire de la Société; 1955: 17.
26. Cet incident fit un certain bruit à l'époque. Radiologue parisien respecté, le Pr Dioclès avait apporté un perfectionnement important à l'appareillage radiologique. Sa visite un peu inopinée au Canada, fruit des avances non sollicitée et sans consultation préalable du regretté docteur Dubé, avait pris par surprise les radiologistes canadiens. Les constructeurs se

réjouissaient de l'effet-propagande escompté, mais les radiologistes français...et canadiens faisaient grise mine. Ce voyage, mal amorcé au départ, cristallisait une sorte d'antipathie de prestige entre constructeurs et radiologistes... Au nom de l'éthique, Pariseau voulait que la Société s'abstînt de participer à l'accueil. En fait le premier contact fut plutôt froid, mais, grâce à Perron et Gagnier, père, tout finit par s'arranger (voir lettre de Pariseau à Perron, papiers personnels de Perron, Archives de la Société canadienne-française d'Electro-Radologie).
27. Journal de l'Hôtel-Dieu, oct. 1935.
28. Jeanne Anctil, décédée vers 1930, était directrice des Écoles ménagères provinciales.
29. Laval Médical, oct. 1954.
30. Lettre Gagnier-Perron, docteur J-E. Perron, papiers personnels.
31. Ibidem.

VI *La Réception des Rayons X au Québec: Radiographie des Pratiques Scientifiques* 107

1. Lamarche Y. Position sociale des intellectuels et nationalisme: le cas de l'Action française. La Philosophie au Québec. Montréal: Bellarmin, 1976.
2. Galarneau C. Les collèges classiques au Canada-francais. Montréal: Fides, 1978.
3. Duchesne R. Problèmes d'histoire des sciences au Canada français. dans Jarrell RA et Ball NR (ed), Les sciences, la technologie et l'histoire canadienne. Waterloo: Wilfrid Laurier University Press, 1980
4. Galarneau C. op cit: 221
5. Bourdieu P. Système d'enseignement et système de pensée. Rev Int Sci Soc 1967; 19: 381.
6. Plusieurs auteurs ont abordé l'histoire des rayons X au Québec: Bureau R. La physique et l'électricité à l'Université Laval au temps de Monseigneur J-C-K Laflamme. Le Naturaliste canadien. 1952; 79: 330; Boissonnault Chs-M. Histoire de la Faculté de médecine de Laval, Québec 1953: 282; Perron J-E. La merveilleuse découverte des rayons X et son écho au Canada français. Annales de l'ACFAS 1940; 6: 145; et Bonenfant J-L. Comment les chanoines au Québec sont devenus transparents au XIX siècle. La Société canadienne d'histoire de la médecine, Nouvelles du printemps 1983: 1
7. Cité par Wheaton BR. The tiger and the shark. Cambridge: Cambridge University Press, 1983.
8. Les informations sur les découvertes des rayons sont tirées de Glasser O. Dr WC Röntgen. Illinois: Thomas, 1945.
9. Forman P, Heilbron JL et Weart S. Physics circa 1900. Personnel, Funding and Productivity of the Academic Establishments. Historical Studies in the Physical Sciences. 1975; 5: 92.
10. Pyenson L. The incomplete transmission of a European image: physics at greater Buenos Aires and Montréal, 1890–1920. Proc Am Phil Soc 1978; 122: 104.
11. The Montréal Daily Star, 6 février 1896.
12. Cox J and Kirkpatrick RC. The new photography with report of a case in which a bullet was photographed in the leg. The Montréal Medical Journal. 1896; XXIV: 661.
13. The Montréal Medical Journal 1896; XXIV: 7: 38.
14. L'Union médicale du Canada 1897; 26:46; et ibid: 118. Voir aussi Lipinski JK. Original Publications in Diagnostic Radiology by Canadian Physicians 1896–1929. La Société canadienne d'histoire de la médecine, Nouvelles du printemps 1938: 8.
15. Cox J and Callendar HL. Some experiments on the x-rays. Mémoires de la Société royale du Canada 1896; 2(section 111): 171.
16. L'Union médicale du Canada 1897; 26: 377.
17. Pour plus de détails sur l'expérience de Fizeau, on consultera Taton R (ed) Histoire générale des sciences. Paris: Presses universitaires de France, 1961
18. Archives de l'Université de Toronto, Papiers McLennan, Scrapbook ; 1: 185.
19. Langton HH. Sir John Cunningham McLennan, A Memoir. Toronto: University of Toronto Press, 1939.
20. Une liste est présentée dans Brecher R et E. The rays. A history of radiology in the United States and Canada. Baltimore: Williams and Wilkins, 1969; Sur la réception des rayons X en Australie, voir Hamersley H, Radiation science and Australian medicine 1896–1914 Hist Rec Austr Sci 1982; 5: 41–63. Sur la sociologie des découvertes simultanées, voir Merton RK. The sociology of science. Chicago: University of Chicago Press, 1973.
21. Monseigneur Thomas-Etienne Hamel. Mémoires de la Société royale du Canada 1914; 8(3e série): IV.
22. Monseigneur J-C-K . Mémoires de la Société royale du Canada 1911; 5(3e série) IV; Simard H. Mgr J-C-K Laflamme. Annuaire de l'Université Laval 1911–1912: 209–223.
23. Le titre même des communications porte la marque des cours de rhétorique: Essai sur la constitution atomique (prononcé en 1884) et De la certitude dans les sciences d'observation (présenté en 1891). A cette époque en effet, les titres des communications scientifiques sont plutôt de la forme: "Notes sur...", "Contribution à...", etc. D'ailleurs la structure des textes de Hamel, où fourmillent les interrogations et les exclamations, s'oppose en tout point à l'exposé plutôt terne et linéaire des "faits" scientifiques. Son intérêt pour les discours se reflète d'ailleurs dans son Cours d'éloquence parlée d'après Delsarte publié à Québec en 1906.
24. Bureau R. op cit: 331.
25. Annuaire de l'Université Laval pour l'année académique 1904–1905, Québec 1904:121. On retrouve la même description jusqu'en 1915.
26. Cite par Boissonnault. op cit: 285.
27. Annual Report of the Principal. McGill University 1892–1893: 28.
28. Archives du Séminaire de Québec, U. 60: 90.
29. Journal du Séminaire; IV: 625.
30. La Vérité, 25 avril 1896.
31. Journal du Séminaire 1896; IV: 642.
32. Bachelard G. La formation de l'esprit scientifique. Paris: Vrin, 1972
33. L'Union médicale du Canada 1897; 26: 271.
34. Annual Report of the President of McGill University 1896: 23.
35. Wilson DB. Experimentalists Among the Mathematicians: Physics in the Cambridge Natural Sciences Tripos, 1851–1900. Hist Stud Phys Sci 1982; 12:338; Sviedrys R. The Rise of Physical Laboratories in Britain. Hist Stud Phys Sci 1976; 7: 405–436.
36. Wilson R. op cit: 350.
37. Thomson JJ. Recollections and reflections. New York:

Macmillan, 1937
38. Snelders HAM. Hugh L Callendar. Dictionary of scientific biography 1973; IV: 19.
39. Sur Rutherford, voir Eve AS. Rutherford. Cambridge: London University Press, 1939.
40. Cox J. Mechanics 2nd ed. Cambridge: Cambridge University Press 1909; Cox J. Beyond the atom, Cambridge: Cambridge University Press, 1913.
41. Heilbron JL. Physics at McGill in Rutherford's time. Bunge M et Shea WR (ed). Rutherford and physics at the turn of the century. New York: Science History Publications, 1979.
42. John Cox. Nature 1923; 111: 817.
43. Sur l'évolution du mode de fonctionnement de la Société royale du Canada, voir Yves Gingras. Croissance de la recherche scientifique et transformation de la section III de la Société royale du Canada. Scientia Canadensis 1986; 10: 53.
44. Henri Simard. Mémoires de la SRC 1928; 22(3e série) IV.
45. Sur les carrières de Provancher, Brunet et Laflamme, on pourra consulter Duchesne R. Science et société coloniale: les naturalistes du Canada français et leurs correspondants scientifiques (1860–1900). HSTC Bulletin 1981; 5(nº 2):99 et, du même auteur La bibliothèque scientifique de l'abbé Provancher. RHAF 1981; 34(nº 4): 535.
46. Porter R. Gentlemen and Geology: The emergence of a scientific career, 1660–1920. The Historical Journal 1978; 21 (nº 4): 809.
47. A propos de son séjour à la Harvard Summer School of Geology à l'été 1877, il écrit a Mgr Hamel: "Je ne sais pas plus distinguer les terrains les uns des autres que je ne le savais avant mon départ: ceci exigerait une connaissance de la paléontologie que je ne possède pas. Il y a un point sur lequel je crois être très bien renseigné. C'est le grand nombre d'hypothèses plus ou moins hardies, plus ou moins solides sur lesquelles reposent les connaissances géologiques. Toutes ces théories sonnent presque toujours le creux." Cité par Duchesne R Science et Société coloniale op cit; 115.
48. Ibid: 116.
49. Rumilly R. Le Frère Marie-Victorin et son temps. Montréal: Les Frères des Écoles chrétiennes, 1949.
50. Duchesne R. La science et le pouvoir au Québec, 1920–1965. Québec: Éditeur officiel, 1978; Ouellet C. La vie des sciences au Canada français. Québec: ministère des Affaires culturelles, 1964.
51. Home RW. Origins of the Australian physics community Historical studies 1983; 20:383; Koizumi K. The emergence of Japan's first physicists: 1868–1900. Hist Stud Phys Sci 1975; 6:3. Gingras Y. Physics and the Rise of Scientific Research in Canada. Montréal: McGill-Queen's University Press, 1991.
52. Bourdieu P. Le sens pratique. Paris: Minuit, 1980.

VII *The Adoption and Effects of X-rays in Ontario* 119

1. For general discussions of these developments see Youngson AJ. The scientific revolution in Victorian Medicine. London: Croom Helm, 1979; Pernick MS. A calculus of suffering: pain, professionalism and anaesthesia in 19th century America. New York: Columbia University Press, 1985.
2. See Roland CG. The early years of antiseptic surgery in Canada. J Hist Med 1967; 380; Connor JTH. Joseph Lister's system of wound management and the Canadian medical practitioner, 1867–1900. MA thesis, University of Western Ontario, 1980; and Connor JTH. To be rendered unconscious of torture. Anaesthesia in Canada, 1847–1920. MPhil thesis, University of Waterloo, 1983.
3. See for example: Godfrey C. Medicine for Ontario. Belleville: Mika, 1979. Heagerty JJ. Four centuries of medical history in Canada, 2 vols. Toronto: Macmillan, 1928. MacDermot HE. One hundred years of medicine in Canada, 1867–1967. Toronto: Macmillan 1967. Brecher E and R. The rays: a history of radiology in the United States and Canada. Baltimore: Williams and Wilkins, 1959. Grigg ERN. The trail of the invisible light. Springfield: Charles C. Thomas, 1965.Jones WA. Gordon Earle Richards—a little about his life and times. Canad Assoc Radiol J 1955; 6: 1. Angus M. Kingston General Hospital: a social and institutional history. Montreal: McGill-Queens University Press, 1973. Cosbie WG, The Toronto General Hospital 1819–1965: A Chronicle. Toronto: Macmillan, 1975.
4. X-rays are short electromagnetic waves (situated in the spectrum between ultraviolet waves and gamma rays) that are emitted when cathode rays hit some solid object. Cathode rays, in turn, are emissions of electrons produced in an evacuated tube when an electrical discharge is passed through it. The primary means of generating cathode and x-rays was through the use of the Crookes' tube, a specially evacuated glass tube that has a cathode and anode located within it; this instrument was invented by the British physicist Sir William Crookes in the 1870s.
For additional information on x-rays see Grigg, op. cit.; Brecher, op. cit.; Dibner B. Wilhelm Conrad Röntgen and the discovery of X-rays. New York: Franklin Watts, 1968.
Specific information on the development of radiology in America is found in Pfahler GE. The early History of Röntgenology in Philadelphia. Part 1:1899–1920. Am J Roentgenol (AJR) 1956; 75: 14; Bromer RS. The history of Radiology in Philadelphia, Part 11: 1920–1954. AJR 1956; 75: 23; Christie AC. The American Röntgen Ray Society. AJR 1956; 76: 1; Fulton H. Sixty years of cardiovascular Röntgenology. AJR 1956; 76: 657; Caffey J. The first sixty years of pediatric Röntgenology in the United States—1896 to 1956. AJR 1956; 76: 437.
5. See the following papers for the month of February 1896: (London) Daily Free Press; Stratford Evening Herald; Ottawa Daily Free Press; Fort William–Port Arthur Daily Journal.
6. For details of the popular response to x-rays in Montréal, see the Daily Star for the month of February and the Gazette for February and March 1896. Generally speaking, the situation in this city was similar to that in Toronto.
7. See Photographing the invisible. Daily Mail and Empire. Feb 7. 1896:8; Tried in Toronto. Globe. 1896 Feb 11: 9.
8. The cathode photography Globe. 1896 Feb 11: 4.
9. The new photography. Daily Mail and Empire. 1896 Feb 11: 4.
10. Cathode rays. Daily Mail and Empire. 1896 Feb. 12:6. See also A Discovery at Varsity. Evening Star 1896 Feb. 12:4; Focusing the rays. Globe. 1896 Feb 13: 6.
11. Another minor feature originated from Toronto when the chemist and analyst for the Grand Trunk Railway, Alexander Roy, proposed a theory to explain the nature of x-rays, the central concept of which was that "all matter consists of

vortex rings of ether." To a 20th-century scientific mind Roy's theory may seem bizarre, and, indeed, to at least one 19th-century scientific mind it appeared a curious explanation. In an anonymous commentary on the novel idea, one contemporary critic remarked that while Roy spoke of vortex rings, he made no use of them; nor did he "appear to weave them in his theory in a sufficiently clear manner to carry conviction at once." In all fairness to Roy it must be borne in mind that the notion of an all-pervasive atmospheric fluid substance known as the aether, as well as the images of vortices in this aether to explain various phenomena, were part of the conventional scientific wisdom of the age.
See Roy's Theory. Daily Mail and Empire. 1986 Feb. 11: 8.

12. Examples of such illustrations are found in the following papers for 1896: Evening Telegram. Feb 18:5; Globe. Feb 12: 6; Feb 22 (supplement): 1; Mail and Empire. Feb 7: 8; Feb 8: 16; Feb 11: 6; Feb 15: 5; Feb 22 (supplement): 1.
13. Kesterton WH. A history of journalism in Canada. Toronto: McClelland and Stewart, 1967.
14. Such advertisements appeared in several issues of newspapers, but see, for example, the Globe 1896 Feb 27: 6.
15. See Editorial Notes. Daily Mail and Empire. 1896 Mar 12:4; Apr 30:6. This paper also contained a column entitled "Local Snap-shots" that relayed information of local news and events in Toronto and which was written by "Röntgen Rae"; see for example the issue of May 25, 1896, p10.
16. The deficit is hid in the safe. Evening Telegram. 1896 Feb 25: 1.
17. That surplus–cathode photography and the Ontario Treasury. Daily Mail and Empire. 1896 Feb 26: 7.
18. By the x-rays. Evening Star. 1896 Feb 20: 7.
19. See Rutherford P. A Victorian authority: The daily press in late nineteenth-century Canada. Toronto: University of Toronto Press, 1982.
20. See announcements and reports pertinent to these meetings in the following papers for 1896: Globe Feb 8: 20; Feb 10: 9; Feb 11: 8; Feb 27: 10; Daily Mail and Empire Feb 10: 7; Feb 11: 5; Feb 18: 6; Feb 27: 6; Mar 9: 3; Evening Telegram. Feb 8: 3.
21. In contrast to the attention given to x-rays, there was no newspaper coverage of other "great 19th-century developments" in medicine such as antiseptic and aseptic surgery or anaesthesia, notwithstanding the published reports of those patients who fatally succumbed to the power of chloroform or ether. On the latter, see Connor, "Torture," passim.
22. Rutherford, op. cit., p157.
23. Bovey HT. Presidential address. Transactions of The Royal Society of Canada 1896:2 (Section 111): 24.
24. In: Re Röntgen's x-rays. Canada Lancet 1895–6; 28: 251
25. The Röntgen rays. Canadian Medical Review 1896; 3: 138.
26. Cathode surgery. Dominion Medical Monthly and Ontario Medical Journal 1896: 59.
27. See Röntgen rays. Canadian Medical Review. 1896: 3: 165; Röntgen rays Canadian Medical Review 1897; 5: 47; Röntgen's Photography. Canadian Medical Review 1896: 4: 10; Skiagraphs. Canadian Medical Review 1897; 6: 13.
28. Advertisement. X-rays. Canadian Medical Review 1896; 4: xxi; Röntgen x-rays. Canadian Practitioner 1896; 21: inside back cover. X-ray kits usually included a Ruhmkorff coil, Crookes' tube and holder, fluoroscope, battery, and photographic apparatus and chemicals.
29. For details of this case see The new photography. Homeopathic Messenger 1895; 3:21. Information on homoeopathy may be found in Kaufman M , Homoeopathy in America: the rise and fall of a medical heresy. Baltimore: Johns Hopkins University Press, 1971; Coulter HL. Homeopathic science and modern medicine: the physics of healing with microdoses. Richmond, Calif: North Atlantic Books, 1981; and Gidney RD and Millar WPJ. The origins of organized medicine in Ontario. 1850–1869 in Health, Disease and Medicine: Essays in Canadian History, Roland CG ed Toronto: Hannah Institute, 1984.
30. See for example bullet wound of thorax. Canadian Medical Review 1897; 5: 126; and Toronto Clinical Society. Canadian Medical Review 1897; 6: 189.
31. King EE. Skin, hair, and nail lesions produced by the action of x-rays. Canadian Practitioner. 1896; 21: 789. While injuries were caused by x-rays, the evidence suggests that the attention given such cases tended to overstate the matter. For example, one Harvard surgeon reviewed the North American and European medical literature from 1896 to 1902 and identified a total of eighty-six cases (there was a maximum of fifty-five cases in 1896, a figure which declined year by year until there was only one case reported in 1901); see Brecher, op. cit., pp161–74. This decline may be attributed in part to more cautious use of the rays as well as the many safeguards that were later developed. These included screens on the x-ray tubes, filters, lead aprons and so on. For further details of these improvements see Brecher, op. cit., pp175–88; Kathren RL. William H Rollins (1852–1929): x-ray protection pioneer. Journal of the History of Medicine and Allied Sciences 1964; 19:287
32. Third J. Some of the diagnostic and therapeutic uses of the Röntgen rays, Canada Lancet 1901–2; 35: 526.
33. Calder RM. Static electricity and x-rays in general practice. Dominion Medical Monthly and Ontario Medical Journal [DMMOMJ] 1907; 29: 47; McMaster J. Some results that are being attained by the use of x-rays, with exhibition of patients. DMMOMJ 1902; 19: 61; Dickson CR. Some uses of the x-ray other than diagnostic. DMMOMJ 1902; 19: 72; McMaster J. X-Ray therapy and skiagraphy. Canada Lancet 1904; 38: 365; Hett FW. The use of x-rays in cancer, Lupus and Hodgkin's Disease. DMMOMJ 1902; 19: 76–80.
Regarding the role of photography in dentistry, one Port Hope dentist made the prophetic statement that "X Ray photography, will, in the future, work a revolution in dental diagnosis." While the truth of this statement is readily apparent today, it does not appear that Ontario dentists embraced the use of x-ray technology immediately; it was not until the 1930's that x-ray equipment came to be considered truly important in dental practice. See Sangster WA. Photography in dentistry. Dominion Dental Journal 1897; 9: 365.
34. For more details about x-rays in dentistry see Price WA. The Röntgen rays in dentistry—illustrated. Dominion Dental Journal 1901; 13: 203.
Price, originally from Ontario, practised in Cleveland, Ohio and became a pioneer in dental x-ray photography. For a more detailed analysis of such improvements see Grigg, op. cit.; Brecher, op. cit.; Otto Glasser, Technical developments of

radiology. AJR 1975; 75: 7; Krabbenhoft KL. A history of Röntgen therapy AJR 1956; 76: 859; Fuchs AW. Evolution of Röntgen film AJR 1956; 75: 30. For details concerning the new radiotherapy, see Report of the Royal Commission on the Use of Radium; Cosbie WG. George Richards and the Ontario Cancer Foundation. Canad Assoc Radiol J 1958; 9: 1; Quimby EH. The background of radium therapy in the United States. 1906–1956. AJR 1956; 75: 443; Eggleston W Canada's Nuclear Story. London: Harrap Research, 1966

35. See G Harvey Agnew. Canadian hospitals 1920 to 1970: a dramatic half Century. Toronto: University of Toronto Press, 1974; and Kerr RB, History of the Medical Council of Canada. Ottawa: Medical Council of Canada, 1979.
Concurrent with these professional developments were others in the medico-academic milieu. At the University of Toronto, George Richards became lecturer in radiology; by 1923 he and JC McLennan of the university's physics department had mounted a post-graduate course in radiology (Cosbie, Toronto General Hospital, p190). Similarly, by 1930 Queen's University, in connection with the Kingston General Hospital, offered a course in medical radiology (Angus, Kingston General Hospital, pp 120–21).
36. For further details of this development see Shortt SED. Before the age of miracles: the rise, fall, and rebirth of general practice in Canada, 1890–1940 in Roland. Health, disease and medicine, pp 123–52.
37. Sarnia General Hospital. Canadian Practitioner 1896; 21: 771.
38. Wingham General Hospital. Dominion Medical Monthly and Ontario Medical Journal 1907; 29: 64.
39. See Angus, op. cit., p 76; Cosbie, op. cit., pp185–85; Braithwaite M, Sick Kids: The story of the Hospital for Sick Children in Toronto. Toronto: McClelland and Stewart, 1974; Runnals JL. A Century with the St Catherines General Hospital. St Catharines: St Catharines General Hospital. 1974; Victoria General Hospital London: Annual Report for the year 1915.
41. Agnew notes that by 1933 about five hundred public hospitals out of six hundred in Canada had radiology departments (p5). In addition to stationary apparatus, many travelling clinics were formed that allowed mass x-ray screening to detect sufferers of tuberculosis. For example, by 1942 all teachers had to be x-rayed for tuberculosis; and the Globe and Mail instituted an examination program for its workers. For further details see Wherrett GJ. The miracle of the empty beds. Toronto: University of Toronto Press, 1977.
42. Cosbie, op. cit., p184.
43. See Hospitals of Ontario, pp 19–21.
44. Runnals, op. cit., p 48.
45. Angus, op. cit., pp71, 109.
46. Ibid. p 115.
47. See Hospitals of Ontario.
48. The noted medical historian Charles Rosenberg states that around the turn of the century hospitals began "to capitalize on their [new] image as temples of science." He further explains that hospital administrators, when appealing for money for their institutions, impressed private patients and others with displays of the technical capability of the hospital such as "the gleaming walls and intimidating apparatus in their operating rooms and laboratories, the startling photographs taken by the x-ray." Rosenberg's interpretation is based on American practices, but there is no reason to suppose a similar situation did not exist in Ontario (Inward vision & outward glance; the shaping of the American hospital, 1880–1914. Bulletin of the History of Medicine 1979; 53:34).
49. See Thompson JD and Goldin G. The hospital: a social and architectural history. New Haven: Yale University Press, 1975.
50. Hospital and the Lamp, pp 70–71.
51. A guide to hospital building in Ontario. Toronto: Minister of Health for Ontario and University of Toronto Press, 1954.

VIII *Early History of Radiology in Manitoba* **127**

1. Tait R, Stevenson JD, MacEwan DW. The first Western Canadian x-ray specialist. Manitoba Medical Journal 1975; 45: 57.

IX *History of Imaging in Manitoba* **131**

1. Tait R, Stevenson JD, MacEwan DW. The first Western Canadian x-ray specialist. Manitoba Medical Journal 1975; 45: 57.
2. Houston CS, DA Stewart 1874–1937: Western tuberculosis pioneer. Annales CRMCC, 1992; 25: 36.

XI *The History of Radiation Therapy in Saskatchewan* **141**

1. Taylor MG. Health insurance and Canadian public policy. The seven decisions that created the Canadian health insurance system. McGill-Queen's University Press, Montréal, 1978.
2. Houston CS. RG Ferguson, crusader against tuberculosis, Canadian Medical Lives No. 17. Hannah Institute & Dundurn Press, Toronto, 1991.
3. Watson TA. Results of treatment of cancer in Saskatchewan 1932–44 (inclusive). King's Printer, Regina, 1951.
4. Feather Joan. From concept to reality: Formation of Swift Current health region. Prairie Forum, 1991; 16:59–80. Impact of the Swift Current Region. Experiment or model? Prairie Forum 1991; 16: 225.
5. Acker MS, Watson TA. Saskatchewan's experience with a comprehensive public cancer program. Am J Publ Health 1960; 50: 65.
6. Saskatchewan Archives Board, M6. Premier CA Dunning papers Y–16–0, pp. 25 914–25 917 (unpublished letters). Murray to Dunning, October 6, 1922.
7. Saskatchewan Archives Board, M6. Premier CA Dunning papers, Y–16–0, pp. 25 918–25 919 (unpublished letters). Dunning to Murray, October 11, 1922.
8. Currie BW. Ertle Leslie Harrington, 1887–1956. Proc and Trans Roy Soc Canad 1956; 50: 91.
9. Davison RO. Saskatchewan's programme for cancer control. Can Publ Health J 1933; 24: 566.
10. Hawkes J. Clarence M Henry, MD. The Story of Saskatchewan and its people. SJ Clarke Publishing, Regina, 1924; p 1720.
11. Obituaries–Dr Clarence Henry. Canad Med Ass J 1954; 70: 701.
12. Becker A. A sketch of radiology at St Paul's Hospital. Saskatchewan Medical Quarterly 1970; 34: 34.
13. Cormack DV. The Saskatchewan radon plant, 1931–1962. Physics in Canada 1985; 41: 3.
14. Anonymous. 400 K.V. x-ray therapy unit now available in this

province. Saskatchewan Medical Quarterly 1935; 2: 22.
15. Obituaries. Dr Allan Walker Blair. Canad Med Ass J 1949; 60: 100.
16. Obituaries. Thomas Alastair Watson. Canad Med Ass J 1987; 137: 245.
17. Watson TA. Incidence of cancer in Saskatchewan in 1948. Can Publ Health J 1950; 41: 308.
18. Watson TA. Diagnosis of cancer in Saskatchewan, 1932–1949. Can Publ Health J 1951; 42: 427.
19. Watson TA. Results of treatment of cancer in Saskatchewan, 1932–1944 (inclusive). Saskatchewan Cancer Commission, Regina, 1951.
20. Watson TA. Results of treatment of cancer in Saskatchewan 1945–52 (inclusive). Saskatchewan Cancer Commission, Regina, 1958.
21. Anonymous. Portraits in radiology: Harold Elford Johns, PhD. Applied Radiology 1978; 25.
22. Taylor Lauriston S. Transcript of interview with Harold Johns, Rockville, Maryland, October 17, 1979.
23. Johns HE. AAPM Coolidge Award, 1976. Medical Physics 1976 ; 3: 375.
24. Houston CS, Fedoruk SO. Saskatchewan's role in radiotherapy research. Canad Med Ass J 1985; 132: 854.
25. Kerst DW. Development of the betatron. Sigma XI lecture, 1946, Am Sci 1947; 35: 57.
26. Watson TA, Burkell CC. The betatron in cancer therapy. Part I. J Can Assoc Radiol 1951; 12: 60.
27. Watson TA, Burkell CC. The betatron in cancer therapy. Part II. J Can Assoc Radiol 1952; 3: 25.
28. Watson TA. 20 million volt x-ray therapy. Acta Radiol Interamerican 1956; 6: 102.
29. Harrington EL, Haslam RNH, Johns HE, Katz L. The betatron building and installation at the University of Saskatchewan. Science 1949; 110: 283.
30. Johns HE, Darby EK, Haslam RNH, Katz L, Harrington EL. Depth dose data and isodose distributions for radiation from a 22 Mev betatron. Am J Roentgenol 1949; 62: 257.
31. Johns HE, Darby EK, Watson TA, Burkell CC. Comparison of dosage distributions obtainable with 400 KVP X-rays and 22 Mev X-rays. Br J Radiol 1950; 23: 290.
32. Johns HE, Darby EK, Kornelson RO. Radiotherapeutic physics. 1. The physical aspects of treatment of cancer by 22 Mev x-rays. Br J Radiol 1951; 24: 355.
33. Schulz MD. The supervoltage story. Am J Roentgenol 1975; 124:541.
34. Harrington EL. The expanding role of physics in biology and in medicine. Trans Roy Soc Canad 1947; 41: 1.
35. Johns, Sybil. At home with the atom. Mayfair Magazine, July 1955; 30: 30 and 53.
36. Johns HE, Bates LM, Epp ER, Cormack DV, Fedoruk SO. 1,000-curie Cobalt-60 units for radiation therapy. Nature 1951; 168: 1035.
37. Morrison A, Dixon WR, Garrett C, Johns HE, Bates LM, Epp ER, Cormack DV, Fedoruk SO. Multicurie cobalt 60 units for radiation therapy. Science 1952; 115: 310.
38. Johns HE. Physical characteristics of the radiation in cobalt-60 beam therapy. Can Assoc Radiol J 1952; 3: 2.
39. Watson TA. The clinical possibilities of the cobalt-60 beam unit. Can Assoc Radiol J 1952; 3: 7.
40. Johns HE, Darby EK, Kornelson RO. Radiotherapeutic physics. I. The physical aspects of treatment of cancer by 22 Mev x-rays. Br J Radiol 1951; 24: 355.
41. Johns HE, Bates LM and Watson TA. 1000 curie cobalt units for radiation therapy. I. The Saskatchewan cobalt 60 unit. Br J Radiol 1952; 25: 296.
42. Johns HE, Epp ER, Cormack DV and Fedoruk SO. 1000 curie cobalt units for radiation therapy. II. Depth dose data and diaphragm design for the Saskatchewan 1000 Curie cobalt unit. Br J Radiol 1952; 25: 302.
43. Johns HE, Fedoruk SO, Kornelson RO, Epp ER, Darby EK. Depth dose data 150 KVP, 150 KVP–22 Mev. Br J Radiol 1952; 25: 542.
44. Fedoruk SO, Johns HE, Watson TA. Isodose distributions for a 1100 curie cobalt 60 Unit. Radiology 1953; 60: 348.
45. Fedoruk SO, Johns HE, Watson TA. An improved clinical dosimeter for the measurement of radiation. Radiology 1954; 62: 177.
46. Watson TA, Johns HE, Burkell CC. The Saskatchewan 1000-curie cobalt 60 unit. Radiology 1954; 62: 165.
47. Johns HE, MacKay JA. A collimating device for cobalt 60 teletherapy units. J Fac Radiol 1954; 5: 239.
48. Johns HE, Morrison MT, Whitmore GF. Dosage calculations for rotation therapy; with special reference to cobalt 60. Am J Roentgenol 1956; 75: 1105.
49. Johns HE, Morrison MT, Watson TA. Radiation distribution from a 1000 curie cobalt unit using conventional and rotation techniques. Acta Radiol 1954; Supp 116: 550.
50. Burkell CC, Watson TA, Johns HE, Horsley RJ. Skin effects of cobalt 60 telecurie therapy. Br J Radiol 1954; 27: 171.
51. Johns HE, Cormack DV, Whitmore GF. Calibration of cobalt units using absolute ionization measurements. J Can Assoc Radiol 1955; 6: 37.
52. Watson TA. The use of the cobalt 60 unit. J Int Coll Surgeons 1954; 22: 219.
53. Watson TA. Co–60 telecurie therapy–after five years, Can Assoc Radiol J 1957; 8: 22.
54. Johns HE. The Gordon Richards memorial lecture. Impact of physics on therapeutic and diagnostic radiology. Can Assoc Radiol J 1979; 30: 192.
55. Cassels D. Brave new worlds for nuclear medicine. Ascent 1979; 1: 8.
56. McKinnon Eleanor. "Open Door Policy" in: Touched by Tommy: Stories of hope and humour in the words of men and women whose lives Tommy Douglas touched. Ed and Pemrose Whelan, editors, Whelan Publications, Regina, 1990.

XIV *Radiology at Vancouver Hospital and Health Sciences Centre* **167**

1. Harrison P, Harrison C. Dr Bede J Harrison. In: Aldrich JE, Lentle BC, editors. A new kind of ray: The radiological sciences in Canada 1895–1995. Montréal: The Canadian Association of Radiologists, 1995.
2. Garrow DG. Life's like that. Diagnostic radiology in Vancouver 1950–1991. Vancouver: Garrow, 1991.
3. Burhenne HJ. The history of interventional radiology of the biliary tract. Radiol Clin N Amer 1990; 28: 1139 (and reprinted in this volume).

XVI *The Evolution and Development of Radiation Oncology in BC* **175**

1. Lam GKY, Goodman GB, Harrison RW, Skarsgard LD, Kornelson RO. Cancer radiotherapy using negative pi-mesons. Nucl Instr Methods Phys Res 1985; B10/11: 1096.

Part Four: Regions and the Canadian Academic Departments of Radiology

I *University of Alberta: The Department of Diagnostic Imaging* **184**

1. Macdonald J. The history of the University of Alberta 1908–1958. Edmonton: The University of Alberta, 1958.

II *Department of Radiology: University of British Columbia* **188**

1. Logan HT. Tuum est. A history of the University of British Columbia. Vancouver: The University of British Columbia, 1958, p1.
2. Ibid, p 222.
3. Turnbull F. The curtain wouldn't rise: Starting a medical school in British Columbia. BC Medical Journal 1987; 29: 82.
4. Logan HT. Tuum est. A history of the University of British Columbia. Vancouver: The University of British Columbia, 1958, p 188.
5. Wylie E, Lentle B. Radiology at Vancouver Hospital and Health Sciences Centre. In: Aldrich JE, Lentle BC, editors. A new kind of ray: The radiological sciences in Canada 1895–1995. Montréal: The Canadian Association of Radiologists, 1995.

V *Les pionniers de la radiologie à l'Université Laval de Québec* **195**

1. Le Journal du Séminaire de Québec 1896; IV: 605
2. Ibid, p 606.
3. Ibid, p 633.
4. Ibid, p 634.
5. Ibid, p 664.
6. Annuaire de la Faculté de médecine, édition 1956–1957.

XII *The Early Story of Radiology at Queen's University* **211**

1. Third J. The Roentgen ray. Early diagnosis of tubercular and other lesions. Kingston Medical Quarterly 1899.
2. Jones WA. The teaching of undergraduate radiology at Queen's. Canad Med Ass J 1954; 70: 302.

XIV *Medical Imaging at Royal University Hospital and the University of Saskatchewan* **216**

1. Wheeler D, Spencer EW. Simplified planigraphy. Radiology 1940; 134: 499.
2. Spencer EW, Johns HE. A radium dosage calculator. Am J Roentgenol 1947; 57: 711.

XV *A Century of Radiology at the University of Toronto* **220**

1. Obituary of Dr EE King. Toronto Telegram, April 30, 1930.
2. The new photography. [Toronto] Globe, February 11, 1896: 8.
3. Anonymous note. Canadian Medical Review 1897; 5: 47.
4. Roentgen rays. Canadian Medical Review 1896; 3: 165.
5. King EE. Skin, hair, and nail lesions, produced by the action of "X" rays. Canadian Practitioner 1896; 21: 789.
6. Connor JTH. The adoption and effects of X-rays in Ontario. Ontario History 1987; 79: 92 (and reprinted above).
7. Bruwer AJ. Classic descriptions in diagnostic roentgenology, vol. 1. Springfield, IL: Charles C Thomas, 1964: 53.
8. [Toronto] Daily Mail and Empire, February 7, 1896: 8.
9. Cathode rays. Toronto Evening Star, February 5, 1896: 1.
10. Uses of the new "X" rays. Evening Telegram, February 18, 1896.
11. Editorial. Canada Lancet 1896; 28: 251.
12. Focusing the rays. Globe, February 12, 1896: 6.
13. Twenty-first annual report of the hospital for sick children, College Street, Toronto, 1896. Toronto: Archives of the Hospital for Sick Children, 1896: 31.
14. Obituary of Dr Samuel Cummings, Evening Telegram, December 19, 1933.
15. Obituary of Dr Samuel Cummings, Daily Mail and Empire, Dec. 19, 1933.
16. Minutes of meetings, Board of Trustees, November 2, 1896. Toronto Hospital-General Division, Archives, 1896: 548.
17. Minutes of meetings, Board of Trustees, April 5, 1911, November 1, 1911. Toronto Hospital General Division, Archives, 1911: 546.
18. Jones WA. Gordon Earle Richards—A little about his life and times. Canad Assoc Radiol J 1955; 6: 1.
19. Richards GE. Localization of foreign bodies. Brit Med J 1916; 2: 15.
20. Minutes of meetings, Board of Trustees, February 17, 1917, Toronto Hospital–General Division, Archives, 1917: 240.
21. Grigg ERN. The trail of the invisible light. Springfield, IL: Charles C Thomas, 1965: 5.
22. Cosbie WG. The Gordon Richards memorial lecture. Canad Assoc Radiol J 1958; 9: 1.
23. Ghent P. Dr William Howard Dickson. Univ of Toronto Med J 1933; 11: 46.
24. Richards GE. Obituary of Dr WH Dickson. Canad Med Assoc J 1933; 29: 690.
25. Minutes of special meeting of Board of Trustees, March 6, 1918, Toronto Hospital—General Division, Archives, 1918: 2.
26. Cosbie WG. The Toronto General Hospital 1819–1965: a chronicle. Toronto: Macmillan, 1975: 190.
27. Holmes RB. Radiology. Report of the Dean of the Faculty of Medicine, University of Toronto, session 1970–1971. Toronto: Faculty of Medicine, 1971: 156.
28. Shorter E. A century of radiology at the University of Toronto. Am J Roentgenol 1994; 163: 1508.

Part Five (a): The Founders

I *Dr James Third* 234

1. Angus, Margaret. Kingston General Hospital: a social and institutional history. Montréal:McGill–Queen's University Press, 1973.

II *Gordon Earle Richards—A Little About His Life and Times* 235

1. Jones WA. Gordon Earle Richards—a little about his life and times. Canada Assoc Radiol J 1955; 6: 1.

Dr Gordon Richards' entire bibliography is recorded in Appendix 2.

Dr AC Singleton wrote of Dr Richards in an editorial following Dr Richards' death.[1] Part of that editorial reads as follows:

That he did greatly serve suffering mankind in one of its most grievous afflictions, the record of his more than thirty years of unremitting fight against cancer bears tribute. It was the grand aim and purpose of his life. Into that fight he threw all the zest of a crusader. All the knowledge, skill, originality and persistence with which he was so richly blessed, were devoted to that cause. It was the concentration of these qualities into his technique for the treatment of malignant disease that brought results of outstanding excellence and carried his fame abroad. He had an infinite capacity for detail and thoroughness. One example of this alone, the records of progress in countless numbers of cases treated, and illustrated with superb color photography, won admiration which was wide and sincere. His originality shone forth in the many special methods and devices he developed for the more efficient application of radium and röntgen rays in cancer treatment. In 1920, following studies in Britain and Germany, he established Canada's first high voltage center for cancer therapy, and every year the number of his patients extended into thousands. Some years ago he was the guest of honor at a dinner where one hundred women, all former cancer patients with no recurrence in periods from five to seventeen years, celebrated most happily. But the price Dr Richards paid for those years of service to others was the sacrifice of a serene old age in rural surroundings of which he had dreamed. In a confidential letter to a friend written in October, 1948 he spoke of the aplastic anemia due to radium from which he suffered, and he intimated that his remaining days on earth would be few. His death, three months later, removed a figure of world renown in the profession of Radiology, and he will be sadly missed by his co-workers in that field. In 1947 Dr Richards was selected to deliver the Skinner Lecture of the Faculty of Radiologists of London, on cancer of the breast. It was the first occasion since the lectureship was inaugurated that any authority on cancer outside Europe was so honored. He was Founder of the Canadian Association of Radiologists, Fellow of the Toronto Academy of Medicine, member of the Ontario and Canadian Medical Associations, member of the American Roentgen Ray Society and of the Radiological Society of North America, and also Councillor of the American College of Radiology. He will be sadly missed by his fellow Radiologists, the profession at large and by a host of patients he has benefited.

1. Singleton AC. Gordon E Richards 1885–1949. Am J Roentgenol 1949; 61: 409.

III *Dr William Alfred Jones: First President of the Canadian Association of Radiologists* 242

1. Jones WA. Familial multilocular disease of the jaws. Am J Cancer 1933; 17: 946.
2. Jones WA. Further observations regarding familial multilocular cystic disease of the jaws. Brit J Radiol 1938; 11: 227.
3. Jones WA, Gerrie J, Pritchard J. Cherubism: a familial fibrous dysplasia of the jaws. J Bone Jt Surg 1950; 32B: 334.
4. Jones WA. Cherubism: a thumbnail sketch of its diagnosis and conservative treatment. Oral Surg Oral Med Oral Path 1965; 20: 648.
5. Taybi H, Lachman RS. Radiology of syndromes, metabolic disorders and skeletal dysplasias. Chicago: Year Book Medical Publishers, 1990, 3rd Ed.

VI *From Szechuan to Saskatchewan: A Profile of HE Johns and the Story of the Development of the "Cobalt Bomb"* 247

Bibliography:

Marko AM, Butler G, Myers DK. Biochemistry at Chalk River. Bull Canadian Biochem Soc 1986; 26: 11.

Johns HE. Comments on the physics of radiology: past and future. Med Phys 1988; 15: 487.

Johns HE, Watson TA. The cobalt-60 story. Cancer in Ontario. Toronto: OCTRF, 1989.

Johns HE. Lectures in the Physics of Radiotherapy by Prof WV Mayneord, delivered in Toronto, August 2–5, 1946 and transcribed by Johns.

Johns HE. The physics of radiology. Springfield, Illinois: Charles C. Thomas, 1953.

Johns HE, Bates LM, Epp ER, et al. 1000-curie units for radiation therapy. Nature 1951; 168: 1035.

Johns HE, Bates LM, Watson TA. 1000-curie cobalt units for radiation therapy. 1 The Saskatchewan cobalt-60 unit. Br J Radiol 1952; 25: 296.

Johns HE, Epp ER, Cormack DV, Fedoruk SO. Depth-dose data and diaphragm design for the Saskatchewan 1000-curie cobalt unit. Br J Radiol; 25: 302.

Green DT, Errington RF. Design of a cobalt-60 beam therapy unit. Br J Radiol 1952; 25: 309.

Dixon WR, Garrett C, Morrison A. Radiation measurements with the Eldorado cobalt-60 teletherapy unit. Br J Radiol 1952; 5: 314.

Mitchell JS. Applications of recent advances in nuclear physics to medicine. Br J Radiol 1946; 19: 481.

Mayneord WV, Cipriani AJ. The absorption of gamma-rays from Co-60. Canad J Res 1947; 25: 303.

Mayneord WV. Some applications of nuclear physics to medicine. Br J Radiol 1950 (Suppl 2): 1.

Smith IH, Fetterly JCM, Lott JS, et al. Cobalt-60 teletherapy. Hoeber Medical Division, New York: Harper and Row, 1966.

Johns HE. Science policy's good side: cobalt. Ottawa: AECL, 1971.

Houston CS, Fedoruk SO. Saskatchewan's role in radiotherapy research. Can Med Assoc J 1985; 132: 854.

Birenbaum R. Saskatchewan scientists make their mark. Ascent 1991; 10: 12.

See also the article by CS Houston and SO Fedoruk elsewhere in this volume.[1]

1. Houston CS, Fedoruk SO. The history of radiation therapy in Saskatchewan. In: JE Aldrich, BC Lentle, editors. A new kind of ray: The radiological sciences in Canada 1895–1995. Montréal: The Canadian Association of Radiologists, 1995.

HE Johns Biographical Highlights

1915 Born July 4 in Chengtu, China.
1920–25 Canadian School of West China (Methodist).
1925 Left China on a one-year furlough. Forced to turn back en route to China, not to return until his retirement in 1980.
1936 BSc mathematics and physics, McMaster University.
1937 MA physics, University of Toronto.
1939 PhD physics, University of Toronto. Awarded an 1851 Exhibition Research Scholarship to study Physics under Dr JD Cockcroft at the Cavendish Laboratory, Cambridge University, UK. Unfortunately, Second World War II intervened.
1939–45 Physicist, University of Alberta, Edmonton. Teacher, Commonwealth Training Scheme. Official radiographer for western Canada.
1940 Married on June 15 to Sybil Hawkins in Toronto.
1942 Cyril (Cy) Garrett, first graduate student.
1943 Daughter Gwyneth Dorothy born July 21.
1945 Physicist, University of Saskatchewan, Saskatoon. Daughter Claire Elizabeth born June 18.
1946 Compiled set of notes of the lecture series given by Dr WV Mayneord at the University of Toronto. Dr JS Mitchell suggests the use of cobalt-60 for radiotherapy.
1947 NRX reactor started on July 22 at Chalk River Nuclear Laboratories.
1948 Betatron installed at Saskatchewan Cancer Clinic.
1949 Arrangements made by Drs WV Mayneord and AJ Cipriani to make the first cobalt-60 sources in NRX. First patient treated on the Betatron.
1950 First female graduate student, Sylvia O Fedoruk.
1951 First three 1000-curie cobalt-60 sources made in NRX. First cobalt-60 machines installed in Saskatoon and London, Ontario and first patients treated on November 8 and October 27, respectively. Elected Fellow of the Royal Society of Canada, Montreal
1952 Daughter Marilyn Anne born August 28.
1953 Publication of The Physics of Radiology. Röentgen Award, British Institute of Radiology, London, UK.
1956 Head of Physics, Ontario Cancer Institute, Toronto.
1958 Established Medical Biophysics Department, University of Toronto.
1959 Concept of tissue–air ratios developed. Honorary Doctor of Law, University of Saskatchewan, Saskatoon.
1960 Sabbatical at Cal Tech, Pasadena California, under Dr M Delbruck. HE Johns/AECL Commercial Products Division production Theratron introduced.
1961 Chairman, Department of Medical Biophysics, University of Toronto.
1962 First Annual Boshkung Conference.
1965 Medal, Canadian Association of Physicists, Vancouver.
1966 Charles Mickle Fellowship, University of Toronto.
1967 Centennial Medal, Confederation of Canada, Ottawa.
1970 Honorary Doctor of Science, McMaster University, Hamilton.
1971 Henry Marshall Tory Award, Royal Society of Canada, Ottawa. Sabbatical at Royal Marsden Cancer Research Unit, Sutton, Surrey England, with Professor JW Boag.
1973 Gairdner Foundation Award, Toronto.
1975 Sylvanus Thompson Medal, Roentgen Society, London, UK. RS Landauer Award, Health Physics Society, San Francisco.
1976 William D Coolidge Award, American Association of Physics in Medicine, Ottawa. Honorary Doctor of Science, Carleton University, Ottawa.
1977 Officer of the Order of Canada, Ottawa. Jules Leger Medal, Ottawa. Made Honorary Fellow of the American College of Radiology.
1978 Honorary Doctor of Science, University of Western Ontario, London, Ontario.
1980 Harold F Batho Memorial Award, American Association of Physicists in Medicine, Minneapolis. Medal of the American Society of Therapeutic Radiologists, Dallas. Retirement after publishing over 220 papers with the help of approximately 68 graduate students. Return trip to the place of his birth in China.
1981 Citation of Recognition, Canadian Biophysical Society, Ottawa. Honorary member of the Ontario Medical Association, Toronto.
1982 RM Taylor Medal, National Cancer Institute of Canada.
1983 Medal of Honor, Canadian Medical Association, Toronto. Radiation Industry Award, American Nuclear Society, San Francisco.
1985 WB Lewis Award, Canadian Nuclear Association, Ottawa.
1994 Honorary Doctor of Science. University Toronto, Toronto.
1994 Over 3000 Cobalt-60 teletherapy units in use world-wide, two-thirds of which have been built in Canada.

VII *Claude James Bodle RT ASXT 1891–1980* **252**

1. Quotation in Focal Spot 1994; 1.

Part 5(b): The Builders

IX *A Lady of Vision: A Transcription of Part of the 28th Mary F Cameron Lecture* **255**

1. Surgeon-General of the Army. The United States Army x-ray manual. New York, Paul B. Hoeber, 1918.
2. Gazdic C. A lady of vision. Filter 1991; 26: 6.

XI *William Howard Dickson MD 1878–1933: Canada's First Physician Specializing in Gastrointestinal Radiology* **261**

1. Ghent P. Dr William Howard Dickson. Univ of Toronto Med J 1933; 11: 46.

XIII *Bede J Harrison MB DMRE* **262**

1. Harrison, BJM. A textbook of roentgenology: The roentgen ray in diagnosis and treatment. Baltimore: William Wood and Co, 1936.
2. Harrison, Mary. Letter to my nieces and nephews: a word about their grandparents. Christmas 1979. CAR Archives.
3. Anon. On the banks of the Murrumbidgee River. The story of the Roche family in Australia. Undated. CAR Archives.

XV *Dr A Stanley Kirkland* **264**

1. Stewart WB. Medicine in New Brunswick. Moncton, NB: The New Brunswick Medical Society, 1974.

The following correspondence[1] between Dr EM Crawford and Dr Kirkland casts further light on the early days of organized radiology in Canada:[2]

The Queen Elizabeth Hospital of Montreal
2100 Marlowe Avenue
Montreal 28

March 27, 1961.

Dr. A. Stanley Kirkland,
Rothesay,
New Brunswick.

Dear Kirk:

I wonder if I can call upon your memory for the following:-

(1) Were you aware of any organization of radiologists previous to the founding of the Canadian Association of Radiologists
in January 1937 when the late Dr. Gordon Richards asked a number of senior radiologists to meet him in Toronto? I understand that there was a Radiological Section of the Canadian Medical Association, and you had an official association with this section. Could you give me data regarding its coming into being, and its existence previous to the year 1937?

(2) Were you aware of any Canadian journals that solely published articles on radiology? In 1949 at Halifax the Journal of the C.A.R. was authorized, and it was another year before it actually came into being.

I wonder if you would be good enough to write or type on the back of this sheet any information that comes to mind on the above questions. Enclosed is a stamped and addressed envelope.

Yours sincerely,
[Signed]
E. M. Crawford, M.D.

EMC/rer

Rothesay, NB
30/3/61

Dear Crawford,

Thank you for your compliment to my memory. However, I have some dates absolutely fixed by dated photos etc.

In 1925 the North American Radiological Society met in Cleveland. The Canadian Radiologists had a special car from Toronto. The following men are to be counted as members of the Radiological Section of the C.M.A. Gordon Richards, Charlie [Clarence] Henry (Regina), Dr. Hess (Hamilton, I think), D. Rolph (Toronto), Dr. McGuffin (Calgary). Dr. Currie MacMillan of Winnipeg, Dr. Pirie, Hamish McIntosh and C.W. Prowd of Vancouver, Dr. Pariseau of Montreal, Dr. Quint of Calgary, I think Jones of Kingston and a wild Irishman with a big family (Mooney).

In 1929 I was chairman of the Section and was the official delegate to the Second International Congress of Radiology in Stockholm. I signed for Canada to accept the roentgen as a unit of measurement. I felt very humble when signing with a great man like Pirie looking over my shoulder.
Dr. Gordon Boult [?] the obs and gynaecologist from the Royal Victoria Hospital was some kind of an honorary member of our group. I believe the rad section of the CMA must have been a going concern from 1921–22 and died giving birth to the C.A.R. I believe it should be re-established.

I do not remember any Journal publishing Canadian articles in Radiology. Most of us published in the CMA Journal.

Hope this is of some help.

[Signed]
Kirk

At a meeting of the CMA in Calgary early in the 30's at the Paliser Hotel—the radiologists ran a "smoke room" in a special suite—liquor the only rations—[we] looked after all the distinguished guests who ranked as good fellows—all at no cost to the C.M.A. Pat Burns the meat packer helped us out quite a bit.

K

1. Archives of the Canadian Association of Radiologists.
2. Houston CS. The Canadian Radiological Society. In: Aldrich JE, Lentle BC, editors. A new kind of ray: The radiological sciences in Canada 1895–1995. Montréal: Canadian Association of Radiologists, 1995.

XVI *Albert J Jutras MD 1900–1981* **264**

1. Feddersen P. The industrial factor: technological innovations which changed radiology. In: Aldrich JE, Lentle BC, editors. A new kind of ray: The radiological sciences in Canada 1895–1995. Montréal: Canadian Association of Radiologists, 1995.

Part 5(c): Teachers

XXV *C Stuart Houston: a Radiologist for All Seasons* **274**

1. Lentle BC. Doubly gifted. In: Aldrich JE, Lentle BC, editors. A new kind of ray: The radiological sciences in Canada 1895–1995. Montréal: The Canadian Association of Radiologists, 1995.
2. Anonymous. The editor's passport. Journal of the Irish Medical Association 1958; 42: 31.
3. Houston CS. Chairman's corner: Supper with the chief. Invest Radiol 1988; 23: 775.

XXVI *Dr Leonard Rosenthall: Canada's Ambassador of Nuclear Medicine* **275**

1. Rosenthall L. The application of radioiodinated rose bengal and colloidal radiogold in the detection of hepatobiliary disease. St Louis: Warren H Green, 1968.
2. Rosenthall L, Lisbona R. Skeletal imaging. Norwalk, Conn: Appleton-Century-Crofts, 1984.

XXVIII *Doubly Gifted* **276**

1. Harrison, BJM. A textbook of roentgenology: The roentgen ray in diagnosis and treatment. Baltimore: William Wood and Co, 1936.
2. Harrison P, Harrison C. Bede J Harrison. In: Aldrich JE, Lentle BC, editors. A new kind of ray: The radiological sciences in Canada 1895–1995. Montréal: The Canadian Association of Radiologists, 1995.
3. Fraser RG, Paré JAP. Diagnosis of diseases of the chest. Philadelphia: WB Saunders Co, 2nd ed, 1979.
4. Margulis AR, Burhenne HJ. Alimentary tract radiology. St Louis: CV Mosby Co, 4th Edition, 1989.
5. Johns HE, Cunningham JR. The physics of radiology. Springfield, Ill: Charles C Thomas, 1983, 4th Edition.
6. Houston CS, Fedoruk S. The history of radiation therapy in Saskatchewan. In: Aldrich JE, Lentle BC, editors. A new kind of ray: The radiological sciences in Canada 1895–1995. Montréal: The Canadian Association of Radiologists, 1995.
7. Greenstock C. From Szechuan to Saskatoon: A profile of HE Johns and the history of the development of the cobalt bomb. Ibid.
8. Harwood-Nash DC, Fitz CR. Neuroradiology in infants and children. St Louis: CV Mosby Co, 1976.
9. Alderson PO, Gilday DL, Wagner HN. Atlas of pediatric nuclear medicine. St Louis: CV Mosby Co, 1978.
10. Lentle BC. Leonard Rosenthall: Canada's ambassador of nuclear medicine. In: JE Aldrich and BC Lentle, editors. A new kind of ray: The radiological sciences in Canada 1895–1995. Montréal: The Canadian Association of Radiologists, 1995.
11. Seeram E. X-ray imaging equipment. Springfield, Ill: Charles C Thomas, 1985.
12. Houston CS. To the arctic by canoe, 1819–1821, the journal and paintings of Robert Hood. Montréal: McGill–Queen's University Press, 1974.
13. Houston CS. Arctic ordeal, the journal of John Richardson, surgeon-naturalist with Franklin, 1820–1822. Montréal: McGill–Queen's University Press, 1984.
14. Houston CS, editor. Arctic artist. The journal and paintings of George Back, midshipman with Franklin, 1819–1822. Montréal: McGill–Queen's University Press, 1994.
15. Houston CS, Street MG. Birds of the Saskatchewan River, Carlton to Cumberland. Regina: Saskatchewan Natural History Society, 1959.
16. Burhenne HJ. Sierra spring ski touring. San Francisco: Mountain Press, 1971.
17. Lapointe J. Naval Officers Association of British Columbia: a record of achievement 1919–1994. Vancouver: Naval Officers Association of BC, 1994.
18. Lentle B. Orest Semchishen: Photographer. In: Aldrich JE, Lentle BC, editors. A new kind of ray: The radiological sciences in Canada 1895–1995. Montréal: The Canadian Association of Radiologists, 1995.
19. Semchishen O. In plain view—Voir Clair. Ottawa: Canadian Museum of Contemporary Photography, 1994.

Part Six: Organizations of those Specialty Groups Working in the Radiological Sciences

I *The Canadian Radiological Society* **284**

1. Anonymous. Tuberculosis prints signs on children: Dr Ferguson gives radiological convention result of survey in Weyburn area. Valley Echo 1925; 6(5): 30.
2. Anonymous. The annual meeting of the Association in Regina in 1925. Can Med Ass J 1924; 14: 1251.
3. Obituary, Dr Clarence Milwood Henry. Can Med Ass J 1954; 70: 701.
4. Obituary, Dr James Victor Connell. Physician dies at 71. Regina Leader-Post, May 4, 1951.
5. Stewart DA. Annual meeting at Regina (Editorial). Can Med Ass J 1925; 15: 842.
6. Association Notes: Annual meeting of the Canadian Medical Association, Victoria, BC, June 21–25, Can Med Ass J 1926; 16: 722.
7. Dickson WH. Duodenal ulcer: The radiological aspect. Can Med Ass J 1927; 16: 1053.
8. McGuffin WH. Goitre from a radiologist's viewpoint. Can Med Ass J 1926; 16: 1182.
9. MacKay H. Radium in dermatology. Can Med Ass J 1926; 16:1352.
10. Association Notes. The fifty-eighth annual meeting of the Canadian Medical Association to be held in Toronto on June 13–18, 1927. Can Med Ass J 1927; 17: 729.
11. Ibid, p 730.
12. Ibid, pp 734–735.
13. Editorial. The Canadian Radiological Society. Can Med Ass J 1927; 17: 830.
    See also the correspondance following: Stewart WB. Dr A Stanley Kirkland. In: Aldrich JE, Lentle BC, editors. A new kind of ray: The radiological sciences in Canada 1895–1995. Montréal: The Canadian Association of Radiologists, 1995.

II *The Canadian Association of Radiologists* **287**

1. Material in the first section of this article is taken from the minutes and other archival material stored in the head office of CAR.
2. Houston CS. The Canadian Radiological Society. In: Aldrich JA, Lentle BC, editors. A new kind of ray: The radiological sciences in Canada 1895–1995. Montréal: The Canadian Association of Radiologists, 1995.
3. MacDermot HE. One hundred years of medicine in Canada (1867–1967). Toronto: McClelland and Stewart Ltd, 1967: 166.
4. Jack D. Rogues, rebels and geniuses. The story of Canadian medicine. Toronto: Doubleday, 1981: 416.
5. CAR Committee on Inter-relations. Minimum acceptable standards for hospital radiologic departments or laboratories. Canadian Hospital 1943 (July); –: 23 and 32.
6. Dufresne O. Roentgentherapy of pain. Can Med Ass J 1949; 227 (and reprinted 1991; 144: 1636–1639).
7. Shephard DAE. The Royal College of Physicians and Surgeons of Canada 1960–1980. Ottawa: The Royal College of Physicians and Surgeons of Canada, 1985: 4.
8. Ibid, p 16.
9. MacDermot HE. One hundred years of medicine in Canada (1867–1967). Toronto: McClelland and Stewart Ltd, 1967: 132.
10. Shephard DAE. The Royal College of Physicians and Surgeons of Canada 1960–1980. Ottawa: The Royal College of Physicians and Surgeons of Canada, 1985: 219.
11. American College of Radiology Newsletter, September 1962:2A.
12. St Louis EL. The Canadian Radiological Foundation. J Canad Assoc Radiol 1993; 44: 421.

ANNEX A: LETTER TO ALL CANADIAN RADIOLOGISTS CONTAINING THE MINUTES OF THE MEETING AT WHICH THE CANADIAN ASSOCIATION OF RADIOLOGISTS WAS CREATED

CANADIAN ASSOCIATION OF RADIOLOGISTS

March 25th, 1937.

Dear Doctor:

The following communication is being addressed to all full-time Radiologists in the Dominion of Canada and deals with the steps and proceedings leading up to the formation of the recently organized Canadian Association of Radiology.

In December of 1936 Dr. G. E. Richards sent invitations to all full-time Radiologists in the Dominion to attend a meeting to be held in the Toronto General Hospital on January 4 & 5, 1937. Because of the distances involved and the rather short notice of the meeting, the majority of the men [sic] present were from the Province of Ontario though there were some men present from Quebec and one from New Brunswick.

Certain matters which concerned Ontario Radiologists only were dealt with but the major portion of the discussion was on matters concerning Radiology in the Dominion and problems of our specialty with regard to such broad problems as fees allowed by the Department of Pensions and National Health, Workmen's Compensation Board fees in the various Provinces and particularly with phases of inter-relationship of Radiologists with Hospitals and with various health insurance organizations.

I feel that the matter will be best explained by including in the present letter a synopsis of transactions of this meeting which now follows:

SYNOPSIS OF THE MINUTES OF THE MEETING OF THE CANADIAN RADIOLOGISTS HELD ON JANUARY 4 AND 5, 1937, AT TORONTO GENERAL HOSPITAL.

Full-Time Radiologists Present:

Dr. E.A. Petrie	Dr. W.C. Kruger
Dr. L.C. Hacking	Dr. W.J. Cryderman
Dr. W.M. Gilmore	Dr. E.H. Shannon
Dr. G. McNeil	Dr. Arnold Morgan
Dr. M.C. Morrison	Dr. C. Liebman
Dr. R.A. Macpherson	Dr. W.H. Borron
Dr. W.L. Harwood	Dr. R.A. Thomas
Dr. A.E. Walkey	Dr. A.R. McGee
Dr. H.M. Tovell	Dr. K.P. Bonner
Dr. W.L. Ritchie	Dr. A.H. Rolph
Dr. O. Dufresne	Dr. P.T. Howell
Dr. G.E. Richards	Dr. R.X. Patterson
Dr. A.C. Singleton	Dr. H.Y. Bell-Milburn
Dr. M.R. Hall	Dr. G.L. Case
Dr. A.D. Irvine	Dr. L.A. Gagnier
Dr. Vera Peters	Dr. H. Perron

January 4th 1937

Dr. M. C. MORRISON, Chairman of the Section of Radiology of the Canadian Medical Association in the Chair.

Dr. Morrison reported that, in reply to a letter sent out by him as Chairman of the Section of Radiology of the Canadian Medical Association, there were a number of letters enthusiastically supporting the proposal for the formation of a new association of Radiologists. Letters were read from Drs. Shepley, Henry, Prowd, McGuffin, Whitelaw and Kirkland.

Dr. W. A. Jones, of Kingston, presented a general review of the steps leading up to the proposal for the formation of the Canadian Association of Radiologists.

A GENERAL REVIEW OF THE STEPS LEADING UP TO THE PROPOSAL FOR THE FORMATION OF A CANADIAN ASSOCIATION OF RADIOLOGISTS.

1.The Canadian Radiological Society.

Demobilized about seven or eight years ago to form the Section on Radiology Of the Canadian Medical Association.

2.The Section of Radiology of the Canadian Medical Association.

(a) Its Advantages.

As members of this Section, we have behind us the backing of the C.M.A., and when the C.M.A. speaks for us, it speaks with the voice of the entire profession and not with the voice of the comparatively few Radiologists of the country.

Our Canadian Medical Association fee covers our sectional activities as well as our general medical association activities.

Notices, etc. are sent out at the expense of the C.M.A.

(b) Its Limitations.

There is no standard of membership in the Section as at present constituted. Any member Of the Canadian Medical Association may attend the meetings of the Section and presumably take part in the business and vote.

The Constitution of the C.M.A. limits the activities of a section to scientific pursuits and other matters which come under the purview of a section and the C.M.A. jointly and severally, but does not permit a section to interest itself in activities beyond the borders of the C.M.A. We are, therefore, obliged as a section to abide entirely by the decisions of the Canadian Medical Association.

The Need for a Canadian Association of Radiologists.

It is still imperative that all Radiologists should be members of the Section on Radiology of the C.M.A. for purposes of joint action with the main body of the C.M.A.

There is also a need for a separate organization that may, as necessity arises, act independently and that may limit its membership to full-time Radiologists or such part-time Radiologists as may be selected.

This Canadian Association of Radiologists, which may be called by this name or some other suitable name, can deal with a number of urgent problems requiring more or less immediate discussion.

SOME PROBLEMS FACING THE PROPOSED CANADIAN ASSOCIATION OF RADIOLOGISTS.

1. The education and qualification of Radiologists and along with this the training and controlling of radiological technicians. (The training and controlling of radiological Technicians, of which more later.)

2. The problem of x-ray fees with regard to the public, the Workmen's Compensation Boards and the Department of Pensions and National Health.

3. Other problems that may arise with regard to our interrelationship with the general public and public bodies and with the rest of the medical profession.

HOW SOME OF THESE PROBLEMS ARE BEING MET AT THE PRESENT TIME

1. Radiological Technicians.

About two years ago there was established the Ontario Society of Radiological Technicians. Charter members were admitted who promised to work only under qualified medical supervision and to not diagnose or treat on their own. A standard of training has been set up and new members will be admitted by examination and after three years' training. A copy of the Bylaws of the organization is available to any Radiologist who will write to Dr. R. H. Bradley, 400 Canada Life Building, Toronto, Ontario.

It is to be hoped that every Radiologist in the Province of Ontario at least will help this organization and will refuse to train technicians on short time courses. Since the organization of technicians, it has been an easy matter to refuse to train those who do not wish to take the full course in as far as my Hospital has been concerned, and we are not training any individual who has not registered as a student technician and is taking the full course. I think we should ask every Radiologist in the Province to stand behind this new Society.

2. Radiologists.

(a) Toronto University has a diploma in Radiology with a course extending over eight months.

(b) Queen's University has recently instituted a course in Radiology extending over a period of three years. One year in the Radiological Department of the Kingston General Hospital and at the Queen's University, instruction covering 1. Radiographic Anatomy. 2. Pathology. 3. Radiobiology. 4. Radiophysics. 5. Radiographic Technique. 6. Diagnostic Radiology. 7. Radiotherapy. 8. General Medicine & Surgery, after which a primary examination is held in the first five subjects. This is followed by two years further training in any Department of Radiology recognized by the University, after which a University examination is held in Diagnostic Radiology, Radiotherapy, General Medicine and Surgery. At the conclusion of the course, the candidate, if successful, is given a Diploma in Medical Radiology (D.M.R).

An arrangement has been made with the University whereby men already doing full-time Radiology may qualify for the Diploma in Medical Radiology without having to put in the year in residence in Kingston, providing that their local centre affords the proper facilities for the carrying out of the necessary experiments, etc. that are required in this course. This was done with the object of stimulating further study in Radiology amongst men already practising the specialty.

3. Most of you are familiar with the requirements of the American Board of Radiology. Details regarding this can be obtained from Dr. B. R. Kirklin of the Department of Radiology of the Mayo Clinic, Rochester, Minnesota.

4. British Association of Radiologists

It may not be a matter of general knowledge that there has been organized a British Association of Radiologists and that the Association has established a Fellowship with a very high standard of training and examinations. A diploma in Radiology is necessary to enable anyone under forty to qualify for the Fellowship. Further particulars regarding this may be obtained from the Secretary, Dr. S. Cochrane Shanks, 68 Harley Street, London, W.I.

5. The Proposed Canadian College of Radiology

At a meeting of the Section on Radiology of the Canadian Medical Association held in Victoria last June, it was decided to proceed with the establishing of the Canadian College of Radiology or, in lieu of this, to try to get the C.M.A. or the Royal College of Physicians and Surgeons in Canada to do something about the matter.

There are certain difficulties that are met with in this connection. For instance it is necessary, in order to obtain a Dominion Charter, for this purpose, to have an Act put through each Provincial Legislative Assembly in Canada, in addition to an Act to be Legislated by the Canadian parliament. The failure to get this through any one province would negative the whole arrangement.

We would likely meet with some degree of opposition from the present recognized bodies in medicine if this were attempted at this time. Some years from now it is possible that something of this nature will be feasible, but just now it would seem best to make haste slowly in this matter.

6. Royal College of Physicians and Surgeons of Canada

The Committee on Specialists of the C.M.A. have persuaded the Royal College of Physicians and Surgeons of Canada to establish Boards for the purpose of overseeing the training, qualification and examination of specialists in Canada. It is likely that the Radiologists will be asked shortly to form a Board for this purpose.

WHAT IS IT POSSIBLE FOR US TO DO TO FURTHER MEET THESE PROBLEMS AND WHAT SHOULD WE GUARD AGAINST?

1. We must establish our own standard of what we consider necessary for the training and examination of Radiologists. Our standard should agree with the standard of the American Board of Radiology and of the British Association of Radiologists.

2. We should encourage graduates to take courses in Radiology at the Universities and we should strive to see that the Universities give courses that will fulfil the requirements of training and examination as outlined by us. The whole field of Radiology should be thoroughly covered in these courses and the accent not placed on any particular branch of Radiology to the detriment of the other branches.

3. All Radiologists should require that their assistants, as they come into the department, should have had their preliminary training for a diploma in Radiology.

4. The question as to how many universities should give courses leading to a diploma in Radiology is debatable. Should it be two or a half-dozen in the Dominion? It would seem best to keep the number down as low as possible. By limiting the number of interns going through according to the law of supply and demand, we can see to it that those men who train with us do not go out into an over-crowded field.

We can also select our men and there is a provision in the announcement of the course for a diploma in Medical Radiology at Queen's, that the course is limited to not more than two students in any one academic session, and that the selection of candidates will rest with a Board appointed by the medical faculty. This means that we will not accept any and every individual who wishes to take up Radiology, and we can pick out men who are likely to make good in the future.

5. We must take care that a man undergoing training is not exploited by the hospitals and, that just because he happens to be required to take three years' training, there is no excuse for treating him as though he were an intern all that time. By keeping the supply within reasonable limits, this matter will adjust itself.

6. The question of whether any of us should allow men to come into our laboratories and look on for a few weeks and then go out and practice Radiology is a point for discussion. In general this plan is obviously unsound and, if we refuse to allow anyone to come into our laboratories except those who are taking the prescribed course in Radiology, or our own members brushing up on certain points, we will be doing a great deal to stop the trend toward mediocre Radiology. On the other hand there is a question as to whether or not in doing so we would be working against the best interests of some sections of the country which cannot support full-time Radiologists. A letter is to hand from Dr. Agnew of the C.M.A. on this point.

7. It would appear that the time is at hand for us to approach the hospitals of the country with an outline of Radiological services. We could offer consulting service in the reading of X-ray films at a flat rate for the smaller hospitals, insisting that such things as gastro-intestinal examinations, barium enemas and other screen examinations, except in cases of emergency, should not be done in the smaller hospitals where a qualified Radiologist is not employed. We could then, as the field opens out and we have new men trained for the job, arrange with the hospitals to have their departments looked after by travelling Radiologists.

8. A letter is to hand from Dr. B.J. Harrison, Radiologist of the Vancouver General Hospital, regarding Radiological organization.

9. Another letter is to hand from Dr. Gilmore of Stratford.

A PLAN FOR THE ORGANIZATION OF RADIOLOGISTS

1. The Section on Radiology of the C.M.A.

The Chairman and Secretary to be elected from the Province where the next meeting of the C.M.A. is to be held.

2. Canadian Association of Radiologists or Canadian Radiological Society, or whatever name may be chosen.

Officers:

President: Elected annually, but usually to hold position for three years.

Vice Pres.: Elected annually from the Province where the next meeting of the C.M.A. is to be held.

Sec.-Treas.: Elected annually, usually to hold position for three years or more.

The President and Secretary-Treasurer, during their terms of office should attend the annual meeting of the Society which should be held when the C.M.A. meets, and the railroad expenses of these two officers should be met out of the funds of the Society. If these two officers attend three meetings in succession, there will be a continuity of interest which will keep the organization alive.

Counsellors: One each from British Columbia, Alberta, Saskatchewan, Manitoba, Maritimes (New Brunswick, Nova Scotia, P.E.I.), Western Ontario, Central Ontario, Eastern Ontario, English-speaking Québec, French-speaking Québec. These counsellors to be nominated and elected by the Radiologists in their district.

The association business meeting to be held annually before the business meeting of the Section on Radiology of the C.M.A.

3. A Committee on education and qualification should be appointed. A Committee on inter-relations to deal with fees and other matters should be appointed.

4. A sheet outlining the Workmen's Compensation Board fees for each province and the Department of National Defense fees is distributed to each member for purposes of discussion.

There was also a good deal of discussion by a number of those present, and it was finally moved by Dr. Richards, that those present approve of the idea of the formation of a Canadian Association of Radiologists. It was also agreed that those present were in favour of the organization of an Examining Board through the Royal College of Physicians and Surgeons of Canada.

Moved by Dr. Morrison, seconded by Dr. Walkey, that the meeting approve of the organization of the Society, but be named later, and at this time appoint a committee to draw up a constitution and bylaws of the new Society for the meeting at Ottawa in June. Carried.

Moved by Dr. Richards, seconded by Dr. Petrie, that Dr. Jones be appointed chairman, and Drs. Singleton and Cryderman members of the committee, with a qualification that it be given the power to add as members, such members as will give a proper representation throughout Canada.

Moved by Dr. Richards, seconded by Dr. Petrie, that Dr. Jones be nominated First President of the Association, and that Drs. Morrison and Patterson be appointed a committee for other nominations.

There was also a great deal of discussion with regard to the Ontario Workmen's Compensation Board Radiological fees, and of the fees recognized by the Department of Pensions and National Health. It was also approved that Dr. Kruger be appointed chairman of a committee with power to appoint representatives for the purpose of interviewing the Ontario Workmen's Compensation Board regarding their proposed revision of Radiological fees.

There was also some discussion regarding the fact that the Workmen's Compensation Board are doing Radiological work and as such are practicing medicine.

There was also some discussion of the relations of the Radiologists to group hospitalization, health insurance, and kindred matters. The question of the formation of the Canadian Association of Radiologists Journal was also discussed. The training of technicians was also under discussion.

The meeting adjourned until the following day.

January 5th, 1937

Dr. Morrison in the Chair.

There was some discussion as to whether the proposed association should be formed at once or delayed until the June meeting. It was finally moved by Dr. McNeil that the whole matter be reconsidered, and that the matter of organization be proceeded with at once. Seconded by Dr. Morrison. Carried.

The committee consisting of Drs.Jones, Morrison and Patterson was requested to retire and bring in a slate of nominations. Suggested by Dr. Jones that Drs. Perron, Shannon and Petrie be added to the committee. The committee then retired.

Dr. Richards assumed the chair in the absence of Dr. Morrison.

Dr. Kruger's committee reported that the Workmen's Compensation Board had stated that it was their wish that they meet representatives right away to talk over the matter of (x)-ray fees. There was considerable discussion regarding the question of Workmen's Compensation Board fees and of (x)-ray fees generally.

The nominations committee having returned, Dr. Shannon reported that the committee had nominated the following officers:

President:	Dr. W.A. Jones,	Kingston.
Vice Pres.:	Dr. J.E. Gendreau,	Montréal.
Secretary:	Dr. A.C. Singleton,	Toronto.
Counsellors:	Dr. C.W. Prowd,	Vancouver.
	Dr. W. Herbert McGuffin,	Calgary
	Dr. C.M. Henry,	Regina.
	Dr. Digby Wheeler,	Winnipeg.
	Dr. W.M. Gilmore,	Stratford. Representing Northern Ontario.
	Dr. Paul Bordeur [sic],	Ottawa. Representing Eastern Ontario.
	Dr. E.H. Shannon,	Toronto. Representing Central Ontario.
	Dr. Lloyd Ritchie,	Montréal. English Speaking.
	Dr. L.A. Gagnier,	Montréal. French Speaking.
	Dr. J.E. Perron,	Québec.
	Dr. S.R. Johnston,	Halifax, N.S.
	Dr. A.S. Kirkland,	Saint John, N.B.
	Dr. G.E. Richards,	Toronto. Elected Chairman of the Interrelations committee with power to appoint his own committee.

Moved by Dr. McNeil, seconded by Dr. Harwood, that the report be received. Carried.

Moved by Dr. Kruger, seconded by Dr. Petrie, that the new association be called the Canadian Association of Radiologists. Carried.

It was agreed that, as a guide to the Committee on Constitution and By-laws that would be formed, the following ideas be approved:

(1) That active members be full-time Radiologists according to the definition by the British Association of Radiologists.

(2) That by selection, certain members doing Radiology as the major part of their work, be approved as associate members.

(3) That in order to strengthen our position with the Canadian Medical Association membership in the Canadian Medical Association be a preliminary requisition [sic] for membership in the new association of radiologists.

(4) That the annual meeting of the association be held just previous to the session of Section on Radiology of the Canadian Medical Association.

(5) That the mid-winter meeting be a fixture of the Canadian Association of Radiologists.

There was also some discussion regarding the standardization of Radiologists, and also regarding the Ontario Society of Radiological Technicians. The question was left over until the June meeting.

Dr. Richards, as Chairman of the Interrelations Committee, was asked to take steps to formulate proposals regarding the relations between hospitals and Radiologists, and regarding relations to State Medicine, Health Insurance and so on.

Dr. Patterson moved a very hearty vote of thanks for the magnificent manner in which Dr. Richards entertained his guests.

The meeting then adjourned.

Following this meeting a great deal of correspondence has taken place between the President and Secretary and various members of the counsel [sic] of the newly formed society. The sending out of this letter has been somewhat delayed as we wished to wait until we could establish the date for our next regular meeting.

During this interval a crisis has arisen in the Province of Ontario with regard to fees allowed by the Workmen's Compensation Board of Ontario for X-ray work. This has involved a great deal of time of the Ontario Radiologists. Briefly, the Board issued a new schedule of rates on February 28th cutting all X-ray fees from 33 1/3 per cent to 50 per cent, the rate to be effective March 1. By immediate action of the Radiologists of Ontario acting through the Ontario Medical Association and assisted to some extent by the Ontario Hospital Association we were able to bring about a reconsideration of this tariff. At the present time we are still working under our old tariff rates pending the establishment of a new Workmen's Compensation Board rate.

This crisis has brought about a unity amongst Ontario Radiologists which probably could not have been accomplished in any other way and certainly indicates the necessity for a united stand amongst the Radiologists of the Dominion to safeguard our interest, to prevent exploitation and to assure proper and ethical consideration of Radiology as a specialty.

The dates for the meeting of the Section on Radiology of the C.M.A. have now been set. These meetings will be held on Wednesday afternoon June 23rd and Thursday morning, June 24th. The meeting of the Canadian Asscciation of Radiologists will be held at 9.30 a.m. on Wednesday morning, June 23rd, in the Chateau Laurier, Ottawa.

At this meeting it is proposed to complete the organization of the Society and to discuss very fully, ways and means of bettering Radiology as a specialty throughout the Dominion. The President of the Society, Dr. W.A. Jones, Kingston, has spent a great deal of time in drawing up the constitution formulating the rules and regulations, and it is hoped that prior to the meeting in Ottawa we will be able to forward to each of you a copy of the proposed rules and regulations for your consideration to act as a basis of discussion for the meeting in Ottawa. May we take the liberty of urging you to make every effort possible to be present at this coming meeting and to enter freely into discussion of all subjects which will be brought up at that time.

Any enquiries or suggestions of subjects for discussion, or communication may be addressed to

Dr. W.A. Jones, President

Dr. A.C. Singleton, Secretary,

Canadian Association of Radiologists.

(A postscript noted that a schedule of the Workmen's Compensation Board fees was attached but this is no longer on file–editor's note.)

ANNEX B: LETTER TO ALL MEMBERS OF CAR FROM DR WA JONES CONCERNING SPECIALTY CERTIFICATION

CANADIAN ASSOCIATION OF RADIOLOGISTS

President	Address Reply To
Dr. W.A. Jones, (Kingston)	
Vice-President	General Hospital,
Dr. J.E. Gendreau, (Montreal)	Kingston,Ont.
Hon. Secretary-Treasurer	
Dr. A.C. Singleton, (Toronto)	April 11, 1939.

Dear Doctor:

I am sending a copy of this letter to all members of the Association, in order that they may think about the matter therein contained so that when the annual meeting arrives in June, each member will be able to express a considered opinion about the matter.

As you know, the Royal College of Physicians and surgeons of Canada has undertaken, at the request of the Canadian Medical Association, the onerous task of overseeing the standardization and qualification of specialists in the Dominion. This question of standardization is one which has been to the front in the last ten years. It has been passed around to all the various voluntary and legal medical organizations in the country, to the faculties of the universities and has gone through all the stages of "passing the buck" until finally, in desperation and in the realization that something had to be done, it was passed to the Royal College of Physicians and Surgeons of Canada, which body has reluctantly accepted the duty of doing something about it.

It can be definitely stated that there was no desire on the part of the Royal College to handle this matter and that it has been taken over by the College simply as a matter of duty and an attempt to do something worthwhile for Canadian medicine.

The proposal is that Boards (such is not necessarily the title) are to be set for each specialty. Where a nationally organized section of specialists exists, that section or association will have the right to nominate the members of the Board for the particular specialty it represents. The nominated members shall not necessarily be Fellows of the Royal College, but could be any member of the particular national association of specialists involved.

This Board would draw up the rules and regulations governing the training, experience and examination of candidates for certificates and would also determine the specialist practitioners considered eligible for registration in the first instance without examination. With relation to radiology, therefore, these matters would be considered, of course, by the Canadian Association of Radiologists.

Due to the fact that the Royal College of Physicians and Surgeons of Canada would undertake to establish these registers of the different specialties and would be responsible in the long run for their proper administration, they would necessarily have to reserve the right to approve the nominations of the individual societies and it is possible that under certain circumstances a nominee might be rejected, in which case another nomination would have to be made by the association. It is extremely unlikely that such a circumstance would arise, but it is a possibility.

There are those amongst us who are sincerely convinced that we should have neither truck nor trade with the Royal College and that we should be sufficient to ourselves alone. They say that we are quite capable of handling our own affairs and that, in fact, we have demonstrated our ability to do so in that we have brought our present Association to fulfilment. I cannot agree, however, because I realize only too well how little power a small organization such as ours, with a maximum membership of possibly one hundred and fifty, can wield in a population of eleven million people with a medical population of nearly eleven thousand in a country where our members are so widely scattered as they are in Canada. In fact, the only power which we do possess is that of being a closely knit organization which can act promptly and, we hope, unanimously in the event of certain difficulties which might arise.

We, I think, cannot hope to exercise much effect upon hospitals and governing bodies by ourselves. I am thinking of the appointment to hospitals or government positions of radiologists properly qualified and registered. It is to be expected, however, that registration brought about by the royal College and supported by the Canadian Medical Association and the French speaking Medical Associations could exercise a very useful influence upon hospitals, governmental and other bodies with which we might have dealings in the future. Because I cannot go into the details of personal knowledge of such matters, for various reasons, I can only state that three times during the past year situations have arisen with regard to radiological appointments which were inimical to the best interests of radiologists, the profession generally and the public and, yet, over which we had no control. If these same situations were to arise, say five years from now, under such conditions as we confidently could anticipate would exist under the aegis of the Royal College and the Boards, they could be satisfactorily dealt with to the benefit of all concerned.

As I see it, we are comparatively powerless in these matters ourselves and can only exert the proper influence in conjunction with other specialties and medical organizations as a whole. There are those who tell us that radiologists should be a distinct division in medicine apart from medicine and surgery and that the profession is built up on a tripod of medicine surgery and radiology. We must not forget, however, that there are other divisions of the profession each one of which thinks that it is the third leg of the tripod, for instance, the gynaecologists and obstetricians. These discussions are, I think, largely academic. From my point of view, I think of a surgeon as one who wields a scalpel and of a medical man as one who diagnoses and treats disease by any other means including the use of needles and such like either for lumbar puncture, venesection or other applications of needles such as treatment with radium. These distinctions however, I think, do not matter much and I believe that the ranks of radiologists will continue to be filled with men who may fancy themselves either as physicians or surgeons, or who may be purists in radiology. After all, medicine is the trunk from which we all take our being, but it so happens that barber-surgeons were grafted on to that trunk and tradition and custom has established them as an entity.

I can see no reason why radiologists cannot carry on as radiologists and still be a part of the general system of medicine. I do not believe that in the proposed set-up there is any possible chance of the Royal College being able to dictate the policy of radiologists. I believe that our rights could be perfectly protected in the matter.

What we will want next June is an expression of opinion as to whether or not our association is willing to cooperate in this matter of standardization and qualification of specialists. If so, we can approve of such cooperation, leaving the final details and the actual approval of details for a later date.

If you are not able to attend the annual Meeting, I would appreciate a letter from you giving your opinion of the matter so that we may have a general idea from all over the country how our members stand in this affair.

Cordially yours,

(signed)
W.A. Jones, M.D., President
Canadian Association of Radiologists

Table:

SELECTED ITEMS FROM THE 1937 SCHEDULE OF RADIOLOGY FEES ($)—CANADA

Mr Alan Crawford of the Bank of Canada advises that $100 in 1937 had the purchasing power of $1182 in 1994; the fee quoted is the global fee: no distinction was made in that era between technical and professional costs.

	PROVINCE								
Part	BC	Alta	Sask	Man	Ont	Que	NB	NS	DPNH*
Skull	10.00–15.00	10.00	10.00	10.00	12.00	12.00	10.00	8.00	7.00
Lower Jaw	10.00–15.00	10.00	10.00	10.00	12.00	12.00	10.00	8.00	7.00
Full dental examination	5.00 plus		6.00	6.00	7.50	4.00			7.00
Shoulder girdle	7.50–11.25	8.00	8.00	10.00	9.00	8.00	7.00	7.50	7.00
Clavicle	7.50–11.25	8.00	6.00	10.00	7.50	8.00	7.00	7.50	7.00
Elbow	5.00–7.50	5.00	6.00	5.00	7.50	8.00	7.00	5.00	4.00
Wrist	5.00–7.50	5.00	5.00	5.00	6.50	8.00	6.00	5.00	4.00
Hand	5.00–7.50	5.00	5.00	5.00	6.50	8.00	6.00	5.00	4.00
Fingers	5.00–7.50	5.00	3.50	5.00	5.00	4.00	6.00	5.00	4.00
Thorax (chest)	10.00–15.00	10.00	9.00	10.00	12.00	12.00	10.00	8.00	8.00
Ribs	10.00–15.00	10.00	6.00	10.00	7.50	8.00	10.00	8.00	8.00
Spine (single region)	10.00–15.00	10.00–12.00	10.00	10.00	15.00	12.00	10.00	8.00	7.00
Pelvis	10.00–15.00	10.00	10.00	10.00	15.00	12.00	10.00	8.00	7.00
Femur	7.50–11.25	8.00	6.00	5.00	7.50	8.00	7.00	5.00	4.00
Tibia	5.00-7.50	5.00	5.00–9.00	5.00	6.50	8.00	7.00	5.00	4.00
Ankle	5.00–7.50	5.00	5.00–9.00	5.00	6.50	8.00	7.00	7.50	4.00
Foot	5.00-7.50	5.00	3.50						
-9.00	5.00	6.50	8.00	6.00	5.00	4.00			
Toes	5.00-7.50	5.00	3.50	5.00	5.00	4.00	6.00	5.00	4.00
Stomach and duodenum (barium)	25.00	25.00		20.00	20.00	24.00	20.00	12.50	15.00
Barium Enema	15.00	10.00			10.00		10.00		7.00
Abdomen KUB	10.00			15.00	10.00	16.00–24.00	15.00	10.00	10.00
Gall Bladder	15.00	15.00			15.00	16.00–24.00	15.00	10.00	10.00

*DPNH = the Department of Pensions and National Health.

III *The Canadian Association of Medical Radiation Technologists: Historical Aspects* **301**

1. Evans WA The science of radiology. Springfield; Chas C Thomas 1933:23.
2. Brown P. American martyrs to science through Roentgen rays. Springfield: Charles C. Thomas, 1936:40.
3. Surgeon-General of the Army. The United States Army x-ray manual. New York: Paul B. Hoeber, 1918.
4. MacEachern MT. Hospital organization and management. Chicago, Physicians' Record Co, 1946:4000.
5. Prince NC. Roentgen technic. St Louis: Mosby, 1918.
6. Clark KC Positioning in radiography. London: Lund Humphries, 1939.
7. Book review. Radiography 1939; 5:46.
8. Pugen E Dominion organization. Ontario Radiographer 1940; II:40.
9. Editorial. Meet your president. Focal Spot 1944; I:9.
10. —— Report of Annual Meeting. Ontario Radiographer 1939; I:32.
11. Editorial. Ontario Radiographer 1943; IV:9.
12. David Sister Mary. Address of the President, Nova Scotia Society of Radiographers. Focal Spot 1944; I:137.
13. Hunt PE Corporation. Focal Spot 1946; III:152.
14. —— Dominion organization. Ontario Radiographer 1941; II:37.
15. Minutes of Meeting, Board of Directors, CSRT. September 1942.
16. —— Report on certain revisions in the rules and regulations of the Board of Examiners, CSRT Focal Spot 1947; IV:940.
17. —— Memorandum of Agreement. CSRT. May 16, 1943.
18. —— Minutes of Annual Meeting. Focal Spot 1944; I:188.
19. —— Minutes of Fourth Annual Meeting, CSRT. Focal Spot 1948; V:34.

In preparing her record the following other sources were used by Sister Crowley:

1. Correspondence with Percy E Hunt, Secretary-Treasurer of CSRT.
2. Correspondence with Dr EA Petrie, who was chairman of the Board of Examiners for CSRT, a former member of the Board of Directors of this society, and a member of the Education Committee on X-ray Technicians of the Canadian Association of Radiologists.
3. Questionnaires sent to the secretary of each provincial society.
4. The official journal of the Canadian Society of Radiological Technicians: The Canadian Journal of Radiography, Radiotherapy and Nucleography, formerly The Focal Spot.
5. The official journals of the American Society of X-ray Technicians and the British Society of Radiographers.

In addition, an earnest effort has been made by the compiler of this history to contact the early members of the society, as well as others who might contribute pertinent information. Any omissions are unintentional. It is hoped that credit and honour have accurately and justly been bestowed.

ANNEX:
BOARDS OF DIRECTORS AND EXAMINERS OF CSRT

Boards of Directors–CSRT

1942–43	Felix G Reason, Chairman
	Mrs Mary F Cameron, Secretary
	Sadie Storm, Treasurer
	Dr W H McGuffin
	Dr W K Colbeck
	Rosemary O'Hagan
1943–44	Dr W H McGuffin
	Dr W K Colbeck
	Dr E L Petrie
	Claude J Bodle, President CSRT
	Mrs Mary Cameron, Vice-President and Secretary-Treasurer CSRT
1944–45	Dr J Perron
	Dr W K Colbeck
	Dr E A Petrie
	Rosemary O'Hagan
	Thomas B Hurst
	Claude J Bodle, President CSRT
	Mrs Mary Cameron, Vice-President and Secretary-Treasurer CSRT
1945–46	Dr J Perron
	Dr W K Colbeck
	Dr E A Petrie
	Rosemary O'Hagan
	Herbert M Welch
	Thomas B Hurst, President CSRT
	Percy E Hunt, Vice-President and Secretary Treasurer CSRT
1946–47	Dr A C Singleton
	Dr Bill H Cheney
	Herbert M Welch
	Henry C J Simkins, President CSRT
	Percy E Hunt, Vice-President and Secretary Treasurer CSRT

Boards of Examiners CSRT

1943–44	Dr M Morrison	London
	Dr W L Ritchie	Montréal
	Dr A D Irvine	Edmonton
	Dr M Morrison, Chair	London
1944–45	Dr W L Ritchie	Montréal
	Dr E A Petrie	Saint John
	Mr T B Hurst	Toronto
	Dr M Morrison, Chair	London
1945–46	Dr B J Harrison	Vancouver
	Mr T B Hurst	Toronto
	Dr E A Petrie, Chair	Saint John
1946–47	Dr A Comtois	Montréal
	Mr T B Hurst	Toronto
	Dr A E Petrie	Sainto John
1947–48	Dr A Comtois	Montréal
	Mr Claude J Bodle	Winnipeg

ANNEX A: SYLLABUS OF TRAINING FOR TECHNICIANS OF CSRT (1948)

1. PHYSICS (Elementary)
   Heat, Light, Electricity, Fundamental Electrical Concepts, Electric Currents and Potentials, Direct and Alternating Currents, Electro-Magnetism and Induction.
2. ELECTRON THEORY AND X-RAY TUBES
   Electron Emission and Acceleration, X-ray Tubes and Valve Tubes (all types), X-rays–Nature and Place in Electromagnetic Spectrum and Properties of, Wave Length, Basic Factors, Voltage, Milliamps, Time, Distance.
3. X-RAY APPARATUS
   Types of Generators, Half Wave, Three Phase etc. Transformers (All types). Rectification, Valve Tube and Mechanical Rectifiers, Meters, Voltmeters, Ammeters, Milliammeters.
4. ELECTRICAL AND RADIATION DANGERS
   Protection, Radiation tolerance, Dose, Radiography, Fluoroscopy, Therapy.
5. ANATOMY AND PHYSIOLOGY
   Development and Morphology of Human Skeleton (Elementary), Different Types of Joints. Upper and Lower Extremities, Spinal Column, Ribs, Pelvis, Surface Markings and Position of Principal Organs.
6. TERMINOLOGY AND NOMENCLATURE
7. RADIOGRAPHIC TECHNIQUE
   Effect of Basic Factors, Density, Contrast, Detail, Distortion etc. Uses of Intensifying Screens, Uses of Cones and Diaphragms. Use of Bucky Diaphragm and Stationary Grid, Effect of Motion, Measurement of Focal Spot of Tube.
8. PRACTICAL RADIOGRAPHY
   Positioning of Patients for Radiography of Various Parts of the Body. Slow and Rapid Techniques, Soft Tissue Work, Voltage and Thickness Technique, Milliamperes and Thickness Technique (with Optimum Voltage), Stereoscopy. Calibration of Machines, Care of Apparatus. Preparation of Technique Chart.
9. PROCESSING PROCEDURES
   Dark Room, Chemistry of Same. Time. Temperature. Care of intensifying screens.

VII *The Canadian Association of Nuclear Medicine and the Society of Nuclear Medicine in Canada* ***332***

1. Brucer, MA. Chronology of nuclear medicine. St Louis, Mo: Heritage Publications; 1990.
2. Lentle BC. Nuclear medicine: the Rutherford legacy. In: Aldrich JE, Lentle BC, editors. A new kind of ray: the radiological sciences in Canada 1895–1995. Montréal: The Canadian Association of Radiologists, 1995.

ANNEX A: *THE ROYAL COLLEGE OF PHYSICIANS AND SURGEONS OF CANADA*

1976 Examination in **NUCLEAR MEDICINE**
Paper no. 1: Monday, September 13, 1976, 9:00 a.m.
SUBJECT: BASIC SCIENCES AS APPLIED TO NUCLEAR MEDICINE
Three Hour Paper. Candidates must answer *ALL FIVE QUESTIONS.*

The first four questions have been sub-divided into ten equal parts (10 marks each; if listed as 2.4 + 2.5–then equal to 20 marks). The value of each part is listed in brackets in the right hand column. The fifth question is an essay question worth 100 marks. Each full question is worth 100 marks. The total value of the paper is 500 marks.

Please be brief, answering where possible with one word or a short sentence. If not, use diagrams and outlines where possible.

You will receive an envelope containing four books. Answer questions 1 to 4 in sequence in one or more of the books (indicating the numbers of the questions on the front cover) and *ANSWER QUESTION 5* in a book by itself.

1. *RADIOPHARMACY* — Marks

1.1.(a)In the majority of commercial "kits" which chemical agent is used to obtain the reduction of pertechnetate to a preferential level?
(b)Which oxidation level is probably necessary for "complexing" to carrier molecules? (10)
(c)Which oxidation state is ^{99m}Tc pertechnetate ion in?
1.2(a)What is the HVL of lead for ^{99m}Tc?
(b) What approximate attenuation factor is obtained shielding ^{99m}Tc with 4 mm.of lead? (10)
(c) To which chemical functional group does reduced 99mTc probably complex to in the commonly used renal and bone scanning agents?
1.3 Quality control of a rapid nature is essential for pre-injection analysis of radiopharmaceuticals.
(a) List the method(s) utilized to determine the ratio of free pertechnetate and bound ^{99m}Tc in a Tc phosphate bone scanning kit.
(b) List the methods for testing for the presence or absence of pyrogens (official and non-official). (10)
(c) What method(s) can be employed to remove unwanted free pertechnetate from a radiopharmaceutical kit?
(d)Many sulfur colloid kits contain a small amount of perrhenate. What is the reason for the addition of this chemical?
1.4 (a) What is a radiochemical impurity?
(b) What is a radionuclidic impurity?
(c) What is meant by the term "alumina breakthrough"? (10)
(d) List at least two impurities found in fission Mo.
(e) List at least two impurities found in n,gamma ^{99}Mo.
1.5 (a) Many radiopharmaceuticals are prepared under vacuum or sterile nitrogen. If this atmosphere is not maintained what would happen to the radio-pharmaceutical? (10)
(b) According to the current literature which of the condensed phosphates has the most rapid plasma clearance?
1.6 ^{99m}Tc DTPA has been proposed and utilized for renal

function imaging and for measurement of glomerular filtration rates. When used (10)
(a) How does it compare with inulin clearance?
(b) What corrections may have to be incorporated and why?
1.7 Other than radioiodinated rose-bengal there have been a number of new radiopharmaceuticals proposed for biliary system imaging. Name two such radiopharmaceuticals and discuss briefly the accumulation pattern, excretion and limitations of one of these agents. (10)
1.8 Various radiolabelled-bleomycins have been proposed for tumour imaging. What natural characteristics of bleomycin does the labelling technique depend on? (10)
1.9 Describe at least two methods for the localization of abscesses. (10)
1.10(a)After the injection of InC13, a characteristic in vivo distribution is noticed. What is the mechanism and final fate of this radio-pharmaceutical? (10)
(b) List the physical characteristics of ^{111}In, ^{67}Ga, ^{3}H, ^{14}C.

2. *PHYSICS*
2.1 A patient is injected with 15 mCi of ^{99m}Tc for a brain scan. Assuming that 10% of the injected dose goes to the head, how many 140 Kev gamma ray photons/second will originate from the head? (10)
2.2 Assuming only physical decay, what will be the photon flux 24 hours later? (10)
2.3 Describe briefly the structure and functioning of the following components on an imaging system.
(a) Photomultiplier tube
(b) Sodium iodide crystal detector (10)
(c) Pulse height analyser.
2.4+2.5 One milllcurie of ^{32}P is administered to a 70kg. patient. Phosphorus has a biological half life of 257 days and ^{32}P has a physical half life of 14.3 days.
(a) What is the effective half life in this case?
^{32}P has an average beta energy of 0.7 Mev and
1 rad = 6.24 x 10^7Mev (20)
(b) What is the absorbed radiation dose to the patient? (The final equation will suffice–do not complete the arithmetic.)
2.6 Describe briefly the following physical process.
(a) positron emission
(b) beta (-) decay (10)
(c) internal conversion
(d) electron capture.
2.7 Describe how you would simply measure
(a) the amounts of H and C in a biological fluid sample. (10)
(b) the fraction of administered 131 I in a patient's thyroid.
2.8 Describe briefly the various mechanisms of photon interaction with matter. (10)
2.9+2.10 Describe the basic principles of a ^{99}Mo-^{99m}Tc radionuclide generator. Include in your discussion the decay scheme of ^{99m}Tc and the essential relationships between parent and daughter radionuclide. Show graphically the ^{99}Mo and the ^{99m}Tc activity in the generator over a 5 day period assuming that the ^{99}Tc is eluted once per day. (20)

3. *RADIOBIOLOGY PROTECTION AND STATISTICS*
3.1(a) List four methods of disposal allowed under an AECB licence.
(b) List the quantities of radioactive materials that can be disposed of by each method. (10)
(c) At autopsy what precautions should be taken with a cadaver containing radionuclides?
3.2 What are the maximal permissable radiation doses per year for
(a) Technologist working in nuclear medicine laboratory:
(i) Whole body.
(ii) Bone marrow.
(iii) Hands and feet.
(iv) Gonads.
(b) Secretary in the office of a nuclear medicine laboratory. (10)
(c) Casual visitor to the hospital.
(d) What may the cumulative whole body dose be for a radiation worker?
3.3 (a) List and briefly explain the three principal methods by which one may keep the external radiation exposure to a minimum when handling gamma-emitting radionuclides.
(b) How may one reduce the external radiation exposure of beta emitters to a minimum. (10)
(c) Which are better shields, high or low atomic numbers for beta and gamma emitters? Explain.
3.4 What is meant by:
(a) r, (b) rad, (c) LET, (d) RBE, and (e) Rem. (10)
3.5 t 3.6 Discuss the biological effects of radiation utilizing these headings:
(a) List and briefly describe two physical theories. (20)
(b) The genetic effects, including the chromosomal changes and changes at the various stages of cell division (mitosis).
3.7 List the properties of the ideal gamma-emitting isotope which will produce a good image with the gamma camera and at the same time keep the patient dose to a minimum. (10)
3.8 List five mechanisms of localization of radiopharmaceuticals in clinical organ imaging and one example of each. (10)
3.9 and 3.10 (a) Calculate the following:
The total number of counts which must be collected so that the standard deviation in the number is:
(i) one per cent.
(ii) five per cent.
(b) The following sequential background count rates (c.p.m.) were measured for a scintillation probe:
16, 22, 20, 23, 21, 13, 20, 29, 18, 22, 16
(i) what is the mean count rate, and
(ii) the standard deviation of the count rate. (20)

4. *INSTRUMENTATION*
4.1 (a) What may be the effects on a scan of an instrument which is improperly calibrated? (10)
(b) List procedures which should be regularly carried out to ensure proper operation of (a) a gamma camera, and (b) a rectilinear scanner.
4.2 Explain: (a) resolving time
(b) dead time (10)
(c) recovery time.

4.3 Why is the count rate from a source being counted in a well counter not equal to the disintegrations per minute? (10)

4.4 (a) How does volume of a sample in a well counter affect counter efficiency? (10)

(b) How is the optimum counting volume determined?

4.5 What is the purpose of each of the following components of a gamma camera:

(a) Dynodes

(b) pre-amplifier (10)

(c) photo-cathode

(d) x,y,z circuitry

4.6 (a) What is the purpose of collimation? (10)

(b) How does collimation affect spatial resolution and sensitivity?

4.7 What are the design parameters of a conventional focussed collimator? (10)

4.8 What considerations should be taken into account when choosing a collimator for imaging procedures?

4.9 (a) What are the components of a typical liquid scintillation "cocktail"?

(b) State the purpose of each to the liquid scintillation procedure?

4.10 What is the arrangement of photomultiplier tubes in liquid scintillation counting? Why is this arrangement used? (10)

5. *RADIOIMMUNO-ASSAY*

(Answer this question in a book by itself.)

5. Assuming the availability of a pure substance, list in outline form the basic principles of radioimmunoassay. The following headings may be useful: (100)

(a) Labelling of antigen with radioiodine. (b) Production of antibody. (c) Choosing the method of separation of bound and free ligand. (d) Assessing specificity. (e) Assessing accuracy and reproducability.

Tuesday, September 14, 1976 9:00 a.m.

SUBJECT: THE CLINICAL PRACTICE OF NUCLEAR MEDICINE

Three Hour Paper. Candidates *MUST ANSWER ALL FIVE QUESTIONS.*

The first four questions have been sub-divided into ten equal parts (10 marks each; if listed as 4.9 and 4.10, then equal to 20 marks). The value is listed in brackets in the right hand column. The fifth question is divided into two parts. (50 marks each). Each full question is worth 100 marks. The total value of the paper is 500 marks.

Please be brief, answering where possible with one word or a short sentence. If not, use diagrams and outlines where possible.

You will receive an envelope containing four books. Answer questions 1 to 4 in sequence in one or more of the books (indicating the numbers of the questions on the front cover) and *ANSWER QUESTION 5* in a book by itself.

1. *CENTRAL NERVOUS SYSTEM* Marks

1.1 List five causes for the "crescent" sign as seen on a brain scintiscan. (10)

1.2 Describe and/or roughly illustrate the normal anatomy of a brain scan utilizing pertechnetate. (10)

1.3 List the scintigraphic features of a cerebral infarct paying attentionto flow, early (blood pool) and delayed studies. Include discussion of (10)
timing of studies in relation to clinical onset of symptoms. Can any prognostic significance be derived from these features?

1.4 What may the cerebral blood flow study look like in:

(a) Superior vena caval obstruction.

(b) AV malformation. (10)

(c) Subdural haematoma.

(d) Cerebral death.

1.5 Given a delayed scintiscan of the head, what features would differentiate a scan utilizing Pertechnetate from one done with:

(a) Technetium–99m diphosphonate (10)

(b) Technetium–99m DTPA

(c) In-113 DTPA

1.6 In brain scanning, what is the dose, the purpose, and physiological activity of using

(a) Perchlorate (10)

(b) Atropine

1.7 List five conditions which may produce a doughnut sign on a brain scan. (10)

1.8 What do we find on a single or repeat scintiscan of the brain in:

(a) Multiple Sclerosis (b) Encephalitis (c) Cerebral metastases (d) Abscess (e) Asphyxia.

1.9 Given the fact that the normal brain scan is a "non-brain" scan (no cerebral activity):

(a) List the pathophysiological factors which produce an abnormal scan.

(b) What effects does the recent intracarotid administration of contrast material have? (10)

(c) Approximately what is the accuracy (percentage) of the brain scintiscan in detecting brain tumours?

1.10 (a) What radiopharmaceuticals are presently used in cerebro spinal fluid scanning?

(b) List the normal pathway for the radiopharmaceutical, when injected into lumbar subarachnoid space and detail time intervals. (10)

(c) List the conditions in which CSF scanning is useful both in adults and children.

(d) List the pathway and time sequence of one of these which is found in a patient with dementia, incontinence and ataxia.

2. *LUNG, CARDIOVASCULAR AND FACIAL STRUCTURES*

2.1 (a) What is the ideal size of the albumin particles used in perfusion scanning of the lung?

(b) Approximately how many are usually injected?

(c) What is the minimal number of albumin particles that would produce an adequate study? (10)

2.1 (d) Why is there no perceptible change in lung function following a perfusion scan?

(e) What is the biological half life of the albumin particles in the lungs?

2.2 (a) List in outline form the radiopharmaceutical used,

the dose given and scan procedure of doing a perfusion lung scan.
(b) Given a patient with sudden onset of cough and chest pain, what other (10)
parameters do you use to evaluate a perfusion defect or defects on the scintiscan.
(c) Under what circumstances may one see a liver image when performing a lung scan? List at least two possibilities.
2.3 (a) What is the most frequently used radionuclide for ventilation scanning?
List its physical characteristics.
(b) Briefly list the changes in each portion of the ventilation scanning sequence–in evaluating chronic obstructive pulmonary disease. (10)
(c) Given a perfusion defect, will there usually be a ventilation defect with it?
(d) Given a patient with a ventilation defect, will there usually be an associated perfusion defect?
(e) 11 the answer to (c) and/or (d) are yes, explain why.
2.4 (a) Under what circumstances does one see the radiopharmaceutical for ventilation scanning accumulate in the right upper quadrant of the abdomen? (10)
(b) During the performance of a liver scan one may occasionally see accumulation radionuclide within the lung. List the possible explanations for this phenomenon.
2.5 Given a good history and normal chest radiograph, what are the statistical chances (percentages) of patients having a pulmonary embolus within the previous 48 hours?
(a) Normal perfusion scan. (b) Subsegmental defect.
(c) Segmental defect. (10)
(d) Lobar defect.
(e) Lobar defect and normal ventilation scan.
2.6 (a) What are the currently most useful radiopharmaceuticals for imaging myocardial infarcts?
(b) How soon may the scintiscan be positive in acute myocardial infraction? (10)
(c) How long may it remain positive?
2.7 (a) What radioisotope methods are used to measure
(i) left ventricular volume
(ii) ejection fraction (10)
(iii) regional wall motion.
(b) How can one confirm, utilizing scanning methods, a suspected left ventricular aneurysm?
2.8 List and briefly discuss how one detects venous thrombosis by isotopic methods. (10)
2.9 Briefly discuss the methodology, dose, radiopharmaceutical and anatomy of tear duct scanning, indicating the clinical value. (10)
2.10 (a) Briefly discuss salivary gland scanning indicating the radiopharmaceutical used, the method of assessing the glands. (10)
(b) Are the neoplasms of the salivary glands detected as hot or cold on scintiscans?

3. *LIVER, BONE AND KIDNEY*
3.1 (a) List the radiopharmaceuticals currently used in liver scanning.
(b) How do these localize in the liver and what information can one derive from these?
(c) Is there a place for flow studies? (10)
(d) Can one utilize specific radiopharmaceuticals which will help evaluate mass lesion or lesions found on routine scanning?
3.2 (a) Describe the normal superior, anterior, posterior and lateral impressions on the liver — how may these extrinsic impressions affect the liver in case of disease processes? (10)
(b) What does a liver scan look like following radiation therapy when one port is directly over the liver?
3.3 (a) List the changes seen on a liver.scan in hepato-cellular disease.
(b) On occasion one sees a hot spot on a liver scan. Usually it is in the area at the junction of the right and left lobes or in the caudate lobe. List three causes for this occurrence. (10)
(c) What procedures can one use to evaluate the subdiaphragmatic space?
3.4 Radionuclide scan of the scrotal sac in a patient with acute pain and severe tenderness of the testicle may show:
(a) Increased flow and increased uptake on the scrotal scan; or
(b) Decreased flow and subsequent diminished activity within a portion of the scrotal sac. (10)
What conditions may these instances represent and how may the radionuclide study help in the management of these patients?
3.5 (a) List the current radiopharmaceuticals most frequently used in bone scanning.
(b) Describe and/or illustrate a normal bone scan utilizing one of these radiopharmaceuticals in an adult. (10)
(c) Recent reports have shown diffuse uptake of bone-seeking radionuclides in the lungs. What clinical conditions may cause this appearance?
3.6 (a) List five conditions without evidence of calcification in which there are extra osseous accumulations of the current bone scanning agents. (10)
(b) Discuss briefly the imaging of arthritis and how different radiopharmaceuticals can help in the evaluation of this process.
3.7 (a) The bone scan of the jaws shows increased uptake in which of the following:
(i) Peridontal disease.
(ii) Uncomplicated impacted teeth. (10)
(iii) Uncomplicated dental cyst.
(iv) Periapical infection.
(b) In chronic gum chewers or in patients with malocclusion, what part of the facial bone scan shows increased uptake?
3.8 (a) The bone scan shows increased uptake in which of the following:
(i) Osteoporosis circumscripta
(ii) Suedek's atrophy
(iii) Osteomalacia
(iv) Chronic renal failure (10)
(v) Renal transplant.
(b) Briefly list the normal localizatlon of the radiopharmaceutical in a bone marrow scan.

3.9 (a) Gallium-67 citrate. List its normal distribution, excretion and biological half life- (10)
(b) List the main uses of this radiopharmaceutical in clinical scanning.
3.10 Very briefly describe the current in-vivo method of investigation of the kedney. (10)

4. *IN-VIVO NON~IMAGING*
4.1 (a) In outline form describe the rationale of the classical Schilling test.
(b) What conditions can cause abnormal findings? (10)
(c) Name and briefly describe the in-vitro test that has replaced the first stage of this test in many laboratories.
4.2 If one finds 5% of the administered dose in a 24 hour urine sample during the performance of a Schilling test:
(a) List the possible causes of this. (10)
(b) Would a second 24 hour urine sample be useful?
4.3 Following intravenous injection of 59Fe citrate:
(a) Draw a graph of the normal curve for incorporation of this radiopharmaceutical into red blood cells. (10)
(b) Contrast this with the curve for incorporation into red blood cells in a patient with hemolytic anemia, polycythemia vera, and aplastic anemia.
4.4 (a) Describe in outline form the labelling of red blood cells with Na25 CrO_4. (10)
(b) Is ascorbic acid added during the labelling of red blood cells with Na25 CrO_4. If it is , then for what reason.
(c) Under what conditions may one observe labelling of red blood cells following injection of 99m$Tc0_4$?
4.5 (a) Outline a method for testing red cell survival.
(b) Describe the method measuring splenic and hepatic Cr activity. (10)
(c) What is a significant spleen:liver ratio which gives a good prognosis for a response to splenectomy?
4.6 (a) Radioactive tracers used to measure blood volume must meet certain criteria. List at least five.
(b) Give a formula for blood volume measurement. (10)
(c) Why is the use of a single labelled tracer not considered absolutely accurate?
4.7 When studying gastrointestinal protein loss:
(a) Briefly list the relative merits of radioiodinated serum proteins versus 51Cr-labelled serum proteins.
(b) Which is more widely used? (10)
(c) Outline the procedure.
(d) How much of the injected dose will be excreted in a normal person?
4.8 List and discuss briefly the newer methods of studying gastrointestinal dysfunction utilizing 14C as a label, resulting in the production of 14CO_2 .
4.9 and 4.10 (a) List four radiopharmaceuticals used in therapy and indicate the conditions that are treated.
(b) Discuss the advantages and adverse sequelae that may ensue with each.
(c) In the case of bone malignancy, has there been any recent promising development in radionuclide therapy (unsealed sources)? Briefly discuss.

5. *THYROID*
5.1 Discuss thyroid carcinoma under the following headings, listing wherever possible: (100)
(a) classification and spread.
(b) importance, if any, of previous radiation.
(c) the use of radionuclide imaging in the differential diagnosis.
(d) the use of other imaging procedures.
(e) indications for, and use of ^{131}I for treatment and follow-up.
5.2 (a) Draw a diagram of the hormonal control of thyroid function.
(b) List the advantages and disadvantages of imaging of the thyroid gland with:
i) Na ^{123}I ii) Na ^{131}I iii) Na $^{99m}TcO_4$
(c) List and indicate briefly the clinical importance of the various in vitro tests available when evaluating thyroid function.

ANNEX B:
MINUTES OF THE AD-HOC COMMITTEE ON CANADIAN MEMBERSHIP OF THE SOCIETY OF NUCLEAR MEDICINE

Thursday, May 30, 1985 8:00 p.m.
Benbrook Room, Four Seasons Hotel, Houston, Texas

Present:

	Chapter
Dr. A. Driedger (Chairman)	Eastern Great Lakes
Dr. P. Cohen	Pacific Northwest
Dr. D. Greeberg	Prairie Provinces
Dr. R. Hooper	Prairie Provinces
Dr. E. LeBel	Eastern Canada
Dr. D. Lyster	Pacific Northwest
Dr. W. Spiers	Eastern Great Lakes

Dr. Driedger opened the meeting with a review of the precirculated material (attached), and summarized his concerns regarding Canadian participation within the Society of Nuclear Medicine (SNM). He and others agreed that the SNM serves both as an international scientific and educational nuclear medicine society, and as an American professional society with several domestic concerns. This presents Canadian members and chapters with certain difficulties, notably:
– Canadian chapter officers are involved in various society structures (e.g., Chapter Presidents Committee, Board of Trustees) which handle, predominantly, American domestic issues. Such involvement is difficult for the multinational chapters (EGL and PNW) where a Canadian may represent American members of his or her chapter, and may be inappropriate for the all- Canadian chapters (PP and EC).
– The SNM is certainly the foremost international scientific and educational nuclear medicine society, and as such most Canadians involved in the discipline are members of it. The SNM is the only nuclear medicine society in Canada with multidisciplinary representation (i.e., physicians, physicists, radiopharmacists), and in fact nuclear medicine community has no other organization with comparable representation to deal

with its own domestic issues. Canadian SNM members therefore find themselves supporting American domestic issues while neglecting their own.

There was considerable discussion of the need for a multidisciplinary structure to respond to domestic Canadian affairs. Dr. Driedger cited recent examples where such a body would have been useful.

There was some discussion of the multidisciplinary (conjoint) nuclear medicine meeting proposed by the Canadian Association of Nuclear Medicine.

The possibility of chapter realignment was considered. Representatives from the two multinational chapters felt that, for scientific, educational and social functions, they would like to continue meeting with their American neighbours. They did feel that they should meet with other Canadian representatives to discuss domestic issues.

The relationship of Canadian technologists to individual chapters, the Society, and the Technologist Section was briefly discussed. It was generally felt that Canadian technologists saw little benefit in joining the SNM Technologist Section.

In light of these discussions, the following suggestions were made:

1.That a new structure, superimposed on the chapter structure, be created within the SNM to handle Canadian domestic affairs. This structure could take many forms;

–a council of Canadian chapter representatives,

–a Canadian socioeconomic committee.

–separate incorporation of a Canadian region (similar to the existing Western region).

2.That all chapters in Canada have representation on the structure noted above, and that one Canadian representative from this structure be sent as a voting member to the SNM Board of Trustees meetings. Multinational chapters would send an American representative to the Board of Trustees meetings, while all Canadian chapters would forfeit their Board positions.

3.That funding through the existing SNM dues structure be negotiated with society representatives for this new structure.

The question arose whether Canadian members would have adequate representation with only one member on the Board. It was noted that Canadians are now over represented (by percentage of membership) on the Board, and that the suggested changes would lead to a fairer representation by population. It was also noted that most of the scientific and educational functions of the society are carried out at the committee rather than board level. Canadians would still be free to serve on most society committees.

It was decided that Dr. Driedger would rework the suggestions listed above and, in consultation with other members of the committee, enter into discussions regarding their implementation with Society representatives.

The meeting adjourned at 9:50 p.m.

R.H.

ANNEX C: MEMORANDUM TO MEMBERS OF THE SOCIETY OF NUCLEAR MEDICINE AD-HOC COMMITTEE ON CANADIAN MEMBERSHIP

Dear Member:

Only a few of you were able to attend the mid winter meeting of the SNM.

The purpose of this memorandum is to advise those who are not able to attend that the Board of Trustees adopted the following motion:

"Resolved that the Board of trustees approve in principle the formation of the Society of Nuclear Medicine in Canada and that the matter be referred to the ad-hoc Committee on Canadian membership which will develop appropriate changes in the by-laws of the Society of Nuclear Medicine."

In the subsequent discussion the motion was modified to include simultaneous referral to the Finance Committee which will examine the financial impact.

The vote was unanimous in support of the motion.

I think it would be appropriate that each of the Canadian Chapters should select its delegates to the Executive Committee on the assumption that there will be a meeting of the Executive Committee in June. While the ad-hoc Committee will be responsible to deal with the By-Laws and Finance Committee of the SNM, it is probably reasonable to begin formation of what should turn into the Executive Committee and to define appropriate agenda items to be brought before it. Therefore, Chapters that will have their annual meeting prior to June ought perhaps to consider the selection of their representatives in accordance with the proposed by-laws. Until the Committee has met and selected its officers I am willing to act as the ad-hoc lighting rod. Please send me any material that your Chapter would like to see on the agenda.

Sincerely Yours,

A.A. Driedger, M.D., F.R.C.P.
Chairman and Ad-hoc Committee on
Canadian Membership SNM

IX *The Journal of the Canadian Association of Radiologists* **337**

1. Lipinski JK. Some observations on early diagnostic radiology in Canada. Canad Med Ass J 1983; 129: 766 (and reprinted here).
2. Grigg ERN. The trail of the invisible light. Springfield, Ill: Charles C Thomas, 1965: 266.
3. Saucier J. Un Med Canada 1936; 65: 1039.
4. MacDermot HE. One hundred years of medicine in Canada (1867–1967). Toronto: McClelland and Stewart, 1967: 161.
5. Ibid: 166.
6. Lentle BC. Canadian Association of Radiologists, Annex A. In: Aldrich JE, Lentle BC, editors. A new kind of ray: The radiological sciences in Canada 1895–1995. Montréal: Canadian Association of Radiologists, 1995.
7. Frontispiece. J Can Assoc Radiol 1950; 1: ii.
8. Editorial. Untitled. J Can Assoc Radiol 1950; 1: 58.
9. Notice. New funds available for radiological research. Can Assoc Radiol J 1950; 1: 37.
10. Sowby FD. The regulation of shoe fitting fluoroscopes. Can Assoc Radiol J 1956; 7: 18.
11. Aubé L. Fabrication d'un appareil à insufflation péritonéale pour pneumopelvigraphie. J Can Assoc Radiol 1965; 16: 234.
12. Belisle LP. The appendix: a study comparing radiological diagnosis with operative, anatomical and pathological findings and subsequent clinical results. Can Assoc Radiol J 1951; 2: 16 (et en français: L'Union Medicale du Canada 1949; 78: 1045).
13. Johns HE. Physical characteristics of the radiation in cobalt-60 beam therapy. 1952; 3:2 et seq, and Watson TA. Co-60 telecurie therapy–after five years. Canad Radiol Assoc J 1957; 8: 22 et seq.
14. Taylor KW, Patt NL, Johns HE. Variations in x-ray exposures to patients. Canad Radiol Assoc J 1979; 30: 6.

X *History of Radiation Oncologists in the Royal College of Physicians and Surgeons* **341**

1. Lougheed MN. Therapeutic radiologists. Canad Med Assoc J 1968; 98: 464.

ANNEX A: PROPOSAL TO CHANGE THE NAME OF THE SPECIALTY FROM THERAPEUTIC RADIOLOGY TO RADIATION ONCOLOGY

The word "Oncology", meaning the "study of tumours" was used by Mayne in 1897. In recent years there has been a proliferation of its use on a universal basis to identify the field of endeavour and to unify the efforts of clinical and allied professionals in the field.

The term Radiation Oncology is suggested to qualify a specific component of the clinical contribution. It is not the intent to usurp the term Oncology for a given discipline on the one hand, nor is it the intent to reject historical associations, on the other.

It is appreciated that the new term has a focus which is disease oriented, but this should not prove to be a serious objection to its adoption since accepted classifications of specialties follow no uniform pattern. Thus, some specialties are age oriented (Paediatrics), sex oriented (Obstetrics and Gynaecology), systems oriented (Cardiology) and some largely technique oriented (Pathology and Radiology).

Therapeutic Radiology is a descriptive term pertaining to the specific use of "Ionising Radiation" in the "Radiological Sciences." The evolution of "radiological sciences" has progressed such that this term inappropriately describes modern practice in both diagnosis and therapy. (The diagnostic radiologist may use ultrasonics in diagnostic imaging, while the therapeutic radiologist may use chemotherapy and other agents in treatment.)

Basic deficiencies of the term Therapeutic Radiology are:
1. The predominant use, namely the treatment of cancer patients, is not apparent. The primary associates of therapeutic radiologists are clinical colleagues in surgery, gynaecology and internal medicine involved in the multidisciplinary delivery of medical care to cancer patients.
2. The clinical potential of this specialty is not sufficiently widely recognized. Even today, in many of our universities there is a tendency inherent in the name, to regard the specialty as technically or laboratory oriented. This lack of appreciation of what is essentially clinical pharmacology has led to inadequate sharing of undergraduate curriculum time which has adverse effects on education and manpower recruitment.

The potential advantages of the term radiation oncologist are:
1. Radiation oncology indicates the clinical nature of the specialty and the term suggests that other disciplines are involved in the care of cancer patients. It may thereby promote greater effort in formulating interdisciplinary approaches to the management of these patients.
2. The clinical implications of the term radiation oncology may lead to a greater interest in this field by clinically oriented, well-qualified students, thus enhancing both education, undergraduate and postgraduate, and recruitment into the specialty.
3. The term radiation oncology will align Canadian terminology with that of other international bodies.
4. The Royal College of Radiologists, UK (June 1975), conducts an examination in "Radiotherapy and Oncology."
5. Conforms to the designation "Department of Radiation Oncology" in current use in major university centres in the USA.

Royal College of Physicians and Surgeons of Canada

February 5th, 1976

Dr. George B. Goodman
Chairman,
Royal College Committee in Therapeutic Radiology,
Cancer Control Agency of British Columbia
2656 Heather Street
Vancouver, BC
V5Z 3J3

Dear Dr. Goodman:

At a recent meeting the Council of the Royal College of Physicians and Surgeons of Canada considered the proposal that you submitted to the College that the name of the Royal College qualification in Therapeutic Radiology be changed to "Radiation

Oncology". This submission was the one that accompanied your letter of November 28, 1975 addressed to Dr. J.B. Firstbrook, Director of our Division of Training and Evaluation, and had been given preliminary consideration at a meeting of the Executive Committee of our Council. From the statements in your letter to Dr. Firstbrook it is our understanding that the proposal for the change in name has the support of the Council of the Canadian Association of Radiologists and your specialty Committee in Therapeutic Radiology.

The Council of the College agreed that the name of the specialty can be changed to "Radiation Oncology." I expect that this change can be implemented almost immediately and on the appointment of the advisory committee in this specialty for the two-year term 1976 to 78 the committee will be known as the "Committee in Radiation Oncology." It is likely that there will be a few candidates at the springtime oral and clinical examinations and it has seemed to us that probably that examination could be conducted as the last certifying examination in therapeutic radiology with the new terminology being utilized for the examinations in the autumn of 1976. It would be my view that for a year or so we should regularly use the older designation in brackets following the use of the new name in various College documents in order to minimize any confusion or misunderstanding.

One of the important matters that must be settled promptly is the appropriate French version for the new terminology. I have discussed this unofficially with one or two people whose first language is French, and there was no immediate agreement as to what the appropriate French terminology should be. Perhaps the difficulty that was evident arises out of the fact that the English name utilized two nouns, the word "radiation" being used in the fashion designated by Fowler and others as a "noun-adjective". Dr. Jacques Letourneau of Quebec City who is a member of your committee undoubtedly can advise on this particular matter.

I expect that our Council would feel that those physicians who are certificated currently in the specialty of Therapeutic Radiology would retain the present certificate and that we would not issue new certificates bearing the changed name of the specialty. On the other hand in our data bank I expect that we will use the same coding for Radiation Oncology as has been assigned up to now for the specialty of Therapeutic Radiology.

I expect that you will be pleased that the Council acted promptly and favourably to your proposal. We will communicate with the Canadian Association of Radiologists to infirm that association about the change in the name of the specialty so that this will become generally known amongst the profession in Canada.

Yours sincerely,

(signed)
JAMES H. GRAHAM, F.R.C.P.(C)
Secretary

ANNEX 2 : SPECIALTY COMMITTEES IN RADIATION ONCOLOGY

Nucleus Members:		
Basco, Vivian E	Vancouver, BC	1987–90
Bush, Raymond	Toronto, Ont	1976–82 *1982–86
Carson, John	Saint John, NB	1989–90
Cummings, Bernard J	Toronto, Ont	*1987–90
Freeman, Carolyn R	Montréal, PQ	1987–90
Goodman, George B	Vancouver, BC	*1976–82
Hong, Kim E	St John's, Newfoundland	1976–78
Letourneau, Jacques M	Québec, PQ	1976–82
McGowan, DG	Saskatoon, Sask	1987–90
Raymond, Paul-Emile	Québec, PQ	1982–86
Simpson, William JK	Toronto, Ont	1976–80 1982–86
Smith, Douglas G	Saint John, NB	1978–82
Starreveld, AA	Edmonton, Alberta	1982–86
Thomson, Dugald H	Halifax, NS	1982–88
Urtasun, Raul	Edmonton, Alta	1976–78
* indicates Chairman of the Board		
Ex-Officio Members–Chairmen of Examining Boards–Radiation Oncology		
Bush, Raymond	Toronto, Ont	1976–78
Cummings, Bernard J	Toronto, Ont	1982–84
Fairey, Randall N	Vancouver, BC	1984–88
Goodman, George B	Vancouver, BC	1978–80
Laverdiere, Jacques	St-Nicolas, PQ	1986–90
Letourneau, Jacques M	Québec, PQ	1976–78
Madore, Paul RM	Montréal, PQ	1978–80
Mercier, Jean Phillipe	Montréal, PQ	1982–86
Raymond, Paul EM	Québec, PQ	1980–82
Simpson, WJK	Toronto, Ont	1980–82
Thomas, Gilliam M	Toronto, Ont	1988–90
Corresponding Members:		
Ayoub, Joseph	Montréal, PQ	1989–90
Froud, Peter J	Kingston, Ont	1987–88
Jackson, SM	Vancouver, BC	1989–90
Klassen, David J	Vancouver, BC	1987–88
Pearson, James G	Edmonton, Alta	1980–82
Specialty Committee in Therapeutic Radiology 1975–76 (Royal College of Physicians & Surgeons of Canada)		
Bush, Raymon	Toronto, Ont	1975–76
Goodman, George B	Vancouver,BC	*1975–76
Hong, Kim E	St John's,Newfoundland	1975–76
Letourneau, Jacques M	Québec, PQ	1975–76
Simpson, WJK	Toronto, Ont	1975–76
Urtasun, Raul	Edmonton, Alta	1975–76
Ex-Officio Members		
Bush, Raymond	Chairman, English Board of Examiners	1975–76
Letourneau, Jacques M	Chairman, French Board of Examiners	1975–76
* indicates Chairman of the Board		

XIII *The Sterling-Winthrop Imaging Research Institute* **348**

1. Lentle BC. Financial support of imaging in an academic setting. Invest Radiol 1993; 28 Suppl 3: S116.
2. Potts DG, Stevenson GW. The Sterling-Winthrop Imaging Research Institute. Canad Assoc Radiol J 1990; 41: 258.
3. Ethier R, Fraser D, Hébert G, Hobbs B, Lentle BC, Potts G, Stevenson G. The first Sterling-Winthrop Imaging Research Institute awards. Canad Assoc Radiol J 1991; 42: 86.
4. Ethier R, Fraser D, Herrington M, Hobbs B, Nickel A, Blair H, Lentle BC, Potts G, Stevenson G. New directions for radiological research. J Canad Assoc Radiol 1992; 43: 329.

Part Seven Groups, Programs and Activities

I *The Industrial Factor: Technological Innovations which Changed Radiology* **355**

1. Don C. The 1987 Gordon Richards memorial lecture: The future of radiography—casetteless or filmless, Can Assoc Radiol J 1988; 39:83.
2. Duckett G, Huot L, Bakker G. 70mm. spot film camera–camera automatique 70mm. Canad Med Ass J 1959; 80: 988.
3. Duckett G, Huot L. Retrospective d'un an de Roentgen cinéma et de Roentgen télévision. L'Union Médicale du Canada 1959; 88: 1097.
4. Roy P. Percutaneous catheterization via the axillary artery. Am J Roentgenol 1965; 94: 1.
5. Duckett G. Daylight telefluoroscopy. Am J Roentgenol 1960; 84:566.
6. Roy P. Peripheral angiography in ischemic arterial diseases of the limbs. Radiol Clin N Am 1967; 5: 467.
7. Roy P, Jutras A, Longtin M. Extra large field angiography: technique and results. Canad Assoc Radiol J 1961; 12.

II *The History of Interventional Radiology of the Biliary Tract* **362**

1. O'Malley M. Doctors. Toronto, Canada: Macmillan, 1983.
2. Margulis AR. Interventional diagnostic radiology—a new subspecialty. Am J Roentgenol 1967; 99: 761.
3. Nordentoft JM, Hansen H. Treatment of intussusception in children: brief survey based on 1,830 Danish cases (I. 1,042 cases 1928–1935. II. 796 cases 1944–1949). Surgery 1955; 38: 311.
4. Burckhardt H, Müller W. Versuche uber die Punktion der Gallenblase und ihre Röntgendarstellung. Deutsche Zeitschrift fur Chirurgie 1921; 162: 168.
5. Pribram BOC. Zur Beseitigung eingeklemmter Choledochuspapillensteine. Dtsch Med Wochenschr 1932; 58: 1167.
6. Pribram BOC. Ether treatment of gall-stones impacted in the common duct. Lancet 1939; 1: 1311.
7. Lamis PA, Letton HJ, Wilson JP. Retained common duct stones: new nonoperative technique for treatment. Surgery 1969; 66: 291.
8. Halsted WS, Finney JMT. Excision of the gallbladder. Johns Hopkins Hospital Bulletin 1902; 13: 54.
9. Longmire WP Jr. The treatment of retained gallstones. West J Med 1979; 130: 422.
10. Mondet A. Técnica de la extracción incruenta de los cálculos en la litiasis residual del colédoco. Bol Soc Cir B Aires 1962; 46: 278.
11. Mazzariello R. Removal of residual biliary tract calculi without reoperation. Surgery 1970; 67: 566.
12. Lagrave G, Plessis JL, Pougeard-Dulimbert G, et al. Lithiase biliaire résiduelle: Extraction à la sonde de Dormia par le drain de Kehr. Mem Acad Chir (Paris) 1969; 95: 431.
13. Mahorner H, Bean WJ. Removal of residual stone from common bile duct without surgery. Ann Surg 1971; 173: 857.
14. Burhenne HJ. Extraktion von Residualsteinen der Gallenwege ohne Reoperation. Fortschr Röntgenstr 1972; 117: 425.
15. Bean WJ, Mahorner H. Removal of residual stones through the T-tube tract. South Med J 1972; 65: 377.
16. Burhenne HJ: Garland Lecture. Percutaneous extraction of retained biliary tract stones: 661 patients. Am J Roentgenol 1980; 134: 88.
17. Way LW: Retained common duct stones. Surg Clin North Am 1973; 53: 1139.
18. Seldinger SI. Catheter replacement of needle in percutaneous arteriography: New technique. Acta Radiol (Stockh) 1953; 39: 368.
19. Remolar J, Katz S, Rybak B, et al. Percutaneous transhepatic cholangiography. Gastroenterology 1956; 31: 39.
20. Kaude JV, Weidenmier CH, Agee OF. Decompression of bile ducts with the percutaneous transhepatic technic. Radiology 1969; 93: 69.
21. Hoevels J, Lunderquist A, Ihse I. Percutaneous transhepatic intubation of bile ducts for combined internal-external drainage in preoperative and palliative treatment of obstructive jaundice. Gastrointest Radiol 1978; 3: 23.
22. Mori K, Misumi A, Sugiyama M, et al. Percutaneous transhepatic bile drainage. Ann Surg 1977; 185: 115.
23. Ring EJ, Oleaga JA, Freiman DB, et al. Therapeutic applications of catheter cholangiography. Radiology 1978; 128: 333.
24. Ring EJ, Husted JW, Oleaga JA, et al. A multihole catheter for maintaining longterm percutaneous antegrade biliary drainage. Radiology 1979; 132: 752.
25. Burhenne HJ. Nonoperative roentgenologic instrumentation technics of the postoperative biliary tract: Treatment of biliary stricture and retained stones. Am J Surg 1974; 128: 117.
26. Molnar W, Stockum AE. Relief of obstructive jaundice through percutaneous transhepatic catheter—a new therapeutic method. AJR 1974; 122: 356.
27. Pereiras RV Jr, Owen JR, Hutson D, et al. Relief of malignant obstructive jaundice by percutaneous insertion of a permanent prosthesis in the biliary tree. Ann Intern Med 1978; 89: 589.
28. Dotter CT, Bilbao MK, Katon RM. Percutaneous transhepatic gallstone removal by needle tract. Radiology 1979; 133: 242.
29. Burhenne HJ. Dilatation of biliary tract strictures: A new roentgenologic technique. Radiologica Clinica 1975; 44: 153.
30. Grüntzig A. Die perkutane Rekanalisation chronischer arterieller Verschlusse (Dotter-Prinzip) mit einem doppellumigen Dilatations-katheter. ROFO 1976; 124: 80.
31. Molnar W, Stockum AE. Transhepatic dilatation of

choledochoenterostomy strictures. Radiology 1978; 129: 59.
32. Burhenne HJ, Morris CD. Biliary stricture dilatation: Use of the Gruntzig balloon catheter. Can Assoc Radiol J1980; 31: 196.
33. Herskovic A, Heaston D, Engler MJ, et al. Irradiation of biliary carcinoma. Radiology 1981; 139: 219.
34. Nagai N, Toli F, Oi J, et al. Continuous endoscopic pancreatocholedochal catheterization. Gastrointest Endosc 1976; 23: 78.
35. Soehendra N, Reynders-Frederix V. Palliative Gallengangdrainage: Eine neue Methode zur endoskopischen Einfuhrung eines inneren Drains. Dtsch Med Wochenschr 1979; 104: 206.
36. Yamakawa T, Mieno K, Noguchi T, et al. An improved choledochofiberscope and non-surgical removal of retained biliary calculi under direct visual control. Gastrointest Endosc 1976; 22:160.
37. Classen M, Demling L: Endoskopische Sphinkterotomie der Papilla Vateri und Steinextraktion aus dem Ductus choledochus. Dtsch Med Wschr 1974; 99: 496.
38. Mason RR, Cotton PE. Combined duodenoscopic and transhepatic approach to stenosis of the papilla of Vater. Br J Radiol 1981; 54: 678.
39. Fernström I, Johansson B. Percutaneous pyelolithotomy: A new extraction technique. Scand J Urol Nephrol 1976; 10: 257.
40. Goodwin WE, Casey WC, Woolf W. Percutaneous trocar (needle) nephrostomy in hydronephrosis. JAMA 1955; 157: 891.
41. Bartley O, Chidekel N, Rådberg C. Percutaneous drainage of the renal pelvis for uraemia due to obstructed urinary outflow. Acta Chir Scand 1965; 129: 443.
42. Huard P, Do-Xuan-Hop. La ponction transhepatique des canaux biliares. Bull Soc Med Chir de l'Indochine 1937; 15: 1090.
43. DeMasi CJ, Akdamar K, Sparks RD, et al. Puncture of the gallbladder during percutaneous transhepatic cholangiography. JAMA 1967; 201: 225.
44. Hogan MT, Watne A, Mossburg W, et al. Direct injection into the gallbladder in dogs, using ultrasonic guidance. Arch Surg 1976; 111: 564.
45. Bean WJ, Calonje MA, Aprill CN, et al. Percutaneous catheterization of the gallbladder with ultrasonic guidance. South Med J 1979; 72: 612.
46. Elyaderani M, Gabriele OF. Percutaneous cholecystostomy and cholangiography in patients with obstructive jaundice. Radiology 1979; 130: 601.
47. Burhenne HJ, Hamilton S. Nonoperative transcholecystic removal of common duct stones [Abstract]. Gastrointest Radiol 1982; 7: 92.
48. Burhenne HJ, Hamilton S. Percutaneous cholecystostomy for entry into the canine gallbladder and common bile duct. Radiology 1983; 149: 844.
49. Mazzariello RM. Transcholecystic extraction of residual calculi in the common bile duct. Surgery 1974; 75: 338.
50. Kerlan RK, LaBerge JM, Ring EJ. Percutaneous cholecystolithotomy: preliminary experience. Radiology 1985; 157: 65.
51. Cope C, Burke DR, Meranze SG. Percutaneous extraction of gallstones in 20 patients. Radiology 1990; 176: 19.
52. vanSonnenberg E, D'Agostino HB, Casola G, et al. The benefits of percutaneous cholecystostomy for decompression of selected cases of obstructive jaundice. Radiology 1990; 176: 15.
53. Gibney RG, Fache JS, Becker CD, et al. Combined surgical and radiologic intervention for complicated cholelithiasis in high-risk patients. Radiology 1987; 165: 715.
54. Kellett MJ, Wickham JEA, Russell RCG. Percutaneous cholecystolithotomy. Br Med J 1988; 296: 453.
55. Riches E. The history of lithotomy and lithotrity. Ann Roy Coll Surg Eng 1968; 43: 185.
56. Büttger B. Zur elektro-hydraulischen Lithotripsie von Blasensteinen mit Urat 1. Zschr Urol 1969; 62: 495.
57. von Gasteyer KH. Die Ultraschall-Lithotripsie. Fortschr Med 1971; 89: 363.
58. Burhenne HJ. Electrohydrolytic fragmentation of retained common duct stones. Radiology 1975; 117: 721.
59. Bean WJ, Davies H, Barnes F. Ultrasonic fragmentation of a large residual biliary tract stone. J Clin Ultrasound 1977; 5: 188.
60. Sauerbruch T, Delius M, Paumgartner G et al. Fragmentation of gallstones by extracorporeal shock waves. N Eng J Med 1986; 314: 818.
61. Fache JS, Rawat B, Burhenne HJ. Extracorporeal cholecystolithotripsy without oral chemolitholysis. Radiology 1990; 177: 719.
62. Miller FJ, Kensey KR, Nash JE. Experimental percutaneous gallstone lithotripsy: Results in swine. Radiology 1989; 170: 985.
63. Allen MJ, Borody TJ, Bugliosi TF, et al. Cholelitholysis using methyl tert-butyl ether. Gastroenterology 1985; 88: 122.
64. Becker CD, Fache JS, Malone DE, et al. Ablation of the cystic duct and gallbladder: first clinical observations. Radiology 1990; 176: 687.
65. Dubois F, Icard P, Berthelot G, et al. Coelioscopic cholecystectomy: Preliminary report of 36 cases. Ann Surg 1990; 211: 60.

IV *Imaging Research at the Montréal Neurological Institute* **371**

1. Reid WB Johns HE. An automatic brain scanner. Int J Applied Rad Isotopes 1958; 3: 1.
2. Cowan GAB, Fedoruk SO, Feindel WH, Stratford JG. Localization of intracranial lesions using radioactive iodinated serum albumin and an automatic scanner. Canad Assoc Radiol J 1960; 11: 15.
3. Wrenn FR Jr, God ML, Matthews WB. Use of positron emitting isotopes for localization of brain tumours. Science 1951; 113: 525.
4. Thompson CJ Yamamoto YL Meyer E. A positron imaging system for measurement of cerebral blood flow. Proc Soc Photo Opt Inst Eng 1976; 96: 263.

VI *Radiation Protection* **376**

1. King EE. Skin, hair and nail lesions produced by the action of x-rays. The Canadian Practitioner 1896; 21: 789.
2. Eggleston W. Canada's Nuclear Story. London (Eng): George G Harrap, 1966.
3. Mitchell JS. Memorandum on some aspects of the biological action of radiations, with especial reference to tolerance problems. Document I-17, National Research Council, Atomic Energy Project, Montréal, 1945.

4. LeBourdais DM. Canada and the atomic revolution. Toronto: McClelland and Stewart Ltd, 1959: 56. [Although erroneously naming Dr CJ Mackenzie as the first president of AECB].
5. Sims GHE. A history of the Atomic Energy Control Board. Ottawa: Government of Canada, 1981: 217.
6. Recommendations of the ICRP, Dec 1954. Brit J Radiol 1955; Supplement No 6.
7. Bird PM. Radiation protection in Canada, parts I to III. Canad Med Assoc J 1964; 90: 1024, 1075 and 1114.
8. ICRP Publication 1. Recommendations of the International Commission on Radiological Protection. Oxford: Pergamon Press, 1959.
9. Cowper G. Radiation exposure records in AECL; G1. External radiation. Appendix G in: A study of the health of the employees of Atomic Energy of Canada Limited by JL Weeks. Atomic Energy of Canada Limited, Report AECL-6813, 1981.
10. Ontario Hydro Radiation Protection Regulations 1962. Toronto: Ontario Hydro, 1962.
11. Wilson R et al. The application of ALARA in Ontario Hydro. Paper presented at Health Physics Society Annual Meeting, Chicago, 1985. Report HSD-IR-85-6. Toronto: Ontario Hydro, 1985.
12. Wilson R et al. Occupational dose reduction experience in nuclear power stations. Report HSD-IR-85-1. Toronto: Ontario Hydro, 1985.
13. Anderson TW. Ontario Hydro Mortality 1970–1982. Health and Safety Division. Toronto: Ontario Hydro, 1983.
14. ICRP Publication 34. Protection of the patient in diagnostic radiology. Annals of the ICRP 1982; 9: nos 2 and 3.
15. Consultative Document C-83. Proposed general amendments to the Atomic Energy Control Regulations. Ottawa: Atomic Energy Control Board, 1986.
16. ICRP Publication 60. 1990 Recommendations of the International Commission on Radiological Protection. Annals of the ICRP, 1991; 21: nos 1 and 3.

VII *Profile of the Founding Members: Canadian Association of Radiologists, 1937–1938* **380**

1. Lipinski JK. Profile of the founding members: Canadian Association of Radiologists, 1937–1938. Ann Roy Coll Physicians Surg Canad 1988; 21: 519 (and reprinted immediately above).

VIII *Profile of the Founding Members of the Canadian Association of Radiation Oncologists* **383**

1. Lipinski JK. Profile of the founding members: Canadian Association of Radiologists, 1937–1938. Ann Roy Coll Physicians Surg Canad 1988; 21: 519 (and reprinted immediately above).

X *Cancer Radiotherapy Using Negative Pi-Mesons* **388**

1. Rosen L. Physics Today 1966; 19: 21.
2. Blazer VJP. Atomikernenergie 1976; 27: 146.
3. Richardson R. Nucl Instr and Meth 1963; 24: 493.
4. Poon M. MSc Thesis, University of British Columbia 1977.
5. Lewis CA, O'Leary K, Jackson DF and Lam GKY. Phys Med Biol 1982; 27: 683.
6. Smith A, Hilco R, Dicello J et al. In: Pion and heavy ion radiotherapy: preclinical and clinical studies, Skarsgard LD (ed). New York: Elsevier/NorthHolland, 1982.
7. Lam GKY. Rev Sci Inst 1982; 53: 1067.
8. Lam GKY, Henkelman RM, Harrison RW, Skarsgard LD, Palcic B. Phys Med Biol 1979; 24: 1243.
9. Skarsgard LD, Palcic B, Lam GKY. In: Pion and heavy ion radiotherapy: preclinical and clinical studies, Skarsgard LD (ed). New York: Elsevier/NorthHolland, 1982.
10. Lam GKY, Henkelman RM, Douglas BG, Eaves CJ. Int J Radiat Oncol Biol Phys 1981; 7: 1689.
11. Douglas BJ. In: Pion and heavy ion radiotherapy: preclinical and clinical studies, Skarsgard LD (ed). New York: Elsevier/NorthHolland, 1982.
12. Goodman GB, Douglas BG, Jackson SM, Ludgate CM. In: Pion and heavy ion radiotherapy: preclinical and clinical studies, Skarsgard LD (ed). New York: Elsevier/NorthHolland, 1982.
13. Goodman GB, Douglas BG, Jackson SM et al. Int J Radiat Oncol Biol Phys 1982; 8: 2187.

XI *The Saskatchewan Radon Plant 1931–1962* **391**

1. Harrington EL. A redetermination of the absolute value of the coefficient of viscosity of air. Phys Rev 1916; 8: 738.
2. Millikan RA. A redetermination of the value of the electron and of related constants. Proc Nat'l Acad Sci 1917; 3: 231.
3. Harrington EL. Radium: Radon Plants. In: Glasser O, editor. Medical physics. Chicago: Year Book Publishers, 1944.
4. Cormack DV. The Saskatchewan radon plant 1931–1962. Physics in Canada 1985; 41: 3.

XII *A Radioactive Gold Ring* **395**

1. Miller RAW, Aldrich JE. Radioactive gold ring dermatitis. J Am Acad Dermatology 1990; 23: 360.

Part Eight: Radiological Sciences and the Graphic Arts

Preamble **400**

1. Lommel A. Shamanism: the beginnings of art. New York: McGraw-Hill, 1967.
2. Gunn SWA. Medicine in primitive Indian and Eskimo art. Canad Med Ass J 1970; 102: 513.
3. Jordan Betty A. ff . Canadian Art 1991; Winter: 36.
4. Bronowski J. The ascent of man. London:British Broadcasting Corporation, 1973.
5. Semchishen O. In plain view–Voir clair. Ottawa: The Canadian Museum of Contemporary Photography, 1994.
6. Lentle BC. Doubly gifted. In: Aldrich JE, Lentle BC, editors. A new kind of ray: The radiological sciences in Canada 1895–1995. Montréal: The Canadian Association of Radiologists, 1995.

II *Dr Orest Semchishen* **403**

1. Semchishen O. In plain view—Voir clair. Ottawa: The Canadian Museum of Contemporary Photography, 1994.

III *Canadian Stamps and the Radiological Sciences* **407**

Individual stamps are referenced to the Scott catalogue by catalogue number and year. The Scott numbering system is the one most widely used in North America. The stamps referenced are Canadian issues unless it is otherwise stated.[9]

1. Dunlop JM. Medical Nobels—stamp of genius. Brit Med J 1988; 297: 1674.
2. Williams FH. The 'x'-ray in medicine. Med Rec NY 1896; 49: 665.
3. Houston CS, Fedoruk SO. In: Aldrich JE, Lentle BC, editors. A new kind of ray: The radiological sciences in Canada 1895–1995. Montréal: The Canadian Association of Radiologists, 1995.
4. Praestholm J, Dissing I, Herning M. Radiology on postage stamps. Radiographics 1988; 8: 981 and 1203, 1989; 9: 341 and 1990; 10: 157.
5. Taub M. Cancer stamps: 50 years in the crusade against cancer through stamps. Ca—a cancer journal for clinicians 1978; 28: 164.
6. Mitchell C. Slide set IV. A philatelic history of radiology. Reston, Virginia: Radiology Centennial Inc. Available from Center for the American History of Radiology, 1891 Preston White Drive, Reston, Virginia 22091.
7. Cohen M. Ernest Rutherford at McGill University, in: Aldrich JA, Lentle BC, editors. A new kind of ray: the radiological sciences in Canada 1865–1965. Montréal: Canadian Association of Radiologists, 1995.
8. Donizetti P. Shadow and substance. The story of medical radiography. Trans A Ellis. trans. Oxford: Pergamon Press, 151.
9. Aldrich JA. Alexander Graham Bell, in: Aldrich JA, Lentle BC, editors. A new kind of ray: The radiological sciences in Canada 1865–1965. Montréal: Canadian Association of Radiologists, 1995.
10. Cummings WW (ed.). Scott 1995 standard postage stamp catalogue. Sidney, Ohio: Scott Publishing Co, 1994.

Postscript **411**

1. Feynman RP. What do you care what other people think? Further adventures of a curious character. New York: Bantam Books, 1989.
2. Galvin JR, D'Alessandro MP, Erkonen WE, et al. The virtual hospital: a new paradigm for lifelong learning in radiology. RadioGraphics 1994; 14: 875.

Destiny is not a matter of chance,
it is a matter of choice;
it is not a thing to be waited for,
it is a thing to be achieved.
— William Jennings Bryan

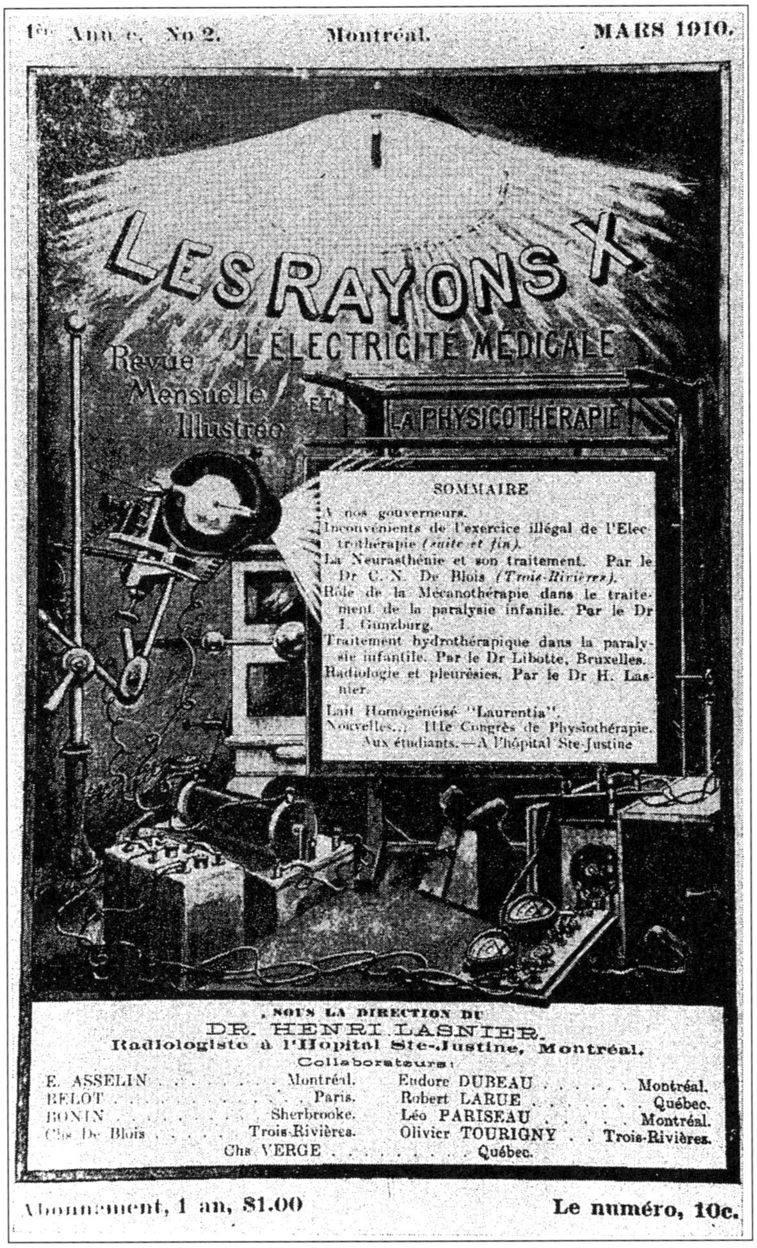

1re Année, No 2. Montréal. MARS 1910.

LES RAYONS X

L'ÉLECTRICITÉ MÉDICALE

Revue Mensuelle Illustrée

ET

LA PHYSICOTHÉRAPIE

SOMMAIRE

A nos gouverneurs.
Inconvénients de l'exercice illégal de l'Electrothérapie (suite et fin).
La Neurasthénie et son traitement. Par le Dr C. N. De Blois (Trois-Rivières).
Rôle de la Mécanothérapie dans le traitement de la paralysie infanile. Par le Dr I. Gunzburg.
Traitement hydrothérapique dans la paralysie infantile. Par le Dr Libotte, Bruxelles.
Radiologie et pleurésies. Par le Dr H. Lasnier.
Lait Homogénéisé "Laurentia".
Nouvelles... IIe Congrès de Physiothérapie. Aux étudiants.—A l'hôpital Ste-Justine

SOUS LA DIRECTION DU
DR. HENRI LASNIER.
Radiologiste à l'Hopital Ste-Justine, Montréal.
Collaborateurs:

E. ASSELIN . . . . Montréal.
BELOT . . . . Paris.
BONIN . . . . Sherbrooke.
Chs De Blois . . . . . . Trois-Rivières.
Eudore DUBEAU . . . . . . Montréal.
Robert LARUE . . . . Québec.
Léo PARISEAU . . . . . . Montréal.
Olivier TOURIGNY . . Trois-Rivières.
Chs VERGE . . . . Québec.

Abonnement, 1 an, $1.00 Le numéro, 10c.

Appendices

Appendix 1

Early Publications in Diagnostic Radiology by Canadian Physicians

(COLLECTED BY J KENNETH LIPINSKI)

Cox J, Kirkpatrick RC. The new photography with report of a case in which a bullet was photographed in the leg. Montréal Medical Journal 1896; 24:661–665.

King EE. Skin, hair and nail lesions produced by the action of x-rays. The Canadian Practitioner 1896; 21:789–793.

Currie M. A method of making x-ray observations on hollow organs. Dominion Medical Monthly 1898; 11:9–10.

Girdwood GP. Stereoskiagraphy. Montréal Medical Journal 1899; 28:193–198.

Verge C. Observations d'examens aux rayons-X. Le Bulletin Medical de Québec 1899–1900; 1:120–121.

Third J. The Roentgen ray. Early diagnosis of tubercular and other lesions. Kingston Medical Quarterly 1900; 99–106.

Verge C. Radiodiagnostic d'un cas de periostite traumatique. *Ibid* 1901–1902; 3:26.

Girdwood GP. On stereoskiagraphy. American X-ray Journal 1901; 8:861–864.

Hamilton WF. The value of x-rays as a diagnostic agent in thoracic disease. Montréal Medical Journal 1902; 933–940.

McMaster J. Some results that are being attained by the use of x-rays with exhibition of patients. Dominion Medical Monthly 1902; 19:61–72.

McMaster J. The use and limitations of the x-rays in the treatment of diseases. Canada Lancet 1902–1903; 36:708–711.

Girdwood GP. On the use of Roentgen rays in medicine and surgery. Montréal Medical Journal 1903; 32:161–171.

Bond JHR. Some forms of electrical application with illustrative cases. Winnipeg Medico-Chirurgical Society 1904; 1:33–41.

Galloway HPH. Coxa vara, with report of a case. *Ibid* 1906–08; 3:115–121.

Nelson HR. The Roentgenrays in general practice. Dominion Medical Monthly 1906; 27:130–135.

Corbert CG. Roentgen rays—use and abuse. Maritime Medical News 1907; 19:14–17.

Calder RM. Static electricity and x-ray in general practice. Dominion Medical Monthly 1907; 29:47–52.

Cummings S. The Roentgenographic diagnosis of bone tuberculosis. Trans American Roentgen Ray Society 1907; 131–137.

Of these publications seven were contributed by Montreal physicians, five from Toronto, two from Winnipeg and one each from Kingston, Petrolia, Saint John and Vancouver.

In a larger survey (Lipinski—unpublished) twenty-three publications appeared between 1896 and 1920 in British, French and American journals. Of these publications, eighteen were by five Montreal authors and the remaining five by two Toronto physicians and one from Victoria. Publications of radiological observations in Canadian periodicals in the same period reflect a similar trend with there being seventeen papers by fourteen Montréalers and nine by nine Torontonians. Of the remaining articles four were from other centres in Ontario, three were from Winnipeg, two from Saskatchewan and one each from Québec and Vancouver.

Appendix 2

Publications by Dr Gordon E Richards

Localization of foreign bodies. Brit Med J 1916; 2: 15.

X-ray reports. J Royal Army Medical Corps 1917; 2: 428–431.

(with Bigham GH) Co-relation of results of goiter treatment by surgical and x-ray methods. Canad Med Ass J 1920; 10: 988.

Diagnosis of gastric ulcer. Canad Med Ass J 1921; 10: 18.

Possibilities of roentgen-ray in cancer of pancreas. Am J Roentgenol 1922; 9: 150–152.

Use of x-rays in diseases of the skin. Canad Med Ass J 1922; 12: 478–480.

Some of less common uses of x-ray therapy. J Radiol 1922; 3: 271–273.

X-ray technique in examination of chest. Canad Med Ass J 1924; 14: 1077–1080.

Radiation in treatment of benign diseases of female pelvis. Canad Med Ass J 1925; 15: 382–387.

X-rays and radium in management of breast carcinoma. Canad Med Ass J 1926; 16: 358–366.

Localization of foreign bodies in the eye. Am J Roentgenol 1927; 18:378–379.

(with Caulfield AHW) Systematic study and classification of stereograms of chest. Canad Med Ass J 1927; 17: 794–797.

Osteochondritis dissecans. Am J Roentgenol 1928; 19: 278–284.

Chronic infections of maxillary antra in systemic disease—radiological study. Brit J Radiol 1931; 4: 120–126.

Radium—its proven uses and limitations in therapy. Canad Pub Health J 1931; 3: 25–387.

Role of radiology in the prevention of cancer. Canad Pub Health J 1933; 24: 29–39.

Value of roentgen method in diagnosis and control of treatment of tuberculosis. J Michigan M Soc 1933; 32: 75–85.

Treatment of external cancer by radiotherapy. Canad Med Ass J 1933; 28: 246–255.

Interpretation of triangular basal shadows in roentgenograms of chest. Am J Roentgenol 1933; 30: 289–295.

Treatment of chest wall secondaries in breast carcinoma; preliminary report of new radium technique. Radiology 1934; 23: 280–284.

(with Peters MV) Nembutal in the treatment of radiation sickness. Am J Roentgenology 1936; 25: 522–525.

Radiological treatment of cancer; methods and results, 1928–35; biological conception of dosage in radiotherapy. Canad Med Ass J 1936; 35: 299–305.

Radiological treatment of cancer; methods and results, 1928–35: malignant lesions of tonsil and its pillars. Canad Med Ass J 1936; 35: 285–290.

Radiotherapy in lesions about eye. Am J Roentgenol 1936; 36: 588–602.

Radiological treatment of cancer, 1929–1935; carcinoma of tongue. Can Med Ass J 1936; 35: 593–598.

(with Cosbie WG) Radiological treatment of cancer; methods and results, 1928–1935; carcinoma cervix uteri. Canad Med Ass J 1936; 35: 381–385.

(with Singleton AC) Giant cell tumours of spine, with report of 3 cases. Radiology 1938; 30: 43–51.

Contribution of radiology to cancer problem. Can Pub Health J 1938; 29: 425–433.

Treatment of cancer of tongue. Am J Roentgenol 1942; 47: 191–206.

Radiation therapy of carcinoma of buccal mucosa (cheek). In: Treatment of cancer and allied diseases. Pack GT, Livingstone EM eds, 1942; 1: 327–344.

Hopeful aspects of the fight against cancer, Queen's Review 1947; 21(4): 93–96.

Hopeful aspects in the fight against cancer. Canad Hospital 1947; 24: 25–27, 68, and 72

The radiological treatment of carcinoma of the cervix uteri. Proceedings of the Royal Society of Medicine 1947; XL: 14: 911–917.

Analysis of technical factors and results of treatment in carcinoma of the cervix uteri; description of improved radium applicator. Am J Roentgenol 58: 783–796.

Mammary cancer; the place of surgery and of radiotherapy in its management. Part I. Brit J Radiol 1948; 21: 109–127.

Idem Part II. Brit J Radiol 1948; 21: 249–258.

Appendix 3

Gordon Richards Memorial Lecturers

Dr Arthur C Singleton, Toronto	1953
Dr Carleton B Peirce, Montréal	1954
Dr WA Jones, Kingston	1955
Dr William Boyd,Toronto	1956
Dr WG Cosbie, Toronto	1957
Dr GE Hall, London	1958
Dr Robert W Begg, Saskatoon	1959
Dr Robert Spencer Stone, San Francisco	1960
Dr Edward BD Newhauser, Boston	1961
Dr Clifford Ash, Toronto	1962
Dr Arthur E Childe, Winnipeg	1963
Dr JWJ Carpender, Chicago	1964
Dr C Allen Good, Rochester	1965
Dr Juan A Del Regato, Colorado Springs	1966
Dr John A Evans, New York City	1967
Dr M Vera Peters, Toronto	1968
Dr Donald L McRae, Toronto	1969
Dr Jean Bouchard, Montréal	1970
Dr JR Cunningham, Toronto	1971
Dr J Scott Dunbar, Vancouver	1972
Dr Lucien Campeau, Montreal	1973
Dr TA Watson, London	1974
Dr WD Rider, Toronto	1975
Dr W Duncan	1978
Dr Harold Johns, Toronto	1979
Dr JG Pearson, Edmonton	1982
Dr J Papillon, Lyon, France	1984
Dr Theodore L Phillips, San Francisco	1986
Dr Conway Don, Ottawa	1987
Dr Brian Lentle, Vancouver	1988
Dr Daniel Vanel,Villejuif, France	1989
Dr Charles B Higgins, San Francisco	1990
Dr Michel Osteaux, Brussels, Belgium	1991
Dr Christopher Flower, Cambridge, England	1992
Dr Claude Manelfe, Toulouse, France	1993
Dr William H Straub, Westport, CT	1994

Appendix 4

Liste des Anciens Présidents de la Société Canadienne Française

Dr Léglius-A Gagnier Sr	1928–1932
Dr J-E Perron	1932–1934
Dr Eugène Panneton	1934–1936
Dr Rosario Potvin	1936–1938
Dr E Gendreau	1938–1940
Dr Albert Comtois	1940–1944
Dr Jules Gosselin	1944–1947
Dr Hervé Lacharité	1947–1950
Dr Henri Lapointe	1950–1951
Dr Origène Dufresne	1951–1953
Dr Léglius-A Gagnier Jr	1953–1955
Dr Albert Jutras	1955–1957
Dr Mathieu Samson	1957–1958
Dr Paul Brodeur	1959–1960
Dr Léo Payer	1961–1962
Dr Louis Ivan Vallée	1963
Dr Robert Lessard	1964
Dr Louis-Philippe Bélisle	1965
Dr Jean-Louis Léger	1966
Dr Luc Audet	1967–1968
Dr Arthur Vallée	1969
Dr Maurice Dufresne	1970
Dr René Drouin	1971
Dr Jean-Pierre Jean	1972
Dr Robert Fortin	1973
Dr Jacques Saltiel	1974–1975
Dr Laurent Aubé	1976
Dr Jean-L Vézina	1977–1978
Dr Jacques Sylvestre	1979
Dre Denise Ouimet-Oliva	1980–1981
Dr Hugues Archambault	1982–1983
Dr Michel Lafortune	1984–1986
Dre Heidi Patriquin	1987–1989
Dr Denis Melançon	1990–1992
Dre Lucie Brazeau-Lamontagne	1993–1994

Appendix 5a

The Canadian Association of Radiologists

PRESIDENTS AND SITES OF ANNUAL MEETINGS

Dr W A Jones	1937, Toronto
Dr W A Jones	1938, Kingston
Dr J E Gendreau	1939, Calgary
Dr J E Gendreau	1940, Québec
Dr W H McGuffin	1941, Ottawa
Dr W H McGuffin	1942, London
Dr W H McGuffin	1943, Hamilton
Dr J E Perron	1944, Toronto
Dr M C Morrison	1945, Montréal
Dr C W Prowd	1946, Vancouver
Dr Digby Wheeler	1947, Québec
Dr A C Singleton	1948, Kingston
Dr E W Spencer	1949, Halifax
Dr E A Petrie	1950, Montréal
Dr Origene Dufresne	1951, Niagara Falls
Dr Origene Dufresne	1952, Winnipeg
Dr R A Macpherson	1953, Toronto
Dr J W McKay	1954, Québec
Dr R C Burr	1955, Ottawa
Dr Andrew Turnbull	1956, Vancouver
Dr Jean Bouchard	1957, Montréal
Dr A R McGee	1958, London
Dr E M Crawford	1959, Saskatoon
Dr A E Childe	1960, Toronto
Dr Donald L McRae	1961, Saint John
Dr Guillaume Gill	1962, Winnipeg
Dr W L Sloan	1963, Québec
Dr R A Lobb	1964, Vancouver
Dr Henri Lapointe	1965, Toronto
Dr Norman S Skinner	1966, Montréal
Dr Jean-Louis Leger	1967, Toronto
Dr John G Stapleton	1968, Québec
Dr Robert G Fraser	1969, Vancouver
Dr K D Symington	1970, Montréal
Dr L R Harnick	1971, Calgary
Dr Maurice Dufresne	1972, Toronto
Dr R B Holmes	1973, Montréal
Dr John D Stevenson	1974, Vancouver
Dr D James Sieniewicz	1975, Toronto
Dr Jean-Pierre Jean	1976, Québec
Dr D W MacEwan	1977, Winnipeg
Dr W M Roy	1978, Toronto
Dr George B Goodman	1979, Vancouver
Dr Ross O Hill	1980, Montréal
Dr Bernard J Reilly	1981, Toronto
Dr Gordon Bray	1982, Winnipeg
Dr Max J Palayew	1983, Québec
Dr Gwilym H Evans	1984, Vancouver
Dr Edward L Lansdown	1985, Toronto
Dr David B Fraser	1986, Halifax
Dr Walter M Little	1987, Ottawa
Dr W James Knickerbocker	1988, Edmonton
Dr Jacques Sylvestre	1989, Québec
Dr Carl J Zylak	1990, Vancouver
Dr Barry B Hobb	1991, Hamilton
Dr Guy Hebert	1992, Halifax
Dr Stephanie Wilson	1993, Québec
Dr JB (Ian) Sutherland	1994, Toronto
Dr W Mason	1995, Montréal

Appendix 5b

Canadian Association of Radiologists Journal

CHAIRMEN OF THE EDITORIAL BOARD AND EDITORS

Dr Joseph W McKay	1950–1953
Dr Jean Bouchard	1953–1955
Dr Origène Dufresne	1955–1957
Dr Donald McRae	1957–1960
Dr J Scott Dunbar	1960–1971
Dr Douglas W MacEwan	1971–1976
Dr C Stuart Houston	1976–1981
Dr Brian C Lentle	1981–1990
Dr Michel Azouz	1991–

Appendix 6a

Canadian Society of Radiological Technicians

PRESIDENTS

George Reason, Ontario	1942
Claude J Bodle, Manitoba	1943–1944
Mary F Cameron, Ontario	1944–1945
TB Hurst, Ontario	1945–1946
Percy E Hunt,Saskatchewan	1946–1947
Henry CJ Simkins, Québec	1947–1948
Percy E Hunt, Saskatchewan	1948–1949
Herbert M Welch, Alberta	1949–1950
William Doern, Manitoba	1950–1951
William Q Stirling, British Columbia	1951–1952
Percy E Hunt, Saskatchewan	1952–1953
John Collins, Ontario	1953–1954
Albert R Chefins, Québec	1954–1955
S Mel Smith, British Columbia	1955–1956
David Sage, Ontario	1956–1957
William Doern, Manitoba	1957–1958
Mary A McMillan, British Columbia	1958–1959
Irwin Fisher, Ontario	1959–1960
Katherine McKeen (Creelman), New Brunswick	1960–1961
Archie Wilkinson, Québec	1961–1962
M Jane Martin, Ontario	1962–1963
Frank Callaway, Alberta	1963–1964
John Leatherdale, Saskatchewan	1964–1965
John S Flanagan, Ontario	1965–1966
George Hall, Alberta	1966–1968
Colin Maxwell, Manitoba	1968–1970
Paul Poitras, Québec	1970–1971
Lewis Edwards, Ontario	1971–1973
W Ray Hansen, Alberta	1973–1974
James D Clark, Nova Scotia	1974–1976
Paul Schmidt, Alberta	1976–1977
Jacob Enns, Alberta	1977–1978

Appendix 6b

Canadian Association of Medical Radiation Technologists

PRESIDENTS

Richard Walton, Manitoba	1979
Larry Wight, Ontario	1980–1981
Nestor Shinkewski, Saskatchewan	1982
Anthony Burgess, Nova Scotia	1983
Denis Poulin, Ontario	1984–1985
Ian Fleming, Alberta	1986–1987
Robin Hesler, Ontario	1988
Richard Wharf, Manitoba	1989–1990
Donna Hateley, Alberta	1991–1992
Rita Eyer, Manitoba	1993
Larry Curtis, Alberta	1994

Appendix 6c

Canadian Association of Medical Radiation Technologists

LIFE MEMBERS

Percy Ghent, Toronto, Ontario	1943
ES Hoare, Calgary, Alberta	1943
Henry Simpkins, Montréal, Québec	1943
Sadie Colbeck, Welland, Ontario	1946
C James Bodle RT, Winnipeg, Manitoba	1950
Mary F Cameron RT, Hamilton, Ontario	1953
Percy E Hunt RT, Regina, Saskatchewan	1954
William Q Stirling RT, Vancouver, BC	1959
Albert Perry RT, Bridgewater, Nova Scotia	1960
William Doern RT, Winnipeg, Manitoba	1967
Ellen I Hood RN RT, Vancouver BC	1970
Leslie Cartwright RT, Winnipeg, Manitoba	1974
George C Hall ACR, Edmonton Alberta	1975
Sr Marie-Flore Gagné FACTRMT, Québec PQ	1976
G Archie Wilkinson RT, Prescott, Ontario	1977
Katherine McKeen RT, Nashwasksis, NB	1978
Lewis Edwards RT, Niagara Falls, Ontario	1984
Sr Noreen Hammill RT, Charlottetown, PE	1988
John S Flanagan RT, London Ontario	1990
Brenda Clark RTNM & T, Surrey, BC	1992
Terry West RTT, Toronto, ON	1994

HONORARY LIFE MEMBERS

Dr E Petrie, Saint John New Brunswick	1944
Dr AC Singleton, Toronto, Ontario	1944
Dr WK Colbeck, Welland Ontario	1946
Frederick Melville FSR, London, England	1951
Alfred Greene BSc RT, Florida USA	1951
Erminda Clark, Lincoln NEB, USA	1953
Dr Guillaume Gill, Tracy, PQ	1957
Margaret Hoing RT, Fort Wayne, Ill. USA	1957
Dr Marshall Mallett, Edmonton, Alberta	1958
Arthur Fuchs RT, Rochester, New York, USA	1959
Dr Chester H Warfield, Fort Wayne, Ind, USA	1961
Dr Jean-Pierre Jean, Montréal, PQ	1967
Dr Delbert G Wollin, Kingston, Ontario	1980

Appendix 7

Atomic Energy Control Board

PRESIDENTS

General AGL McNaughton	1946–1948
Dr CJ Mackenzie	1948–1961
Dr GC Laurence	1961–1970
Dr DG Hurst	1970–1974
Dr AT Prince	1975–1978
JH Jennekens	1978–1987
Dr R Levesque	1988–1993
Dr A Bishop	1994–

Appendix 8

Division of Medical and Biological Physics and of the Canadian Organization of Medical Physicists

CHAIRPERSONS

Dr HE Johns	1955
Dr LS Stephens-Newsham	1956
Dr HF Batho	1957
Dr AF Holloway	1958
Dr DV Cormack	1959
Dr JCF MacDonald	1960
Dr DB Scott	1961
Dr HE Johns	1962
Dr GF Whitmore	1963
Dr R Beique	1964
Dr WR Inch	1965
Dr RJ Horsley	1966
Ms SO Fedoruk	1967
Dr J Cunningham	1968
Dr P Bird	1969
Dr P Pfalzner	1970
Dr RO Kornelsen	1971
Dr R Mathieu	1972
Dr W Reid	1973
Dr N Aspin	1974
Dr JR Cunningham	1975
Dr JCF MacDonald	1976
Dr ME Repacholi	1977
Dr JE Aldrich	1978
Dr PF O'Brien	1979
Dr PMK Leung	1980
Dr M Cohen	1981
Ms K Breitman	1982
Dr DWO Rogers	1983
Dr A Rainbow	1984
Dr JW Andrew	1985
Dr JJ Battista	1986
M RL Carrier	1987
Dr RM Henkelman	1988
Dr C Thompson	1989
Dr M Yaffe	1990
Dr E El-Khatib	1991
Dr JE Aldrich	1992
Dr A Fenster	1993
Ms Sherry Connors	1994

Appendix 9

Canadian Association of Nuclear Medicine

PRESIDENTS

Dr DonaldWoods	1971–1973
Dr Leonard Rosenthall	1973–1975
Dr JB (Ian) Sutherland	1975–1977
Dr Frederick Heagy	1977–1979
Dr Brian Lentle	1979–1981
Dr Michael Chamberlain	1981–1983
Dr Raymone Chartrand	1983–1985
Dr Albert Driedger	1985–1989
Dr Alex Wilkinson	1987–1989
Dr Adel Mattar	1989–1991
Dr Georges Dupras	1991–1993
Dr Reihard Kloiber	1993–1995

Appendix 10

The Canadian College of Physicists in Medicine

PRESIDENTS

Dr HE Johns	1979–1980
Dr AF Holloway	1981
Dr DV Cormack	1982–1983
Dr MJ Bronskill	1984–1986
Dr EB Podgorsak	1987–1988
Dr FS Prato	1989–1990
Mr J Van Dyk	1991–1992
Dr A Fenster	1992–1993

Appendix 11

Canadian Radiation Protection Association

PRESIDENTS

Roch DesRochers	1980–1981
Dr Art Marko	1981–1982
Don Watson	1982–1983
WayneGreene	1983–1984
John Johnson	1984–1985
Dave Grogan	1985–1986
JohnWetherill	1986–1987
William Bush	1987–1988
Dr Ernest Letourneau	1988–1989
John Tai-Pow	1989–1990
Robi Chatterjee	1990–1991
Brian Phillips	1991–1992
Jean-Pierre Gauvin	1992–1993
Murray Walsh	1993–1994

Appendix 12

Canadian Association of Radiation Oncologists

PRESIDENTS

Stewart M Jackson	1987–1989
Bernard Cummings	1989–1991
Caroline R Freeman	1991–1993
David G Payne	1993–1995

Appendix 13
Canadian Association of Radiopharmaceutical Scientists

PRESIDENTS

Mervyn W Billinghurst (Founding President)	1981
William J Welsh	1982
Antoine A Noujaim	1983
Donald Lyster	1984
Iain C Trevena	1985
Ann Warbick-Cerone	1986
John R Scott	1987–1988
Pamela Zabel	1989–1990
Douglas N Abrahams*	1991–1994
Gilbert Matte	1995–1996
Raymond M Reilly	1997–1998

* The President-Elect, Kerry Logan-Smith was unable to start her term as President and the position was filled by the new President-Elect, who served for two terms.

Appendix 14
The Society of Nuclear Medicine in Canada

CHAIRPERSONS

Dr Albert A (Al) Driedger	1887–1989
Mr John Scott	1989–1991
Ms Pamela Zabel	1991–1993
Dr Brian Lentle	1993–1995

Appendix 15

University Academic Radiology Departments

CHAIRMEN

University of Alberta

Dr Hector Duggan	1957–1965
Dr Fleming McConnell	1965–1970
Dr JDR (Jack) Miller	1970–1983
Dr D Russell	1986–1991
Dr AJB (Sandy) McEwan	1992–

University of British Columbia

Dr Scott Dunbar	1971–1974
Dr Joachim Burhenne	1978–1990
Dr Brian Lentle	1991–

University of Calgary

Dr Hector Duggan*	1969–1978
Dr Hugh Morrish	1978–1990
Dr Bob Johns	1990–1992
Dr Chen Fong	1994–

* see also the University of Alberta

Dalhousie University

Dr JS Manchester	1955–1975
Dr James Standen	1975–1979
Dr David B Fraser	1979–

L'Université Laval

Dr Mathieu Samson	1955–1961
Dr Henri Lapointe	1961–1967
Dr Luc Audet	1969–1972
Dr Robert J Fortin	1972–1985
Dr Réginald Langelier	1985–1992
Dr Jean-Marc Turcotte	1992–

University of Manitoba

Dr Robert A Macpherson	1945–1965
Dr Douglas W MacEwan	1966–1982
Dr JB(Ian) Sutherland	1982–1990
Dr E(Ted) Lyons	1990–

Université de Montréal

Dr Jean-Louis Léger	1964–1969
Dr Roger Maltais	1969–1977
Dr Jacques Saltiel	1977–1988
Dr Guy Hébert	1988–

McGill University

Dr WL Ritchie	1942–1943
Dr Carlton Bernhart Pierce	1943–1964
Dr JJL Bouchard	1964–1969
Dr J Scott Dunbar	1969–1972
Dr Robert G Fraser	1972–1976
Dr JI Fabrikant (acting)	1976–1978
Dr Max J Palayew	1978–1987
Dr Roméo Ethier	1987–1992
Dr Patrice M Bret	1992–

McMaster University

Dr Peter Cockshott	1969–1977
Dr Carl Zylak	1977–1987
Dr Giles Stevenson	1987–

Memorial University

Dr CJ Hodson	1968–1977
Dr EA MacLoughlin	1977–1989
Dr PJ McManamon	1989–

University of Ottawa

Dr Conway Don	1958–1988
Dr Peter McDonald	1988–1992
Dr Ian Hammond	1992–

Queen's University

Dr WA Jones	1946–1960
Dr SL Fransman	1960–1980
Dr Thomas W Challis	1980–1991
Dr Robert Nolan	1992–

University of Saskatchewan

Dr Earle W Spencer	1954–1963
Dr Henry Peter Kent	1963–1982
Dr Stuart Houston	1982–1987
Dr Stanley Tchang	1987–1990 and 1991–1994
Dr JA Loewy	1994–

Université de Sherbrooke

Dr Domenico Dilinge	1968–1977
Dr Bertil G Ström	1977–1984
Dr Réjean-Yves Lévesque	1984–1990
Dr Bertil G Ström	1990
Dr Gérard R Schmutz	1990–

University of Toronto

Dr Gordon Richards*	1917–1949
Dr AC Singleton	1949–1962
Dr Malcolm Hall	1962–1965
Dr Brian Holmes	1965–1973
Dr E(Ted) Lansdown	1974–1984
Dr D Gordon Potts	1985–1991
Dr Walter Kucharczyk	1991–

* It is not clear if or when Dr Richards was formally made academic head of radiology at the University of Toronto although this fact is alluded to. Dr Singleton was so appointed (information courtesy of Dr Walter Kucharczyk).

University of Western Ontario

Dr H Wismer	1942–1949 (acting)
Dr M Morrison	1949 (July 1 to Nov 27)
Dr A Bartelink	1949–1953
Dr Paul New	1953–1958
Dr Gerald Copestake	1958–1968
Dr W Wilkins	1968–1971 (acting)
Dr Lewis Carey	1971–1986
Dr Barry B Hobbs	1986–

Appendix 16

Canadian Heads of Academic Radiology (CHAR)

PRESIDENTS

Dr H Joachim Burhenne (Founding president)	1979–1980
Dr Max Palayew	1980–1981
Dr Ted Lansdown	1981–1982
Dr Douglas MacEwan	1982–1983
Dr Robert Fortin	1983–1984
Dr Gordon Potts	1984–1985
Dr David Fraser	1985–1986
Dr Roméo Ethier	1986–1988
Dr Don Russell	1988–1990
Dr David Fraser	1990–1992
Dr Barry Hobbs	1992–1994
Dr Brian Lentle	1994–

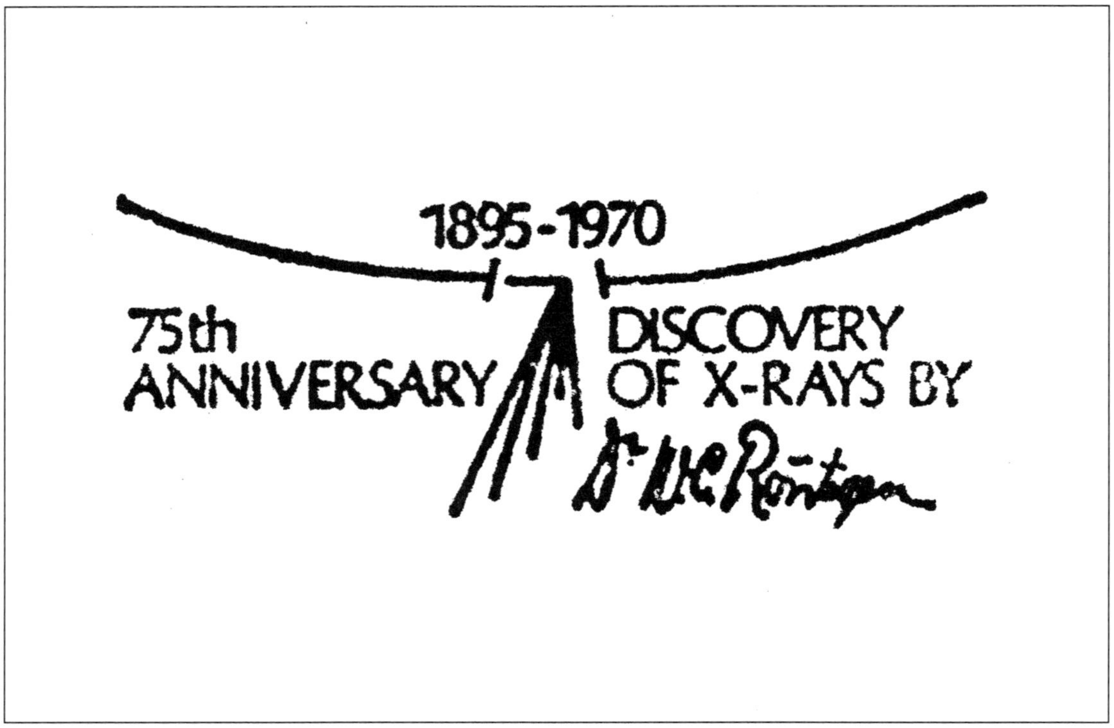
1895-1970
75th
ANNIVERSARY
DISCOVERY
OF X-RAYS BY

Photographic Credits

Archives of the Canadian Association of Medical Radiation Technologists (courtesy of Ms Rita Hudek); Archives of the Canadian Association of Radiologists (courtesy of Ms Suzanne Charette); Biomedical Communications, University of British Columbia; Ms Helen Blair; Canadian Museum of Health and Medicine at the Toronto Hospital; Dr Guy Duckett; Glenbow Museum and Archives, Calgary; Dr Robert Fraser; Dr Sylvia Fedoruk; General Electric Medical System, Canada; Dr George Goodman; Dr David Hynes; Dr Stuart Houston; Karsh of Ottawa; Dr Étienne LeBel; Dr Brian Lentle; National Film Board; Dr John Radomsky, Röntgen Kuratorium, Würtzburg; Saskatchewan Cancer Commission; Dr Orest Semchishen; Dr Stephanie Wilson; and the Stirling-Winthrop Imaging Research Institute.

Index

About the typeface

The letterforms used throughout this book were selected from the Stone family of typefaces, both for its legibility and to symbolize the historical and contemporary aspects of radiological sciences. For even though the letterforms look traditional they were designed in the late 1980s for computerized technology.

About the artwork

The series of paintings separating the parts of this volume were inspired by its title—A New Kind of Ray—and by the beauty of radiographic images.

The diagonal strokes represent rays—although radiological rays are invisible, they are suggested visually in an abstract style. Since the artwork is black and white, textures are used to add detail and interest.

The layered technique is intended to produce transparency, depth, and a sense of the mystery and promise of further discoveries that the illustrator perceives in the fields of radiological sciences.